Controversies
in Lung Cancer

BASIC AND CLINICAL ONCOLOGY

Editor

Bruce D. Cheson, M.D.

National Cancer Institute
National Institutes of Health
Bethesda, Maryland

1. Chronic Lymphocytic Leukemia: Scientific Advances and Clinical Developments, *edited by Bruce D. Cheson*
2. Therapeutic Applications of Interleukin-2, *edited by Michael B. Atkins and James W. Mier*
3. Cancer of the Prostate, *edited by Sakti Das and E. David Crawford*
4. Retinoids in Oncology, *edited by Waun Ki Hong and Reuben Lotan*
5. Filgrastim (r-metHuG-CSF) in Clinical Practice, *edited by George Morstyn and T. Michael Dexter*
6. Cancer Prevention and Control, *edited by Peter Greenwald, Barnett S. Kramer, and Douglas L. Weed*
7. Handbook of Supportive Care in Cancer, *edited by Jean Klastersky, Stephen C. Schimpff, and Hans-Jörg Senn*
8. Paclitaxel in Cancer Treatment, *edited by William P. McGuire and Eric K. Rowinsky*
9. Principles of Antineoplastic Drug Development and Pharmacology, *edited by Richard L. Schilsky, Gérard A. Milano, and Mark J. Ratain*
10. Gene Therapy in Cancer, *edited by Malcolm K. Brenner and Robert C. Moen*
11. Expert Consultations in Gynecological Cancers, *edited by Maurie Markman and Jerome L. Belinson*
12. Nucleoside Analogs in Cancer Therapy, *edited by Bruce D. Cheson, Michael J. Keating, and William Plunkett*
13. Drug Resistance in Oncology, *edited by Samuel D. Bernal*
14. Medical Management of Hematological Malignant Diseases, *edited by Emil J Freireich and Hagop M. Kantarjian*
15. Monoclonal Antibody-Based Therapy of Cancer, *edited by Michael L. Grossbard*
16. Medical Management of Chronic Myelogenous Leukemia, *edited by Moshe Talpaz and Hagop M. Kantarjian*
17. Expert Consultations in Breast Cancer: Critical Pathways and Clinical Decision Making, *edited by William N. Hait, David A. August, and Bruce G. Haffty*
18. Cancer Screening: Theory and Practice, *edited by Barnett S. Kramer, John K. Gohagan, and Philip C. Prorok*

ADDITIONAL VOLUMES IN PREPARATION

Controversies in Lung Cancer

A Multidisciplinary Approach

edited by

Benjamin Movsas
Corey J. Langer
Melvyn Goldberg

Fox Chase Cancer Center
Philadelphia, Pennsylvania

MARCEL DEKKER, INC.   NEW YORK · BASEL

ISBN: 0-8247-0274-3

This book is printed on acid-free paper.

Headquarters
Marcel Dekker, Inc.
270 Madison Avenue, New York, NY 10016
tel: 212-696-9000; fax: 212-685-4540

Eastern Hemisphere Distribution
Marcel Dekker AG
Hutgasse 4, Postfach 812, CH-4001 Basel, Switzerland
tel: 41-61-261-8482; fax: 41-61-261-8896

World Wide Web
http://www.dekker.com

The publisher offers discounts on this book when ordered in bulk quantities. For more information, write to Special Sales/Professional Marketing at the headquarters address above.

To my wife, Tammy, my children, Shoshana, Avielle, Shira, and Aviva, and my parents, Sam and Sonia.   *Benjamin Movsas*

To my wife, Mindy, my children, Adina and Micah, and my parents, Leon and Rita.   *Corey Langer*

To my wife, Judith, and my children, Jennifer, Joanna, and Heather.   *Melvyn Goldberg*

Series Introduction

The current volume, *Controversies in Lung Cancer: A Multidisciplinary Approach*, is Volume 25 in the Basic and Clinical Oncology series. Many of the advances in oncology have resulted from close interaction between the basic scientist and the clinical researcher. The current volume follows, expands on, and illustrates the success of this relationship as demonstrated by new therapies and promising areas for scientific research.

As editor of the series, my goal has been to recruit volume editors who not only have established reputations based on their outstanding contributions to oncology, but also have an appreciation for the dynamic interface between the laboratory and the clinic. To date, the series has consisted of monographs on topics such as chronic lymphocytic leukemia, nucleoside analogs in cancer therapy, therapeutic applications of interleukin-2, retinoids in oncology, gene therapy of cancer, and principles of antineoplastic drug development and pharmacology. *Controversies in Lung Cancer* is certainly a most important addition to the series.

Volumes in progress include a work on chronic lymphoid leukemias. I anticipate that this and future volumes will provide a valuable contribution to the oncology literature.

Bruce D. Cheson, M.D.

Foreword

Although progress is being made in the treatment of lung cancer, the long-term survival rate for lung cancer patients remains disappointing. In order to effect a major impact on lung cancer survival, the paradigm must shift. Currently, too many people develop lung cancer, too many people present with locally advanced or disseminated disease, and too many people have tumors that are refractory to available systemic treatment. Fortunately, there are potential ways to influence the frequency of lung cancer, the stage of the disease, and responsiveness to systemic therapy. First, optimism exists that educational efforts directed toward children will result in a decline in the prevalence of smoking. Second, low-dose rapid spiral CT scans of the chest may detect disease earlier in persons at risk and reduce the percentage of patients who present with advanced disease. Lastly, treatments directed at novel targets—including autocrine growth factors, angiogenesis, and defective programmed cell death—may provide new venues to treat locally advanced and disseminated disease and ultimately lead to less toxic, more effective adjuvant therapy.

Although we anticipate a favorable shift in the lung cancer paradigm, we must urgently confront our current challenge—to provide the most effective available treatment now for hundreds of thousands of lung cancer patients, who will be diagnosed in the next five years and who cannot wait for theoretical therapies. The editors of *Controversies in Lung Cancer* have carefully identified key areas where real progress has been achieved and where continued work is likely to result in further improvement. Equally important, they have gathered an impressive group of recognized experts in the field who are themselves directly involved in this task.

The book begins with a refreshing discussion on lung cancer staging. TNM staging was adopted for lung cancer more than three decades ago, and the staging system has since been refined twice (1986 and 1997). The authors of Chapter 1 highlight the current inadequacies of the staging system and discuss possibilities for improving it. The next two chapters focus on the results achieved in limited-stage small cell lung cancer. In the year 2000, more than 25% of limited-stage small cell lung cancer patients treated with concurrent chemotherapy and radiation had survived for at least five years; this has truly "raised the bar" compared to results only 10 to 20 years ago. Using evidence-based medicine, the authors of subsequent chapters meticulously address dilemmas regarding local therapy (including the proper timing, volume, and fractionation schedule for radiation therapy) and revisit the heretofore dormant issue of surgical treatment. The potential drawbacks and benefits of prophylactic cranial radiation and chemotherapy dose intensification are also discussed in detail. The relative pros and cons are presented in a balanced manner that enables the reader to fully appreciate the subtleties behind each position.

Other topics in the book include novel strategies to improve outcome in selected groups of locally advanced non–small cell lung cancer patients; the role of adjuvant postoperative chemotherapy and radiation therapy; surgery versus chemoradiation in patients with marginally resectable stage III disease; and opposing viewpoints on a recently emerging controversy—three-dimensional conformal radiation therapy versus conventional radiation in lung cancer. In addition to providing information in a pro/con format for the most controversial issues, this text presents comprehensive, state-of-the-art discussions of supportive care, chemoprevention, endobronchial therapy, economic and resource analyses, and the role of chemotherapy dose intensification in non–small cell lung cancer.

For the clinician involved in the management of lung cancer, this book is an invaluable resource. Because of our increasing workloads, we have considerable difficulty in collecting and assimilating, on our own, the critical information necessary to provide the best possible care for patients. The well-organized and thoughtful presentations in *Controversies in Lung Cancer* will help the multidisciplinary team of lung cancer physicians and nurses to achieve their primary objectives—to improve not only the quantity, but also the quality, of life for patients with lung cancer.

Philip Bonomi, M.D.
Director, Section of Medical Oncology
Rush-Presbyterian-St. Luke's Medical Center
Chicago, Illinois

Preface

Lung cancer is the leading cause of cancer death in the United States for both men and women. Indeed, the number of deaths per year from lung cancer exceeds that of the second, third, and fourth leading causes of cancer death (viz., breast, prostate, and colorectal cancer) combined. It is not surprising, then, that many exhaustive textbooks have been written on this subject, encompassing a vast amount of intricate details about pathological factors, molecular markers, staging workup, and so forth. Despite the wealth of information available on lung cancer, many controversies and dilemmas still exist. Rather than focus on what is already known and accepted, we have decided to tackle challenging issues that remain unresolved.

In this light, we have divided the chapters into ''controversies'' and ''dilemmas.'' For the chapters centering on controversies, both ''pro'' and ''con'' viewpoints are presented. Although similar material is sometimes presented in the opposing chapters, the key difference between the two lies in the interpretation of and emphasis placed on the studies discussed. We believe that it is important for the reader to be exposed to the subtleties behind both arguments in such controversies. Other topics do not lend themselves as readily to this format, but still constitute an ongoing dilemma worthy of discussion. For example, the opening chapter addresses current issues regarding staging. How are new techniques, such as PET scanning, to be incorporated into our staging algorithms?

Leading national and international authorities on particular subjects have been selected to present their views. For example, a heated controversy still exists regarding the timing of thoracic radiotherapy for patients with limited-stage small cell lung cancer. Arguing for early administration of radiotherapy in Chapter 2 is Nevin Murray, first author of the NCI Canada randomized trial favoring early over delayed radiotherapy. The opposing argument is presented in Chapter 3 by Mark Bryer and Michael C. Perry, the lead author of the CALGB randomized trial suggesting a benefit to delayed radiotherapy. The authors (pro and con) of each chapter use evidence-based medicine to support the "bottom line" of why they favor one of two contrary approaches.

Chapter 4 leads the reader through the ongoing dilemmas regarding radiotherapy fractionation and volume in small cell lung cancer. Chapter coauthor Andrew Turrisi was first author of the pivotal randomized trial (recently published in the *New England Journal of Medicine*) on radiation fractionation in lung cancer patients. Throughout this volume, not only are the authors leading experts in the treatment of lung cancer, but they have been specifically chosen to address issues about which they feel passionate. This applies not only to the chapters on small cell lung cancer, but also to the subsequent section on non–small cell lung cancer. The final section of the book investigates more global issues that apply to all patients with lung cancer.

This book is geared toward the clinician who encounters these challenging problems in everyday oncologic practice. The management of lung cancer has become a multidisciplinary effort, requiring cooperation and communication among practitioners from various fields. Indeed, the specialization of the editors represent the three major modalities of treatment—radiation, medical, and surgical oncology. In our weekly Multidisciplinary Thoracic Oncology Tumor Board at Fox Chase Cancer Center, we have attempted to share our observations and thus highlight many of the dilemmas that confront us within and across disciplines.

Controversies in Lung Cancer will prove a valuable resource, not only for oncologists and thoracic surgeons, but also for pulmonologists and general practitioners, who share the burden of caring for this large group of patients. Pulmonologists will find several chapters devoted to the supportive care of patients with lung cancer. These chapters include discussions of the preoperative pulmonary evaluation of patients, as well as the management of the key side effects of thoracic radiation and chemotherapy, pneumonitis, and esophagitis.

In the current era of second opinions, patients often lose their direction on the ''information superhighway'' and look toward their primary physician for guidance and assurance. This book helps crystallize the reasoning behind the opinions that patients often face, and it enables their physicians to make this information more understandable and accessible. The book will also be an indispensable reference for oncology nurses who are instrumental in taking care of patients with lung cancer. Finally, residents and medical students can glean countless insights regarding the management of lung cancer patients, and observe how evidence-based medicine can be used to formulate cogent arguments at chart rounds or tumor boards.

We would like to take this opportunity to thank the many contributors who have worked diligently to present their perspectives in the prescribed format. We would also like to acknowledge Sandra Beberman and Michael Deters of Marcel Dekker, Inc., for their tireless efforts and Louise Marcewicz for her excellent secretarial support. We are deeply grateful to our families, who supported us wholeheartedly in this worthwhile project. Finally, we are forever indebted to our patients, whose courage and determination continue to inspire us.

Benjamin Movsas
Corey J. Langer
Melvyn Goldberg

Contents

Contributors

Rodrigo Arriagada, M.D.   Department of Radiation Oncology, Instituto de Radiomedicina, Santiago, Chile

Mark D. Bergman, M.D., Ph.D.   Department of Hematology/Oncology, Beth Israel Deaconess Medical Center, Boston, Massachusetts

Eugene H. Blackstone, M.D.   Department of Thoracic and Cardiovascular Surgery, Department of Epidemiology and Biostatistics, Cleveland Clinic Foundation, Cleveland, Ohio

Mark Bryer, M.D.   Radiation Oncology, University of Missouri/Ellis Fischel Cancer Center, Columbia, Missouri

Roger W. Byhardt, M.D.   Radiation Oncology, Medical College of Wisconsin, Milwaukee, Wisconsin

Desmond N. Carney, M.D., Ph.D. Department of Medical Oncology, Mater Hospital, and University College Dublin, Dublin, Ireland

J. Donald Chapman, Ph.D. Department of Radiation Oncology, Fox Chase Cancer Center, Philadelphia, Pennsylvania

Douglas Coyle Department of Medicine, University of Ottawa, Ottawa, Ontario, Canada

Jeffrey Crawford, M.D. Director of Clinical Research, Duke Comprehensive Cancer Center, Durham, North Carolina

Russell F. DeVore III, M.D.* Thoracic Oncology, Vanderbilt-Ingram Cancer Center, Vanderbilt University School of Medicine, Nashville, Tennessee

Jan Dombrowski, M.D. Department of Radiation-Oncology, Genesee Hospital, Rochester, New York

Craig C. Earle, M.D. Dana-Farber Cancer Institute, Harvard Medical School, Boston, Massachusetts

Anthony Elias, M.D. Adult Oncology, Dana-Farber Cancer Institute, Harvard University, Boston, Massachusetts

William K. Evans, M.D. Oncology Program, University of Ottawa, Cancer Care Ontario, Ottawa, Ontario, Canada

David R. Gandara, M.D. Department of Internal Medicine, Division of Hematology and Oncology, University of California Davis Cancer Center, Sacramento, California

Sunil Gandhi, M.D. University of Texas M. D. Anderson Cancer Center, Houston, Texas

Eli Glatstein, M.D. Vice Chairman, Department of Radiation Oncology, The University of Pennsylvania Medical Center, Philadelphia, Pennsylvania

Elizabeth M. Gore, M.D. Radiation Oncology, Medical College of Wisconsin, Milwaukee, Wisconsin

---

* Current affiliation: East Tennessee Oncology/Hematology, Knoxville, Tennessee.

Mary V. Graham, M.D. Director, Radiation Oncology, Phelps County Regional Medical Center, Rolla, Missouri

Mark R. Green, M.D. Hollings Cancer Center, Medical University of South Carolina, Charleston, South Carolina

Richard I. Inculet, M.D. Division of Thoracic Surgery, London Health Sciences Centre, London, Ontario, Canada

Daniel D. Karp, M.D. Director, Cancer Clinical Trials Office, Department of Hematology/Oncology, Harvard Medical School, Boston, Massachusetts

Steven M. Keller, M.D.* Chief, Division of Thoracic Surgery, Beth Israel Medical Center, New York, and Cardiothoracic Surgery, Albert Einstein College of Medicine, Bronx, New York

Earl King, M.D. Director, Pulmonary Medicine and Respiratory Care, Fox Chase Cancer Center, Philadelphia, Pennsylvania

Ritsuko Komaki, M.D. Department of Radiation Oncology, University of Texas M. D. Anderson Cancer Center, Houston, Texas

Primo N. Lara, Jr., M.D. Department of Internal Medicine, Division of Hematology-Oncology, University of California Davis Cancer Center, Sacramento, California

Derick Lau, M.D., Ph.D. Department of Internal Medicine, Division of Hematology-Oncology, University of California Davis Cancer Center, Sacramento, California

Thierry Le Chevalier, M.D. Department of Medicine, Institut Gustave-Roussy, Villejuif, France

Cécile Le Péchoux, M.D. Department of Radiotherapy, Institut Gustave-Roussy, Villejuif, France

Swan S. Leong, M.D. Department of Medical Oncology, National Cancer Center, Singapore, Republic of Singapore

---

* Current affiliation: Montefiore Medical Center, Bronx, New York.

Chong Hee Lim, M.D.   Department of Thoracic and Cardiovascular Surgery, Cleveland Clinic Foundation, Cleveland, Ohio

Sandra McDonald   Department of Radiation Oncology, Genesee Hospital, Rochester, New York

Nevin Murray, M.D.   Department of Medical Oncology, University of British Columbia and British Columbia Cancer Agency, Vancouver, British Columbia, Canada

Michael C. Perry, M.D.   Division of Hematology/Oncology, University of Missouri/Ellis Fischel Cancer Center, Columbia, Missouri

Thomas W. Rice, M.D.   Department of Thoracic and Cardiovascular Surgery, Cleveland Clinic Foundation, Cleveland, Ohio

Philip Rubin, M.D.   Radiation Oncology, University of Rochester Cancer Center, Rochester, New York

Alan Sandler, M.D.   Department of Hematology/Oncology, Vanderbilt University, Nashville, Tennessee

Frances A. Shepherd, M.D.   Division of Medical Oncology, Princess Margaret Hospital, Department of Medicine, University of Toronto, Toronto, Ontario, Canada

Zvi Small, M.D.   Albert Einstein College of Medicine, Bronx, New York

Burton L. Speiser, M.D.   Medical Director, Department of Radiation Oncology, St. Joseph's Hospital and Medical Center, Phoenix, Arizona

Charles Thomas, Jr., M.D.*   Radiation Oncology, Medical University of South Carolina, Charleston, South Carolina

Andrew T. Turrisi III, M.D.   Chairman, Department of Radiation Oncology, Medical University of South Carolina, Charleston, South Carolina

---

* Current affiliation: University of Texas Health Science Center at San Antonio, San Antonio Cancer Institute, San Antonio, Texas.

Michael Unger, M.D.   Pulmonary Cancer Detection and Prevention Program, Fox Chase Cancer Center, and Thomas Jefferson Medical College, Philadelphia, Pennsylvania

R. C. Urtasun, M.D.   Professor Emeritus, Oncology, Cross Cancer Institute, Edmonton, Alberta, Canada

Garrett L. Walsh, M.D.   Department of Thoracic and Cardiovascular Surgery, University of Texas M. D. Anderson Cancer Center, Houston, Texas

William H. Warren, M.D.   Departments of Cardiovascular-Thoracic Surgery and Pathology, Rush-Presbyterian-St. Luke's Medical Center, Chicago, Illinois

Jacqueline Williams, Ph.D.   Radiation Oncology, University of Rochester Cancer Center, Rochester, New York

Todd Williams, M.D.   Radiation Oncology, Medical University of South Carolina, Charleston, South Carolina

1

Staging Dilemmas in Lung Cancer

Swan S. Leong
National Cancer Center, Singapore, Republic of Singapore

Mark R. Green
Hollings Cancer Center, Medical University of South Carolina,
Charleston, South Carolina

INTRODUCTION

The goals of a cancer staging system are to standardize the description of disease based on extent and severity; to reflect the different prognoses of each stage group; to direct management; and to facilitate conduct and comparison of clinical and translational research.

Lung cancer staging, built upon this template, has undergone significant changes over the last two decades as more data on the behavior and outcome of disease have been accumulated and different management strategies, based on patterns of failure and treatment endpoints for different groups of patients, have been implemented. The accuracy of staging investigations has also improved as new tools and techniques have become available, enhancing the validity and usefulness of the lung cancer staging system.

Issues and questions remain however. These issues continue to fuel discussion and reexamination of the International Lung Cancer Staging System.

EVOLUTION OF LUNG CANCER STAGING

Several classifications for lung cancer staging were proposed but none became widely accepted until the 1970s, when the American Joint Committee for Cancer Staging and End Results Reporting (AJCC) put forth an evidence-based proposal for staging. In 1973, the AJCC Task Force on Carcinoma of the Lung, adopting the TNM classification scheme as described by Denoix (1), recommended criteria for clinical staging of lung cancer. This staging system was based on information collected from 2155 patients with bronchogenic carcinoma (2). Variables such as size, location, and extent of primary tumor; association with obstructive pneumonitis, atelectasis, and pleural effusion; spread of tumor to different lymph node stations; and involvement of distant organs were analyzed against survival data. The T (T_{0-3}), N (N_{0-2}), and M (M_{0-1}) categories were developed based on these data. In the 1973 system, the presence of pleural effusion (either with or without malignant cells) and the involvement of mediastinal structures by direct tumor invasion were placed in a heterogeneous T_3 category. This grouping also included much more limited tumors, for example those involving only the chest wall. This arrangement was based on survival data that were available at the time and reflected the inadequate radiographic staging tools in use at the time. We now know that this diverse T_3 category includes several subgroups with different treatment options and important outcome differences (3–6).

Stage groupings were formed from analysis of more than 300 survival curves plotted for various combinations of T, N, and M descriptors. Three stage groups were defined, with stage I disease demonstrating the best outcome and stage III the worse. Stage I disease included $T_{1-2}N_0M_0$ and $T_1N_1M_0$ tumors. Stage II disease, the smallest category, included just $T_2N_1M_0$ tumors. Stage III disease included all T_3, N_2, or M_1 tumors. The stage III disease category, like the T_3 category, was very broad and had patients ranging from those with locally infiltrative disease to patients with systemic metastasis. This staging system reflected the limited treatment options of that era. Essentially all of the stage III patients, with the exception of those with T_3N_0 disease, had a dismally poor outlook. Even in this early analysis, the survival estimates of patients with $T_3N_0M_0$ disease, including some with superior sulcus tumors, demonstrated some chance for long-term survival (2,4). Yet in the 1973 staging system no stage III subgroups were defined to acknowledge that fact.

Survival for patients with small cell carcinoma was also recognized to be exceptionally poor regardless of the demonstrated extent of disease. The proposed TNM guidelines were viewed as inappropriate for staging of small cell lung cancer.

The 1973 staging system's three stages generally reflected prognoses as appropriate for that period. However, with improvements in imaging techniques and treatment approaches, the deficiencies of the system became increasingly apparent. Various meetings held during 1985 by members of AJCC, Union Internationale Contre Cancer (UICC), and Japanese and German representatives culminated in the proposal for a revised International Staging System for Lung Cancer, published in 1986 (7). The database for this revision comprised records of 3753 lung cancer patients from M.D. Anderson Hospital and the North American Lung Cancer Study Group's Reference Center for Anatomic and Pathologic Classification of Lung Cancer. Changes from the 1973 system were intended to better reflect prognoses and provide more meaningful guidelines for directing management. Tumors with invasion of mediastinal structures or vertebral bodies and tumors associated with a malignant pleural effusion were moved from T_3 to a new category of T_4 tumors. Malignant effusion was more fully defined to exclude pleural fluids that were cytologically negative, nonbloody, and not exudative. A footnote to the staging system defined superficial tumors limited to the bronchial wall as T_1, irrespective of the distance of involvement along the bronchial mucosa and proximity to the main bronchus.

Mediastinal nodes were divided into two categories. N_2 disease was now limited to ipsilateral mediastinal and subcarinal lymph node involvement while a new N_3 descriptor, including supraclavicular, contralateral hilar (previously designated M_1), and contralateral mediastinal lymph nodes, was added. Although the prognosis of patients with contralateral hilar and supraclavicular lymph nodes (N_3) was recognized to be very poor, these areas of involvement were readily included in the field of radiation treatment and were considered regional spread by radiation oncologists.

In the 1986 system, the stage groupings were also revised. Patients with $T_1N_0M_0$ tumors, with 5-year survival rates of more than 60%, were recognized as a particularly favorable subgroup. The possibility of having a totally separate stage group was considered but ultimately this was not implemented. $T_1N_1M_0$ disease, having a poorer prognosis than N_0 patients because of lymph node involvement (8,9), was combined with $T_2N_1M_0$ disease as stage II. The heterogeneous stage III category of the first AJCC system was now separated into locally advanced disease (stage III) and disseminated disease (stage IV). Surgery was clearly the primary treatment approach for stage I and II disease while palliative management was indicated for stage IV disease. The new stage III category was too complex from the outset to uniformly define prognosis and direct therapy. Therefore, it was further subdivided into IIIA (T_3 and/or N_2), where complete resection might still be feasible, and IIIB (T_4 and/or N_3), where it usually was not feasible.

The second major revision in the lung cancer staging system was implemented in 1997 (10), following a decade of working with the 1986 system. The 1997 revision was again based on patient data, an analysis of records from 5319 lung cancer patients treated at the M.D. Anderson Cancer Center from 1975 to 1988, and by the North American Lung Cancer Study Group from 1977 to 1982.

TABLE 1 Primary Tumor (T)

	1974	1986	1997
T_x	Tumor proven by malignant cells in bronchopulmonary secretions but not visualized by imaging or bronchoscopically	Same as 1974 + primary tumors that cannot be assessed	Same as 1986
T_0	No evidence of tumor	Same as 1974	Same as 1974
T_{is}	—	Carcinoma in situ	Same as 1986
T_1	Tumor 3 cm or less, surrounded by lung or visceral pleura, without invasion proximal to a lobar	Same as 1974	Same as 1974
T_2	Tumor with any of the following: >3 cm; involves main bronchus but $\geq$2 cm distal to carina; invades visceral pleura; assoc. with atelectasis or obstructive pneumonitis which involve <1 lung	Same as 1974	Same as 1974
T_3	Tumor that invades all adjacent structures including mediastinum *and its contents*; or <2 cm from carina; or assoc. with atelectasis or obstructive pneumonitis that involves the whole lung; or *pleural effusion*	Tumor that invades: chest wall; diaphragm, mediastinal pleura, parietal pericardium; main bronchus <2 cm from carina but not involving it; assoc. with atelectasis or obstructive pneumonitis that involves the whole lung	Same as 1986
T_4	—	Tumor that invades: mediastinal structures including heart, great vessels, trachea, esophagus; vertebral body; or presence of malignant effusion	Same as 1986 + *satellite tumor nodule(s) within ipsilateral primary-tumor lobe of lung*

Source: Leong et al. Chest 1999; 115:242–248.

Among the issues addressed by the 1997 revision were the varying prognoses of resectable tumors based on tumor diameter or the presence of multiple synchronous tumor "satellite" lesions in the same lung at diagnosis. In this most recent revision, stage I was divided into IA and IB, based on tumor size of 3 cm or less (T_1) versus greater than 3 cm (T_2) and the presence (T_2) or absence (T_1) of visceral pleural invasion. Stage II was also divided into IIA and IIB subgroups based on the same criteria. In addition, $T_3N_0M_0$ patients were regrouped as stage IIB. Tumors with satellite nodules in the same lobe as the primary were designated T_4 (stage IIIB). Synchronous lesions in a different lobe of the same lung as from the primary tumor were considered M_1 disease (Tables 1–4).

Patients with $T_1N_0M_0$ tumors have a significantly better outcome after complete resection compared to patients with $T_2N_0M_0$ tumors. This had already been clear from the database of the 1986 staging proposal. In that database, the 5-year survival rate of patients with pathological $T_1N_0M_0$ disease was 68.5% versus 59% for patients with $T_2N_0M_0$ disease (7). Other series had also demonstrated the same finding. For example, of 461 patients with $T_1N_0M_0$ or $T_2N_0M_0$ disease treated with curative surgical resection between April 1972 and March 1978 at the Mayo Clinic, Williams et al. showed a 5-year survival rate of 80% for $T_1N_0M_0$ disease compared to about 62% for $T_2N_0M_0$ disease (8). Similar findings were noted by Naruke et al. (11) and Harpole et al. (12). Given the volume of data demonstrating a substantially superior survival outcome, $T_1N_0M_0$ disease was given a separate subgroup heading of stage IA in the 1997 staging revisions,

TABLE 2 Regional Lymph Nodes (N)

	1974	1986	1997
N_x	—	Regional lymph nodes cannot be assessed	Same as 1986
N_0	No regional lymph node metastasis	Same as 1974	Same as 1974
N_1	Metastasis to ipsilateral hilar lymph nodes	Metastasis to ipsilateral peribronchial and/or ipsilateral hilar lymph nodes	Same as 1986
N_2	Metastasis to *mediastinal lymph nodes*	Metastasis to ipsilateral mediastinal and/or subcarinal lymph nodes	Same as 1986
N_3	—	Metastasis to *contralateral mediastinal, contralateral hilar, ipsilateral/ contralateral supraclavicular nodes*	Same as 1986

Source: Leong et al. Chest 1999; 115:242–248.

TABLE 3 Distant Metastasis (M)

	1974	1986	1997
M_x	—	Presence of distant metastasis cannot be assessed	Same as 1986
M_0	No distant metastasis	Same as 1974	Same as 1974
M_1	Distant metastasis including *involvement of scalene, cervical, and contralateral hilar lymph nodes*	Distant metastasis excluding scalene, cervical, and contralateral hilar nodes	Same as 1986

Source: Leong et al. Chest 1999; 115:242–248.

emphasizing the distinction from $T_2N_0M_0$ disease. Watanabe et al. have demonstrated a continuous effect of tumor size on survival, finding not only a difference in 5-year survival between $T_1N_0M_0$ disease (77.6%) and $T_2N_0M_0$ disease (60.1%), but also a difference when comparing survival rates of patients with tumors measuring 3–5 cm in diameter (61%) and those with tumors greater than 5 cm (46%)

TABLE 4 Stage Grouping (TNM Combinations)

1974		1986		1997	
Occult	$T_xN_0M_0$	Occult	$T_xN_0M_0$	Occult	$T_{xs}N_0M_0$
Stage 0	$T_{is}N_0M_0$	Stage 0	$T_{is}N_0M_0$	Stage 0	$T_{is}N_0M_0$
Stage I	$T_1N_0M_0$	Stage I	$T_1N_0M_0$	Stage IA	$T_1N_0M_0$
	$T_2N_0M_0$		$T_2N_0M_0$	Stage IB	$T_2N_0M_0$
	$T_1N_1M_0$				
Stage II	$T_2N_1M_0$	Stage II	$T_1N_1M_0$	Stage IIA	$T_1N_1M_0$
			$T_2N_1M_0$	Stage IIB	$T_2N_1M_0$
					$T_3N_0M_0$
Stage III	T_3, any N, any M	Stage IIIA	$T_3N_0M_0$	Stage IIIA	$T_3N_1M_0$
	Any T,N_2, any M		$T_3N_1M_0$		$T_1N_2M_0$
	Any T, any N,M_1		$T_1N_2M_0$		$T_2N_2M_0$
			$T_2N_2M_0$		$T_3N_2M_0$
			$T_3N_2M_0$		
		Stage IIIB	T_4, any N,M_0, any T,N_3,M_0	Stage IIIB	T_4, any N,M_0, any T,N_3,M_0
—		Stage IV	Any T, any N,M_1	Stage IV	Any T, any N,M_1

Source: Leong et al. Chest 1999; 115:242–248.

(13). However, only two subgroups of stage I disease are designated in the current staging scheme.

In the 1997 staging revision, stage II disease has also been divided into stage IIA and stage IIB subgroups based on T characteristics. A difference in prognosis is demonstrable between patients with $T_1N_1M_0$ disease and those with $T_2N_1M_0$ disease (7,11). However, the available data do not show as great a survival disparity between the two stage II subgroups as is seen in stage IA and IB patients. For example, Naruke et al. demonstrated a 5-year survival rate of 43.6% for patients with $T_1N_1M_0$ disease and 37.6% for patients with $T_2N_1M_0$ disease (11). Mountain found survival rates of 54.1% and 40%, respectively (7). In the current revision, $T_3N_0M_0$ disease, which has shown a survival comparable to $T_2N_1M_0$ disease, was also added to the stage IIB category. The 5-year survival rate for T_3N_0 patients was 31.6% in the Naruke series (11) and 44.2% in data presented by Mountain (7).

Significant differences in survival rates following complete surgical resection have been shown between patients with T_3N_{0-1} and $T_{1-3}N_2$ disease (14,15). Patients with T_3N_0 disease due to chest wall invasion do especially well after complete resection of their tumor (3,4). In such individuals, McCaughan et al. were able to show a 5-year survival rate of 56% (3). In retrospect $T_3N_0M_0$ patients had been recognized as having a superior outcome at least since the 1974 staging system was proposed (2). In the survival data of the 1997 staging proposal, the 5-year survival rate for T_3N_0 patients was almost identical to that of patients with $T_2N_1M_0$ disease (10), in contrast to the much poorer outcome for patients with N_2 disease (16,17), cementing the move of the T_3N_0 group from stage IIIA to stage IIB, where surgery represents the primary treatment approach.

AREAS OF CONTROVERSY

While the 1997 staging revision addressed several important issues already discussed, other compelling issues were either incompletely addressed or ignored. This means that the international lung cancer staging scheme will remain dynamic. Within a decade, as a broad experience with the 1997 system becomes available, additional discussion will inevitably lead to yet further revision of the current TNM staging classification. Some of the important questions less than fully addressed in the current staging system are discussed below.

Pulmonary Nodules

The 1986 staging system did not provide strong, evidence-based information for categorizing patients with synchronous satellite lesions or pulmonary nodules in the ipsilateral lung. However, in the footnotes of the fourth edition of the AJCC staging manual published in 1993, satellite lesions in the same lobe led to upstaging of the primary by one T category while the presence of a synchronous ipsilateral lesion in a separate lobe was categorized as T_4. The notion that ipsilateral synchronous nodules in a separate lobe should be considered T_4 (stage IIIB) rather than hematogenous M_1 disease was questioned by many investigators. Some considered them as locally advanced disease while others considered them metastases.

Deslauriers et al. retrospectively reviewed the records of 84 patients with primary lung cancer accompanied by one or more satellite nodules, and 1021 patients who had a primary lung cancer but no satellite nodules. All had undergone pulmonary resection between January 1969 and December 1986 (18). In most of the patients, the satellite nodule(s) occurred in the same lobe as the primary tumor (68 of 84). Disease was staged according to the 1974 guidelines, and survival was compared, stage for stage, in patients with and without satellite nodules. For patients without satellite nodules, the 5-year survival rates were 54.4% for stage I, 40.4% for stage II, and 20.3% for stage III disease. For patients with satellite nodules, the 5-year survival rates were 32%, 12.5%, and 5.6%, respectively, for stages I, II, and III disease. Since over 80% of the patients had their satellite nodules in the same lobe as the primary, no exploratory subset analysis of nodules occurring in the same lobe as the primary tumor versus those occurring in a different lobe was carried out. The work of Deslauriers did demonstrate that the presence of satellite nodules connoted a poorer prognosis. However, it also showed that some patients with satellite lesions in the same lobe as the primary tumor were able to achieve long-term survival with resection.

In another retrospective review by Shimizu et al., 42 patients with lung cancer were found to have intrapulmonary satellite nodules in the pathology specimen obtained at the time of pulmonary resection (19). The 2-year survival rate was significantly better in patients with satellite lesions in the same lobe as the primary tumor (41.5%) than in patients with lesions in different lobes (20%). The presence of satellite nodules in the same lobe as the primary tumor did not necessarily preclude long-term survival following surgery.

Watanabe et al., in an evaluation of 49 patients with ipsilateral intrapulmonary lesions, suggested that the survival of patients with satellite lesions was similar to that of stage IIIA patients without satellite lesions and superior to that of stage IIIB patients without satellite lesions (13). There was no breakdown as to how many of these individuals had lesions in the same lobe as the primary tumor and how many had them in different lobes, but clearly, the survival following surgery was better than would be expected from M_1 disease.

In the 1997 revision of the staging system, satellite lesions in the same lobe as the primary tumor are categorized as T_4 stage IIIB disease. Synchronous lesions outside the primary tumor lobe but in the ipsilateral lung are considered metastatic spread (M_1). This distinction is based in part on the proposed difference in the mechanisms of disease, with lesions in the same lobe thought to represent tumor emboli and lesions in different lobes considered hematogenous metastases. However, the T_4 designation for satellite lesions in the same lobe suggests a poorer prognosis than appears warranted by the available data. Many surgeons continue to offer surgery to patients with T_4 satellite lesions if the N and M status of their presentation do not preclude curative surgery.

Pleural Effusion

In the 1986 staging system, a malignant pleural effusion was defined as one containing malignant cells and/or one that was either bloody or exudative. In patients with lung cancer, the presence of a malignant pleural effusion confers a poor prognosis. Naruke et al. (11) compared the postoperative survival of 1298 lung cancer patients without a pleural effusion, 112 patients with a nonmalignant effusion, and 48 patients with malignant pleural fluid at surgery. Five-year survival rates for the three groups were 40%, 39.2%, and 10.7%, respectively. In the Naruke series, the survival of the patients with malignant pleural effusion was similar to that of all operated patients with T_4 disease (8.4%) seen in the database for the 1986 staging system. This suggested at the time that it was reasonable to include malignant pleural effusion within the T_4 stage IIIB category.

As management strategies have evolved to include multimodality treatment for T_4 stage IIIB disease, the inclusion of malignant pleural effusion in the T_4 category has become more problematic. The substantial advances made over the last decade for managing patients with stage III disease all involve local or regional treatment modalities designed to eradicate intrathoracic disease (20,21). The presence of a malignant effusion implies involvement of the pleural cavity, limiting the curative potential of radiotherapy or surgery.

Recent data demonstrate that the survival of patients with malignant pleural effusion approximates that of stage IV disease. Sugiura et al. investigated the impact of pleural effusion in patients with advanced non–small cell lung cancer (6). A total of 197 patients with stage IIIB or IV non–small cell lung cancer were studied. The median survival for patients with stage IIIB disease without pleural effusion, stage IIIB disease with pleural effusion, and stage IV disease was 15.3, 7.5, and 5.5 months, respectively. The survival of patients with stage IIIB disease with effusion was significantly worse than that of IIIB patients without effusion, but not significantly different from that of stage IV patients. In this study, there was no significant difference in survival between patients with cytologically positive and cytologically negative pleural effusions provided the effusion was as exudate. Mountain (22) also came to a similar conclusion when he found no difference in survival for patient with malignant cells present in the pleural fluid, those with negative cytology, and those with clinically evident pleural fluid not further analyzed but thought to be the result of the underlying malignancy. These data suggest that patients with malignant pleural effusion should be considered to have stage IV disease, perhaps stage IVA versus stage IVB for those with frank metastatic disease, to reflect the current incurability of such patients and the palliative nature of treatment.

Pleural Nodules

Pleural nodules in the absence of pleural effusion constitute a vexing staging problem. Nodular pleural involvement was classified as T_4 disease in the footnotes to the 1986 staging classification. However, information on the outcome of patients with pleural dissemination without pleural effusion is scarce. Might there not be a distinction between a more limited involvement of visceral pleura overlying the primary tumor, suggesting spread by tumor emboli, versus extensive, multifocal, visceral, and/or parietal pleural involvement suggesting true metastasis? Such an approach would be analogous to the current categorization of ipsilateral pulmonary nodules.

Akaogi et al. (23) retrospectively assessed the distribution of pleural nodules in 23 patients with pleural dissemination but no distant metastasis who underwent pleuropulmonary resection. Thirteen patients had small pleural nodules but either no effusion or only a small amount of effusion. All 13 had involvement of the visceral pleura and 10 of these 13 also had involvement of the parietal pleura. In 10 of 13 patients, visceral involvement was considered "local and limited," while in the majority (6 of 10) with parietal pleural involvement, the parietal disease was extensive. Although it is difficult to draw any definite conclusions from these findings, they suggest different patterns of spread leading to different distributions of pleural involvement. Whether this translates into survival differences cannot be discerned from this small series. Of interest, all 13 patients with pleural involvement did poorly except for those who did not have N_2 node involvement.

In another small series reported by Shimizu et al., 38 patients with pleural dissemination without pleural effusion were studied (24). The overall 5-year survival rate was found to be 19.4%. This survival outcome is better than would have been expected from patients with pleural dissemination with effusion. Once again, the survival rate of the patients appeared to correlate with nodal stage and tumor size. The correlation of survival with the extent of pleural involvement was not discussed. Clearly, more data will be required before an evidence-based classification of visceral and parietal pleural involvement can be provided within the staging system.

NEW STAGING INVESTIGATIONS

Improvement in staging investigations have complemented the development of the staging system for lung cancer. Since the 1970s, staging of lung cancer patients has relied heavily on computed tomography (CT) of the chest and upper abdomen. Though invaluable for the evaluation of the primary tumor, staging of lymph nodes with CT has its limitations (25). Glazer et al., after studying CTs of 56 normal subjects and reviewing a previous set of data on patients with non–small cell lung cancer, suggested a measurement of 1.0 cm in the short axis of a lymph node as the threshold for defining pathological enlargement (26,27). McLoud et al. studied 143 patients prospectively with CT using the same criteria and compared the results with surgical staging (28). The sensitivity of CT was found to be 64% and specificity 62%. Thirteen percent of normal-sized lymph nodes and 25% of lymph nodes measuring 1–1.9 cm in short-axis diameter were found to contain metastatic disease. The likelihood of lymph nodes being involved with tumor increased with increasing nodal size. However, Gallardo et al. found, in a series of 167 patients, that only 23% of enlarged lymph nodes had neoplastic involvement (29). This high false positive rate dictates the need for an adjunctive staging instrument or procedure to further assess enlarged lymph nodes shown on chest CT. The current procedure of choice for this additional assessment is mediastinoscopy. European investigators have recently reported the sensitivity and specificity of mediastinoscopy to be 89% and 100%, respectively, in the staging of 100 consecutive patients with non–small cell lung cancer. In the same series the sensitivity and specificity of CT among the same patients were 63% and 57%, respectively (30). Such data have led to routine use of mediastinoscopy (cervical or parasternal) prior to thoracotomy, to evaluate enlarged lymph nodes found on chest CT.

The role of mediastinoscopic staging when lymph nodes are normal in size on a staging chest CT is more controversial. In this setting the false negative rate ranges from approximately 10 to 13% (25,28). Some have suggested that microscopic involvement of a normal-sized lymph node may not have the same prognostic significance as nodes enlarged with tumor. Daly et al. reviewed data on 681 patients who had both CT and surgical staging (31). A total of 501 patients had normal-sized mediastinal lymph nodes. Thirty-seven of these were subsequently found to have positive lymph nodes at mediastinoscopy or thoracotomy. Thirty-one patients underwent definitive resection. For these 31 patients, the 5-year survival was 31%. Among patients with negative CT scans later found to have mediastinal lymph node involvement, prognosis was worse if the primary tumor was central rather than peripheral. The authors concluded that definitive thoracotomy without mediastinoscopy is justified in most patients with a normal mediastinum on CT. For central tumors, however, mediastinoscopic examination may prove helpful (15,31).

Endoscopic ultrasound (EUS) examination of mediastinal lymph nodes has improved staging accuracy in centers where expertise with the technique is available. It has the advantage of being able to evaluate lymph nodes based on thickness, contour, and internal architecture rather than size alone. Kondo et al. tested the sensitivity and specificity of EUS mediastinal staging in 101 Japanese patients with lung cancer (32). The sensitivity was found to be 53.6% and specificity 97.5%. Endoscopic ultrasound can also be used to perform fine-needle aspiration biopsies of abnormal lymph nodes either poorly accessible or completely inaccessible to cervical mediastinoscopy, especially the level 5 and 7 lymph nodes. Silvestri et al. evaluated the sensitivity of EUS in 27 patients with lung cancer (33). Twenty-two of the 27 patients had mediastinal lymph node enlargement on chest CT. Only 16 had a positive EUS evaluation. In 15 of the 16, the positive EUS was confirmed by FNA. Of the remaining 12 patients, two had lymph nodes found to be involved at operation. Overall sensitivity was 89%. One limitation of endoscopic ultrasound is that it can only be used to assess lymph nodes adjacent to the esophagus. Clearly it can complement, but does not replace, chest CT and mediastinoscopy in the staging of lung cancer.

Small pulmonary nodules are frequently detected during CT staging for lung cancer. This is especially true with the newest generation of spiral scanners. If these lesions are not calcified, it is often difficult to distinguish between malignant disease and benign changes. For example, among 551 patients with lung cancer who underwent preoperative CT scanning, Keogan et al. reported that 88 patients (16%) had small, noncalcified nodules separate from the lung primary (34). Of the 88 patients, 25 had adequate radiological follow-up of at least 24 months or pathological examination of the nodules at surgery. Seventy percent were eventually determined to be benign, 11% malignant, and 19% remained indeterminate.

The development of positron emission tomography (PET) is an exciting advance in radiological imaging. However, its true effectiveness in diminishing staging ambiguity in lung cancer is still being defined. Nonetheless, in the United States the Health Care Financing Administration (HCFA) has recently authorized Medicare to pay for PET scans in the staging of patients with non–small cell lung cancer (35). Glycolysis is increased in tumor tissue and PET detects increased uptake of ^{18}F-fluoro-2-deoxy-D-glucose (FDG), a glucose analog radiopharmaceutical, in malignant tissue. It can be useful in evaluating both parenchymal lung nodules and mediastinal nodes. It has stronger negative than positive predictive value because nonmalignant diseases may also result in an increase in FDG uptake. However, small parenchymal lesions ($<$7–10 mm) may be falsely negative with PET scanning. Sazon et al. have reported that PET is 100% sensitive and 52% specific in predicting the malignant nature of radiographic abnormality (36). Others have reported less impressive findings but a 90% or greater sensitivity for PET in detecting primary lung cancer is well accepted. Positron emission tomography has also been found to be superior to CT in both sensitivity and specificity in the staging of mediastinal lymph nodes (37–39). A sensitivity of 93% and specificity of 97% have been reported (39) when combined CT-PET scanning was used for evaluation, versus 91% and 86%, respectively, with PET alone (38).

Whole-body PET may also be useful in detecting distant metastasis (37). Nabi et al. reported their experience with PET in 12 patients deemed resectable for cure after conventional workup (40). Eight patients showed increased mediastinal uptake, confirmed by mediastinoscopy or thoracotomy; one showed increased uptake in the thoracic vertebrae, confirmed later by bone scan; and one showed increased uptake in the liver, borne out later by clinical course. In contrast, two patients found to have adrenal enlargement radiologically turned out to have negative PET scans. In a recent study with 102 patients, PET scanning resulted in a different stage than the one determined by standard imaging (e.g., CT, ultrasound, bone scan, needle biopsy) in 62 patients; the stage was lowered in 20 and raised in 42 (38). In time, PET may prove to be the most cost-effective method for detecting both intrathoracic disease extent and the presence of extrathoracic metastasis.

The potential that PET has, not just for staging, but in guiding management as well, is encouraging. With the advent of combined modality management in stage III non–small cell lung cancer, prethoracotomy evaluation of response to induction chemotherapy or combined chemotherapy and radiotherapy may give important predictive information for resectability and outcome. The difficulty in assessing patients who have been treated with chemo/RT has long been appreciated, as it can be impossible to distinguish between persistent/recurrent disease and fibrosis. In a prospective study, FDG-PET response (but not CT response) was a powerful predictor of survival (p = 0.0004) (41). Eberhardt et al. have advocated repeat mediastinoscopy in guiding further management after induction chemotherapy and radiation (42). Positron emission tomography is being evaluated as an alternative approach for this restaging. Venugopal et al. have shown a significant correlation between the final pathological status and the differential uptake ratios of preoperative PET scans in 11 patients treated with chemoradiation followed by surgery (43). These provocative studies suggest that functional imaging may become a critical component of treatment algorithms, not only in defining the target, but also in assessing its response to therapy. Clearly, further defining the true capabilities of PET scanning in each of these settings is critically important.

SUMMARY

Over the past quarter century, the staging system for non–small cell lung cancer has evolved into a widely employed structure for defining prognosis, directing therapy, and facilitating communication and further clinical investigation. However, several issues remain incompletely addressed by the current staging scheme. The designation T_4 (stage IIIB) for satellite nodules in the same lobe as the primary tumor suggests a worse prognosis for these lesions than may be warranted. Long-term survival following definitive surgery can be achieved in some such patients (18,19) and they should not be excluded from consideration of surgery. Conversely, the designation of T_4 (stage IIIB) for malignant pleural effusion may not adequately convey the adverse prognosis of this extent of disease. Treatment of such patients is usually palliative, with symptomatic treatment of the effusion and systemic chemotherapy as appropriate for advanced disease. In addition to these concerns with the 1997 staging revision, rational staging of visceral and parietal pleural studding without effusion has yet to be defined.

New staging procedures such as EUS and PET are expanding the prethoracotomy options for defining the true extent of disease in patients with lung cancer. Each has great potential to help guide management. However, like any new technology, more experience will be required before we can understand their true role in standard staging approaches to patients with lung cancer.

REFERENCES

1. Denoix PF. Enquete permanent dans les centres anticancereux. Bull Inst Nat Hyg 1946; 1:70–75.
2. Mountain CF, Carr DT, Anderson WAD. A system for the clinical staging of lung cancer. Am J Roentgenol 1974; 120:130–138.
3. McCaughan BC, Martini N, Bains MS, et al. Chest wall invasion in carcinoma of the lung: therapeutic and prognostic implications. J Thorac Cardiovasc Surg 1985; 89:836–841.
4. Paul DL. Carcinomas in the superior pulmonary sulcus. J Thorac Cardiovasc Surg 1975; 70(6):1095–1104.
5. Martini N, Yellin A, Ginsberg RJ, Bains MS, Burt ME, McCormack PM, Rusch VW. Management of non–small cell lung cancer with direct mediastinal involvement. Ann Thorac Surg 1994; 58:1447–1451.
6. Sugiura S, Ando Y, Minami H, Ando M, Sakai S, Shimokata K. Prognostic value of pleural effusion in patients with non–small cell lung cancer. Clin Cancer Res 1997; 3:47–50.
7. Mountain CF. A new International Staging System for Lung Cancer. Chest 1986; 89(4):225s–231s.
8. Williams DE, Pairolero PC, Davis CS, Bernatz PE, Payne WS, Taylor WF, Uhlenhopp MA, Fontana RS. Survival of patients surgically treated for stage I lung cancer. J Thorac Cardiovasc Surg 1981; 82:70–76.
9. Pairolero PC, Williams DE, Bergstralh EJ, Piehler JM, Bernatz, PE, Payne WS. Postsurgical stage I bronchogenic carcinoma: morbid implications of recurrent disease. Ann Thorac Surg 1984; 38:331–336.
10. Mountain CF. Revisions in the International System for Staging Lung Cancer. Chest 1997; 111:1710–1717.
11. Naruke T, Goya T, Tsuchiya R, Suemasu K. Prognosis and survival in resected lung carcinoma based on the new International Staging System. J Thorac Cardiovasc Surg 1988; 96:440–447.
12. Harpole DH, Herndon JE, Wolfe WG, Iglehart JD, Marks JR. A prognostic model of recurrence and death in stage I non–small cell lung cancer utilizing presentation, histopathology, and oncoprotein expression. Cancer Res 1995; 55:51–56.
13. Watanabe Y, Shimizu J, Oda M, Hayashi Y, Iwa T, Nonomura A, Kamimura R, Takashima T. Proposals regarding some deficiencies in the New International Staging System for non–small cell lung cancer. Jpn J Clin Oncol 1991; 21:160–168.
14. Mountain CF. Expanded possibilities for surgical treatment of lung cancer. Survival in stage IIIa disease. Chest 1990; 97:1045–1051.

15. Watanabe Y, Shimizu J, Oda M, et al. Results of surgical treatment in patients with stage IIIA non–small-cell lung cancer. Thorac Cardiovasc Surgeon 1991; 39:44–49.

16. Martini N, Flehinger BJ. The role of surgery in N2 lung cancer. Surg Clin North Am 1987; 67(5):1037–1049.

17. Pearson FG, Delarue NC, Ilves R, Todd TRJ, Cooper JD. Significance of positive superior mediastinal nodes identified at mediastinoscopy in patients with resectable cancer of the lung. J Thorac Cardiovasc Surg 1982; 83:1–11.

18. Deslauriers J, Brisson J, Cartier R, Marcien F, Gagnon D, Piraux M, Beaulieu M. Carcinoma of the lung: evaluation of satellite nodules as a factor influencing prognosis after resection. J Thorac Cardiovasc Surg 1989; 97:504–512.

19. Shimizu N, Ando A, Date H, Teramoto S. Prognosis of undetected intrapulmonary metastases in resected lung cancer. Cancer 1993; 71(12):3868–3872.

20. Albain KS, Rusch VW, Crowley JJ, Rice TW, Turrisi AT, Weick JK, Lonchyna VA, Presant CA, McKenna RJ, Gandara DR et al. Concurrent cisplatin/etoposide plus chest radiotherapy followed by surgery for stage IIIA(N2) ad IIIB non–small-cell lung cancer: mature results of Southwest Oncology Group Phase II Study 8805. J Clin Oncol 1995; 13(8):1880–1892.

21. Dillman RO, Hercon J, Seagren SL, Eaton WL Jr, Green MR. Improved survival in stage III non–small-cell lung cancer: seven-year follow-up of Cancer and Leukemia Group B (CALGB) 8433 Trial. J Natl Cancer Inst 1996; 88(17):1210–1215.

22. Mountain CF. Prognostic implications of the International Staging System for Lung Cancer. Semin Oncol 1988; 15(3):236–245.

23. Akaogi E, Mitsui K, Onizuka M, Ishikawa S, Tsukada H, Mitsui T. Pleural dissemination in non–small cell lung cancer: results of radiological evaluation and surgical treatment. J Surg Oncol 1994; 57:33–39.

24. Shimizu J, Oda M, Morita K, Hayashi Y, Arano Y, Matsumoto I, Kobayashi K, Nonomura A, Watanabe Y. Comparison of pleuropneumonectomy and limited surgery for lung cancer with pleural dissemination. J Surg Oncol 1996; 61:1–6.

25. Broderick LS, Tarver RD, Conces DJ Jr. Imaging of lung cancer: old and new. Semin Oncol 1997; 24:411–418.

26. Glazer GM, Gross BH, Quint LE, Francis IR, Bookstein FL, Orringer MB. Normal mediastinal lymph nodes: number and size according to American Thoracic Society mapping. Am J Roentgenol 1985; 144:261–265.

27. Glazer GM, Orringer MB, Gross BH, Quint LE. The mediastinum in non–small cell lung cancer: CT-surgical correlation. Am J Roentgenol 1984; 142:1101–1105.

28. McLoud TC, Bourgouin PM, Greenberg RW, Kosiuk JP, Templeton PA, Shepard JO, Moore EH, Wain JC, Mathisen DJ, Grillo HC. Bronchogenic carcinoma: analysis of staging in the mediastinum with CT by correlative lymph node mapping and sampling. Radiology 1992; 182:319–323.

29. Gallardo JFM, Naranjo FB, Cansino MT, Rodriguez-Panadero F. Validity of enlarged mediastinal nodes as markers of involvement by non–small cell lung cancer. Am Rev Respir Dis 1992; 146:1210–1212.

30. Gdeede A, Van Schil P, Corthouts B, Van Mieghem F, Van Meerbeeck J, Van Marck E. Prospective evaluation of computed tomography and mediastinoscopy in mediastinal lymph node staging. Eur Respir J 1997; 10:1547–1551.

31. Daly BDT, Mueller JD, Faling LJ, Diehl JT, Bankoff MS, Karp DD, Rand WM. N2 lung cancer: outcome in patients with false-negative computed tomographic scans of the chest. J Thorac Cardiovasc Surg 1993; 105(5):904–911.

32. Kondo D, Imaizumi M, Abe T, Naruke T, Suemasu K. Endoscopic ultrasound examination for mediastinal lymph node metastases of lung cancer. Chest 1990; 98:586–593.

33. Silvestri GA, Hoffman BJ, Bhutani MS, Hawes RH, Coppage L, Sanders-Cliette A, Reed CE. Endoscopic ultrasound with fine-needle aspiration in the diagnosis and staging of lung cancer. Ann Thorac Surg 1996; 61:1441–1446.

34. Keogan MT, Tung KT, Kaplan DK, Goldstraw PJ, Hansell DM. The significance of pulmonary nodules detected on CT staging for lung cancer. Clin Radiol 1993; 48:94–96.

35. McCann J. PET scans approved for detecting metastatic non–small-cell lung cancer. J Natl Cancer Inst 1998; 90(2):94–96.

36. Sazon DA, Santiago SM, Soo Hoo GW, Khonsary A, Brown C, Mandelkern M, Blahd W, Williams AJ. Fluorodeoxyglucose-positron emission tomography in the detection and staging of lung cancer. Am J Respir Crit Care Med 1996; 153:417–421.

37. Wahl RL, Siegal BA. Positron emission tomography imaging in cancer staging and therapy assessment: basic principals and clinical applications. ASCO Educational Book Spring 1999; 604–613.

38. Pieterman RM, van Putten JWG, Meuzelaar JJ, Mooyaart EL, Vallburg W, Koeter GH, Fidler V, Pruin J, Groen HJM. Preoperative staging of non-small-cell lung cancer with positron-emission tomography. N Eng J Med 2000; 343:254–261.

39. Vansteenkiste JF, Stroobants SG, De Leyn PR, Dupont PJ, Verschakelen JA, Nacckaerts KL, Mortelmans LA, Leuven Lung Cancer Group. Mediastinal lymph node staging with FDG-PET scan in patients with potentially operable non–small cell lung cancer: a prospective analysis of 50 cases. Chest 1997; 112:1480–1486.

40. Nabi HA, Steinbrenner L, Lamonica D, Spaulding M. The use of positron emission tomography. Proc Ann Meet Am Soc Clin Oncol 1996; 15:A1204.

41. MacManus MP, Hicks RJ, Wada M, Hogg A, Matthews J, Wirth A, Rischin D, Ball DL. Early F-18 FDG-PET response to radical chemoradiotherapy correlates strongly with survival in unresectable non–small cell lung cancer. Proc Am Soc Clin Oncol 2000; 19:483a.

42. Eberhardt W, Wilke H, Stamatis G, Stuschke M, Harstrick A, Menker H, Krause B, Mueller MR, Stahl M, Flasshove M, Udach V, Greschuchna D, Konietzko N, Sack H, Seeber S. Preoperative chemotherapy followed by concurrent chemoradiation therapy based on hyperfractionated accelerated radiotherapy and definitive surgery in locally advanced non–small-cell lung cancer: mature results of a phase II trial. J Clin Oncol 1998; 16(2):622–634.

43. Venugopal P, Bonomi P, Ali A, Patel S, Faber LP, Lincoln S, LaFollette S, Priesler H. Correlation of positron emission tomography (PET) scan, computerized tomographic (CT) scan and histologic response to combined modality chemo-radiotherapy (CT/RT) in stage III non–small cell lung cancer (NSCLC). Proc Ann Meet Am Soc Clin Oncol 1997; 16:A1750.

2

Early Timing of Radiotherapy Is Critical in Limited-Stage SCLC: Pro

Nevin Murray

University of British Columbia and British Columbia Cancer Agency, Vancouver, British Columbia, Canada

INTRODUCTION

> Cancer treatment is many things. It is not just biochemistry, cell population kinetics, pharmacology, or sophisticated therapeutics in model systems and man. It is all these things and many more, but most of all it is discovery, development, cooperation across disciplines, and application to man with a prevailing sense of urgency. We want and need and seek better guidance and are gaining it, but we cannot sit and wait for the promise of tomorrow so long as stepwise progress can be made with the tools at hand today.
>
> —Howard Skipper, 1979 (1)

For patients with limited-stage small cell lung cancer (LS-SCLC), it is usually easy to produce an impressive improvement in symptoms and chest radiographs within a short period of time with multiagent chemotherapy or thoracic irradiation. Unfortunately, the natural history of LS-SCLC is that despite impressive

17

tumor regression, the majority of patients harbor resistant elements of disease that persist after induction therapy and cause an incurable relapse. The challenge in the treatment of LS-SCLC is to combine chemotherapy and thoracic irradiation in an optimal fashion resulting in an improvement in median survival and the proportion of long-term survivors. A consensus on the most effective sequence of chemotherapy and thoracic irradiation (early versus delayed thoracic irradiation) has not been reached. This topic is the subject of this debate.

The Veterans Administration Lung Group system (2) that divided patients into either limited or extensive stages has endured for SCLC because of its simplicity, reliable prognostic value, and practical utility (3,4). LS-SCLC is defined as tumor confined to one hemithorax and the regional lymph nodes, whereas extensive-stage small cell lung cancer (ESCLC) patients have disease spread beyond this definition. The original operational definition of limited disease was tumor quantity and configuration that could be encompassed by a "reasonable" radiotherapy treatment volume. Because long-term survival is uncommon (9%) when chemotherapy alone is used to treat LS-SCLC (5,6), the reasonable radiotherapy port rule continues to be a practical guide in the design of combined-modality therapy.

The necessity for accurate staging may be influenced by the sequence of treatment modalities. Since complete staging workup may delay symptom-relieving treatment, and because chemotherapy is recommended for all fit patients anyway, some clinicians may prefer not to bother with standard staging procedures outside the context of clinical trials. This pattern of practice may not be associated with serious negative consequences if the best treatment paradigm consisted of initial treatment with multiple chemotherapy cycles followed sequentially by administration of consolidative thoracic irradiation after drug treatment was finished. However, if patients with bona fide LS-SCLC benefit from early delivery of thoracic irradiation concurrent with combination chemotherapy, the importance of modern staging technology is crucial. The enhanced curative power of such integrated modality protocols would justify their increased complexity and toxicity in LS-SCLC but not ESCLC.

STRATEGIC FACTORS FOR OPTIMAL SEQUENCING OF RADIOTHERAPY AND CHEMOTHERAPY

Arbitrary assembly of chemotherapy and thoracic irradiation is unlikely to yield the best results. Previous experience with treatment protocols for LS-SCLC make it difficult to explore the scientific rationale of combining therapeutic modalities in an unprejudiced manner. Before review of clinical data, it would be useful to examine the fundamental principles for various sequences of therapeutic modalities. The goal of optimal treatment modality assembly is to maximize the probability of elimination of the last cancer stem cell thereby attaining a durable complete remission.

A simplified overview of strategic considerations for combined-modality therapy would identify two distinct plans for combining chemotherapy and thoracic irradiation (Table 1). The strategy of the first plan must be to attempt to destroy as many cancer cells as possible in the shortest period of time. Such front-end-loaded therapy would involve using the most effective modalities early in the treatment program. Four concepts support early chemoradiation including decreased probability of metastatic events, lower probability of development of chemotherapy resistance, lower probability of development of resistance to radiotherapy, and diminished accelerated repopulation.

The alternative method would require rationalization of the strategic superiority of deploying modalities in a more sequential fashion, via delayed administration of thoracic radiation (after chemotherapy) (Table 1). Sequential rather

TABLE 1   Conceptual Basis for Early Integration Versus Sequential Delivery of Therapeutic Modalities in the Assembly of Multimodality Cancer Treatment Programs

A. Early integration of modalities
   Characteristics
      Eliminate as many cancer cells as possible in the shortest period of time
      Deploy multiple modalities quickly
      More complex logistically: requires early multidisciplinary involvement
      More toxic
   Scientific rationale
      1. Decreased probability of metastatic events
      2. Lower probability of chemotherapy resistance
      3. Lower probability of resistance to radiotherapy
      4. Minimize accelerated repopulation
B. Sequential assembly of therapy
   Characteristics
      Modalities deployed with temporal separation
      Tumor burden destroyed in phases
      Logistically less complex: disciplines involved sequentially
      Chemotherapy nonresponders spared toxicity of radical local therapy
      Less toxic
   Scientific rationale
      1. Originally impossible local therapy made feasible in subset with good response to neoadjuvant chemotherapy
      2. Requires treatment modality (chemotherapy or radiotherapy) resistance to reverse at time of planned modality deployment

than concurrent use of modalities in oncology has been prevalent for obvious logistical reasons including simplicity and diminished toxicity. Existence of reversible resistance is a concept that could support sequential therapy. If a definitive local therapy was originally impossible but was rendered feasible by neoadjuvant therapy, this concept would also support the sequential therapy model.

Concepts that Favor Early Integrated Combined-Modality Therapy

The concepts that scientifically favor early integration of effective therapeutic modalities have clear-cut characteristics. The probability of treatment failure events associated with these concepts occurring must increase fairly quickly with the elapse of time. Therefore, the chance of avoiding treatment failure should be minimized with elimination of as many tumor cells as possible in the shortest period of time. Rapid eradication of tumor cells requires the early integration of definitive local treatment(s) with systemic chemotherapy.

Decreased Probability of Metastatic Events

Experimental work by Hill et al. (7,8) indicates that tumor cells mutate spontaneously and randomly to acquire metastatic potential. Moreover, once tumors reach a critical size or volume, metastatic phenotypes are generated ''explosively.'' The cumulative probability of the existence of metastases and the number of metastases increase in proportion to elapsed time. The best way to decrease metastatic events is to quickly eliminate as much tumor as possible.

Lower Probability of Chemotherapy Resistance

A large body of experimental and clinical data exists that support the observation that variability exists for chemosensitivity within tumor cell populations (9,10). Moreover, tumor cells display a capacity to be resistant to many drugs concurrently (11). The biological basis of this evolution of resistance originates during tumor growth from mutations in the cancer genome (12). The development of resistant mutants is a random process, and the probability of their appearance increases with time in proportion to the total number of cell divisions the neoplastic burden has undergone. The somatic mutation theory of drug resistance (13) predicts that once a tumor has reached a critical size, the probability of cure is lost over a small additional size increase in a short time period. The best way to minimize the probability of chemotherapy resistance is to eliminate as many cancer cells as possible in the shortest time.

Lower Probability of Resistance to Radiotherapy

Local control rates with radiotherapy are inversely related to tumor size (14,15). Although microenvironmental effects such as hypoxia (16) may be relevant, increasing evidence indicates that tumor cell populations are heterogeneous with respect to inherent radiosensitivity, and like chemotherapy resistance, resistance to ionizing radiation may be genetically determined and a stochastic process (17). Epigenetic mechanisms for radiotherapy resistance also exist including up-regulation of DNA repair enzymes (17). Induction of DNA repair enzymes by chemotherapy is a plausible reason why thoracic irradiation delivered after chemotherapy may be less effective. SCLC is less responsive to irradiation when recurrent after chemotherapy and mechanisms of resistance may overlap; however, cross-resistance is not complete (18). The probability of mutation to radiotherapy resistance or radioresistance as a consequence of enhanced DNA repair efficiency secondary to previous chemotherapy should be minimized by the early deployment of both modalities.

Diminished Accelerated Repopulation

Accelerated proliferation of tumors undergoing radiotherapy has been proposed (19,20) to explain the clinical observation that extended therapy regimens often require increased radiation dosages to achieve an isoeffective result (21,22). Accelerated tumor growth has been reported after surgery (23) and chemotherapy (24) in animal models. Accelerated repopulation will decrease local control, but additionally increased mitotic activity with larger burden of residual tumor may also hasten the tempo of metastatic events and increase the probability of developing drug and radiation resistance.

Noncurative perturbation of the primary tumor may have detrimental effects (possibly mediated by cytokines) on existing metastatic lesions (25). Accelerated repopulation is independent of modalities and an obvious form of cross-resistance. This phenomenon has not been mathematically modeled but it appears to be well established within a few weeks after initiation of therapy (19). Rapid destruction of tumor by early integration of chemoradiation should minimize the amount of tumor capable of repopulation.

Concepts that Favor Sequential Application of Radiotherapy and Chemotherapy

Simplicity has great appeal. The model of a medical oncologist administering a series of chemotherapy treatments, assessing response, and subsequently referring the LS-SCLC patient for consolidative thoracic irradiation when toxicity has subsided is undoubtedly simple. This approach is also associated with less toxicity. However, is sequential or delayed administration of thoracic irradiation after chemotherapy credible scientifically?

The strategic concepts favoring *early* combined modality have a simple rule for the timing of effective modalities: any delay is potentially detrimental because the probability of treatment failure increases as a function of time. The rules are more arcane for concepts that favor sequential modalities because an additional element of information is required. It is necessary to know the most advantageous amount of delay required for the optimum sequence of modalities. This crucial knowledge must be supplied by the concept itself or learned by the conduct of controlled clinical trials. Other than simplicity and diminished toxicity, there are two strategic concepts that may favor sequential therapy.

Originally Impossible Local Therapy Rendered Feasible by Neoadjuvant Therapy

An unambiguous scenario where sequential therapy would offer an advantage would be when a locally advanced tumor was originally untreatable by a definitive local therapy but such therapy was rendered feasible by downstaging. This is a classic rationale for neoadjuvant chemotherapy before surgery. However, LS-SCLC is rarely considered for surgery and the definition of this stage indicates that all original tumor should be encompassable within a reasonable radiotherapy treatment volume at the outset. There is no obvious scientific reason why chemotherapy-resistant residual tumor should be confined to the postchemotherapy tumor volume.

Reversible Resistance

Sequential application of modalities could be strategically superior if resistance to a particular therapy (chemotherapy or radiotherapy) was present at one point in the treatment program, but the resistance reversed later allowing successful use of that modality. Once genetically determined resistance to chemotherapy has been acquired by a tumor, it is improbable that such elements would disappear by spontaneous mutation (12). However, resistance to chemotherapy with an epigenetic basis could occur and would be a possible form of reversible resistance. Kinetic resistance is another type of reversible resistance. The potential superiority of sequential therapies as predicted by the Norton-Simon hypothesis (26) is based on the possible existence of kinetic resistance.

The arguments supporting either early integration of chemoradiation or sequential utilization of chemotherapy and thoracic irradiation are hypothetical and must be supported by clinical data. Clinical data to be examined will be classified under the following categories: meta-analysis of randomized trials of chemotherapy versus chemoradiation and randomized trials of thoracic irradiation timing.

META-ANALYSES OF PHASE III TRIALS OF CHEMOTHERAPY WITH OR WITHOUT THORACIC IRRADIATION

Thirteen randomized studies investigated this question. Two meta-analyses have been published that examine the trials to determine the role of thoracic radiotherapy in LSCLC (5,6). One was based on published data (1911 patients) and looked at 2-year survival rates, local control, and toxicity (5). The other (6) included 2140 patients and examined survival at 3 years and prognostic factors for survival. Because most data in each meta-analysis were derived from the same studies, the conclusions are consistent and complementary despite differences in the methods used in the meta-analyses. Both show a modest improvement in survival rates in those patients given thoracic radiotherapy. The survival benefit becomes evident at about 15 months after start of treatment and persists beyond 5 years. At 3 years, 8.9% of the chemotherapy-only group are alive, compared with 14.3% of the combined-modality group. The relative rate of death in the combined-modality group as compared with the chemotherapy group was 0.86 (95% confidence interval, 0.78–0.94; $p = 0.001$), corresponding to a 14% reduction in the mortality rate. The analysis of local control was based on 1521 patients for whom data were reported and showed a marked reduction in the absolute 2-year local failure rate comparing the irradiated patients (23%) to the nonirradiated patients (48%) ($p = 0.0001$). These benefits were obtained at the cost of an increase in treatment-related deaths of 1%.

Most of these studies were designed to permit a chemotherapy response evaluation, which allows the possibility of a reduction in the radiotherapy field size. The timing of thoracic irradiation was most often after three to six cycles of chemotherapy but was concurrent with the first cycle of chemotherapy in four studies. Treatment factors, such as radiotherapy timing and chemoradiation integration (sequential, concurrent, or alternating), were not significant in the meta-analyses, but the heterogeneity of trial design did not allow a precise assessment of these issues. An additional explanation for not demonstrating the importance of timing or integration of thoracic irradiation may be found in the shape of the survival curve and the statistical methodology used in this analysis. Initially, the overall survival graph begins in favor of chemotherapy but the curves cross at about 1 year and later demonstrate a long-term survival advantage for chemoradiation. The initial separation of the curves is not large, but many events occur on this steep portion of the curves. Because thoracic irradiation adds toxicity that may diminish chemotherapy delivery, the relative risk of death is not constant over time. The short-term mortality increase may cancel out the long-term survival gain as measured by relative risk. Reexamination of this data set for an effect of thoracic irradiation timing on long-term survival rather than relative risk of death may be useful.

Most studies in the meta-analyses were initiated before 1981 and did not deliver cisplatin and etoposide concurrently with thoracic irradiation. The safety and efficacy of early concurrent chemoradiation has been markedly improved with the administration of etoposide/cisplatin chemotherapy rather than cyclophosphamide-, nitrosourea-, or doxorubicin-based regimens. From the earliest report (27), it was clear that etoposide and cisplatin could be delivered concurrently with thoracic irradiation without dire normal tissue toxicity or the need to compromise the dose of either modality. Concurrent etoposide plus cisplatin or carboplatin with thoracic irradiation has become a prevalent theme in current LSCLC regimens. Lack of data of this type in the meta-analyses (5,6) reduces the capacity of these reports to provide guidance on optimal integration of chemoradiation that is relevant to the modern era.

RANDOMIZED TRIALS OF THE TIMING OF THORACIC IRRADIATION

The highest standard of evidence for the optimal timing of chemotherapy and thoracic irradiation for LSCLC comes from prospective randomized trials directly addressing this question. To date, five trials (28–33) of thoracic irradiation timing have been performed; four trials are published in peer-reviewed journals (28–32) and one is currently available as an abstract (33). Because of the importance of these trials, each study is discussed separately and summarized in Table 2.

The Cancer and Leukemia Group B Trial

This large trial (28,29) performed from 1981 to 1984 included 399 evaluable LSCLC patients distributed between three arms including chemotherapy alone (cyclophosphamide, etoposide, vincristine, and doxorubicin), initial chemoradiation (50 Gy thoracic irradiation and whole-brain irradiation concurrently with the initial cycle of chemotherapy), and delayed chemoradiation (chest and brain irradiation concurrently with the fourth cycle of chemotherapy at week 9). Both arms that included thoracic irradiation had significantly superior response rates, time to progression, and overall survival rates compared with chemotherapy alone. However, no significant differences were found between the initial and delayed thoracic irradiation arms; an insignificant trend favored the delayed thoracic irradiation arm. The rationale of a randomized trial is to hold all variables constant, except the experimental one. Unfortunately, the interpretation of the CALGB study is confounded by the fact that potential differences in outcome from thoracic irradiation timing may be obscured by unequal chemotherapy delivery. Myelosuppression from initial thoracic irradiation, brain irradiation, and concurrent CEV chemotherapy resulted in an unplanned attenuation (50% reduction) in the doses of cyclophosphamide, etoposide, and doxorubicin after the first cycle. This trial clearly supports the addition of thoracic irradiation to chemotherapy in LS-SCLC, but the utility of the study to provide guidance for optimal integration of chemoradiation is doubtful. The long-term survival rates for chemoradiation in the CALGB study are low (<13%) (29).

TABLE 2 Randomized Trials of Thoracic Irradiation Timing in Limited-Stage Small Cell Lung Cancer

Study	Drugs	Thoracic irradiation			Number of patients		Survival, median (mo.)		Survival 5-year (%)		p-Value
		Dose	Start time								
			Early	Late	Early	Late	Early	Late	Early	Late	
1. CALGB (28,29)	CEVA	50 Gy/25F/5 wk	Week 1	Week 9	125	145	13.04	14.54	6.6	12.8	NS
2. Aarhus (31)	CAV/EP	40–45 Gy/22F/6 wk[a]	Week 1	Week 18	99	100	10.7	12.9	10.0	10.0	NS
3. NCIC (30)	CAV/EP	40/15F/3 wk	Week 3	Week 15	155	153	21.2	16.0	22.0	13.0	0.013
4. Yugoslavian (32)	Carbo/EP	54 Gy/36F/3 1/2 wk[b]	Week 1	Week 6	52	51	34	26	30	15	0.027
5. JCOG (33)	EP	45 Gy/30F/3 wk[b]	Week 1	Week 15	114	114	31.3	20.8	30	15	<0.05

CALGB = Cancer and Leukemia Group B; NCIC = National Cancer Institute of Canada; JCOG = Japan Clinical Oncology Group; C = cyclophosphamide; E = etoposide; V = vincristine; A = doxorubicin; P = cisplatin; Carbo = carboplatin.
[a]Split course.
[b]1.5 Gy twice daily.

The Aarhus Lung Cancer Group Trial

In this Danish trial (31) performed between 1981 and 1989, 199 patients with LSCLC were randomly allocated to initial chest irradiation or late chest irradiation delayed by 18 weeks. Both groups received nine cycles of combination chemotherapy: three cycles of EP and six cycles of CAV. The timing of radiotherapy (40–45 Gy) had no significant effect on the median survival (about 1 year) or long-term survival (about 10%). However, thoracic irradiation was delivered sequentially rather than concurrently with EP. In addition, the thoracic radiation was administered as a split course. Radiobiologically, this is a disadvantage in tumors that have the potential for accelerated repopulation.

The National Cancer Institute of Canada Trial

In 1993, the NCIC published results of a randomized trial (30) (accrual period 1985–88) comparing early versus late thoracic irradiation (Figure 1) that demonstrated a significant improvement in survival for early thoracic irradiation in the combined modality therapy of LS-SCLC. All 308 eligible patients received CAV alternating with EP for three cycles of each regimen. Patients randomized to early thoracic irradiation received 40 Gy/15F to the primary site concurrent with the

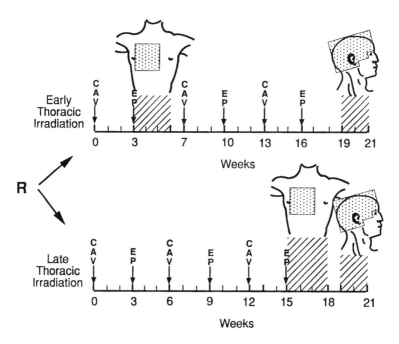

FIGURE 1   Schema of the National Cancer Institute of Canada BR6 trial (30).

first cycle of EP (week 3), and the late thoracic irradiation arm received the same radiation concurrent with the last cycle of EP (week 15). Dose intensity and total dose of chemotherapy were uniform in both arms (85–90% delivery according to protocol).

Although complete response rates were not significantly different (CR early arm 64%, CR late arm 56%, $p = 0.14$), the overall survival was significantly superior ($p = 0.013$) in the early thoracic irradiation arm (Figure 2). Median survival was 21.2 months in the early arm and 16.0 months in the late arm; actual survival at 5 years was 22% in the early arm and 13% in the late arm. A delay of thoracic irradiation by 12 weeks was associated with a 50% decrease in the probability of long-term survival. This was the first phase III study to demonstrate that actual 5-year survival rates of over 20% were achievable using early integrated chemoradiation in LS-SCLC.

The Yugoslavian Trial

This extraordinary phase III study (32) performed between 1988 and 1992 has achieved outcomes in LS-SCLC that are not only superior to any other phase III study, but survival is also better than in any published phase II trial. All patients received accelerated hyperfractionated thoracic irradiation with 1.5 Gy twice

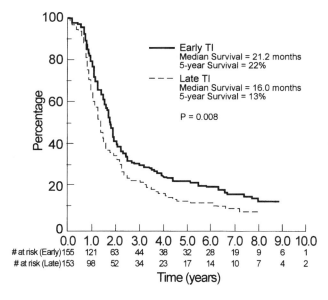

FIGURE 2   Final analysis for overall survival of the National Cancer Institute of Canada BR6 study (30).

daily to 54 Gy plus concurrent daily carboplatin/etoposide and four sequential cycles of EP. Early thoracic irradiation was delivered between weeks 1 and 4 and late thoracic irradiation patients received concurrent chemoradiation between weeks 6 and 9. The difference in timing of the initiation of thoracic irradiation between the two arms was only 5 weeks.

The median survival was 34 months for initial chemoradiation versus 26 months for delayed chemoradiation; 5-year survival was 30% and 15%, respectively. The difference was significant on multivariate analysis ($p = 0.027$). This study by Jeremic and colleagues (32) shows that early integration of chemotherapy with intensive radiation for LS-SCLC may generate median survival times of almost 3 years and long-term survival rates may approach 30%.

The Japan Clinical Oncology Group Trial

This study (33) also examined the optimal sequence of chemoradiation for LSCLC by randomizing patients to initial concurrent versus delayed sequential chemoradiation. The chemotherapy prescription was EP (four cycles) and thoracic irradiation consisted of 45 Gy over 3 weeks (two daily fractions of 1.5 Gy). A total of 228 patients were entered between 1991 and 1995.

Initial concurrent chemoradiation was significantly superior ($p < 0.05$) to sequential therapy with median survivals of 31.3 months and 20.8 months and projected 5-year survival rates of 30% and 15%, respectively. These results strengthen the conclusion that long-term survival rates of >20% for LS-SCLC are obtainable with early chemoradiation.

Why Are the Randomized Trials of Thoracic Irradiation Timing Discordant?

Of the five controlled trials of thoracic irradiation timing performed, three [NCIC (30), Yugoslavian (32), JCOG (33)] support the concept that the optimal integration of chemotherapy and thoracic irradiation is early concurrent chemoradiation; the CALGB (28,29) and the Aarhus (31) studies suggest that the timing of thoracic irradiation does not influence outcome. Why are the results discordant? There are three possible reasons:

1. The timing of thoracic irradiation is unimportant and the discordant results are due to the play of chance.
2. Delivery of chemotherapy or thoracic irradiation was inadequate in the negative trials.
3. The patient populations differ.

The influence of chance cannot be discounted, but other explanations may be more plausible. The CALGB study (28,29) and the Aarhus trial (31) were associated with issues related to the adequate delivery of chemotherapy or thoracic radiotherapy, respectively. Thoracic irradiation can improve the long-term prognosis of LSCLC only in those cases in which the systemic therapy successfully controls distant subclinical disease, but fails to eliminate regional residual tumor. Suboptimal systemic therapy (e.g., secondary to marked dose attenuation in the CALBG trial) will unavoidably decrease the impact of a change in the timing of local therapy for a systemic disease. Similarly, suboptimal radiotherapy (e.g., split-course as in the Aarhus trial) may dampen the benefit of this modality.

However, the most important reason for discordance of results probably is associated with differences in the trial patient populations. The prevalence of metastatic drug-resistant tumor outside the thoracic irradiation volume in the study population strongly affects the likelihood that thoracic irradiation or an innovation of it (timing or dose) will be associated with a survival advantage. If a poor prognosis LS-SCLC population (as evidenced by short median survival) is studied, the proportion of cases that can have their prognosis improved by better integration of chemoradiation will be low and the benefit of early thoracic irradiation timing will be diluted out by the presence of incurable cases. That the study populations in the CALGB (28,29) and Aarhus (31) trials, which fail to show superiority of early chemoradiation, were a poor prognostic group is strongly suggested by the short median survivals reported (Table 2). Long-term survival in these reports is also low. Adverse prognostic factors in these studies that commenced in 1981 may have been due to staging procedures that were less accurate than more recently reported trials. Median survival in the early chemoradiation arms of the NCIC (30), Yugoslavian (32), and JCOG (33) trials ranges from 21.2 to 34 months, which is two to three times longer than the median survival times in the CALGB (28) and Danish (31) studies. Median survival in the delayed chemoradiation arms of the trials that support early chemoradiation (30,32,33) ranges from 16 to 21 months, indicating that all patients in these trials had better prognostic factors than the negative trials (28,31). More importantly, long-term survival for early chemoradiation in the positive trials consistently exceeds 20% at 5 years (30,32,33). Delayed chemoradiation has never approached the 20% long-term survival milestone, which should be considered the minimum standard for LS-SCLC at this time. Delayed chemoradiation usually is associated with a long-term survival rate of approximately 10% (Table 2), which is not much different than the 9% rate expected from chemotherapy alone, as reported in the meta-analysis (6) of randomized trials performed in a similar era.

CONCLUSION

The available data from modern randomized trials of thoracic irradiation timing indicate that the typical patient with LS-SCLC staged with modern technology has a median survival expectation of 16–26 months and long-term survival of 10–13% when treated with standard chemotherapy and *late* thoracic irradiation.

Combining *early* thoracic irradiation concurrently with etoposide-cisplatin chemotherapy improves that median survival expectation to 21–34 months and long-term survival to more than 20%.

The addition of more intensive thoracic irradiation has recently been associated with improved outcome in LS-SCLC when such radiotherapy is delivered with early concurrent etoposide-cisplatin (34). Turrisi et al. (34) demonstrated that 45 Gy delivered twice daily in 3 weeks (5-year survival 26%) was superior to 45 Gy once daily over 5 weeks (5-year survival 16%). Notably, twice-daily thoracic irradiation had no impact on median or long-term survival in a randomized trial by Bonner et al. (35) that delivered radiotherapy in a delayed fashion (beginning concurrently with the fourth etoposide-cisplatin chemotherapy cycle).

An increase in long-term survival from 10% to >20% is a modest, albeit worthwhile, advance in a common condition such as LS-SCLC. This gain is a least as large as the improvement in stage III NSCLC outcome associated with integrated chemoradiation (36) that changed the treatment paradigm for this condition. Moreover, a consensus (37) now exists that patients with stage III NSCLC, who may benefit from combined modality therapy, must be carefully staged and have good prognostic factors. It is unlikely that similar guidelines for accurate staging and patient selection can be relaxed when innovations of local therapy (timing or dose of radiotherapy) are tested in a systemic disease such as LS-SCLC. That survival improvement from early chemoradiation in LS-SCLC is difficult to detect in inadequately staged patient populations with adverse prognostic factors should not be interpreted as either surprising or particularly relevant to the question of whether early chemoradiation is more efficacious.

Now that early concurrent chemoradiation has been demonstrated superior to delayed chemoradiation for stage III NSCLC (38), persistence of controversy on this therapeutic principle should not be acceptable to physicians who treat local-regional small cell or non–small cell lung cancer. More randomized trials of local and systemic treatment modality sequencing are urgently needed. Such investigations probe fundamental issues in cancer biology and are likely to be relevant to other common malignancies where local and systemic therapies are combined with curative intent.

REFERENCES

1. Skipper HE. Historic milestones in cancer biology: a few that are important in cancer treatment (revisited). Semin Oncol 1979; 6:506–513.
2. Green RA, Humphrey E, Close H, et al. Alkylating agents in bronchogenic carcinoma. Am J Med 1969; 46:516–525.
3. Albain KS, Crowley JJ, LeBlanc M, et al. Determinants of improved outcome in small cell lung cancer: an analysis of the 2,580-patient Southwest Oncology Group data base. J Clin Oncol 1990; 8:1563–1574.

4. Rawson NSB, Peto J. An overview of prognostic factors in small cell lung cancer: a report from the Subcommittee for the Management of Lung Cancer of the United Kingdom Coordinating Committee on Cancer Research. Br J Cancer 1990; 61:597–604.
5. Warde P, Payne D. Does thoracic irradiation improve survival and local control in limited-stage small-cell carcinoma of the lung? A meta-analysis. J Clin Oncol 1992; 10:890–895.
6. Pignon JP, Arriagada R, Ihde DC, et al. A meta-analysis of thoracic radiotherapy for small cell lung cancer. N Engl J Med 1992; 327:1618–1624.
7. Hill RP, Chambers AF, Ling V. Dynamic heterogeneity: rapid generation of metastatic variants in mouse B 16 melanoma cells. Science 1984; 224:998–1001.
8. Hill RP, Young SD, Ling V, et al. Metastatic cell phenotypes: quantitative studies using the experimental metastasis assay. Cancer Rev 1986; 5:118–151.
9. Claes Trope. Different susceptibilities of tumor cell subpopulations to cytotoxic agents and therapeutic consequences. In: Owens AH, Coffey DS, Baylin SB, eds. Tumor Cell Heterogeneity: Origins and Implications. New York: Academic Press, 1982:147.
10. Young RC. Drug Resistance: the clinical problem. In: Ozols RF, ed. Drug Resistance in Cancer Therapy. Norwell, MA: Kluwer Academic Publishers, 1989:1.
11. Cole SP, Bhardwaj G, Gerlach JH, et al. Overexpression of a transporter gene in a multidrug-resistant human lung cancer cell line. Science 1992; 258:1650–1654.
12. Goldie JH, Coldman AJ. Genetic origin of drug resistance in neoplasms. Cancer Res 1984; 44:3643–3653.
13. Goldie JH, Coldman AJ. A mathematical model for relating the drug sensitivity of tumors to their spontaneous mutation rate. Cancer Treat Rep 1979; 63:1727–1733.
14. Tubiana M. The role of local treatment in the cure of cancer. Eur J Cancer 1992; 28:2061–2069.
15. Suit H. Local control and patient survival. Int J Radiat Oncol Biol Phys 1992; 23: 653–660.
16. Tomlinson RH, Gray LH. The histological structure of some human lung cancers and the possible implications for radiotherapy. Br J Cancer 1955; 9:539–549.
17. Yaes RJ. Tumor heterogeneity, tumor size, and radioresistance. Int J Radiat Oncol Biol Phys 1989; 17:993–1005.
18. Ochs JJ, Tester WJ, Cohen MH, et al. "Salvage" radiation therapy for intrathoracic small cell carcinoma of the lung progressing on combination chemotherapy. Cancer Treat Rep 1983; 67:1123–1126.
19. Withers HR, Taylor JMG, Maciejewski B. The hazard of accelerated tumor clonogen repopulation during radiotherapy. Acta Oncol 1988; 27:131–146.
20. Trott KR. Cell repopulation and overall treatment time. Int J Radiat Oncol Biol Phys 1990; 19:1071–1075.
21. Maciejewski B, Preuss-Bayer G, Trott KR. The influence of the number of fractions and of overall treatment time on local control and late complication rate in squamous cell carcinoma of the larynx. Int J Radiat Oncol Biol Phys 1983; 9:321–328.
22. Holsti LR, Mantyla M. Split-course versus continuous radiotherapy. Analysis of a randomized trial from 1964 to 1967. Acta Oncol 1988; 27:153–161.
23. Simpson-Herren L, Sanford AH, Holmquist JP. Effects of surgery on the cell kinetics of residual tumor. Cancer Treat Rep 1976; 60:1749–1760.

24. Stephens TC, Steel GG. Regeneration of tumors after cytotoxic treatment. In: Meyn RE, Withers HR, eds. Radiation Biology in Cancer Research. New York: Raven, 1980:385–395.
25. Fisher B, Gunduz N, Coyle J, et al. Presence of a growth stimulating factor in serum following primary tumor removal in mice. Cancer Res 1989; 49:1996–2002.
26. Norton L, Simon R. Tumor size, sensitivity to therapy and design of treatment schedules. Cancer Treat Rep 1977; 61:1307–1317.
27. Murray N, Hadzic E, Shah A, et al. Alternating chemotherapy and thoracic radiotherapy with concurrent cisplatin-etoposide for limited stage small cell lung cancer. Proc Am Soc Clin Oncol 1984; 3:214 (abstr 835).
28. Perry MC, Eaton WL, Propert KJ, et al. Chemotherapy with or without radiation therapy in limited small-cell carcinoma of the lung. N Engl J Med 1987; 316:912–918.
29. Perry MC, Herndon JE, Eaton WL, et al. Thoracic radiation therapy added to chemotherapy for small-cell lung cancer: an update of cancer and leukemia group B study 8083. J Clin Oncol 1998;16:2466–2467.
30. Murray N, Coy P, Pater J, et al. Importance of timing for thoracic irradiation in the combined modality treatment of limited-stage small-cell lung cancer. J Clin Oncol 1993; 11:336–344.
31. Work E, Nielsen O, Bentzen S, et al. Randomized study of initial versus late chest irradiation combined with chemotherapy in limited-stage small cell lung cancer. J Clin Oncol 1997; 15:3030–3037.
32. Jeremic B, Shibamato Y, Acimovic L, Milisavljevic S. Initial versus delayed accelerated hyperfractionated radiation therapy and concurrent chemotherapy in limited small-cell lung cancer: a randomized study. J Clin Oncol 1997; 15:893–900.
33. Takada M, Fukuoka M, Furuse K, Ariyoshi Y, Ikegami H, Kurita Y, Nishiwaki Y, Nishikawa H, Wantanabe K, Noda K, Saijo N. Phase III study of concurrent versus sequential thoracic radiotherapy in combination with cisplatin and etoposide for limited-stage small cell lung cancer: preliminary results of the Japan Clinical Oncology Group (JCOG). Proc Am Soc Clin Oncol 1996; 15:372 (abstr 1103).
34. Turrisi AT, Kim K, Blum R, Sause WT, Livingston RB, Komaki R, Wagner H, Aisner S, Johnson DH. Twice daily compared with once daily thoracic radiotherapy in limited small-cell lung cancer treated concurrently with cisplatin and etoposide. N Eng J Med 1999; 340(4):265–271.
35. Bonner JA, Sloan JA, Shanahan TG, Brooks BJ, Marks RS, Krooks JE, Gerstner JB, et al. Phase III comparison of twice-daily split-course irradiation versus once-daily irradiation for patients with limited stage small-cell lung cancer. J Clin Oncol 1999; 17(9):2681–2691.
36. Dillman RO, Seagren SL, Herndon J, et al. Improved survival in stage III non–small cell lung cancer: seven year follow-up of CALGB 8433. J Natl Cancer Inst 1996; 88:1210–1215.
37. Non–small Cell Lung Cancer Expert Panel: Clinical practice guidelines for the treatment of unrespectable non-small cell lung cancer. J Clin Oncol 1997; 15:2996–3018.
38. Furuse K, Fukuoka M, Kawahara M, Nishikawa H, Takada Y, et al. Phase III study of concurrent versus sequential thoracic radiotherapy in combination with mitomycin, vindesine, and cisplatin in unresectable stage III non–small-cell lung cancer. J Clin Oncol 1999; 17(9):2692–2699.

3

Early Timing of Radiotherapy Is Critical in Limited-Stage SCLC: Con

Mark Bryer and Michael C. Perry
University of Missouri/Ellis Fischel Cancer Center, Columbia, Missouri

INTRODUCTION

The decade of the 1970s recognized the uniqueness of small cell lung cancer (SCLC) and saw the adoption of combination chemotherapy as a standard therapy (1). In the 1980s, the primary topic of debate was the need for thoracic radiation therapy in limited stage SCLC (2,3). Two meta-analyses were published in the 1990s evaluating the role of thoracic radiation therapy in addition to chemotherapy in the management of limited-stage SCLC (4–6). These two meta-analyses showed an improvement in 3-year survival rates of about 5% in those receiving chemotherapy and radiotherapy compared to those receiving chemotherapy alone. The Pignon et al. meta-analysis involved 13 randomized trials including 2140 patients (4,6). At 3 years, the survival advantage for the addition of radiation therapy was 5.4% $\pm$ 1.4%. The improvement in survival was even greater for patients < 55 years of age who received thoracic irradiation, but was not observed in patients > 70 years of age.

Thoracic radiation therapy offered the possibility of more complete responses, reduced recurrences at the primary site and improved survival, but at a potential cost of increased toxicity. Many questions remain to be answered with regard to the optimal sequencing, timing, dose, treatment volume, and fractionation of thoracic radiation therapy in the management of limited stage SCLC. An in-depth review of the radiation fractionation and volume issues is found in another chapter. Certainly, there is no consensus at this time regarding these factors. Many investigators have championed the cause of early thoracic radiation therapy in limited-stage SCLC, but analysis of the data suggests that delayed thoracic radiation therapy may be equally efficacious.

EARLY STUDIES

In 1980, the Cancer and Leukemia Group B addressed both the role and optimal timing of thoracic radiation in a randomized, prospective trial of chemotherapy with or without radiation therapy in limited-stage SCLC (7). After stratification for gender and performance status, patients were randomly assigned to receive initial chemotherapy and thoracic radiation therapy starting on day 1, chemotherapy with radiation therapy starting with cycle 3 (day 63), or chemotherapy alone. The chemotherapy was the same in all three arms: cyclophosphamide, vincristine, and etoposide every 3 weeks for 18 cycles. Starting at cycle 7 for odd-numbered cycles, doxorubicin replaced the 3 days of etoposide. The radiation therapy was directed at the primary tumor at a dose of 4000 cGy in 4 weeks, followed by a 1000-cGy ''boost'' directed against residual disease as demonstrated on a midcourse chest film taken after the first 2 weeks of initial therapy. The initial field included the primary disease site with a 2-cm margin around the mass and the ipsilateral hilum, the whole width of the mediastinum, and both supraclavicular fossae. The whole brain was simultaneously treated prophylactically with 3000 cGy in 10 fractions.

A total of 399 patients were enrolled, and at the conclusion of the study, there was a statistically significant difference in the frequency of complete responses in favor of the two thoracic radiation therapy arms ($p = 0.0013$). These two regimens also yielded better failure-free survival ($p < 0.001$), treatment failure-free interval in the chest ($p < 0.001$), and overall survival ($p = 0.0099$). As anticipated, toxicity was worse in the combined-modality arms, but was generally tolerable. In regimen 1, in which radiation therapy and chemotherapy both started on day 1, the incidence of neutropenia and neutropenic fever prompted reductions of the chemotherapy that were maintained throughout treatment, resulting in less chemotherapy being administered in this arm. For this reason, CALGB adopted the second arm (with radiation therapy starting with cycle 4) as its standard.

These findings were confirmed in a recent update (8). It should be noted, however, that the staging and chemotherapy used in this study are not what we would choose in the 1990s. More aggressive staging would likely produce better results as more patients with extrathoracic disease would be identified. The results of more modern chemotherapy would likely be better as well.

RECENT STUDIES

Investigators in Aarhus, Denmark have also evaluated the timing of thoracic irradiation in a phase III trial in patients with limited-stage SCLC (9). From 1981 to 1989, 199 patients with limited-stage SCLC were randomized to early chest irradiation ($n = 99$) or delayed chest irradiation ($n = 100$) starting at week 18 of chemotherapy. All patients received the same chemotherapy, consisting of three cycles of cisplatin, etoposide (PE), and six cycles of cyclophosphamide, doxorubicin, and vincristine (CAV). The patients received 40 or 45 Gy of radiation to the chest. Chest irradiation was given as a split-course treatment of two treatment courses (of 20 or 22.5 Gy in 11 fractions) separated by an interval of 21 days, during which PE chemotherapy was administered. In the early thoracic radiation therapy group, irradiation was started prior to the first cycle of PE chemotherapy. Prophylactic cranial irradiation (PCI) was initially given to patients randomized to early radiation therapy, but after the first 42 patients were treated in the delayed-radiation-therapy arm, the protocol was amended so that all patients received PCI. Based on the recent meta-analysis showing a survival advantage to PCI, excluding PCI from the treatment of the first 42 patients in the delayed-radiation-therapy arm may have biased the results in favor of the early-radiation-therapy arm. However, at 2 years, the timing of radiation therapy did not significantly affect the overall survival, in-field recurrence rate, or median survival durations (Table 1).

While bone marrow toxicity was felt to be acceptable with 15% of patients in both groups developing World Health Organization (WHO) grade 4 leukopenia

TABLE 1 Results of Randomized Trial of Timing of Thoracic Radiation Therapy in 199 Patients with Limited-Stage SCLC (Aarhus Lung Cancer Group)

	Early RT	Late RT	p
2-year overall survival	20%	19%	0.4
2-year in-field recurrence	72%	68%	0.2
Median survival	10.5 m	12.0 m	

and 4% grade 4 thrombocytopenia, grade 4 leukopenia was noted to be more pronounced in the early-radiation-therapy group. The authors concluded that the timing of chest irradiation did not influence survival or local control in the chest. Since grade 4 leukopenia was higher in the early-radiation-therapy group, this study also suggests that delayed radiation therapy may be preferable.

A third randomized trial examining the timing of thoracic irradiation in patients with limited-stage SCLC has been reported by Shultz et al. (10). Patients were treated with alternating cycles of etoposide, cisplatin, and cyclophosphamide, doxorubicin (Adriamycin), vincristine chemotherapy. Patients were randomized between early thoracic irradiation starting day 1 and delayed thoracic irradiation starting day 120. The thoracic radiation therapy given was 40 Gy in 22 fractions or 45 Gy in 22 fractions using a split-course technique. These doses and the use of a split-course technique would not be considered standard therapy in the United States. There was a nonstatistically significant trend toward improved median survival in patients receiving late thoracic radiation therapy (Table 2). Results for local control and toxicity were not reported.

A phase III randomized trial performed by the European Organization for Research and Treatment of Cancer (EORTC) and the United Kingdom Coordinating Committee on Cancer Research compared cyclophosphamide, doxorubicin, and etoposide chemotherapy with either thoracic radiation therapy (10 Gy in four fractions over 1 week) alternating between chemotherapy cycles 2, 3, 4, and 5 or postchemotherapy radiation in patients with limited-stage SCLC (11). At 3 years, survival was not significantly different between the two treatment arms (Table 3). Severe acute hematological toxicity was observed in the alternating chemotherapy/radiotherapy arm resulting in about a 25% reduction in chemotherapy dose intensity. Ninety-three percent of the patients in the sequential arm completed their radiation, versus only 77% in the alternating arm.

The most commonly quoted phase III randomized trial on the timing of thoracic radiation therapy in patients with SCLC showing a benefit to early thoracic radiation therapy was published by Murray et al. from the National Cancer Institute of Canada (NCIC) (12). The NCIC treated 308 eligible patients with six cycles of alternating cisplatin, etoposide (PE), and cyclophosphamide, doxorubi-

TABLE 2 Results of Randomized Trial of Timing of Thoracic Radiation Therapy for Patients with Limited-Stage SCLC (10)

	Early RT	Late RT
Median survival	10.7 m	12.9 m

TABLE 3 Survival Results from EORTC
Randomized Trial Comparing Sequential
to Alternating Chemo/radiotherapy for
Limited-Stage SCLC

	Alternating	Sequential
3-year survival	12%	15%

cin (Adriamycin), etoposide chemotherapy. Patients were randomized to concurrent thoracic irradiation starting with the first cycle of PE chemotherapy (week 3) or the third cycle of PE (week 15). Thoracic irradiation consisted of 40 Gy in 15 fractions. Thoracic irradiation was administered in 149 of 155 (96.1%) patients on the early-radiation-therapy arm and 133 of 153 (86.9%) patients on the late-thoracic-radiation-therapy arm. Overall survival was improved in patients receiving early-thoracic-radiation therapy (Table 4).

When patterns of failure were analyzed, however, there was no difference in local control or the overall metastatic rate. There was a reduction in the frequency of brain metastases in the early-radiation-therapy group (18%) versus the late-radiation-therapy group (28%). PCI was delayed for 19 weeks in this trial and was only given if there was no progression at any site. Thus, 85.8% of the early-thoracic-radiation-therapy patients and 79.7% of the late-thoracic-radiation-therapy patients received PCI. With no differences in local control or overall metastatic failure rate, it is difficult to explain the observed differences in survival in the two groups.

Jeremic et al. treated 107 limited-stage small cell lung cancer patients with accelerated hyperfractionated radiation therapy with 1.5 Gy twice daily to 54 Gy plus concurrent daily carboplatin/etoposide and four sequential cycles of cisplatin/etoposide on days 1–3 (13). One-half of the patients received concurrent chemoradiation at weeks 1–4 (group 1) and the other half (group 2) at weeks 6–9. Median survival was better in group 1 (34 months versus 26 months, $p =$ .027 on multivariate analysis), and local control was better, but there was no

TABLE 4 NCIC Study of Radiation Therapy
Timing in Patients with Limited-Stage SCLC

	Early RT	Late RT
Overall median survival	21.2 m	16 m
4-year survival	25%	15%

difference in distant metastasis rate or toxicity. This is a small study of an unusual regimen and the results must be confirmed in a larger trial.

The meta-analysis by Pignon et al. of trials of chemotherapy with or without radiation therapy could not identify the optimal timing for thoracic irradiation (4). A direct comparison of early to late radiotherapy and of sequential to nonsequential radiotherapy did not demonstrate any significant differences. The relative risk of early thoracic irradiation (defined as < 60 days after starting chemotherapy) was not significant.

While many phase II trials have reported excellent results with combined-modality therapy utilizing early-thoracic-radiation therapy (14,15), equally good results have been reported by other groups utilizing thoracic irradiation starting later in the chemotherapy course. The Mayo Clinic reported the results of a phase II trial for the treatment of limited-stage SCLC patients with three cycles of cyclophosphamide, etoposide, and infusion cisplatin chemotherapy followed by concurrent cyclophosphamide and etoposide chemotherapy and hyperfractionated radiation therapy (4800 cGy in 32 fractions of 150 cGy twice daily) and PCI (16). Twenty-nine patients with limited-stage SCLC were treated with this regimen. Median survival was 26.5 months and 2-year survival was 55%. Only seven of the 29 patients failed in the chest. These excellent results are similar to the best single-institution studies using early thoracic irradiation.

There remains considerable uncertainty regarding the optimal timing of thoracic irradiation in patients with limited-stage SCLC. Review of the literature shows that regimens utilizing late thoracic irradiation with concurrent chemotherapy produce results as good as those seen with early radiation therapy. While most studies favor concurrent administration of chemotherapy and radiation, alternative regimens, including alternating chemo/radiation therapy, have produced very good results. However, overall survival remains poor with late relapses occurring after 5 years and long-term survivors experiencing a high rate of new lung cancers (17,18).

The above studies have mixed results regarding the timing of thoracic radiotherapy. While a few of the studies suggest a benefit to early rather than delayed radiation, others do not substantiate this advantage. Without a clear benefit in terms of efficacy, the next critical issue relates to the impact of timing regarding toxicity. There is a benefit in delaying thoracic radiotherapy after several cycles of chemotherapy that is not often addressed. This benefit directly relates to the size of the radiotherapy field that is required. While limited-stage disease may be confined to one hemithorax, patients often present with bulky disease. As the required radiation dose for small cell lung cancer exceeds lung tolerance, encompassing the initial volume of disease can lead to more radiation fibrosis and increase the risk of radiation pneumonitis. Yet, there is compelling evidence that there is no need to treat such large prechemotherapy volumes. Indeed, in a randomized trial, there was no difference in outcome whether prechemotherapy volume was treated versus the postchemotherapy volume (19). Other studies also support this strategy (20,21). This issue is discussed in further detail in another chapter. While the use of smaller postchemotherapy volumes has not translated into more local failures or compromised outcome, it clearly has the potential to reduce toxicity, not only in terms of sparing normal lung tissue, but also by reducing the length of the esophageal irradiation. Prior studies have documented that the length of esophagus in the radiotherapy field significantly impacts on the rate of radiation esophagitis (22). Thus, an argument can be made that delayed radiotherapy, by allowing reduced field sizes, has the potential to substantially reduce toxicity and thereby enhance the therapeutic ratio. The shrinkage of disease in small cell lung cancer with chemotherapy is often dramatic and the benefit in terms of reducing radiation exposure to normal tissue can be significant.

This strategy of delayed radiotherapy has other important advantages. Despite the current staging workup, there is still a significant percentage of patients deemed ''limited stage'' who harbor metastatic disease. Delaying the radiotherapy will select out a proportion of these patients who will not benefit from intensive combined-modality therapy and can be spared the toxicity of this aggressive approach. There is nothing more upsetting than having to counsel a patient who is still suffering from chemoradiation esophagitis that there is now evidence of metastatic disease, not previously appreciated. Rather, several cycles of chemotherapy has the advantage of a ''tincture of time'' to test the natural history of the disease and ensure that the patient continues to have limited-stage disease and actually benefits from the thoracic radiation. Even the best results reported to date utilizing concurrent chemotherapy and early radiotherapy have 5-year survival rates of only 20–25%, with the majority of the failures being due to distant metastatic disease. Better prognostic indicators and improved systemic therapy are needed before we mandate early intensive thoracic radiotherapy to all patients. Delayed radiotherapy also benefits another cohort of patients whose disease is initially too bulky or locally extensive for a ''tolerable'' radiotherapy field, but then responds well to chemotherapy, thereby facilitating combined-modality treatment. In summary, delayed radiotherapy allows both those who respond poorly to chemotherapy and those who respond well to chemotherapy to benefit from this strategy.

During the first half of the 1990s, new agents have been identified with activity in SCLC, including Gemcitabine, Irinotecan, Topotecan, Docetaxol, and Paclitaxel. Studies will need to be performed to determine the role of these agents in the management of SCLC compared to currently used agents. Several of these agents, including Gemcitabine, are potent radiation sensitizers and combining them with radiation will need to proceed carefully to limit toxicity, while hopefully improving the results currently obtained. The timing of radiation therapy will continue to be an important issue in the management of these patients. It is likely that specific issues, such as treatment volume, dose, fractionation, and timing of thoracic irradiation, as well as the chemotherapy used, will prove important in providing optimal results. In addition, newer radiation planning techniques, such as conformal radiation therapy, which can limit the volume of normal tissues (e.g., esophagus, lung, and heart) irradiated, may further improve the results of treatment by limiting toxicity and allowing treatment to be delivered with fewer interruptions and dose reductions. It may also be important for treating physicians and patients to accept severe acute toxicities without interrupting radiation treatments or reducing the doses of chemotherapy to produce optimal survival results.

CONCLUSION

These authors conclude, that at the current time, the optimal timing of thoracic radiation therapy in limited-stage SCLC is unknown. Early administration of thoracic radiation, with the likelihood of resultant reduced chemotherapy doses, has no clear advantage. What is important is finding the optimal combination of chemotherapy for distant disease and optimal dose and schedule of thoracic radiotherapy for local disease.

REFERENCES

1. Weiss RB. Small cell carcinoma of the lung: therapeutic management. Ann Intern Med 1978; 88:522–531.
2. Cohen MH. Is thoracic radiation therapy necessary for patients with limited stage small cell lung cancer? No. Cancer Treat Rep 1983; 67:217–221.
3. Byhardt RW, Cox JD. Is thoracic radiation therapy necessary for patients with limited stage small cell lung cancer? Yes. Cancer Treat Rep 1983; 67:209–215.
4. Pignon JP, Arriagada R, Ihde DC, Johnson DH, Perry MC, Souhami RL, Brodin O, Joss RA, Kies MS, Lebeau B, Onoshi T, Osterlind K, Tattersall MHN, Wagner H. A meta-analysis of thoracic radiotherapy for small cell lung cancer. N Engl J Med 1992; 327(23):1618–1624.
5. Warde P, Payne D. Does thoracic irradiation improve survival and local control in limited stage small cell carcinoma of the lung? A meta-analysis. J Clin Oncol 1992; 10(6):890–895.
6. Arriagada R, Pignon JP, Ihde DC, Johnson DH, Perry MC, Souhami RL, Brodin O, Joss RA, Kies MS, Lebeau B, Onoshi T, Osterlind K, Tattersall MHN, Wagner H. Effect of thoracic radiotherapy on mortality in limited small cell lung cancer. A meta-analysis of 13 randomized trials among 2,140 patients. Anticancer Res 1994; 14:333–335.
7. Perry MC, Eaton WL, Propert KJ, Ware JH, Zimmer B, Chahinian AP, Skarin A, Carey RW, Kreisman H, Faulkner C, Comis R, Green MR. Chemotherapy with or without radiation therapy in limited small cell lung carcinoma of the lung. N Engl J Med 1987; 316:912–918.
8. Perry MC, Herndon JE III, Eaton WL, Green MR. Thoracic radiation therapy added

to chemotherapy for small-cell lung cancer: an update of Cancer and Leukemia Group B study 8083. J Clin Oncol 1998; 16:2466–2467.

9. Work E, Nielsen OS, Bentzen SM, Fode K, Palshof T. for the Aarhus Lung Cancer Group. Randomized study of initial versus late chest irradiation combined with chemotherapy in limited stage small cell lung carcinoma. J Clin Oncol 1997; 15(9): 3030–3037.

10. Shultz HO, Nielson O, Sell A, Steenholdt S, Bentzen S. Timing of chest irradiation with respect to combination chemotherapy in small cell lung cancer, limited disease. Lung Cancer 1988; 4:153 (abstract).

11. Gregor A, Drings P, Sahmoud T, Giaccone G. Sequential versus alternating chemoradiotherapy in limited small cell lung cancer—the EORTC Lung Cancer Cooperative Group experience. International Association for the Study of Lung Cancer, Bruges, Belgium, 1996 (abstr).

12. Murray N, Coy P, Pater JL, Hudson I, Arnold A, Zee BC, Payne D, Kostashuk EC, Evans WK, Dixon P, Sadura A, Feld R, Levitt M, Wierzbicki R, Ayoub J, Maroun JA, Wilson KS for the National Cancer Institute of Canada Clinical Trials Group. Importance of timing for thoracic irradiation in the combined modality treatment of limited stage small cell lung cancer. J Clin Oncol 1993; 11:336–344.

13. Jeremic B, Shibamoto Y, Acimovic L, Milisavljevic S. Initial versus delayed accelerated hyperfractionated radiation therapy and concurrent chemotherapy in limited small cell lung cancer: a randomized study. J Clin Oncol 1997; 15:893–900.

14. Turrisi AT, Glover DJ. Thoracic radiotherapy variables: Influence on local control in small cell lung cancer limited disease. Int J Radiat Oncol Biol Phys 1990; 19: 1473–1479.

15. Johnson DH, Salem C, Nesbitt J. Limited stage small cell lung cancer treated with concurrent BID chest radiotherapy and etoposide-cisplatin followed by chemotherapy selected by in vitro drug sensitivity testing (DST). Proc Am Soc Clin Oncol 1991; 10:240 (abstr).

16. Frytak S, Shaw EG, Jett JR, Richardson RL, Foote RL, Creagan ET, Eagan RT, Su JQ. Infusion cisplatin chemotherapy and hyperfractionated thoracic radiotherapy for small cell lung cancer. Am J Clin Oncol (CCT) 1996; 19:193–198.

17. Wagner H Jr. Thoracic irradiation of limited small cell lung cancer: have we defined optimal dose, time, and fractionation? Lung Cancer 1997; 17(Suppl):S137–148.

18. Wagner H Jr. Radiation therapy in the management of limited small cell lung cancer: when, where, and how much? Chest 1998; 113(Suppl):S92–100.

19. Kies M, Mira J, Crowley J. Multimodal therapy for limited small cell lung cancer: a randomized study of induction combination chemotherapy with or without thoracic radiation in complete responders and with wide-field versus reduced-field radiation in partial responders: a Southwest Oncology Group study. J Clin Oncol 1987; 5: 592–600.

20. Liengswangwong V, Bonner JA, Shaw EG, Foote RL, Frytak S, Eagan RT, Jett JR, Richardson RL, Creagan ET, Su JQ. Limited stage small cell lung cancer: patterns of intrathoracic recurrence and the implications for thoracic radiotherapy. J Clin Oncol 1994; 12(3):496–502.

21. Arriagada R, Pallae-Cosset B, Ladron de Guevara JC, el Bakry H, Benna F, Martin M, de Cremoux H, Baldeyrou P, Cerrina ML, Le Chevalier T. Alternating radiother-

apy and chemotherapy schedules in limited small cell lung cancer: analysis of local chest recurrences. Radiother Oncol 1991; 20(2):91–98.

22. Hudes RS, Langer C, Movsas B, Nicolauo N, Litwin S, Schol J. Keenan E, Curran WJ. Induction paclitaxel-carboplatin followed by concurrent radiotherapy and dose escalation of paclitaxel-carboplatin in unresectable, locally advanced non-small cell lung carcinoma: a report of FCCC 94-001. Int J Radiat Oncol Biol Phys 1999; 45(3): 243.

4

Limited-Stage SCLC: Radiotherapy Fractionation and Volume Issues

Todd Williams, Charles Thomas, Jr.,*
and Andrew Turrisi III
Medical University of South Carolina, Charleston, South Carolina

INTRODUCTION

Thoracic radiotherapy has been demonstrated to be a valuable component in the treatment of limited-stage small cell lung cancer (LS-SCLC) (1,2). Yet the method of its delivery continues to pose challenges to radiation oncologists. Despite high response rates to both radiotherapy and chemotherapy, failure rates remain unacceptably high. In an attempt to improve local control and survival, radiation treatment parameters have been altered. They include treatment volumes and fractionation schedules.

FRACTIONATION

Fractionation refers to the dividing of the total radiation dose into multiple segments. The most frequent schedule utilized in the United States delivers one treatment per day, 5 days a week.

---
*Current affiliation: University of Texas Health Science Center at San Antonio, San Antonio Cancer Institute, San Antonio, Texas.

Generally, tissues in the body can be divided into late responding (slowly or nonproliferating) or early responding (rapidly proliferating). Examples of late-responding, normal tissues include the central nervous system, lung, and kidney. The gastrointestinal tract, skin, and gonads are considered early-responding normal tissues; they behave differently when exposed to ionizing radiation. Early-responding tissue effects are *more* related to overall treatment time and less dependent on fraction size. In contrast, late-responding tissues are *mainly* dependent on the fraction size. Increasing the dose per fraction (>2.5–3.0 Gy) will result in more severe late effects (fibrosis, necrosis, etc.) for equivalent early effects (skin erythema, esophagitis, etc.).

Conceptually, two distinct altered fractionation strategies can be utilized in the hope of improving local control or survival. Hyperfractionation involves smaller-than-conventional RT doses (e.g., 1–1.2 Gy) administered multiple times daily (typically two to three times) to achieve a higher cumulative dose over the course of therapy. Radiobiologically, hyperfractionation yields differential sparing of late-reacting normal tissue compared with acute-reacting malignant tissues. By contrast, with accelerated (hyperfractionated) RT, a more conventional radiation fraction size is utilized (e.g., 1.5–2 Gy), but as multiple fractions are administered daily, the overall treatment time is significantly shorter. Unlike hyperfractionated radiotherapy (HFRT), the aim of accelerated RT is to reduce the tumor cell repopulation in rapidly proliferating neoplasms by shortening the overall treatment time.

The rationale for altered fractionation is based on several radiobiological principles (3). One is that repair of sublethal radiation damage in aerobic cells is essentially complete within 2–4 hr. Therefore, if several treatments per day are delivered, separated by 4–6 hr to allow for normal tissue repair, it would theoretically be more effective on rapidly proliferating tumors (e.g., small cell carcinoma) and improve the therapeutic ratio.

Another observation is that the shape of the dose-response relationships for early- and late-responding tissues is different. The fraction size dependence of most tumors, including small cell carcinoma, mimics that of rapidly proliferating tissues (although there are exceptions, e.g., malignant melanoma). The optimal dose per fraction for cancer in general, as well as small cell lung cancer, continues to be a hotly debated subject. The "standard" regimens vary from institution to institution but are most often in the range of 1.8–2.5 Gy per fraction delivered once a day. There are data that this may not be optimal for small cell lung carcinoma. It has been demonstrated in in vitro studies to exhibit exponential cell killing with small fraction sizes as well as with the "standard" daily doses. As noted previously, the larger the dose per fraction, the greater the chance for long-term side effects (fibrosis, pneumonitis). Accelerated, hyperfractionated treatment would potentially allow continued exponential tumor kill, with lower prospects of long-term side effects. Finally, it is theorized that fractionation allows time for reassortment of tumor cells into more radiosensitive phases of the cell cycle [gap 2 (G2) and mitosis (M)].

Several pilot studies performed in the 1980s and early 1990s tested the hypothesis of using accelerated hyperfractionated radiotherapy along with concurrent chemotherapy in limited-stage small cell lung cancer (4–12). As these studies suggested superior responses and survival rates, this concept was tested in a large, cooperative group, phase III, prospective randomized trial (13). A total of 417 patients with limited-stage disease were randomized. Patients on both arms received four cycles of cisplatin (60 mg/m^2, day 1) and etoposide (120 mg/m^2, days 1, 2, and 3) chemotherapy. The radiotherapy consisted of 45 Gy in both treatment arms and was started on day 1 of chemotherapy cycle 1. The once-daily arm received 1.8 Gy/day, treated Monday through Friday, for 5 weeks. The accelerated, hyperfractionated arm received 1.5 Gy twice a day for 3 weeks. The twice-daily fractions were separated by a 4–6-hr interval. The volume of lung and mediastinum irradiated was defined by chest CT scan. Clinical treatment volumes incorporated gross tumor, mediastinum, and ipsilateral hilum. The contralateral hilum and supraclavicular regions were excluded. Prophylactic cranial irradiation, consisting of 25 Gy in 10 fractions, was recommended for patients achieving a complete clinical response. The primary endpoint of the study was overall survival measured from the date of study entry to the date of death from any cause. The median follow-up was approximately 8 years, with a minimum of 5 years. Final analysis revealed the median survival to be 20 months for all patients. For the once-daily and twice-daily arms, it was 19 and 23 months, respectively. The 2- and 5-year overall survivals are as follows:

	2-year overall survival (%)	5-year overall survival (%)
Once-daily XRT	41	16
Twice-daily XRT	47	26

The survival differences were statistically significant ($p = 0.04$). A pattern of failure analysis divulged a substantial reduction in local failure in the investigational arm, 36%, compared to 52%, in the standard, once-daily treatment arm ($p = 0.06$). There was a statistically significant increase in grade 3 esophagitis in the twice-daily treatment arm, 27% versus 11% for those receiving chest radiotherapy once daily ($p < 0.001$). The duration of esophagitis was not measured, but there were no cases of esophageal stricture or long-term dysphasia.

A criticism of this trial is that the dose of radiotherapy used in the standard arm was too low (14). There are dose-response data for small cell carcinoma suggesting improved local control with higher total doses; likewise, higher doses have recently been shown to be tolerable with concurrent cisplatin-based chemotherapy (15–17). Choi et al. performed a phase I trial to determine the maximum tolerated dose (MTD) of thoracic radiotherapy for both standard and twice-daily schedules in patients with LS-SCLC (18). All patients received concurrent cisplatin/etopside chemotherapy. Esophagitis was found to be the dose-limiting toxicity in both arms. For the field sizes and chemotherapy used, the MTD was 45 Gy and 70 Gy in the twice-daily and standard treatment arms, respectively. These patients received three cycles of PCE chemotherapy (cisplatin, cytoxan, etoposide) prior to receiving the concurrent treatment. Thus, their radiotherapy was delivered as later concurrent (like the CALGB standard) as compared to early concurrent, with cycle 1 or 2. Other investigators have demonstrated superior results with earlier concurrent treatment (19,20). It is yet unproven whether higher doses delivered with a standard once-daily regimen are superior to 45 Gy delivered twice daily. Higher total doses (60 and 70 Gy, delivered with a once-a-day fraction regimen) are now being investigated by several U.S. cooperative groups. It is also unknown whether using smaller treatment volumes, which exclude regions that have historically been treated "prophylactically," will allow further dose escalation or compromise local control. Data for non–small cell lung cancer suggest the dose can be dramatically increased to smaller volumes, without a concordant rise in regional failure (21).

Other investigators have also compared once-daily versus twice-daily therapy. Bonner et al. randomized 262 patients to standard chest radiotherapy (50.4 Gy/1.8 Gy fractions) versus twice-daily (48 Gy/1.5 Gy fractions) (22). Similar to Choi's dose escalation trial, these patients received late concurrent therapy beginning with cycle 4. The chemotherapy consisted of cisplatin (30 mg/m^2, days 1, 2, 3, cycles 1–6) and etoposide (130 mg/m^2, days 1, 2, 3, cycles 1, 2, 3). During the concurrent treatment, the etoposide dose was reduced to 100 mg/m^2. All twice-daily patients had a planned 2-week interruption of the thoracic radiotherapy after receiving 24 Gy. Prophylactic cranial irradiation was administered after the completion of six cycles of chemotherapy, if a complete response had been observed. This consisted of 30 Gy in 15 fractions. Esophageal toxicity was statistically different between the two arms, with the twice-daily patients experiencing 13% ≥ grade 3 esophagitis versus 5% for the once-daily patients ($p = 0.027$). No statistically significant difference in median survival between the two arms was found. Owing to the difference in toxicities, a quality-of-life evaluation was performed (23). Quality-adjusted life-years (QALY) were calculated using the Q-TWiST methodology and found to be greater for the once-daily thoracic radiation arm than for the twice-daily treatment arm. However, the difference was not statistically significant and the benefit was restricted to the time of therapy, not subsequent years. It was the authors' opinion that in evaluating both survival and treatment toxicity, there was no significant difference between the two treatments.

Several caveats should be kept in mind regarding this study. While the split course in the twice-daily arm was intended to decrease esophageal toxicity, it also defeats the purpose of this regimen, which is to combat accelerated tumor repopulation. Such a break does not fit with known radiobiological principles. Moreover, unlike the Intergroup Trial (13), the radiotherapy in this study was delayed until cycle 4. While the timing of radiotherapy remains controversial, many studies support the use of earlier, rather than delayed, radiotherapy (24,25). These key distinctions between these two studies (13,22) may account for the differences reported regarding the benefit of twice-daily radiotherapy.

As this disease often presents in older patients, it is important to assess whether twice-daily therapy is tolerable in this patient population. A retrospective analysis of elderly patients ≥ 70 years of age was performed from data collected from intergroup trial 0096 (26). It was found that severe (grade 4–5) hematological toxicity was more common in this group (85% in the twice-daily arm versus 60% in the daily arm, $p < 0.01$), although no significant difference in the frequency of nonhematological toxicities was observed. In particular, neither esophageal toxicity nor survival was different when compared with younger patients.

Experiences in altered fractionation in both LS-SCLC and non–small cell lung carcinoma (NSCLC) may be useful in defining the current limits of combined therapy. In an Australian study by Ball and colleagues, 50 patients were treated with 2 Gy twice daily to a total of 60 Gy over the 3-week span with or without carboplatin chemotherapy (27). Patients experienced esophagitis lasting a median of 2–3 months. The multivariate analysis showed carboplatin did not influence the duration of symptoms. Locally advanced NSCLC patients received similar therapy in a trial reported by Kelly and colleagues (28). Instead of 2 Gy twice daily, they received 1.5 Gy twice daily, also to a total of 60 Gy.

Esophageal toxicity was significant and was felt to be near the tolerable limits by the authors. In LS-SCLC patients Ali et al. delivered 1.1 Gy three times daily to a total dose of 66 Gy (6). This accelerated hyperfractionated regimen was started on day 1 of chemotherapy. Only 12 patients were treated on this phase II trial with a median survival of 20 months; the 2- and 5-year survival was 50 and 17%, respectively. Toxicity was severe with 65% grade 3–4 esophageal and 85% hematological toxicity. This prompted the early termination of the trial.

Current Recommendations

The addition of thoracic irradiation to systemic therapy significantly improves the local control rates and provides a modest improvement in survival. The optimal dose and fractionation schemes are unknown. However, previously standard doses of 45–50 Gy delivered in a once-daily scheme are known to result in unacceptably high local failure rates ($\geq 50\%$). Hyperfractionated radiotherapy, incorporating biological data in their design, to the same total dose has been shown in recent phase III trials to be tolerable and efficacious (though more toxic). The larger of the two reported trials demonstrated statistically significant improved 5-year survival and local control rates. Is this superior to higher doses of radiotherapy delivered in a once-daily regimen? The answer to that question is unknown and will need to be answered in future prospective randomized trials. The available data do strongly suggest that the current doses used in twice-daily fractionation schemes are close to or at tolerance. It may be possible to escalate doses using smaller volumes. With modern chemotherapy, this may be feasible. There are plans to design a randomized trial comparing 45 Gy twice daily to 66 Gy once daily (each with four cycles of platinum-etoposide chemotherapy).

VOLUME

The irradiated volume is a crucial variable. Limited-stage disease has been defined as the extent of disease that can be incorporated into a tolerable radiation portal. With the doses used at the time (40–45 Gy), this volume included most of the ipsilateral hemithorax and regional lymph nodes. The mediastinal, bilateral hilar, and ipsilateral supraclavicular regions were typically encompassed.

In the 1970s and 1980s, the majority of authors emphasized the need to utilize such large radiation portals. They encompassed not only clinically involved areas, but all regional lymphatic drainage sites, regardless of whether they showed evidence of disease or not. This design likely arose from the treatment of Hodgkin's lymphoma, in which adjacent nodal areas are included, because of its propensity for contiguous spread. Moreover, confidence may have been lacking concerning pre–cisplatin chemotherapy's ability to eradicate subclinical disease.

To counter that presumed deficit, extremely large fields have been attempted, including even hemibody and total-body radiation (29,30). A small trial reported by Byhardt et al. attempted to answer the question: could total-body irradiation (TBI) replace chemotherapy as a more effective systemic treatment? (29). Sixteen patients with limited-stage disease received 30 Gy/10 fractions thoracic radiotherapy and were then randomized to receive 1 Gy/10 fractions TBI versus CAV chemotherapy (cyclophosphamide, Adriamycin, vincristine). Although the toxicity related to the TBI was tolerable, it demonstrated no improvement over chemotherapy. A later trial attempted to incorporate TBI (same regimen) in the treatment of extensive-stage-disease patients (30). In that pilot, 19 patients received induction chemotherapy consisting of four cycles of VOCA (VP-16, vincristine, cyclophosphamide, and Adriamycin) followed by TBI *and* prophylactic cranial irradiation delivered concurrently. "Responding" participants then went on to receive further CMH chemotherapy (cyclophosphamide, methotrexate, and hexamethylmelamine). Owing to toxicity, only eight of 19 patients received the consolidative chemotherapy and four of those required a delay before resuming chemotherapy. No improvement was noted in response or median survival with the addition of the low-dose TBI over chemotherapy alone compared to historical controls. A larger randomized trial compared systemic chemotherapy (pre–cisplatin era) plus locoregional thoracic radiotherapy versus that plus additional upper-abdominal and prophylactic cranial radiation (31). A total of 114 patients were randomized and the final analysis showed no local control or survival benefit to the larger-field radiotherapy, but rather a trend toward worse survival. Toxicity was not statistically different between the treatment arms. These series suggest that large-field radiotherapy for small cell carcinoma appears to be of limited use.

In 1981, Perez and colleagues reported results of a prospective, randomized, combined therapy trial of the Southeastern Cancer Study Group (SECSG) (32). They established decreased intrathoracic failures (32.5%) in patients treated with large portals as compared with those where fields did not include the contralateral hilum or entire mediastinum (69.2%). However, it was not clear if the locoregional failures actually occurred in the unirradiated areas. Pre–cisplatin era chemotherapy was used. Typical radiation fields of the era are shown in Figure 1.

THE LUNG   ·   *Perez et al.*

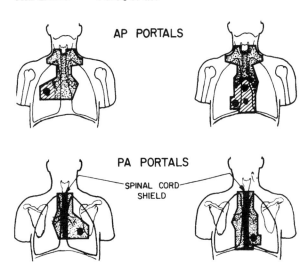

FIGURE 1   Traditional (large) radiotherapy portals used in the past.

Other investigators also found the vast majority of intrathoracic failures occurred in the radiation ports, but suggested inadequate dose and resistant disease may have been the problem, rather than the volume treated (33). More recently, investigators have advocated using smaller postchemotherapy tumor volumes in designing fields rather than prechemotherapy volumes. Mira and Livingston evaluated 17 patients treated with reduced, postchemotherapy volume portals (34). They found that the majority of chest failures were outside the high-dose volume, such as the development of lung parenchymal metastases and/or pleural effusions. They suggested that the systemic therapy might have left subclinical disease that was not included in the radiation portals. Liengswangwong et al. retrospectively compared 31 patients who had been treated with prechemotherapy tumor volumes to 28 patients who had been treated with postchemotherapy volumes (35). Thirty-two percent of patients experienced intrathoracic recurrence; however, the incidence was equally distributed between the two groups. No convincing evidence was found that treating postchemotherapy volumes placed patients at higher risk for intrathoracic or marginal failure.

Investigators at the Institut Gustave-Roussy analyzed the chest recurrences in 72 patients with limited-stage disease treated in several phase II trials of combined modality therapy (36). The in-field recurrence rate was 33% in the group of patients treated with prechemotherapy volumes versus 36% for those treated with postchemotherapy fields. The difference was not statistically significant. Owing to the low number of patients in this analysis, the authors were only able to suggest that postchemotherapy volumes may be adequate and thereby reduce the treatment toxicity. After assessing the local failure in 117 patients with LS-SCLC treated with combined modality therapy (83% receiving cisplatin-containing regimens), Tada and colleagues suggested that treatment volumes should be enlarged for patients with N_2 or N_3 involvement (37). Typical treatment field arrangements included the primary lung lesion with a 1.5-cm margin and all enlarged lymph nodes and the entire mediastinum down to the level of the subcarinal nodes (Figure 2).

Marginal failures were noted in 13% and 27% of patients presenting with N_2 and N_3 disease, respectively. A marginal failure was defined as locoregional relapse (including cervical lymph nodes) outside or on the edge of the initial radiation port. They detected a majority of the marginal failures to occur in the superior mediastinum, supraclavicular, and cervical regions.

Only one prospective, randomized trial has attempted to answer the pre- versus postchemotherapy volume question. The Southwest Oncology Group (SWOG) trial reported by Kies and colleagues randomized 191 patients with partial responses to chemotherapy to receive either wide-volume prechemotherapy or reduced-volume postchemotherapy radiotherapy after several cycles of induction chemotherapy (38). No appreciable difference emerged in either relapse pattern or survival. Patients receiving the wide-field radiotherapy had a slightly

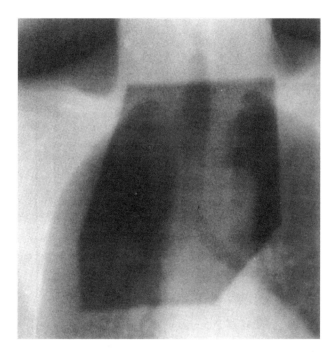

FIGURE 2   Radiotherapy portal of such a classic radiation treatment field (anterior view).

longer median survival and remission duration, but this was not statistically significant ($p = 0.73$ and 0.32, respectively).

It is important to note that in the previously mentioned studies, only the volume around primary disease changed. All these studies treated regional lymphatic sites prophylactically. The literature is silent about treating clinically involved areas alone, without treating radiographically uninvolved nodes. Three dimensional (3D) treatment planning systems are now widely available. Utilizing computerized tomography (CT) imaging, it is possible to better define gross tumor volumes and plan treatments that are no longer confined to two dimensions (Figure 3). One clear advantage of the 3D technique is its ability to treat less normal tissue (Figures 4 and 5). Using multiple noncoplanar beam arrangements, the dose to the surrounding normal tissue can be reduced. With the advent of intensity-modulated radiation therapy (IMRT), even more sophisticated conformal treatments are now possible. Using this new technology it is possible to adjust the radiation flux across the beam to confine the radiation dose tightly around critical structures, while maintaining high doses to the tumor volume. This

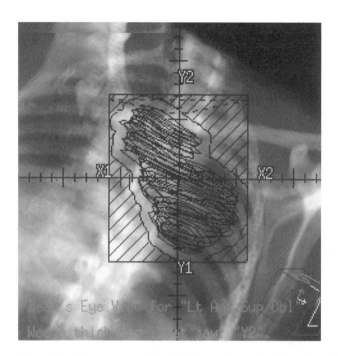

FIGURE 3 Beam's-eye view of a three-dimensional conformal radiotherapy field.

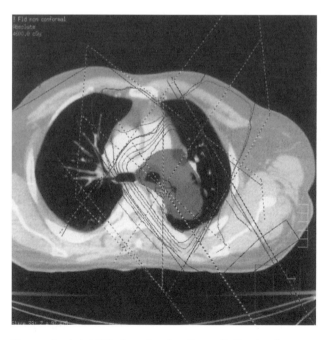

FIGURE 4 Axial CT slice showing the radiation isodose curves conforming to the shape of the target.

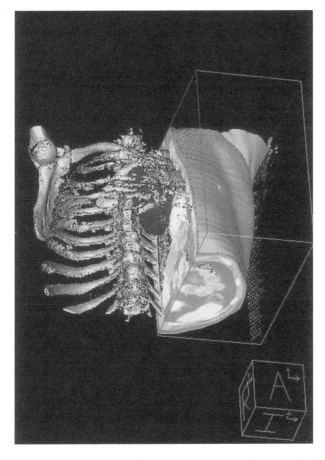

FIGURE 5 Three-dimensional reconstruction demonstrating the location of the tumor in the context of the surrounding anatomy.

technology has shown promise in several body sites, but its use is still considered investigational (39,40).

It is a well-recognized tenet in radiotherapy that treating larger volumes requires a corresponding decrease in the deliverable dose. It is therefore reasonable to hypothesize that by decreasing the treated volume, dose escalation would be allowed, possibly leading to an increase in local control and survival. Supporting data include several studies in which the entire mediastinum was not treated, and the contralateral hilum and supraclavicular fossae were omitted. Excellent local control and survival were verified (8,11,13).

It is also reasonable to hypothesize that as diagnostic capabilities improve, with more effective evaluation of the mediastinum, including esophageal ultrasound (41–43) and positron emission tomography (PET) (44–46), marginal or locoregional failures can hopefully be avoided.

Current Recommendations

Most modern radiotherapy series indicate that failure occurs within the irradiated volume at the primary site, and the problem appears to be intrinsic tumor resistance, rather than marginal miss. Reducing the irradiated volume may allow for significant dose escalation without an attendant rise in toxicity. Recent dose escalation trials in both LS-SCLC and NSCLC have borne this out. Modern chemotherapy will hopefully aid in this goal by sterilizing subclinical disease and allowing omission of lymphatic regions previously treated prophylactically. Field size reduction can be exploited to increase dose and decrease toxicity. Developing technologies, including 3D treatment planning and IMRT, will also assist in this goal and hopefully lead to an improvement in local control and survival.

REFERENCES

1. Pignon JP, Arriagada R, Ihde DC. A meta-analysis of thoracic radiotherapy for small-cell lung cancer. N Engl J Med 1992; 327:1618–1624.
2. Warde P, Payne D. Does thoracic irradiation improve survival and local control in limited stage small-cell carcinoma of the lung? J Clin Oncol 1992; 10:890–895.
3. Choi N. Accelerated radiation therapy in small cell lung cancer: rationale and limitation in its utility. Int Radiat Oncol Biol Phys 1990; 19:1623–1625.
4. Johnson D, Turrisi A, Chang A, Blum A, Bonomi P, Ettinger D, Wagner H. Alternating chemotherapy and twice-daily thoracic radiotherapy in limited-stage small-cell lung cancer: a pilot study of the Eastern Cooperative Oncology Group. J Clin Oncol 1993; 11(5):879–884.
5. Johnson BE, Bridges JD, Sobezeck M, Gray J, Linnoila RI, Gazdar AF, Hankins L, Steinberg S, Edison M, Frame J, Pass H, Nesbitt J, Holden D, Mulshine JL, Glatstein E, Ihde DC. Patients with limited-stage small-cell lung cancer treated with concurrent twice-daily chest radiotherapy and etoposide/cisplatin followed by cyclophosphamide, doxorubicin, and vincristine. J Clin Oncol 1996; 14(3):806–813.
6. Ali M, Kraut M, Valdivieso M, Herskovic A, Du W, Kalemkerian G. Phase II study of hyperfractionated radiotherapy and concurrent weekly alternating chemotherapy in limited-stage small cell lung cancer. Lung Cancer 1998; 22:39–44.
7. Johnson BE, Salem C, Nesbitt J, Gazdar A, Lesar M, Phelps R, Edison M, Linnoila R, Phares J, Pass H, Mulshine J, Minna J, Glatstein E, Ihde D. Limited stage small cell lung cancer treated with concurrent hyperfractionated chest radiotherapy and etoposide/cisplatin. Lung Cancer 1993; 9(suppl. 1):S21–S26.
8. Turrisi AT, Glover DJ, Mason B, Tester W. Long term results of platinum etoposide

(PE) + twice-daily (BID) thoracic radiotherapy (TRT) for limited small-cell lung cancer (LSCLC): results on 32 patients with 48 month minimum F/U. Proc ASCO 1992; 11:292.

9. Turrisi A, Wagner H, Glover D, Mason B, Oken M, Bonomi P. Limited small cell lung cancer (LSCLC): concurrent BID thoracic radiotherapy (TRT) with platinum-etoposide (PE): an ECOG study. Proc ASCO 1990; 9:230.

10. Mornex F, Trillet V, Chauvin F, Ardiet JM, Schmitt T, Romestaing P, Carrie C, Mahe M, Mornex JF, Fournel P, Souquet PJ, Boniface E, Vincent M, Piperno D, Rebattu P, Gerard JP, and the Groupe Lyonnais d'Oncologie Thoracique. Hyperfractionated radiotherapy alternating with multidrug chemotherapy in the treatment of limited small cell lung cancer (SCLC). Int J Radiat Oncol Biol Phys 1990; 19:23–30.

11. Turrisi AT, Glover DJ, Mason BA. A preliminary report: concurrent twice-daily radiotherapy plus platinum-etoposide chemotherapy for limited small cell lung cancer. Int J Radiat Oncol Biol Phys 1988; 15(1):183–187.

12. Armstrong JG, Rosenstein MM, Kris MG, Shank BM, Scher HI, Fass DE, Harrison LB, Leibel SA, Fuks ZY. Twice daily thoracic irradiation for limited small cell lung cancer. Int J Radiat Oncol Biol Phys 1991; 21:1269–1274.

13. Turrisi AT, Kim K, Blum R, Sause WT, Livingston RB, Komaki R, Wagner H, Aisner S, Johnson DH. Twice-daily compared with once-daily thoracic radiotherapy in limited small-cell lung cancer treated concurrently with cisplatin and etoposide. N Engl J Med 1999; 340(4):265–271.

14. Abadir R, Orton C. Radiotherapy for small-cell lung cancer. Correspondence. N Engl J Med 1999; 340(25):2002–2003.

15. Coy P, Hodson I, Payne D, Evans W, Feld R, MacDonald A, Osoba D, Pater J. The effect of dose of thoracic irradiation on recurrence in patients with limited stage small cell lung cancer. Initial results of a Canadian multicenter randomized trial. Int J Radiat Oncol Biol Phys 1987; 14:219–236.

16. Choi N, Carey R. Importance of radiation dose in achieving improved loco-regional tumor control in limited stage small-cell lung carcinoma: an update. Int J Radiat Oncol Biol Phys 1989; 17:307–310.

17. Papac R, Son Y, Bien R, Tiedemann D, Keohane M, Yesner R. Improved local control of thoracic disease in small cell lung cancer with higher dose thoracic irradiation and cyclic chemotherapy. Int J Radiat Oncol Biol Phys 1987; 13:993–998.

18. Choi NC, Herndon JE, Rosenman J, Carey RW, Chung CT, Bernard S, Leone L, Seagren S, Green M. Phase I study to determine the maximum-tolerated dose of radiation in standard daily and hyperfractionated-accelerated twice-daily radiation schedules with concurrent chemotherapy for limited-stage small-cell lung cancer. J Clin Oncol 1998; 16(11):3528–3536.

19. Jeremic B, Shibamoto Y, Acimovic L, Millsavijevic S. Initial versus delayed accelerated hyperfractionated radiation therapy and concurrent chemotherapy in limited small-cell lung cancer: a randomized study. J Clin Oncol 1997; 15(3):893–900.

20. Goto K, Nishiwaki Y, Takada M, Fukuoka M, Kawahara M, Sugiura T, Kurita Y, Watanabe K, Noda K, Yoshimura K, Tamura T, Saijo N. Final results of a Phase III study of concurrent versus sequential thoracic radiotherapy (TRT) in combination with cisplatin (P) and etoposide (E) for limited-stage small cell lung cancer (LD-

SCLC): the Japan Clinical Oncology Group (JCOG) study. Proc ASCO 1999; 18: 468a.

21. Hayman J, Martel M, Ten Haken R, Todd R, Turrisi A, Lichter A, University of Michigan Health System, Ann Arbor, MI. Dose escalation in non-small cell lung cancer (NSCLC) using conformal 3-dimensional radiation therapy (C3DRT): update of a Phase 1 Trial. Proc ASCO 1999; 18:459a.

22. Bonner JA, Shanahan TG, Brooks BJ, Marks RS, Sloan JA. Phase III comparison of once-daily thoracic radiation versus twice-daily thoracic radiation in patients with limited stage small cell lung cancer. Proc ASCO 1998; 17:456a.

23. Bonner JA, Sloan JA, Hillman SH, Shanahan TG, Brooks BJ, Marks RS, Ochsner Clinic CCOP, New Orleans, LA, and North Central Cancer Treatment Group (NCCTG). A quality adjusted re-analysis of a phase III trial comparing once-daily thoracic radiation therapy versus twice-daily thoracic radiation therapy in patients with limited stage small cell lung cancer. Proc ASCO 1999; 18:466a.

24. Murray N, Coy P, Pater J, et al. Importance of timing for thoracic irradiation in the combined modality treatment of limited-stage small-cell lung cancer. J Clin Oncol 1993; 11:336–344.

25. Jeremic B, Shibamato Y, Acimovic L, Milisavljevic S. Initial versus delayed accelerated hyperfractionated radiation therapy and concurrent chemotherapy in limited small-cell lung cancer: a randomized study. J Clin Oncol 1997; 15:893–900.

26. Yuen A, Zou G, Turrisi A, Sause W, Komaki R, Wayner H, Aisner S, Livingston R, Blum R, Johnson D. Similar outcome of elderly patients in intergroup trail 0096: cisplatin (P), etoposide (E), and thoracic radiotherapy (TRT) administered once (QD) or twice daily (BID) in limited stage small cell lung cancer (SCLC). Proc ASCO 1999; 18:467a.

27. Ball D, Bishop J, Smith J, et al. A phase III study of accelerated radiotherapy (RT) with and without carboplatin in non-small cell lung cancer (NSCLC): interim toxicity analysis. Lung Cancer 1994; 11(suppl 2):54–55.

28. Kelly K, Bunn PA, Hazuka MB, et al. A phase I-II study of daily carboplatin in patients with regionally inoperable non-small cell lung cancer (NSCLC). Lung Cancer 1994; 11(suppl):693 (abstr).

29. Byhardt R, Cox J, Wilson J, Libnoch J, Stein R. Total body irradiation vs. chemotherapy as a systemic adjuvant for small cell carcinoma of the lung. J Radiat Oncol Biol Phys 1979; 5:2043–2048.

30. Dillman R, Seagren S, Taetle R. Failure of low-dose, total-body irradiation to augment combination chemotherapy in extensive-stage small cell carcinoma of the lung. J Clin Oncol 1983; 1(4):242–246.

31. Hansen H, Dombernowsky P, et al. Prophylactic irradiation in bronchogenic small cell anaplastic carcinoma: a comparative trial of localized versus extensive radiotherapy including prophylactic brain irradiation in patients receiving combination chemotherapy. Cancer 1980; 46:279–284.

32. Perez C, Krauss S, Bartolucci A. Thoracic and elective brain irradiation with concomitant or delayed multiagent chemotherapy in the treatment of localized small cell carcinoma of the lung. Cancer 1981; 47:2407–2413.

33. Brodin O, Arnbert H, Bergh J, et al. Increased radioresistance of an in vitro transformed human small cell lung cancer cell line. Lung Cancer 1995; 12:183–198.

34. Mira JG, Livingston RB. Evaluation and radiotherapy implications of chest relapse patterns in small cell lung carcinoma treated with radiotherapy-chemotherapy: study of 34 cases and review of the literature. Cancer 1980; 46:2557–2565.

35. Liengswangwong V, Bonner JA, Shaw EG, Foote RL, Frytak S, Eagan RT, Jett JR, Richardson RL, Creagan ET, Su JQ. Limited-stage small-cell lung cancer: patterns of intrathoracic recurrence and the implications for thoracic radiotherapy. J Clin Oncol 1994; 12(3):496–502.

36. Arriagada R, Pallae-Cosset B, Ladron de Guevara JC, el Bakry H, Benna F, Martin M, de Cremoux H, Baldeyrou P, Cerrina ML, Le Chevalier T. Alternating radiotherapy and chemotherapy schedules in limited small cell lung cancer: analysis of local chest recurrences. Radiother Oncol 1991; 20(2):91–98.

37. Tada T, Minakuchi K, Koda M, Masuda N, Matsui K, Kawase I, Nakajima T, Nishioka M, Fukuoka M, Kozuka T. Limited-stage small cell lung cancer: Local failure and chemotherapy and radiation therapy. Radiology 1998; 208:511–515.

38. Kies M, Mira J, Crowley J. Multimodal therapy for limited small cell lung cancer: a randomized study of induction combination chemotherapy with or without thoracic radiation in complete responders and with wide-field versus reduced-field radiation in partial responders: a Southwest Oncology Group study. J Clin Oncol 1987; 5: 592–600.

39. Verhey LJ. Comparison of three-dimensional conformal radiation therapy and intensity-modulated radiation therapy systems. Semin Radiat Oncol 1999; 9(1):78–98.

40. Meeks SL, Buatti JM, Bova FJ, Friedman WA, Mendenhall WM, Zlotecki RA. Potential clinical efficacy of intensity-modulated conformal therapy. Int J Radiat Oncol Biol Phys 1998; 40(2):483–495.

41. Silvestri GA, Hoffman BJ, Bhutani MS, Hawes RH, Coppage L, Sanders-Cliette A, Reed CE. Endoscopic ultrasound with fine-needle aspiration in the diagnosis and staging of lung cancer. Ann Thorac Surg 1996; 61(5):1441–1445.

42. Serna DL, Aryan HE, Chang KJ, Brenner M, Tran LM, Chen JC. An early comparison between endoscopic ultrasound-guided fine-needle aspiration and mediastinoscopy for diagnosis of mediastinal malignancy. Am Surg 1998; 64(10):1014–1018.

43. Hunerbein M, Ghadimi BM, Haensch W, Schlag PM. Transesophageal biopsy of mediastinal and pulmonary tumors by means of endoscopic ultrasound guidance. J Thorac Cardiovasc Surg 1998; 116(4):554–559.

44. Coates G, Skehan SJ. Emerging role of PET in the diagnosis and staging of lung cancer. Can Respir J 1999; 6(2):145–152.

45. Saunders CA, Dussek JE, O'Doherty MJ, Maisey MN. Evaluation of fluorine-18-fluorodeozxyglucose whole body positron emission tomography imaging in the staging of lung cancer. Ann Thorac Surg 1999; 67(3):790–797.

46. Marom EM, McAdams HP, Erasmus JJ, Goodman PC, Culhane DK, Coleman RE, Herndon JE, Patz EF. Staging non-small cell lung cancer with whole-body PET. Radiology 1999; 212(3):803–809.

5

The Role of Prophylactic Cranial Irradiation: Pro

Cécile Le Péchoux and Thierry Le Chevalier
Institut Gustave-Roussy, Villejuif, France

Rodrigo Arriagada
Instituto de Radiomedicina, Santiago, Chile

INTRODUCTION

Small cell lung cancer (SCLC) represents 20% of all lung cancer cases. Specific characteristics distinguish it from other cell types: the risk of early hematogenous dissemination, and its marked radiosensitivity and chemosensitivity (1). About two-thirds of these patients, and particularly those presenting limited disease, and treated with aggressive induction therapy combining multidrug chemotherapy and thoracic radiation therapy, will achieve a complete remission. Yet only 15–20% of complete responders will be long-term survivors. Indeed, the majority of these patients relapse.

A consequence of improved local control is that brain metastases have now become a significant cause of treatment failure (2,3). Even if SCLC is chemosensitive, unless they are highly liposoluble, drugs find it difficult to cross the blood-brain barrier. In the seventies, Hansen proposed central nervous system (CNS) prophylaxis given that the brain was considered a pharmacological sanctuary where metastases could be protected from cytostatic agents due to the blood-brain barrier (4). Here pediatric acute lymphoblastic leukemia (ALL) served as a paradigm of successful CNS prophylaxis; meningeal leukemia had been significantly reduced and the cure rate of ALL improved as a result of such treatment. These observations were part of the rationale underlying a number of clinical trials investigating prophylactic cranial irradiation (PCI) over the last two decades, in an attempt to prevent the development of brain metastases and reduce the risk of CNS relapses. Many of these trials were too small to detect significant benefits in terms of the prevention of brain metastases or enhanced survival. However, by the mid-1980s, PCI had been demonstrated to significantly reduce the incidence of CNS relapses compared to no PCI, although doubts persisted as to whether such treatment would be beneficial for survival. Physicians were also concerned about the best ways to preclude recurrences without generating unacceptable toxicity and without impairing the patient's quality of life. More recent studies have tested PCI in patients achieving a good response to induction therapy, and have confirmed that PCI significantly decreases the likelihood of developing brain metastases by at least 30%. Despite several retrospective and prospective studies, the usefulness of PCI has remained controversial owing to the lack of improvement in survival in individual trials and possible neurotoxicity in long-term survivors (5–8). However, data have recently been published that help clarify the role of PCI in SCLC.

INCIDENCE OF CENTRAL NERVOUS SYSTEM METASTASES IN SCLC

Neurological disorders, either at the time of presentation or during the subsequent clinical course of SCLC, are frequent. They include brain metastases, meningeal carcinomatosis, intramedullary metastases, epidural metastases, and hyponatremia producing CNS symptoms. However, carcinomatous leptomeningitis or spinal cord lesions are usually found in patients who develop recurrent disease (9). Brain metastases are the most common forms of CNS involvement, and are the only lesions shown to be potentially preventable. At initial diagnosis, 10–15% of patients have brain metastases; the incidence varies between 50 and 65% in autopsy series (3,4,10,11). Indeed, brain metastases are present in 50–80% of 2-year survivors (2,3,12). The incidence of brain metastasis as the first site of treatment failure varies between 14 and 45% at 2 years, even in patients who achieve a complete response (13,14). With the improvement in local control in SCLC, brain metastases have become a common cause of treatment failure.

TREATMENT OF BRAIN METASTASES

Historically, cytotoxic agents have played a limited role in the treatment of brain metastases, since cytostatic drugs were generally unable to cross the blood-brain barrier of the normal brain in tumoricidal concentrations. However, more recent studies have reported a better response in brain metastases after treatment with chemotherapy alone, with rates ranging from 40 to 76% (15–18). Although these small studies have shown that brain relapses are quite responsive to systemic therapy, radiation therapy has remained the most widely accepted treatment modality for brain metastases. According to retrospective studies, cranial irradiation significantly improves neurological symptoms in 56–92% of patients with SCLC brain metastases (3,19–22). Both initial and delayed brain metastases are included in most studies, and about 70–75% of patients have some improvement of their symptoms and 40% achieve a complete remission. Success, however, is inversely proportional to the severity of the neurological symptoms; in effect, all patients who had minimal symptoms had complete palliation, whereas only 45% of patients with severe symptoms had complete palliation (19). The response rate for initial metastases (73–74%) is higher than for delayed metastases (56–58%) (19,21). Whereas systemic chemotherapy may be appropriate for patients with brain metastases at initial diagnosis, therapeutic cranial irradiation appears preferable for patients who develop brain metastases after induction treatment.

Although relief of symptoms with therapeutic brain radiation is clearly beneficial, overall survival after development of brain metastases is low, with median survival ranging from 1.5 to 4.5 months (20,22–25). Brain metastases are also associated with considerable morbidity, which has been shown to be worse in terms of days spent in hospital than in patients with SCLC liver involvement (26). As brain metastases are so difficult to treat, and are accompanied by distressing and sometimes life-threatening symptoms, prophylactic treatment seems a reasonable alternative. It has been suggested that prophylactic cranial irradiation could confer an advantage over therapeutic brain irradiation by preserving a better quality of life (QoL) (27). In one early study, the QoL was evaluated with the Karnofsky performance status. The mean survival, with a Karnofsky score of 60 or greater, was superior in patients who had prophylactic cranial irradiation (10 months) compared to patients who had no PCI and who subsequently developed brain metastases (6 months) (27). Thus historically, one of the first arguments of the proponents of PCI was that the development of brain metastases gave rise to considerable morbidity, and such morbidity could be prevented with elective irradiation. Furthermore, brain failure is a rapidly fatal event once CNS metastases have emerged (20,23–25).

Alternatives to prophylactic cranial irradiation have been proposed. Chemoprophylaxis of brain metastases, even with lipophylic agents, has failed in past studies (3,28). Regular follow-up of the brain (CT scan every 3 months for 2 years) was also proposed as an alternative to PCI in a study that included 127 patients (29). There, the objective was to detect brain metastases at an early asymptomatic stage in the hope of achieving long-term control with immediate therapeutic radiotherapy and thus avoid possible long-term morbidity due to PCI. Among the 56 patients (44%) who had a CNS relapse, it emerged between scans in 20 of them. Despite cranial irradiation, about 60% of the patients who developed brain metastases died with active CNS disease. The authors concluded that PCI could not be replaced by regular follow-up with CT scans.

EFFICACY OF PROPHYLACTIC CRANIAL IRRADIATION

Older Trials

Several retrospective studies have shown that PCI could reduce CNS relapse; only 2–5% of patients thus treated would develop brain metastases as the first site of relapse (19,30). Other studies have reported higher rates of CNS relapse. Some of the difficulties in assessing the value of PCI have come from statistical ambiguities in the definition of a brain relapse, i.e., sole site of first relapse, cumulative rate of brain failure at a given time, crude rate of brain metastases or actuarial rate. Furthermore, as the duration of survival has increased due to increasingly effective systemic therapy, combined or not with thoracic radiotherapy in localized disease, so has the frequency of brain metastases (2,3,31). Many investigators have routinely used PCI during the past 20 years, since it was generally accepted that it would delay the onset of symptomatic brain metastases and reduce by 30–50% the lifetime risk of CNS relapse (2,3).

Since then, several randomized trials have been published (32–38). However, they included very heterogeneous patient populations: patients who failed to achieve a complete remission, patients with limited and extensive disease, patients who had concomitant chemotherapy and different PCI doses and fractionation, which may account for the differences observed in the reduction of brain failure. Table 1 summarizes the results of several randomized trials that show that the incidence of CNS metastases varies between 13% and 67% in patients not receiving PCI. Almost all these studies showed a significant two- to threefold decrease in the incidence of brain metastases, but no impact on the survival rate. However, in 1983, Rosen et al. were the first to report that PCI could have an impact on survival in a subgroup of patients. Since then, several retrospective studies have suggested that PCI not only reduced brain failure rates, but could also improve survival in complete responders to induction treatment (12,41–43). In other studies, increased survival with PCI was also observed in patients with other favorable characteristics, such as a good performance status, moderate weight loss, young age, and a serum sodium value that could be predictive of a relatively long life expectancy (44). Furthermore, brain metastases were the only cause of death in only a minority of patients (10%) (45). This may also contribute to the fact that these randomized studies did not show any impact on survival.

Recent Randomized Trials

More recent randomized trials have enrolled only patients considered to be in complete remission, as shown in Table 2 (12,46–49). When PCI is restricted to

TABLE 1 Randomized Trials Evaluating PCI in SCLC Patients

Study	No. of patients	PCI dose, Gy/fraction, timing of PCI	Rate of brain metastases (%)		p value	Median survival	
			PCI(+)	PCI(−)		PCI(+)	PCI(−)
Aroney (40) 1983	29	30/10 CR	0	27	NS	NR	NR
Beiler (32) 1979	54	24/8 3rd week	0	16	<0.05	>104 wk LD	58 wk LD
Cox (33) 1978	45	20/10 D1	17	24	NS	NR	NR
Eagan (23) 1981	30	36/10 20th week	13	73	<0.05	13.6 mo	12.9 mo
Hansen (34) 1980	110	40/20 12th week	9	13	NS	9.2 mo	10.2 mo
Jackson (35) 1983	29	30/10 D1	0	27	<0.05	9.8 mo	7.2 mo
Katsenis (36) 1982	35	40/25 D1	12	44	<0.05	NR	NR
Maurer 1980	163	30/10 9th week	4	18	<0.01	8.4 mo	8.8 mo
Niiranen (37) 1989	51	40/20 4th week	0	26	<0.05	13 mo	10 mo
Seydel (39) 1985	217	30/10 D1	5	21	<0.005	53 wk	52 wk

NS: No significant difference in terms of overall survival; CR: PCI given when patients are in complete remission; D1: PCI given on the first day of induction treatment.

TABLE 2 Randomized Trials Evaluating PCI in SCLC Complete Responders

Study	No. of patients	PCI dose, Gy/fraction, timing of PCI	Rate of brain metastases (%)			Median survival	
			PCI(+)	PCI(−)	p value	PCI(+)	PCI(−)
Arriagada (13) 1995	300	24/8 CR	40	67	$<10^{-13}$	NR	NR
Gregor (46) 1997	314	Various CR	30	54	0.00004	305 days	300 days
Laplanche (47) 1998	211	24/8–30/10 CR	44	51	0.14	NR	NR
Ohonoshi (48) 1993	46	40/20 CR	22	52	<0.05	21 mo	15 mo
Wagner (49) 1996	31	25/10 CR	20	50		15.3 mo	8.8 mo

NS: No significant difference in terms of overall survival; CR: PCI given when patients are in complete remission.

this favorable group of patients, brain metastases appear to be a major cause of failure. Virtually all the oldest randomized trials demonstrated a decreased rate of brain metastases from 22% to 6% for the groups not receiving and receiving PCI, respectively (32–40). These were crude brain metastasis rates. In the more recent trials, the rates seem higher, but are reported as actuarial rates (13,46–49). The overall 2-year actuarial brain failure rates are 40% and 67% (for PCI+ and PCI−, respectively) in the trial reported by Arriagada and colleagues and 30% and 54%, respectively, in the trial reported by Gregor and colleagues (Table 3) (13,46). In both the French and the EORTC trials, a plateau was observed after 2 years in the brain metastasis rate, suggesting that brain metastases can potentially be prevented, and not simply delayed, with PCI. This can be considered a second strong argument for the advocates of PCI. None of these randomized trials were large enough to confirm statistically the survival benefit suggested in retrospective studies (12,42–44). Since the probability that a patient might have the brain as the only site of failure ranges from 5 to 10%, only a small gain in long-term survival could be expected from PCI (19,45).

Meta-Analysis

A meta-analysis of individual patient data collected from seven trials, including a total of 987 patients randomized from 1977 to 1995, compared PCI to no PCI in patients with SCLC in complete remission (Table 4). The primary endpoint was overall survival (50). The results, which have recently been reported, showed PCI led to a 16% reduction in the mortality rate corresponding to an absolute increase of 5.4% in the 3-year survival rate (from 15.3% observed in the control group to 20.7%). PCI, therefore, not only decreased the risk of developing brain metastases significantly (from 58.6% to 33.3% at 3 years), as shown in other individual trials, but also improved overall survival and disease-free survival (50).

Optimal PCI Dose?

Although the dose-response relationships for PCI in SCLC are a fundamental element in planning the optimal treatment schedule, they have not been well established. In most studies, the prescribed PCI dose is about 24–30 Gy. One study has reported interesting results with one fraction of 8 Gy (51). However, large PCI fractions should be avoided because of late neurotoxicity. It has been demonstrated by Withers et al. that the dose-response relationship for subclinical metastatic disease is usually linear and within the 20–50-Gy dose range (52). Only one randomized trial has directly addressed this issue (46). The first part of this three-arm trial compared two PCI doses (24 Gy and 36 Gy) to no PCI. The hazard ratio between the group of patients treated with 24 Gy and the no-PCI group was 0.71 whereas it was 0.16 between the 36-Gy and no-PCI groups, and highly significant. Thus, the higher dose reduced the risk of brain metastasis

TABLE 3   Results at 2 Years (except for the IPC 88) of the Three Main PCI Randomized Studies in SCLC Complete Responders

	No. of patients, PCI+/PCI−	Rate of brain metastases		OS, PCI(+)	OS, PCI(−)
		PCI(+)	PCI(−)		
IPC 85 (13)	149/151	40%	67%	29%	21.5%
ICP 88 (47)	100/111	44% (4 years)	51% (4 years)	22% (4 years)	16% (4 years)
UKCCCR-EORTC (46)	194/120	30%	54%	25%	19%

TABLE 4   Randomized Studies Included in the Meta-Analysis

Study	Stage	PCI dose, Gy/fractions	Number of patients	Years of accrual
Aroney (40)	All	30/10	32	1977–80
Danish/NCI	All	24/8	48	1986–91
Ohonoshi (48)	All	40/20	46	1981–86
Wagner ECOG 3589 RTOG 9201 (49)	All	25/10	32	1991–94
Arriagada IPC 85 (13)	All	24/8	300	1985–93
Laplanche IPC 88 (47)	All	24–30/8–10	211	1988–94
Gregor UKCCCR/ EORTC (46)	Limited	8–40/1–18	314	1987–95

more effectively. In the study by Work et al., among the 199 patients with limited SCLC who were randomized to initial chest irradiation versus late (18 weeks) chest irradiation, 157 received PCI. The PCI dose was 33 Gy in 11 fractions for 45 patients and 25 Gy in 11 fractions for the other 112. The 5-year incidence of CNS recurrences was 15% after 33 Gy and 23% after 25 Gy. Although the difference was not significant, there was a trend toward a dose-response relationship, which was also apparent in the meta-analysis (44). The effect of PCI on brain metastases increased with the total PCI dose when four dose groups (8 Gy, 24–25 Gy, 30 Gy, 36–40 Gy) were analyzed in the meta-analysis (trend $p = 0.02$). Hence the reduction of the relative risk of developing brain metastasis as compared to the control group was 24% in the 8-Gy group, 48% in the 24–25-Gy group, 68% in the 30-Gy group, and 73% in the 36–40-Gy group, but the effect on survival did not differ significantly according to the dose. A dose-response relationship was also found in a recent review that collected data from 12 nonrandomized studies and 12 randomized studies comparing brain relapse rates with and without PCI (53). The dose-response curve was almost linear within the 20–35-Gy dose range.

Optimal Timing?

The optimal timing for PCI in limited-stage SCLC has not been firmly determined either. Many relapses probably reflect an uninterrupted metastatic process, given the tumor doubling time in SCLC and the short life-span. Even if PCI is administered early to avoid reseeding in the brain, it has been recommended that it be administered preferably following documentation of complete remission, after 2–4 months of follow-up, but before 6 months from initiation of chemotherapy (54). Rarely is brain metastasis observed within 6 months from the initiation of chemotherapy (12). In the study by Lee et al., the overall incidence of brain metastasis was higher in patients who received PCI after five to six cycles of chemotherapy than in patients who received PCI after two to three courses of induction and maintenance chemotherapy (54). Only one trial has directly addressed the optimal timing of PCI. In the Perez study, comparing the effectiveness of concomitant versus delayed chemotherapy combined with irradiation to the mediastinum and to the brain in 70 patients with localized disease, PCI was administered either during the first week (early-PCI group) or during the seventh week (late-PCI group). There was no difference in the incidence of brain metastases (7% in both groups). However, the induction treatment would now be considered inadequate as patients in the early-PCI group received chemotherapy only in case of relapse or in case of no response to mediastinal radiotherapy (38). Therefore, no firm conclusions can be drawn from this trial.

In the study by Murray et al., a delay of 12 weeks in the initiation of chest irradiation (PCI being delivered on the nineteenth week at a dose of 25 Gy) was associated with a significant increase in the incidence of CNS recurrences. The total proportion of brain metastases in the early arm (18.1%) was significantly less than in the late-mediastinal-irradiation arm (28.1%) (55). The authors explained that although SCLC is chemosensitive, about 30–40% of patients have a chemoresistant tumor confined to the primary site. Thus, early mediastinal radiotherapy would decrease the probability of growth of a chemoresistant tumor during treatment in sites such as the brain. In the Aarhus Lung Cancer Group study, there was no difference in CNS recurrences whether chest irradiation was given at the beginning of treatment or delayed, but PCI was delivered initially, together with early mediastinal irradiation or with the first cycle of chemotherapy (44).

Recently Suwinski et al. have conducted an interesting analysis of PCI dose response according to its timing (53). They showed that the delay between the initiation of induction treatment and PCI introduces a 20-Gy threshold in the dose-response curve, which would otherwise have been linear. If only studies during which PCI was initiated less than 60 days after the first day of induction treatment are considered, there was almost a linear relationship between the dose delivered in 2-Gy fractions equivalent and the percentage reduction in total brain relapse rates within the 8–30-Gy dose range. In the studies in which PCI was initiated later, higher doses appeared to be necessary to obtain the same prophylactic effect. Effective induction treatment may arrest the development of new metastases to the brain, but it probably does not affect existing brain metastases. Thus, increasing the delay between induction treatment and PCI may increase the burden of metastatic disease to the brain.

The meta-analysis has shown that PCI influences long-term survival of patients who achieve a complete response to therapy (50). However, PCI is directly suspected in the onset of neurotoxicity in long-term survivors. Several studies have reported neurological and intellectual impairment and abnormalities on brain CT scan potentially related to PCI (56–70). However, neurological sequelae are difficult to assess in this subset of patients and there is a wide variety of interpretations regarding the etiology of the morbidity in all of these retrospective studies. This confusion has contributed largely to the controversy regarding PCI. Age, the effects of chronic cigarette abuse, possible paraneoplastic syndromes, and micrometastases may also contribute to neurotoxicity (69,71–73). Several studies, however, have reported that it was dependent on the total dose, the dose per fraction, the timing of chemotherapy (concomitant with PCI), and the type of chemotherapy.

NEUROTOXICITY

In the past, neurotoxicity was the overriding argument against PCI, particularly as no improvement was demonstrated in survival, until now. Early toxicity is minimal with the exception of transitory alopecia, although varying degrees of headache, mild nausea, and fatigue are observed. Most data on late neurotoxicity are based on small retrospective studies (57,58,61–67). There has been much concern about the possible long-term damaging effects of PCI: ataxia, seizures, and even dementia (57,59,62,63,65). Some sequelae are shown in Table 5. Lishner et al. analyzed 58 long-term survivors and found that nine of 48 patients (19%) who had had PCI had neurological complications (66). However, PCI was responsible for progressive dementia in only two patients. Laukkanen et al. evaluated 12 patients who had PCI and who were alive at 2 years for clinical, neuropsychological, and brain CT scan sequelae (65). All were capable of looking after

TABLE 5 Retrospective Studies Reporting Neurotoxicity After PCI

Author	No. of patients	Neuropsychological abnormalities		Brain CT abnormalities	
		PCI(+)	PCI(−)	PCI(+)	PCI(−)
Catane (57)	16	4/13	2/3	9/13	2/3
Cull (60)	64	25%		60%	
Craig (58)	13	4/13		13/13	
Frytak (61)	283	28/160 (17%)	0/123	Present	
Johnson (62)	20	11/17	1/3	10/17	1/3
Lee (64)	25	3/20	0/5	14/20	0/5
Laukkanen (65)	12	8/12		12/12	
Lishner (66)	58	9/48	2/10		
Twijnstra (67)	21	12/14	0/7		

themselves and none had dementia, as described in other studies. As suggested by Johnson, patients who were given high-dose induction chemotherapy while receiving cranial irradiation or large radiotherapy fractions (more than 3 Gy) were more likely to have abnormal neuropsychological tests and abnormal mental status examinations (62,63). Brain CT scan abnormalities are common: cerebral atrophy, ventricular dilatation, and periventricular and subcortical white matter changes, which seem to worsen after completion of treatment (62). These abnormalities seem to occur more frequently in patients with abnormal neuropsychological function (63).

To determine the specific causes of CNS abnormalities occurring in patients with SCLC is difficult: metastases, paraneoplastic syndromes, infections, metabolic effects, a chronic smoking habit, psychological stress, and chemotherapy may contribute to these complications (69–73). PCI has often been delivered with chemotherapeutic agents, some of which are potentially neurotoxic, either due to synergism with PCI or via independent mechanisms. Patients who receive methotrexate, nitrosoureas, and procarbazine after whole-brain irradiation are at high risk for clinical CNS neurotoxicity and for the development of periventricular white matter changes depicted on CT brain scans (64). Methotrexate is known to interact with PCI to produce necrotizing leukoencephalopathy, mineralizing microangiopathy, and cognitive impairment (74). Among 13 patients who received concomitant chemotherapy and PCI, posttreatment scans documented cerebral atrophy (100%), ventricular dilatation (70%), and decreased coefficient of absorption in the white matter (15%) (58). Van Oosterhout et al. reported neurological sequelae in a series of 51 long-term SCLC survivors who were treated with chemotherapy alone (group 1), with sequential PCI (group 2), or with concurrent chemotherapy and PCI (group 3) (75). Mental impairment, motor abnormalities, and visual complaints were observed in 24% of group 1 patients, 42% of group 2 patients, and 73% of patients in group 3. White matter abnormalities were found more frequently in group 3, whereas there was no significant difference in the analysis of brain atrophy. No significant differences existed between groups with respect to their neuropsychological status. The authors concluded that there was no statistical evidence for additional neurotoxicity of PCI. However, they did observe marked neuropsychometric differences between patients and matched controls, so cognitive impairment may be partly related to disease, but also to a deteriorated physical condition and emotional distress (75). A small prospective study has evaluated the magnitude of neuropsychological deficits thoroughly in 30 patients with SCLC who had PCI. Almost all the patients with favorable responses to combination chemotherapy had specific cognitive deficits before receiving PCI (29 of 30 patients) (69).

A recent study by Cull et al., also reported neurological and cognitive impairment in 64 long-term survivors (≥2 years) (60). The authors emphasized how difficult it was to assess these patients, but used validated scales for toxicity and the performance status; 75% of these patients were well, 11% had cognitive deficits, and 16% had ataxia that could be attributed to late neurotoxicity. These data contrast with those reported in older studies where up to 85% of patients were found to have clinically detectable neurological problems (62,64). Several studies have therefore reported neurological and intellectual impairment and abnormalities on brain CT scan potentially related to PCI, but they are all retrospective and have analyzed a small number of patients. Only two recent prospective trials have included a neurological assessment in their study (13,46). Several patients had an initial neuropsychological examination (before PCI could possibly have been administered) that was abnormal (40–60%). The results within the first years of follow-up did not show any significant difference in neuropsychological modifications between treated and untreated patients. Long-term follow-up is, however, necessary to better evaluate late neurotoxicity. PCI seems to have an adverse effect on the quality of life only in a minority of patients, provided smaller fractions are used (<3 Gy) and no concomitant chemotherapy is given.

OTHER INDICATIONS FOR PROPHYLACTIC CRANIAL IRRADIATION

Should PCI be restricted to patients in complete remission? In the study by Nugent et al., PCI seemed to effectively prevent brain metastasis in patients with liver and bone marrow metastasis even if they had a short life expectancy (3). Several studies have indicated that if the aim is to reduce the incidence of brain recurrences, then all patients should receive PCI, whereas if the aim is to improve survival, then only patients with a favorable prognosis should receive PCI (12,44).

CONCLUSION

For many years, PCI was a controversial issue with opponents arguing that none of the published reports of randomized trials on PCI showed an effect on overall survival and that the late-occurring neurological effects would clearly outweigh its benefits. However, a number of studies during the past 20 years have reported a lower incidence of brain metastases with PCI, with an accompanying decrease in the risk of associated morbidity and the social consequences of brain failure. Not only have recent trials shown that brain metastases could really be prevented and not just delayed with PCI in complete responders, but the recent meta-analysis has demonstrated that PCI leads to an absolute increase of 5.4% in the 3-year survival rate (from 15.3% observed in the control group to 20.7%). This benefit conferred on overall survival can be added to the effect of thoracic radiotherapy, which has about the same value.

Selecting the optimal dose for PCI that would lead to a further decrease in the incidence of brain metastasis with minimal toxicity is one of the challenges identified by the meta-analysis as well the ideal timing of PCI. Future trials are therefore warranted that will require cooperation worldwide. Prophylactic cranial irradiation should now be considered as part of the standard treatment of patients with SCLC.

ACKNOWLEDGMENT

The authors wish to thank Lorna de Saint-Ange for editorial assistance.

REFERENCES

1. Ihde DC, Pass HI, Glatstein E. Small cell lung cancer. In: DeVita V, Hellman S, Rosenberg SA, eds. Cancer. Principles and Practice of Oncology. 1997:911–949.
2. Komaki R, Cox JD, Whitson W. Risk of brain metastasis from small cell carcinoma of the lung related to length of survival and prophylactic irradiation. Cancer Treat Rep 1981; 65:811–814.
3. Nugent J, Bunn P, Matthews M, Ihde DC, Cohen MH, Gazdar A, Minna J. CNS metastases in small brochogenic carcinoma. Increasing frequency and changing pattern with lengthening of survival. Cancer 1979; 44:1885–1893.
4. Hansen HH. Should initial treatment of small cell carcinoma include systemic chemotherapy and brain irradiation? Cancer Chemother Rep 1973; 4:239–241.
5. Einhorn LH. The case against prophylactic cranial irradiation in limited small cell lung cancer. Semin Radiat Oncol 1995; 5:57–60.
6. Wagner H. Prophylactic cranial irradiation for patients with small cell lung cancer. An enduring controversy. Chest Surg Clin North Am 1997; 7:151–166.
7. Turrisi AT. Brain irradiation and systemic chemotherapy for small-cell lung cancer: dangerous liaisons? Editorial. J Clin Oncol 1990; 8:196–199.
8. Fleck JF, Einhorn LH, Lauer RC, Schultz SM, Miller ME. Is prophylactic cranial irradiation indicated in small-cell lung cancer? J Clin Oncol 1990; 8:209–214.
9. Sculier JP, Feld R, Evans WK, De Boer G, Sheperd FA, Payne DG, Pringle JF, Yeoh JL, Quirt IC, Curtis JE. Neurologic disorders in patients with small cell lung cancer. Cancer 1987; 60:2275–2283.
10. Hirsch FR, Paulson OB, Hansen HH. Intracranial metastases in small cell carcinoma of the lung. Correlation of clinical and autopsy findings. Cancer 1982; 50:2433–2437.
11. Bunn PA, Nugent JL, Matthews MJ. Central nervous system metastases in small cell bronchogenic carcinoma. Semin Oncol 1978; 5:314–322.
12. Rosen ST, Makuch RW, Lichter AS, Ihde DC, Matthews MJ, Minna JD, Glastein E, Bunn PA. Role of prophylactic cranial irradiation in prevention of central nervous system metastases in small cell lung cancer. Potential benefit restricted to patients with complete response. Am J Med 1983; 74:615–624.
13. Arriagada R, Le Chevalier T, Borie F, Rivière A, Chomy P, Monnet I, Tardivon A,

Viader F, Tarayre M, Benhamou S. Prophylactic cranial irradiation for patients with small cell lung cancer in complete remission. J Natl Cancer Inst 1995; 87:183–190.

14. Ball DL, Matthews JP. Prophylactic cranial irradiation: more questions than answers. Semin Radiat Oncol 1995; 5:61–68.

15. Postmus PE, Sleijfer DT, Haaxma-Reiche H. Chemotherapy for central nervous system metastases from SCLC. A review. Lung Cancer 1989; 5:254–263.

16. Kristjansen PE, Soelberg SP, Skov HM, Hansen HH. Prospective evaluation of the effect on initial brain metastases from small cell lung cancer of platinum-etoposide based induction chemotherapy followed by an alternating multidrug regimen. Ann Oncol 1993; 4:579–583.

17. Lee JS, Murphy WK, Glisson BS, et al. Primary chemotherapy of brain metastases in small-cell lung cancer. J Clin Oncol 1989; 7:916–922.

18. Kristensen CA, Kristjansen PEG, Hansen HH. Systemic chemotherapy of brain metastases from small cell lung cancer. A review. J Clin Oncol 1992; 10:1498–1502.

19. Baglan RJ, Marks JE. Comparison of symptomatic and prophylactic irradiation of brain metastases from oat cell carcinoma of the lung. Cancer 1981; 47:41–45.

20. Cox JD, Komaki R, Byhardt RW, Kun LE. Results of whole brain irradiation for metastases from small cell carcinoma of the lung. Cancer Treat Rep 1980; 64:957–961.

21. Carmichael J, Crane JM, Bunn PA, Glatstein E, Ihde DC. Results of therapeutic cranial irradiation in small cell lung cancer. Int J Radiat Oncol Biol Phys 1988; 14:455–459.

22. Hagerdorn HE, Haaxma-Reiche H, Canrimus AA, Vermey J, Smit EF, Postmus PE. Results of whole-brain radiotherapy for brain metastases of small cell lung cancer. Lung Cancer 1993; 8:293–300.

23. Eagan RT, Frytak S, Lee RE, Creagan ET, Ingle JN, Nichols WC. A case for pre-planned thoracic and prophylactic whole brain radiation therapy in limited small cell lung cancer. Cancer Clin Trials 1981; 4:261–266.

24. Shaw EG, Su JQ, Eagan RT, Jett JR, Maksymiuk AW, Deigert FA. Prophylactic cranial irradiation in complete responders with small-cell lung cancer: analysis of the Mayo Clinic and North Central Cancer Treatment Group data bases. J Clin Oncol 1994; 12:2327–2332.

25. Van Hazel GA, Scott M, Eagan RT. The effect of CNS metastases on the survival of patients with small cell lung cancer. Cancer 1983; 51:933–937.

26. Feletti R, Souhami RL, Spiro SG, Geddes DM, Tobias JS, Mantel BS, Harper PG, Trask C. Social consequences of brain or liver relapse in small cell carcinoma of the bronchus. Radiother Oncol 1985; 4:335–339.

27. Rosenman J, Choi N. Improved quality of life in patients with small cell carcinoma of the lung by elective irradiation of the brain. Int J Radiat Oncol Biol Phys 1982; 8:1041–1043.

28. Neijstrom ES, Capizzi RI, Rudnick SA. High-dose methotrexate in small cell lung cancer: lack of efficacy in preventing CNS relapse. Cancer 1981; 51:1056–1061.

29. Hardy J, Smith I, Cherryman G, Vincent M, Judson I, Perren T, Williams M. The value of computed tomographic (CT) scan surveillance in the detection and management of brain metastases in patients with small cell cancer. Br J Cancer 1990; 62:684–686.

30. Moore TN, Livingstone R, Heilbrun L. The effectiveness of prophylactic brain irradiation in small cell carcinoma of the lung. Cancer 1978; 41:2149–2153.

31. Le Chevalier T, Arriagada R, Dewar JA, Ruffié P, Martin M. Prophylactic cranial irradiation in small cell lung cancer. Lancet 1985; 8430:692–693.

32. Beiler DD, Kane RC, Bernath AM, Cashdollar MR. Low dose elective brain irradiation in small cell carcinoma of the lung. Int J Radiat Oncol Biol Phys 1979; 5:941–945.

33. Cox JD, Petrovich Z, Paig C, Stanley K. Prophylactic cranial irradiation in patients with inoperable carcinoma of the lung. Preliminary report of a cooperative trial. Cancer 1978; 42:1135–1140.

34. Hansen HH, Dombernowsky P, Hirsch FR, Hansen M, Rygard J. Prophylactic irradiation in bronchogenic small cell anaplastic carcinoma. A comparative trial of localized versus extensive radiotherapy including prophylactic brain irradiation in patients receiving combination chemotherapy. Cancer 1980; 46:279–284.

35. Jackson DV, Richards F, Cooper MR, Feree C, Muss HB, White DR, Spurr CL. Prophylactic cranial irradiation in small cell carcinoma of the lung. A randomized study. JAMA 1983; 237:2730–2733.

36. Katsenis AT, Karpasitis N, Giannakakis D, Maragoudakis N, Kiparissiadis P. Elective brain irradiation in patients with small cell carcinoma of the lung: a preliminary report. Lung Cancer Int Congress Series. 558. Amsterdam: Excerpta Medica 1982: 277–284.

37. Niiranen A, Holsti P, Salmo M. Treatment of small cell lung cancer. Two-drug vs four-drug chemotherapy and loco-regional irradiation with or without prophylactic cranial irradiation. Acta Oncol 1989; 28:501–505.

38. Perez CA, Krauss S, Bartolucci AA, Durant JR, Lowenbraun S, Salter MM, Storadoli J, Kellermeyer R, Comas F for the Southeastern Cancer Study Group. Thoracic and elective brain irradiation with concomitant or delayed multiagent chemotherapy in the treatment of localized small cell carcinoma of the lung. Cancer 1981; 47:2407–2413.

39. Seydel HG, Creech R, Pagano M, Salazar O, Rubin P, Concannon J, Carbone P, Mohuiddin M, Perez C, Matthews M. Prophylactic versus no brain irradiation in regional small cell lung carcinoma. Am J Clin Oncol 1985; 8:218–223.

40. Aroney RS, Aisner J, Wesley MN, Whitacre MY, Van Echo DA, Slaeson RG, Wiernik PH. Value of prophylactic cranial irradiation given at complete remission in small cell lung carcinoma. Cancer Treat Rep 1983; 67:675–682.

41. Rosenstein M, Armstrong J, Kris M, Kris M, Shank B, Scher H, Fass D, Harrison L, Fuks Z, Leibel S. A reappraisal of the role of prophylactic cranial irradiation in limited small cell lung cancer. Int J Radiat Oncol Biol Phys 1992; 24:43–48.

42. Rubenstein JH, Dosoretz DE, Katin MJ, Blitzer PH, Salenius SA, Floody PA, Harwin WN, Teufel TE, Raymond MG, Reeves JA. Low doses of prophylactic cranial irradiation effective in limited stage small cell carcinoma of the lung. Int J Radiat Oncol Biol Phys 1995; 33:329–337.

43. Liengswangwong V, Bonner JA, Shaw EG, Foote RL, Frytak S, Richardson RL, Creagan ET, Eagan RT, Su JQ. Prophylactic cranial irradiation in limited-stage small cell lung cancer. Cancer 1995; 75:1302–1309.

44. Work E, Bentzen SM, Nielsen OM, Fode K, Michalski W, Palshof T. Prophylactic

cranial irradiation in limited stage small cell lung cancer: survival benefit in patients with favourable characteristics. Eur J Cancer 1996; 32A:772–778.

45. Pedersen AG, Kristjansen PE, Hansen HH. Prophylactic cranial irradiation and small cell lung cancer. Cancer Treat Rev 1988; 15:85–103.

46. Gregor A, Cull A, Stephens RJ, Kirkpatrick JA, Yarnold JR, Girling DJ, Macbeth FR, Stout R, Machin D. Prophylactic cranial irradiation is indicated following complete response to induction therapy in small cell lung cancer: results of a multicentre randomised trial. Eur J Cancer 1997; 33:1752–1758.

47. Laplanche A, Monnet I, Santos-Miranda JA, Bardet E, Le Péchoux C, Tarayre M, Arriagada R. Controlled clinical trial of prophylactic cranial irradiation for patients with small-cell lung cancer in complete remission. Lung Cancer 1998; 21: 193–201.

48. Ohnoshi T, Ueoka H, Kawahara S, Kiura K, Kamei H, Hiraki Y, Segawa Y, Hiraki S, Kimura I. Comparative study of prophylactic cranial irradiation in patients with small cell lung cancer achieving a complete response: a long-term follow-up result. Lung Cancer 1993; 10:47–54.

49. Wagner HJ, Kim K, Turrisi A, Jiroutek M, Shaw EG, Einhorn LH, Eisert D, Johnson D. A randomized phase III study of prophylactic cranial irradiation vs observation in patients with small cell lung cancer achieving a complete response: final report of an incomplete trial by the ECOG and RTOG. Proc Am Soc Clin Oncol 1996; 15:376.

50. Aupérin A, Arriagada R, Pignon JP, Le Péchoux C, Gregor A, Stephens RJ, Kristjansen PE, Johnson BE, Ueoka H, Wagner H, Aisner J. Prophylactic cranial irradiation for patients with small-cell lung cancer in complete remission. N Engl J Med 1999; 341(7):476–484.

51. Brewster AE, Hopwood P, Stout R, Burt PA, Thatcher N. Single fraction prophylactic cranial irradiation for small cell carcinoma of the lung. Radiother Oncol 1995; 34:132–136.

52. Withers HR, Peters LJ, Taylor JMG. Dose-response relationship for radiation therapy for subclinical disease. Int J Radiat Oncol Biol Phys 1995; 31:353–359.

53. Suwinski R, Lee SP, Withers HR. Dose-response relationship for prophylactic cranial irradiation in small cell lung cancer. Int J Radiat Oncol Biol Phys 1998; 40: 797–806.

54. Lee JS, Umsawasdi T, Barkley HT, Murphy WK, Welch S, Valdivieso M. Timing of elective brain irradiation: a critical factor for brain metastasis-free survival in small cell lung cancer. Int J Radiat Oncol Biol Phys 1987; 13:697–704.

55. Murray N, Coy P, Pater JL, Hodson I, Arnold A, Zee BC, Payne D, Kostashuk EC, Evans WK, Dixon P, Sadura A, Feld R, Levitt M, Wierzbicki J, Ayoub J, Maroun JA, Wilson KS for the National Cancer Institute of Canada Clinical Trials Group. Importance of timing for thoracic irradiation in the combined modality treatment of limited-stage small-cell lung cancer. J Clin Oncol 1993; 11:336–344.

56. Bleehen NM, Bunn PA, Cox JD, Dombernowsky P, Fox RM, Host H, Joss R, White JE, Wittes RE. Role of radiation therapy in small cell anaplastic carcinoma of the lung. Cancer Treat Rep 1983; 67:11–19.

57. Catane R, Schwade JG, Yarr I, Lichter AS, Tepper JE, Dunnick NR, Brody L, Brereton HD, Cohen M, Glatstein E. Follow-up and neurological evaluation in patients

with small cell lung carcinoma treated with prophylactic cranial irradiation and chemotherapy. Int J Radiat Oncol Biol Phys 1981; 7:105–109.

58. Craig J, Jackson D, Moody D, Cruz JM, Pope EK, Powell BL, Spurr CL, Capizzi RL. Prospective evaluation of changes in computerized cranial tomography (CCT) in patients with small cell carcinoma (SCLC) treated with chemotherapy and cranial irradiation. J Clin Oncol 1984; 2:1151–1156.

59. Crossen JR, Garwood D, Glatstein E, Neuwelt EA. Neurobehavioral sequelae of cranial irradiation in adults: a review of radiation-induced encephalopathy. J Clin Oncol 1994; 12:627–642.

60. Cull A, Gregor A, Hopwood P, Macbeth F, Karnicka-Mlodkowska H, Thatcher N, Burt P, Stout R, Stepniseska K, Stewart M. Neurological and cognitive impairment in long-term survivors of small cell lung cancer. Eur J Cancer 1994; 8:1067–1074.

61. Frytak S, Shaw JN, O'Neill BP, Lee RE, Eagan RT, Shaw EG, Richardson RL, Coles DT, Jett JR. Leukoencephalopathy in small cell lung cancer patients receiving prophylactic cranial irradiation. Am J Clin Oncol 1989; 12:27–33.

62. Johnson BE, Becker B, Goff WB, Patronas N, Krehbel MA, Makuch RW, McKenna G, Glastein E, Ihde DC. Neurologic, neuropsychologic, and computed cranial tomography scan abnormalities in 2- to 10-year survivors of small cell lung cancer. J Clin Oncol 1985; 3:1659–1667.

63. Johnson BE, Patronas N, Hayes W, Grayson J, Becker B, Gnepp D, Rowland J, Anderson A, Glastein E, Ihde DC, Frank JA. Neurologic, computed cranial tomographic, and magnetic resonance imaging abnormalities in patients with small cell lung cancer: further follow-up to 6- to 13-year survivors. J Clin Oncol 1990; 8:48–56.

64. Lee JS, Umsawasdi T, Lee YY, Barkley HT, Murphy WK, Welch S, Valdivieso M. Neurotoxicity in long-term survivors of small cell lung cancer. Int J Radiat Oncol Biol Phys 1986; 12:313–321.

65. Laukkanen E, Klonoff H, Allan B, Graeb D, Murray N. The role of prophylactic brain irradiation in limited stage small cell lung cancer: clinical, neuropsychologic, and CT sequelae. Int J Radiat Oncol Biol Phys 1988; 14:1109–1117.

66. Lishner M, Feld R, Payne DG, Sagman U, Sculier JP, Pringle JF, Yeoh JL, Evans WK, Sheperd FA, Maki E. Late neurological complications after prophylactic cranial irradiation in patients with small-cell lung cancer: the Toronto experience. J Clin Oncol 1990; 8:215–221.

67. Twijnstra A, Boon PJ, Lormans ACM, Ten Velde GPN. Neurotoxicity of prophylactic cranial irradiation in patients with small cell carcinoma of the lung. Eur J Cancer Clin Oncol 1987; 23:983–986.

68. Constine LS, Konski A, Ekholm S, McDonald S, Rubin P. Adverse effects of brain irradiation correlated with MR and CT imaging. Int J Radiat Oncol Biol Phys 1988; 15:319–330.

69. Komaki R, Meyers CA, Shin DM, Garden AS, Byrne K, Nickens JA, Cox JD. Evaluation of cognitive function in patients with limited small cell lung cancer prior to and shortly following prophylactic cranial irradiation. Int J Radiat Oncol Biol Phys 1995; 33:179–182.

70. Van Oosterhout AGM, van de Pol M, ten Velde GPM, Twijnstra A. Neurologic

disorders in 203 consecutive patients with small cell lung cancer. Results of a longitudinal study. Cancer 1996; 77:1434–1441.

71. Erlington GM, Murray NM, Spiro SG, Newsom-Davis J. Neurological paraneoplastic syndromes in patients with small cell lung cancer. A prospective survey of 150 patients. J Neurol Neurosurg Psychiatry 1991; 54:764–767.

72. Hill R. Residual effects of cigarette smoking on cognitive performance in normal aging. Psychol Aging 1989; 4:251–254.

73. Komaki R. Prophylactic cranial irradiation for small cell carcinoma of the lung. Cancer Treat Symp 1985; 2:35–39.

74. Bleyer W, Griffin T. White matter necrosis, mineralizing microangiopathy, and intellectual abilities in survivors of childhood leukaemia: associations with central nervous system irradiation and methotrexate therapy. In: Gilbert HA, Kagan AR, eds. Radiation Damage to the Nervous System. New York: Raven Press, 1980:155–174.

75. Van Oosterhout AG, Ganzevles PG, Wilmink JT, De Geus BW, Van Vonderen RG, Twijnstra A. Sequelae in long-term survivors of small cell lung cancer. Int J Radiat Oncol Biol Phys 1996; 34:1037–1044.

6

The Role of Prophylactic Cranial Irradiation: Con

Alan Sandler
Vanderbilt University, Nashville, Tennessee

INTRODUCTION

Lung cancer has become the leading cause of cancer death in the United States and is a leading cause of cancer-related mortality throughout the world. Small cell lung cancer (SCLC) accounts for approximately 20% of all cases of lung cancer. Staging for SCLC divides patients into two groups. The first group is limited-stage patients (LS), defined as patients with disease confined to the ipsilateral chest, including supraclavicular or scalene lymph nodes, without the presence of a malignant pleural effusion. With cisplatin-based chemotherapy and concurrent radiotherapy, these patients can expect a median survival of 20–22 months and a 5-year survival of 20–25%. The second group is those patients with disease outside the chest, and/or a malignant pleural effusion, who are staged as extensive SCLC. These patients are considered incurable and make up the majority of patients with SCLC, representing approximately two-thirds of patients diagnosed with SCLC. Combination chemotherapy has improved median survival from several weeks for the untreated patient to a median survival of approximately 9 months.

Despite improvements in the treatment of SCLC, the vast majority of patients with SCLC will succumb to their disease. As described earlier, SCLC is a disease that has a high degree of systemic dissemination, both at presentation and at subsequent relapse. To postulate that a local prophylactic therapy, such as cranial irradiation, is effective in improving survival, several theories must be true:

1. Evidence that successful eradication of systemic micrometastatic disease has been attained
2. Evidence that isolated central nervous system (CNS) relapse plays a significant role in this setting (i.e., is it merely a "forme fruste" of ultimate systemic failures)
3. Evidence that cranial irradiation can provide successful "sterilization" of the CNS—at least in the micrometastatic setting (i.e., as prophylactic therapy)
4. Evidence that the successful systemic chemotherapy has not already provided CNS sterilization
5. Evidence that prophylactic CNS radiotherapy does not result in significant toxicity, both short-term and long-term
6. Evidence for a survival advantage for prophylactic cranial irradiation in patients with SCLC

I will attempt to address these issues with respect to the role of prophylactic cranial irradiation (PCI) in SCLC. Although some data may be compelling favoring PCI, there are still issues that are not fully addressed.

EVIDENCE FOR SUCCESSFUL ERADICATION OF SYSTEMIC MICROMETASTATIC DISEASE

Perhaps the best results to date in the literature for limited-stage SCLC come from a recently published ECOG/RTOG/SWOG trial (1). The study randomized 419 patients with limited SCLC to receive cisplatin and etoposide with either once-daily thoracic radiation (45 Gy/25 fractions/5 weeks) or twice-daily fractionation (45 Gy/30 fractions/3 weeks). In both arms, thoracic radiotherapy was given concurrently with chemotherapy commencing with the first day of cycle 1 and prophylactic cranial radiation was administered to all patients with a complete response to chemoradiation. The twice-daily radiotherapy arm significantly improved survival when compared with the once-daily arm ($p = 0.04$). With a median follow-up of almost 8 years, the median survival was 23 months for the twice-daily radiotherapy and 19 months for the once-daily arm. The survival rates were 26% at 5 years for the twice-daily arm compared to 16 at 5 years for the once-daily arm. This survival advantage appeared related to improved local failure rates in the twice-daily thoracic radiotherapy arm. Local failure rate was 52%

in the once-daily arm and 36% in the twice-daily arm ($p = 0.06$). The rate of simultaneous local and distant failure was also significantly different in the once-daily arm and 6% in the twice-daily arm, $p = 0.01$. The results of this trial provide evidence that systemic chemotherapy and thoracic irradiation can successfully eliminate micrometastases resulting in long-term survival of 20–25%. Even with state-of-the-art therapy, however, the vast majority (75%) of patients unfortunately succumb to this disease and thus probably do not derive any long-term survival advantage with the addition of PCI.

EVIDENCE THAT ISOLATED CNS RELAPSE PLAYS A SIGNIFICANT ROLE IN THIS SETTING (OR IS IT MERELY A "FORME FRUSTE" OF ULTIMATE SYSTEMIC FAILURE?)

To surmise that PCI can affect survival, there must be evidence that a significant number of patients with SCLC who achieve a complete remission ultimately relapse in the CNS alone.

There is an inherent difficulty in quantifying the incidence of isolated CNS relapse. Patients presenting with symptomatic brain metastases undergo variable degrees of further evaluation. Those patients undergoing more aggressive forms of evaluation (i.e., CT scans and bone scans) will most likely manifest other sites of systemic failure compared to those patients undergoing fewer diagnostic tests. This information is not often specifically reported in the literature and, as such, the available data would appear to reflect this lack of consistency. Ball and Matthews (2) reviewed the data for 17 clinical trials involving 1202 patients who did not receive PCI. There were 655 patients for whom data describing the crude incidence of cerebral relapse as a first or sole site of progression was available. Of these 655 patients, brain metastases occurred in 166 patients (25%). However, when reported as an isolated site of progression, this number decreased to 14%. Firsch et al. (3) reported the results of a large autopsy series in which only 3% of patients with SCLC manifested CNS as the sole site of relapse.

It would appear that the incidence of isolated brain metastases is ≤15% in patients not receiving PCI. Ultimately, based on the effectiveness of PCI, the maximum survival benefit that PCI could achieve would be a fraction of that number.

EVIDENCE THAT PCI CAN PROVIDE SUCCESSFUL "STERILIZATION" OF THE CNS

Having established that there is a small but finite subset of patients who may relapse with isolated CNS metastases, the next logical question is whether cranial irradiation is effective in eradicating micrometastatic disease. Table 1 lists the

TABLE 1 Randomized Trials of PCI in SCLC Achieving a Complete Response to Induction Chemotherapy or Chemoradiation

Author	Patients	CNS failure		Median survival		
		PCI	No PCI	PCI	No PCI	p value
Aroney (4)	32	0	27%	NR	NR	NR
Ohonoshi (5)	46	22%	52%	21 mo	15 mo	0.097
Wagner (6)	32	18%	53%	15.3	8.8	0.249
Gregor (7)	314	Hazard ratio 0.41		NR	NR	NR
Laplanche (8)	211	44% @ 4 yr	51% @ 4 yr	22% @ 4 yr	16% @ 4 yr	0.25
Arriagada (9)	300	40% @ 2 yr	67% @ 2 yr	29% @ 2 yr	21.5% @ 2 yr	0.14

results of randomized trials of PCI that included only patients in complete remission. In all trials, the incidence of CNS relapse is lower in the PCI arm thus providing evidence that PCI can affect the subsequent development of overt CNS metastases (~20–60% absolute reduction in development of CNS metastases).

EVIDENCE THAT PROPHYLACTIC CNS RADIOTHERAPY DOES NOT RESULT IN SIGNIFICANT TOXICITY, EITHER SHORT-TERM OR LONG-TERM

The predominant deleterious effects of cranial radiotherapy typically occur from 9 to 12 months after treatment, but may occur years later (10,11). The most serious of these events is brain necrosis resulting from high doses of radiation therapy. More important in the setting of PCI is a potential decrease in a patient's functional capability following treatment. These effects, seen in long-term follow-up, are manifested by memory impairment, cognitive deficits, and personality changes. Subtle motor effects may occur as well. Late effects on cognitive function are obviously more subtle than the dramatic effects of overt brain necrosis and thus more difficult to document and/or discriminate from other organic processes. These effects may or may not be associated with radiographic findings (12,13). Another problem is that the majority of the data has been generated from retrospective analyses (14,15).

Evaluating a patient with SCLC for potentially subtle cognitive deficits is complicated by a number of potential mitigating factors: (1) Age—The median age of a patient with SCLC is approximately 65 years. These patients may be undergoing subtle personality and psychological changes from aging or other unrelated processes such as Alzheimer's disease. (2) Tobacco use—It is possible that the long-term hypoxemia associated with smoking may contribute to subtle cognitive deficits. (3) Other illnesses—Patients with SCLC typically have other tobacco-related illnesses that may contribute, i.e., chronic obstructive lung disease, coronary artery disease with resultant cardiopulmonary impairment. Clearly, prospective, randomized trials evaluating patient's cognitive function pre- and postradiotherapy are needed.

Fortunately, over the past few years there have been several illustrative trials. Ahles et al. reported on the findings of the Cancer and Leukemia Group B trial 8534 (16). This trial randomized 347 patients with limited SCLC to three cycles of ACE chemotherapy (doxorubicin, cyclophosphamide, and etoposide). This was followed by two cycles of PCE chemotherapy (cisplatin, cyclophosphamide, and etoposide). Concurrent with PCE, all patients received thoracic radiotherapy (RT) and PCI. Following PCE and RT, patients went on to receive an additional three cycles of ACE, but this was discontinued after 179 patients were entered, secondary to excessive pulmonary toxicity. Patients were randomized to receive warfarin or no warfarin starting on day 1 of the induction chemotherapy. Of the 347 patients entered on study, 295 (85%) patients were recruited for the psychological study at baseline, and 224 (65%) and 177 (51%) patients, respectively, completed the pre-RT and post-RT assessments. This study employed the POMS (Profile of Mood States) and Trail Making B Test (Trails B) as psychological and neuropsychological assessment tools (17,18). The authors noted stable POMS scores pre- and post-RT (stable emotional pattern) but decreased Trails B scores (cognitive function), suggesting that the treatment had a negative impact on cognitive function. The results of this study are confounded by at least two factors: (1) The evaluation was only 1 month post-RT, and (2) the patients received chemotherapy and concurrent thoracic RT at the time of their PCI. Another important message from this trial, which emphasizes the need for pre- and post-PCI evaluations, is that all patients evaluated pre-PCI performed in the 25th percentile, when compared with age-matched norms. In other words, three-fourths of the general population in this age range performed better than patients in the SCLC study. Komaki et al. (19) reported on a small study of 30 patients with limited SCLC who underwent neuropsychological testing pre- and post-PCI. They also noted baseline cognitive deficits. Eleven patients underwent testing 6–20 months after PCI. No significant differences were noted.

Only two trials evaluating the role of PCI have prospectively evaluated the potential neurotoxicity associated with the effects of PCI. Arriagada et al. (9) reported on a prospective trial of 300 patients with SCLC in complete remission after induction therapy. In this trial, patients underwent neuropsychological examination and computerized tomography scan of the brain at the time of randomization and at 6, 18, 30, and 48 months. A total of 294 patients were eligible for study and of these, 65 patients (34 patients in the control group and 31 patients in the PCI group) were not fully evaluable for neurotoxicity (no baseline neuropsychological evaluation or the development of brain metastases within 1 month of randomization). Of the 229 patients (115 patients in the control arm and 114 in the PCI arm) who underwent initial neuropsychological testing, only 41% (50 patients/control group and 44 patients/PCI group) had a normal baseline neuropsychological evaluation. Patients were evaluated for cognitive (orientation, memory, judgment, language, and praxis), sensory, mood, walking, cerebellar, and cranial nerve functions; and tendon reflexes. The testing was performed by the same neurologist at each treatment site. Within the first 5 years of follow-up, there was no statistical difference in the 2-year cumulative incidence of abnormalities in any of these parameters. Gregor et al. (7) reported on a large European randomized trial of 314 patients with LS-SCLC in complete remission randomized to PCI at variable doses determined by the individual investigator versus observation. Prospective neuropsychometric and quality-of-life assessments were part of this trial in selected institutions and involved 136 patients (43%). In this trial too, the large majority of patients (78%) undergoing evaluation evidenced some neuropsychological deficit prior to PCI. Patients who underwent repeat testing at 6 and 12 months revealed some new impairments. No evidence of sustained deterioration over time was noted and no statistically significant difference was noted between the two groups. The authors commented on the fact that the number of patients undergoing prospective evaluation was small and that follow-up was limited.

One final word of caution regarding the potential neurotoxicity of PCI must be raised. Looper et al. (20) reported on a series of 120 patients with SCLC treated with CAV-based (cyclophosphamide, doxorubicin, and vincristine) chemotherapy with or without thoracic radiotherapy, all of whom received PCI. The authors noted that of 18 patients (15%) alive and disease-free at ≥ 3 years, 14 patients (78%) experienced significant neurological sequelae felt to be related to PCI. These complications occurred an average of 4–7 years after completing PCI. Indeed, some investigators have suggested that the neurocognitive sequelae of RT may be underestimated in long-term survivors (11).

EVIDENCE FOR A SURVIVAL ADVANTAGE FOR PCI IN PATIENTS WITH SCLC

As discussed earlier, given the relatively low incidence of patients with isolated CNS failures, one can expect a similar small difference in survival when comparing patients treated with PCI to those patients undergoing observation. Table 2 shows the results of recent randomized trials in patients achieving a complete remission with induction therapy. None of these randomized trials demonstrated a survival advantage to PCI. As most of these trials were relatively small, however, a meta-analysis was conducted by the Prophylactic Cranial Irradiation Overview Collaborative Group. This meta-analysis included 987 patients with SCLC in complete remission enrolled in seven randomized trials assessing the role of prophylactic irradiation (21) (Table 2).

The results of this analysis revealed a statistically significant, albeit small, improvement in the relative risk of death favoring PCI (RR = 0.84, $p = 0.01$). This difference resulted in a 5.4% absolute increase in survival at 3 years from 15.3% to 20.7%. The authors again noted a decrease in cumulative incidence of brain metastases (relative risk of 0.46, $p < 0.001$). The authors commented on the fact that higher doses of PCI led to relatively greater decreases in the risk of brain metastases (8 Gy vs. 24–25 Gy vs. 30 Gy vs. 36 Gy, $p = 0.02$) but no additional impact on survival (Table 3).

TABLE 2 Randomized Phase III Trials Included in Meta-Analysis

Trial	Enrollment period	No. of patients	PCI dose/fractions	Survival advantage?	Evaluation for cognitive deficits
UMCC (4)	1977–80	29	30 Gy/10	No	No
Okayama (5)	1981–86	46	40 Gy/20	No	No
PCI-85 (9)	1985–93	300	24 Gy/8	No	Yes
Danish-NCI (21)	1985–91	55	24 Gy/8	No	No
UKCCCR-EORTC (7)	1987–95	314	8–36 Gy/1–18[a]	No	Yes
PCI-88 (8)	1988–94	211	24 Gy/8	No	No
ECOG-RTOG (6)	1991–94	32	25 Gy/10	No	No

[a]Initially designed with three treatment groups (no PCI, 24 Gy/12, and 36 Gy/18; subsequently changed to no PCI versus PCI at variable doses).

TABLE 3   Meta-analysis of Randomized Phase III Trials of PCI

	No. of patients				Rate in control group (%)	Absolute benefit at 3 yr (%)
	PCI	No PCI	Hazard ratio	p value		
Survival	526	461	0.84	0.01	15.3	+5.4
Cumulative rate of brain metastases	524	457	0.46	<0.0001	58.6	−25.3
DFS	526	461	0.75	<0.0001	13.5	+8.8
Cumulative rate of other metastases	325	332	0.89	0.37	45.6	−3.8

SUMMARY

It would appear that while several of the issues surrounding the use of PCI have been addressed, others remain unanswered. Although there appears to be a small percentage of patients with limited SCLC who are cured with chemotherapy and thoracic irradiation and remain at risk for relapse with isolated brain metastases, we are not able, at this time, to identify these patients upfront. Thus, for every 20 patients who receive PCI, only one benefits. Should we perhaps focus our priorities elsewhere, such as on other systemic issues? The potential benefit in survival from PCI is so small (~5%) that a meta-analysis became necessary to identify any impact at all. Although meta-analyses have achieved recent popularity, not all statisticians are convinced of their accuracy (22,23). There are many other unanswered questions. If PCI is to be utilized, what is the optimal dose, schedule, and timing of PCI? Is there any role in patients with extensive disease in complete response? Most importantly, however, is the unresolved issue of the full extent of CNS toxicity. Scant prospective data are currently available and continued follow-up is warranted. This information is critical before we can accurately assess the benefit/risk ratio of PCI. While, based on the current information, PCI should be offered at this time as part of the therapeutic regimen in patients with LS-SCLC who achieve a good response to chemoradiation, it is critical that the full implications of this strategy be reassessed over time as more information regarding long-term neurotoxicity becomes available.

REFERENCES

1.   Turrisi AT III, Kim K, Blum R, et al. Twice-daily compared with once-daily thoracic radiotherapy in limited small-cell lung cancer treated concurrently with cisplatin and etoposide. N Engl J Med 1999; 340:265–271.

2. Ball DL, Matthews JP. Prophylactic cranial irradiation: more questions than answers. Semin Radiat Oncol 1995; 5:61–68.
3. Firsch FR, Paulson OB, Hansen HH, et al. Intracranial metastases in small cell carcinoma of the lung. Correlation of clinical and autopsy findings. Cancer 1982; 50: 2433–2437.
4. Aroney RS, Aisner J, Wesley MN, Whitacre MY, Van Echo DA, Slaeson RG, Wiernik PH. Value of prophylactic cranial irradiation given at complete remission in small cell lung carcinoma. Cancer Treat Rep 1983; 67:675–682.
5. Ohnoshi T, Ueoka H, Kawahara S, Kiura K, Kamei H, Hiraki Y, Segawa Y, Hiraki S, Kimura I. Comparative study of prophylactic cranial irradiation in patients with small cell lung cancer achieving a complete response: a long-term follow-up result. Lung Cancer 1993; 10:47–54.
6. Wagner H. Prophylactic cranial irradiation for patients with small cell lung cancer. An enduring controversy. Chest Surg Clin North Am 1997; 31:353–359.
7. Gregor A, Cull A, Stephens RJ, Kirkpatrick JA, Yarnold JR, Girling DJ, Macbeth FR, Stout R, Machin D. Prophylactic cranial irradiation is indicated following complete response to induction therapy in small cell lung cancer: Results of a multicentre randomised trial. Eur J Cancer 1997; 33:1752–1758.
8. Laplanche A, Monnet I, Santos-Miranda JA, Bardet E, Le Pechoux C, Tarayre M, Arriagada R. Controlled clinical trial of prophylactic cranial irradiation for patients with small-cell lung cancer in complete remission. Lung Cancer 1998; 21:193–201.
9. Arriagada R, Le Chevalier T, Boric F, et al. Prophylactic cranial irradiation for patients with small cell lung cancer in complete remission. J Natl Cancer Inst 1995; 87:183–190.
10. Mahler P, Griffin B, Geyer JR, et al. Chemoradiotherapy interactions and the blood-brain barrier. In: Nieuwalt EA, ed. Implications of the Blood-Brain Barrier and Its Manipulation. New York: Plenum Press, 1989:373–387.
11. Crossen JR, Garwood D, Glatstein E., et al. Neurobehavioral sequelae of cranial irradiation in adults: a review of radiation-induced encephalopathy. J Chin Oncol 1994; 12:627–642.
12. Johnson BE, Becker B, Goff WB, Patronas N, Krehbel MA, Makuch RW, McKenna G, Glatstein E, Ihde DC. Neurologic, neuropsychologic, and computed cranial tomography scan abnormalities in 2- to 10-year survivors of small cell lung cancer. J Clin Oncol 1985; 3:1659–1667.
13. Johnson BE, Patrons N, Hayes W, Grayson J, Becker B, Gnepp D, Rowland J, Anderson A, Glatstein E, Ihde DC, Frank JA. Neurologic, computed cranial tomographic, and magnetic resonance imaging abnormalities in patients with small cell lung cancer: further follow-up to 6- to 13-year survivors. J Clin Oncol 1990; 8:48–56.
14. Catane R, Schwade JG, Yarr I, Lichter AS, Tepper JE, Dunnick NR, Brody L, Brereton HD, Cohen M, Glatstein E. Follow-up and neurological evaluation in patients with small cell lung carcinoma treated with prophylactic cranial irradiation and chemotherapy. Int J Radiat Oncol Biol Phys 1981; 7:105–109.
15. Lee JS, Umsawasdi T, Lee YY, Barkley HT, Murphy WK, Welch S, Valdivieso M. Neurotoxicity in long-term survivors of small cell lung cancer. Int J Radiat Oncol Biol Phys 1986; 12:313–321.

16. Ahles TA, Silberfarb PM, Herndon J II, et al. Psychologic and neuropsychologic functioning of patients with limited small-cell lung cancer treated with chemotherapy and radiation therapy with or without warfarin: a study by the Cancer and Leukemia Group B. J Clin Oncol 1998; 16:1954–1960.

17. McNair DM, Lorr M, Droppleman LF. Profile of Mood States. San Diego, CA: Educational and Testing Service, 1971.

18. Reitan RM, Davison LA. Clinical Neuropsychology: Current Status and Applications. New York: Wiley, 1974.

19. Komaki R, Meyers CA, Shin DM, Garden AS, Byrne K, Nickens KJA, Cox JD. Evaluation of cognitive function in patients with limited small cell lung cancer prior to and shortly following prophylactic cranial irradiation. Int J Radiat Oncol Biol Phys 1995; 33:179–182.

20. Looper JD, Einhorn LH, Garcia SA, et al. Severe neurological problems following successful therapy for small cell lung cancer. Proc ASCO 1984; 3:31.

21. Auperin A, Arriagada R, Pignon JP, Le Pechoux C, Gregor A, Stephens R, Kristjansen PE, Johnson BE, Ueoka H, Wagner H, Aisner J. Prophylactic cranial irradiation for patients with small-cell lung cancer in complete remission. Prophylactic Cranial Irradiation Overview Collaborative Group. N Engl J Med 1999; 341:476–484.

22. LeLorier J, Gregore G, Benhaddad A, et al. Discrepancies between meta-analyses and subsequent large randomized, controlled trials. N Engl J Med 1997; 337:536–542.

23. Bailar JC. The promise and problems of meta-analysis. N Engl J Med 1997; 337:559–561.

7

Dose Intensification of Chemotherapy in SCLC: Pro

Anthony Elias
Harvard Medical School and Dana-Farber Cancer Institute,
Boston, Massachusetts

RATIONALE FOR DOSE-INTENSIVE THERAPY IN SCLC

The principles of dose and combination therapy are strongly supported by preclinical and clinical evidence. Increased dose intensity of certain chemotherapeutic agents can yield greater cytotoxicity against the overall tumor cell population and is more likely to kill drug-resistant tumor cells. Which agents are chosen depends on pharmacology/mode of action and schedule/dose relationships to cytotoxicity. For these reasons, alkylating agents usually form the backbone of most high-dose regimens since near-log-linear dose-response relationships are consistently demonstrated for the alkylating agents and radiation in preclinical in vitro and in vivo experiments (1–4).

Clinical success requires eradication of all clonogenic tumor if solely cytotoxic strategies are employed. The kinetics of tumor regrowth (Gompertzian models) suggest that near-eradication might yield fairly similar clinical outcomes compared with more modest antitumoral effects delivered over longer periods. The ability to detect clinical benefits from high-dose therapy would be greatest in clinical settings with high risk of systemic relapse but low tumor burden. Increased cytotoxicity may be irrelevant if tumor burden is great. Chemosensitivity, particularly the shape of the dose-response relationship for the drug-resistant tumor cell subpopulations, is also critical. Dose escalation of agents inactive against a particular disease is not likely to prove a fruitful strategy in generating significant clinical success.

Many established chemotherapeutic agents including etoposide or teniposide, cisplatin or carboplatin, ifosfamide, cyclophosphamide, vincristine, and doxorubicin have major activity against small cell lung cancer (SCLC). Many of these agents, particularly the oxazaphosphorines, nitrosoureas, and the platinums, have strong preclinical rationales for dose escalation. There is also extensive clinical evidence to support a dose-response relationship with these agents against a variety of tumor types including SCLC. The major controversy surrounding dose-intensive therapy is whether an increase in tumor response can translate into prolonged survival and whether this benefit can outweigh the enhanced toxicities generated. Methods to deliver dose-intensive therapy include shortening cycle length, increasing dose and/or number of agents over multiple cycles, or increasing dose as consolidation of clinical response.

On review of the phase II trials evaluating high-dose therapy with hematopoietic cellular support, outcomes are frequently better than those reported by conventional dose approaches. However, patient selection (low patient comorbidity) and staging biases clearly contribute to these results. Even if randomized data support the use of high-dose therapy, one may still ask whether the benefit is generalizable to the entire population of patients with that disease and/or stage of disease, or if the treatment strategy is applicable only for the most physiologically fit. In most cases, if the treatment is deemed worthwhile, technological advances in supportive therapy will develop to increase feasibility.

A further question concerning dose-intensive strategies is whether they can be combined with other modalities. Assuming dose-intensive therapy improves overall response and complete response rates, this approach may serve as a suitable foundation to generate minimal residual tumor burdens and potentially render other therapeutic strategies more effective. The use of combinations of treatment modalities becomes more compelling given the generic properties of tumors, namely plasticity, adaptability, and heterogeneity.

CONVENTIONAL-DOSE THERAPY IN SCLC

Approximately 15–20% of all bronchogenic carcinomas, SCLC are the fourth leading cause of death from cancer in both men and women in the United States (5). Systemic metastatic disease is present in almost all patients at diagnosis: overt in two-thirds (extensive stage, ED) and subclinical in a third (limited stage, LD). Established chemotherapeutic agents include etoposide, cisplatin, carboplatin, ifosfamide, cyclophosphamide, vincristine, and doxorubicin. By general consensus, conventional dose treatment consists of four to six cycles of platinum/ etoposide alone for extensive-stage disease or with concurrent chest radiation therapy for the third of patients with limited-stage disease (6). Complete response rates are 50–70% for LD and 10–20% for ED patients. However, by 2 years 20–40% of LD and fewer than 5% of ED patients remain alive (7,8). Five-year survival is about half that at 2 years. Although ifosfamide has improved survival in ED patients in conjunction with cisplatin and etoposide (9), this lead has not yet been tested in LD patients. New agents with promising activity include the taxanes, gemcitabine, and the topoisomerase I inhibitors. The role of these new agents is being evaluated in ongoing first-line therapy trials. The underlying cardiovascular and pulmonary comorbidity typical of this population, median age 60–65 years, and enhanced risk of secondary smoking-related malignancies inherent in lung cancer patients contribute to an increased risk when applying dose-intensive therapy.

DOSE INTENSITY: WITHOUT CELLULAR SUPPORT

Klasa et al. analyzed dose intensity (expressed in drug dose administered per square meter per week) of individual agents or regimens delivered in ED SCLC trials (10). Higher dose intensities of cyclophosphamide and doxorubicin with vincristine (CAV) and with etoposide (CAE), but not etoposide and cisplatin (EP), were associated with a longer median survival. The relative range of doses administered and the response and survival advantages were small (10).

Six randomized trials have evaluated dose intensity in ED SCLC with or without cytokine support (11–16). The actual delivered doses, when reported, were significantly less different between the arms than the planned dose intensity differences (1.2–2-fold). Two of these trials showed a modest survival advantage for the higher-dose therapy. Arriagada et al. treated LD patients with six cycles of conventional-dose chemotherapy wherein the first cycle only was randomly assigned conventional dose versus modest intensification (17). A complete response and survival advantage for the patients receiving the intensified chemotherapy was observed. This result was somewhat unexpected, since the relative difference in the two groups was so small. It is possible that dose intensity, particularly if given early in the course of treatment, may be more effective in limited SCLC rather than extensive SCLC. Early intensification and treatment of earlier-stage disease are two themes to consider when designing new trials.

Multidrug cyclical weekly therapy was designed to increase the dose intensity of treatment by taking into account the differing toxicities of the weekly agents. Early phase II results were promising, although patient selection effects were evident (18,19). However, none of the cooperative group randomized trials demonstrated survival benefits (20–23), perhaps owing to the greater morbidity, dose reductions, and delays required for the weekly schedules; thus the actual delivered dose intensities were not that different. Moreover, not only were doses and schedules varied, but so were the regimens, leading to interpretation obstacles (24).

Currently established cytokines (e.g., GM-CSF and G-CSF) were able to maintain dose intensity across multiple cycles (25). Fukuoka et al. documented a statistically significant survival advantage for the use of G-CSF to support the CODE regimen (59 vs. 32 weeks) (26). With cytokine use, a modest increment in dose intensity, limited by cumulative thrombocytopenia, can be achieved (1.5–2-fold). But the effectiveness of various thrombopoietins or other cytokines to increase achievable dose intensity remains uncertain.

DOSE INTENSITY: WITH CELLULAR SUPPORT

Trials reported prior to 1995 of patients with SCLC undergoing autologous bone marrow transplantation (ABMT) were reviewed by Elias and Cohen (27) if specifics about their response status (relapsed or refractory; untreated; or responding to first-line chemotherapy—partial or complete response) and their extent of disease (limited or extensive stage) had been provided. Patients in these various categories were pooled for aggregated relapse-free and overall survival characteristics.

Complete and overall responses in 52 patients with relapsed or refractory disease were 19% and 56% (28–41), respectively, but lasted only 2–4 months. While combination chemotherapy, especially those containing multiple alkylating agents, produced slightly higher response rates, these regimens were more toxic (18% vs. 6% deaths). The high complete response rate substantiated a dose-response relationship, but was insufficient for cure.

Complete and overall responses in 103 patients with untreated SCLC (71% limited disease) who received single- or double-cycle high-dose therapy as initial treatment were 42% and 84%, respectively (42–48). Relapse-free, 2-year, and overall survivals were comparable to those with treatment with conventional multicycle regimens. Transplantation in the newly diagnosed SCLC setting is potentially hazardous because of the frequency of life-threatening complications from uncontrolled disease, and the likelihood of tumor cell contamination in untreated autografts. Theoretically, early intensification may have greater impact on the disease.

High-dose chemotherapy with autologous hematopoietic support as consolidation has been given to approximately 466 patients responding to first-line chemotherapy (49–68). About 40–50% of partial responders converted to complete response, but without durable effect. Of patients with limited disease in complete response at the time of high-dose therapy, about 35% remained progression-free at a median follow-up > 3 years at the time of publication.

Brugger et al. administered two cycles of mobilization chemotherapy to 18 LD patients. Thirteen (72%) received high-dose ifosfamide, carboplatin, and etoposide (ICE) with epirubicin as consolidation (64,65). Event-free survival was 56% (median follow-up 44 months). About 25% had stage I or II SCLC, and surgical resection was performed in seven patients. Peripheral blood progenitor cells (PBPCs) collected after the second cycle of mobilization chemotherapy contained no microscopic tumor cells as measured by immunocytochemistry using keratin and EMA-125 antibodies.

At the Dana Farber Cancer Institute and Beth Israel Deaconess Medical Center, over 55 patients with limited-stage and over 30 with extensive-stage SCLC have been treated with high-dose combination alkylating agents [high-dose cyclophosphamide, carmustine, and cisplatin (CBP), or ICE] following response to conventional dose induction therapy. Of the original cohort of 36 patients with limited-stage SCLC (stages IIIA or B), 29 were in or near CR prior to treatment with high-dose CBP with marrow ± PBPC support and subsequent chest and prophylactic cranial radiotherapy (62,66). For this group, the 5-year event-free survival is 53% (minimum follow-up 40 months, range to 11 years). By multivariate analysis, response to induction was most important (CR/near CR best vs. PR), but short induction ≤ four cycles and the use of ifosfamide during induction also imparted better prognosis. Of the extensive-stage patients, about 17% remain progression free greater than 2 years after high-dose therapy, largely confined to patients with oligometastatic disease.

Humblet et al. performed the only randomized trial to be reported (60). Five cycles of conventional chemotherapy with prophylactic cranial irradiation were given to 101 patients with SCLC. Of these, 45 were randomized to one further cycle of either high- or conventional-dose therapy using cyclophosphamide, etoposide, and carmustine (60). Dose response was demonstrated. Complete response was achieved in 77% of partial responders after high-dose therapy, but in none after conventional-dose treatment. High-dose therapy enhanced disease-free survival and trended to improve survival. However, because overall outcomes were mediocre, with an 18% toxic death rate on the high-dose arm, the investigators concluded that dose-intensive therapy should not be considered a standard therapy in SCLC. In addition, almost all patients experienced disease recurrence in the chest, reflecting the fact that chest radiotherapy was not given in this trial.

Sites of prior tumor involvement, particularly the chest, are most likely to be sites of first relapse owing to a number of factors. These include increased tumor burden and/or drug-resistant clones in the chest; poorer drug delivery; intratumoral resistance factors such as hypoxia in areas of bulk tumor; or, in the case of autograft contamination, the possibility of homing with microenvironmental support for the tumor in local-regional sites (48,56). Chest relapse is reduced by conventional-dose radiotherapy (50 Gy), from 90% to 60%. Thus, high-dose curative treatment approaches should include "consolidative" radiotherapy to sites of bulky disease.

In many of the older trials, doses were attenuated and treatment-related morbidity and mortality was higher than currently expected. Many trials employed either single high-dose chemotherapeutic agents (±low-dose agents in addition) (47–52,67,68) or single alkylating agents (41,44,47,54–57). Combination alkylating agents were employed in a minority of patients (29,32,38,43,58–66).

FUTURE DIRECTIONS

Intensify Involved-Field Radiotherapy

Thoracic radiotherapy (TRT) provides a 25–30% improvement in local-regional control and a 5% increase in long-term progression-free survival for limited-stage SCLC (69,70). Local-regional relapse still remains high (about a 60% actuarial risk of local relapse by 3 years) with the typical 45–50 Gy TRT (71–73), and may be underestimated due to the competing risk of systemic relapse (74). Further enhancement of local-regional control might increase the proportion of long-term survivors.

Dose intensity of chest radiotherapy has not been sufficiently studied. The Eastern Cooperative Oncology Group (ECOG) and the Radiation Therapy Oncology Group (RTOG) compared 45 Gy TRT given either daily over 5 weeks or twice daily over 3 weeks concurrent with cisplatin and etoposide chemotherapy (75). Tumor recurrence in the chest was reduced from 61% to 48% at 2 years with the more intense TRT. A survival advantage for the more intensive radiotherapy has been reported (76). Many investigators have pointed to this trial as establishing a new benchmark for SCLC treatment outcomes. However, similar to high-dose trials, a patient selection bias is evident. Patients who were too sick (not suited for upfront combined modality therapy) or who had bilateral bulky mediastinal adenopathy (too large a radiotherapy port) were not generally enrolled onto the trial. Thus, a full 40% of patients enrolled in this trial had no apparent mediastinal adenopathy on computerized tomography—distinctly unusual for SCLC populations. This observation in no way undermines the demonstrated benefit of more intense radiotherapy, but does require caution before applying this advance to the general population of SCLC, even those with limited SCLC.

Using a shrinking-field technique, Choi et al. gave escalating doses of TRT concurrently with cisplatin and etoposide either as daily 180-cGy fractions or as twice-daily 150-cGy fractions in LD SCLC (77). The maximal tolerated dose defined by acute esophagitis was 45 Gy for twice daily administration and 70+

Gy when given once daily. Intensification of TRT dose is feasible and should be evaluated in a randomized setting. Since most relapses occur in-field, a more focused port may be feasible to reduce morbidity of more intense TRT. Here too, there may be a role for 3-D conformal planning.

Intensify Induction

Induction therapy may reduce tumor burden, stabilize rapidly progressive systemic and local symptoms from SCLC, select patients possessing chemosensitive tumors for subsequent intensification, and diminish micrometastases in the autograft sources. On the other hand, chemoresistant tumor cells might proliferate or even be induced across treatment, and might blunt these putative benefits. The Arriagada trial supports initial intensification of induction (17). A logical extension of this concept is the administration of multicycle dose-intensive combination therapies supported by cytokines and PBPCs (78–85). Pettengell et al. treated good-performance-status SCLC patients with conventional-dose ICE supported by autologous whole blood cells given on day 3 of chemotherapy for six cycles (80). Cycle length could be shortened to 2 weeks using either pheresis products or 750 ml whole blood stored at $4°C$. Cycles were repeated upon platelet recovery to $30,000/\mu l$, rather than the usual $100,000/\mu l$. In this phase I trial of 25 patients, the full planned dose intensity for each of the arms was reached across the first three cycles, and 56% completed all six. Mortality was 12% and complete response rate was 64%. The authors note that the collection of whole blood without cryopreservation reduced the cost and complexity of cellular support for nonablative therapy substantially (80). In a subsequent randomized phase II study, 50 ''good prognosis'' patients were given ICE either every 2 or 4 weeks (79). The median dose intensity delivered over the first three cycles was 1.8 (0.99–1.97) versus 0.99 (0.33–1.02) for the 2-week versus 4-week cycles, respectively. Paradoxically, more hematopoietic and infectious events occurred on the standard-dose 4-week arm. A phase III trial is ongoing.

In the European Bone Marrow Transplant (EBMT) group, 47 patients underwent mobilization with epirubicin and G-CSF followed by three cycles of moderately intensive ICE (81). Radiation to chest and head was recommended. Of 35 evaluable, the complete and near-complete response rate was 69%. Mortality was 14%. A phase III trial is ongoing.

Using an innovative trial design, Humblet et al. treated 37 limited-stage patients with four intensive alternating cycles of etoposide with either ifosfamide or carboplatin with stem cell support (85). To integrate early chest radiotherapy, bursts of 10 Gy TRT in five fractions were given concurrently with each chemotherapy administration (total dose 40 Gy). Mortality was 3%. The median event-free survival was 18 months, and 80% remain alive at 30 months. Eight of 13 relapses occurred in the brain, perhaps because no PCI was given.

Minimal Residual Tumor/Autograft Involvement

Autograft contamination by tumor cells may cause relapse. Gene-marking studies have definitively proven that residual tumor cells directly contribute to relapse in certain hematological malignancies and neuroblastoma (86–88). However, this has not been adequately tested in solid tumors (89). These cells also serve to indicate the patient has increased systemic chemotherapy-resistant tumor burden.

In SCLC, the marrow is a common metastatic site. Subclinical micrometa-static disease is detected in marrow in 13–54% of newly diagnosed limited- and 44–77% of newly diagnosed extensive-stage SCLC (90–94) using immunohisto-chemical techniques with sensitivities of $\sim 1/10^4$ cells. Two-thirds of patients in CR may have subclinical disease in marrow (95,96), and residual tumor appears to predict relapse (96). Brugger et al. detected circulating tumor cells in patients with metastatic SCLC or breast cancer mobilized with G-CSF and IPE chemo-therapy (97), but not after the second cycle of chemotherapy. In the short term, in vivo chemotherapy induction may "purge" the patient and the autologous stem cell source (67). In our unpublished data using a technique with a sensitivity of $1-10/10^6$, up to 77% of limited-disease patients in or near complete response prior to high-dose therapy have detectable tumor cells in their marrow by keratin staining (98).

Molecular and antigenic characterization of these residual cancer cells may guide strategies for further treatment. We are utilizing a fluorescence microscope with automated computerized scanning with one set of fluorescent probes for detection and a second set with different fluorophores for biological characteriza-tion to analyze patterns of coexpression of various markers in these cells (98). Prospective trials to determine the clinical significance of marrow or peripheral blood tumor contamination and the impact of novel stem cell sources to support high-dose therapy are underway.

CONCLUSION

Two major complementary strategies to administer high-dose therapy for SCLC include dose-intensive multicycle approach as initial treatment and "late" inten-sification in responders. Advantages for each approach are evident. The multicy-cle approach can achieve early dose intensity and maintain it for about three to four cycles. Disadvantages to this approach include subtransplant doses, high mortality rates, late administration of chest radiotherapy (except for the recent Humblet trial), and the collection of stem cells early in treatment when they have a higher potential to be contaminated with tumor cells. Advantages to later intensification include a patient with decreased tumor burden and decreased tumor-related symptoms with consequent improved performance status and a partial purge of the autograft. Early-dose intensive thoracic radiotherapy can be given before high-dose therapy. The drawback of later administration of the dose-intense cycles can be surmounted in part by intensification and shortening of induction chemoradiotherapy. The optimum may be to merge the two strategies into one: a brief dose-intensive induction followed by a single or double cycle of stem-cell-supported therapy followed by TRT and PCI. Ultimately, a randomized trial in patients with limited comorbid disease will be necessary to determine whether the increased toxicity is worthwhile and for which subsets of patients this approach is curative.

High-dose therapy has a strong scientific basis: it kills more tumor cells and achieves minimal tumor burden in most. In clinical situations in which toxicity has been acceptable, it typically results in prolonged progression-free survival in a subset of patients. An additional group of patients may be near cure. High-dose therapy may have increased value if additional targets of residual tumor cells can be identified for novel treatment strategies and modalities. Most biological strategies such as active or adoptive immunotherapy, gene function replacement (retinoblastoma gene and/or p53), or interruption of autocrine or paracrine growth loops work best against minimal tumor burden.

REFERENCES

1. Teicher BA. Preclinical models for high-dose therapy. In: Armitage JO, Antman KH, eds. High-Dose Cancer Therapy: Pharmacology, Hematopoietins, Stem Cells. Baltimore, Williams & Wilkins. 1992:14–42.
2. Frei E III. Combination cancer chemotherapy: presidential address. Cancer Res 1972; 32:2593–2607.
3. Frei E III, Canellos GP. Dose, a critical factor in cancer chemotherapy. Am J Med 1980; 69:585–594.
4. Frei E III, Antman KH. Combination chemotherapy, dose, and schedule: section XV, Principles of Chemotherapy. In: Holland JF, Frei E III, Bast RC Jr, Kufe DW, Morton DL, Weichselbaum RR, eds. Cancer Medicine. Philadelphia: Lea & Febiger, 1993:631–639.
5. Boring CC, Squires TS, Tong TT. Cancer statistics, 1993. CA—Cancer Journal for Clinicians 1994; 44:19–51.
6. Johnson DH, Kim K, Sause W, et al. Cisplatin and etoposide plus thoracic radiotherapy administered once or twice daily in limited stage small cell lung cancer: final report of intergroup trial 0096. Proc ASCO 1996; 15:374 (Abstract 1113).
7. Seifter EJ, Ihde DC. Therapy of small cell lung cancer: a perspective on two decades of clinical research. Semin Oncol 1988; 15(3):278–299.
8. Osterlind K, Hansen HH, Hansen M, Dombernowsky P, Anderson PK. Long-term disease-free survival in small-cell carcinoma of the lung: a study of clinical determinants. J Clin Oncol 1986; 4(9):1307–1313.
9. Loehrer PJ, Ansari R, Gonin R, et al. Cisplatin plus etoposide with and without ifosfamide in extensive small-cell lung cancer: a Hoosier Oncology Group study. J Clin Oncol 1995; 13:2594–2599.

10. Klasa RJ, Murray N, Coldman AJ. Dose-intensity meta-analysis of chemotherapy regimens in small-cell carcinoma of the lung. J Clin Oncol 1991; 9:499–508.
11. Cohen MH, Creaven PJ, Fossieck BE, et al. Intensive chemotherapy of small cell bronchogenic carcinoma. Cancer Treat Rep 1977; 61:349–354.
12. Brower M, Ihde DC, Johnston-Early A, et al. Treatment of extensive stage small cell bronchogenic carcinoma: effects of variation in intensity of induction chemotherapy. Am J Med 1983; 75:993–1000.
13. Johnson DH, Einhorn LH, Birch R, et al. A randomized comparison of high dose versus conventional dose cyclophosphamide, doxorubicin, and vincristine for extensive stage small cell lung cancer: a phase III trial of the Southeastern Cancer Study Group. J Clin Oncol 1987; 5:1731–1738.
14. Mehta C, Vogl SE. High-dose cyclophosphamide in the induction therapy of small cell lung cancer: minor improvements in rate of remission and survival. Proc AACR 1982; 23:155.
15. Figueredo AT, Hryniuk WM, Strautmanis I, et al. Co-trimoxazole prophylaxis during high-dose chemotherapy of small-cell lung cancer. J Clin Oncol 1985; 3:54–64.
16. Ihde DC, Mulshine JL, Kramer BS, Steinberg SM, Linnoila RI, Gazdar AF, Edison M, Phelps RM, Lesar M, Phares JC, Grayson J, Minna JD, Johnson BE. Prospective randomized comparison of high-dose and standard-dose etoposide and cisplatin chemotherapy in patients with extensive-stage small-cell lung cancer. J Clin Oncol 1994; 12:2022–2034.
17. Arriagada R, Le Chevalier T, Pignon J-P, Riviere A, Monnet I, Chomy P, Tuchais C, Tarayre M, Ruffie P. Initial chemotherapeutic doses and survival in patients with limited small-cell lung cancer. N Engl J Med 1993; 329:1848–1852.
18. Miles DW, Earl HM, Souhami RL, Harper PG, Rudd R, Ash CM, James L, Trask CWL, Tobias JS, Spiro SG. Intensive weekly chemotherapy for good-prognosis patients with small-cell lung cancer. J Clin Oncol 1991; 9:280–285.
19. Murray N, Gelmon K, Shah A, Grafton C, Tsang V, McKenzie M, Goddard K, Morris J, Karsai H, Page R. Potential for long-term survival in extensive stage small-cell lung cancer (ESCLC) with CODE chemotherapy and radiotherapy. Lung Cancer 1994; 11(suppl 1):99 (377).
20. Furuse K, Kubota K, Nishiwaki Y, et al. Phase III study of dose intensive weekly chemotherapy with recombinant human granulocyte-colony stimulating factor (G-CSF) versus standard chemotherapy in extensive stage small cell lung cancer (SCLC). Proc ASCO 1996; 15:375 (1117).
21. Murray N, Livingston RB, Shepard FA, et al. Randomized study of CODE versus alternating CAV/EP for limited stage small cell lung cancer: an Intergroup Study of the National Cancer Institute of Canada Clinical Trials Group and the Southwest Oncology Group. J Clin Oncol 1999; 17:2300–2308.
22. Sculier JP, Paesmans M, Bureau G, et al. Multiple drug weekly chemotherapy versus standard combination regimen in small cell lung cancer: a phase III randomized study conducted by the European Lung Cancer Working Party. J Clin Oncol 1993; 11:1858–1865.
23. Souhami RL, Rudd R, Ruiz de Elvira MC, et al. Randomized trial comparing weekly versus 3-week chemotherapy in small cell lung cancer: a Cancer Research Campaign trial. J Clin Oncol 1994; 12:1806–1813.

24. Johnson DH, Carbone DP. Editorial. Increased dose-intensity in small cell lung cancer: a failed strategy. J Clin Oncol 1999; 17:2297–2299.

25. Crawford J, Ozer H, Stoller R, et al. Reduction by granulocyte colony-stimulating factor of fever and neutropenia induced by chemotherapy in patients with small-cell lung cancer. N Engl J Med 1991; 325:164–170.

26. Fukuoka M, Masuda N, Negoro S, et al. CODE chemotherapy with or without granulocyte colony stimulating factor in small cell lung cancer. Br J Cancer 1997; 75: 306–309.

27. Elias A, Cohen BF. Dose intensive therapy in lung cancer. In: Armitage JO, Antman KH, eds. High-Dose Cancer Therapy: Pharmacology, Hematopoietins, Stem Cells, 2nd edition. Baltimore: Williams & Wilkins, 1995:824–846.

28. Phillips GL, Fay JW, Herzig GP, et al. Nitrosourea (BCNU), NSC #4366650 and cryopreserved autologous marrow transplantation for refractory cancer: a phase I–II Study. Cancer 1983; 52:1792–1802.

29. Stahel RA, Takvorian RW, Skarin AT, Canellos GP. Autologous bone marrow transplantation following high-dose chemotherapy with cyclophosphamide, BCNU, and VP-16 in small cell carcinoma of the lung and a review of current literature. Eur J Cancer Clin Oncol 1984; 20:1233–1238.

30. Wolff SW, Fer MF, McKay CM, et al. High-dose VP-16-213 and autologous bone marrow transplantation for refractory malignancies: a phase I study. J Clin Oncol 1983; 1:701–705.

31. Pico JL, Beaujean F, Debre M, et al. High dose chemotherapy (HDC) with autologous bone marrow transplantation (ABMT) in small cell carcinoma of the lung (SCCL) in relapse. Proc ASCO 1983; 2:206.

32. Pico JL, Baume D, Ostronoff M, et al. Chimiotherapie a hautes doses suivie d'autogreffe de moelle osseuse dans le traitement du cancer bronchique a petites cellules. Bull Cancer 1987; 74:587–595.

33. Postmus PE, Mulder NH, Elema JD. Graft versus host disease after transfusions of non-irradiated blood cells in patients having received autologous bone marrow. Eur J Cancer 1988; 24:889–894.

34. Rushing DA, Baldauf MC, Gehlsen JA, et al. High-dose BCNU and autologous bone marrow reinfusion in the treatment of refractory or relapsed small cell carcinoma of the lung (SCCL). Proc ASCO 1984; 3:217.

35. Spitzer G, Dicke KA, Verma DS, Zander A, McCredie KB. High-dose BCNU Therapy with autologous bone marrow infusion: preliminary observations. Cancer Treat Rep 1979; 63:1257–1264.

36. Spitzer G, Dicke KA, Latam J, et al. High-dose combination chemotherapy with autologous bone marrow transplantation in adult solid tumors. Cancer 1980; 45:3075–3085.

37. Eder JP, Antman K, Shea TC, Elias A, Teicher B, Henner WD, Schryber SM, Holden S, Finberg R, Critchlow J, Flaherty M, Mick R, Schnipper LE, Frei E III. Cyclophosphamide and thiotepa with autologous bone marrow transplantation in patients with solid tumors. J Natl Cancer Inst 1988; 80:1221–1226.

38. Elias AD, Ayash LJ, Wheeler C, Schwartz G, Tepler I, Gonin R, McCauley M, Mazanet R, Schnipper L, Frei E III, Antman KH. A phase I study of high-dose ifosfamide, carboplatin, and etoposide with autologous hematopoietic stem cell support. Bone Marrow Transplant 1995; 15:373–379.

39. Douer D, Champlin RE, Ho WG, et al. High-dose combined-modality therapy and autologous bone marrow transplantation in resistant cancer. Am J Med 1981; 71: 973–976.
40. Harada M, et al. Combined-modality therapy and autologous bone marrow transplantation in the treatment of advanced non-Hodgkin's lymphoma and solid tumors: the Kanawaza experience. Transplant Proc 1982; 4:733–737.
41. Lazarus HM, Spitzer TR, Creger RT. Phase I trial of high-dose etoposide, high-dose cisplatin, and reinfusion of autologous bone marrow for lung cancer. Am J Clin Oncol 1990; 13:107–112.
42. Lange A, Kolodziej J, Tomeczko J, Toporski J, Sedzimirska M, Jazwiec B, Bochenska J, Mroz E, Bielecka E, Was A, Glejzer O, Tomaszewska-Toporowska B, Jagas M, Zukowska B, Spaltenstein A, Bieranowska D, Klimczak A. Aggressive chemotherapy with autologous bone marrow transplantation in small cell lung carcinoma. Arch Immunol Ther Exp 1991; 39:431–439.
43. Nomura F, Shimokata K, Saito H, Watanabe A, Saka H, Sakai S, Kodera Y, Saito H. High dose chemotherapy with autologous bone marrow transplantation for limited small cell lung cancer. Jpn J Clin Oncol 1990; 20:94–98.
44. Spitzer G, Farha P, Valdivieso M, et al. High-dose intensification therapy with autologous bone marrow support for limited small-cell bronchogenic carcinoma. J Clin Oncol 1986; 4:4–13.
45. Johnson DH, Hande KR, Hainsworth JD, Greco FA. High-dose etoposide as single-agent chemotherapy for small cell carcinoma of the lung. Cancer Treat Rep 1983; 67:957–958.
46. Littlewood TJ, Spragg BP, Bentley DP. When is autologous bone marrow transplantation safe after high-dose treatment with etoposide? Clin Lab Haematol 1985; 7:213–218.
47. Littlewood TJ, Bentley DP, Smith AP. High-dose etoposide with autologous bone marrow transplantation as initial treatment of small cell lung cancer—a negative report Eur J Respir Dis 1986; 68:370–374.
48. Souhami RL, Hajichristou HT, Miles DW, Earl HM, Harper PG, Ash CM, Goldstone AH, Spiro SG, Geddes DM, Tobias JS. Intensive chemotherapy with autologous bone marrow transplantation for small cell lung cancer. Cancer Chemother Pharmacol 1989; 24:321–325.
49. Smith IE, Evans BD, Harland SJ, et al. High-dose cyclophosphamide with autologous bone marrow rescue after conventional chemotherapy in the treatment of small cell lung carcinoma. Cancer Chemother Pharmacol 1985; 14:120–124.
50. Banham S, Burnett A, Stevenson R, ct al. Pilot study of combination chemotherapy with late dose intensification and autologous bone marrow rescue in small cell bronchogenic carcinoma. Br J Cancer 1982; 42:486.
51. Banham S, Loukop M, Burnett A, et al. Treatment of small cell carcinoma of the lung with late dosage intensification programmes containing cyclophosphamide and Mesna. Cancer Treat Rev 1983; 10(suppl A):73–77.
52. Burnett AK, Tansey P, Hills C, et al. Haematologic reconstitution following high dose and supralethal chemoradiotherapy using stored non-cryopreserved autologous bone marrow. Br J Haematol 1983; 54:309–316.
53. Jennis A, Levitan N, Pecora AL, Isaacs R, Lazarus H. Sequential high dose chemo-

therapy (HDC) with filgrastim/peripheral stem cell support (PSCS) in extensive stage small cell lung cancer (SCLC). Proc ASCO 1996; 15:349 (1021).

54. Ihde DC, Diesseroth AB, Lichter AS, et al. Late intensive combined modality therapy followed by autologous bone marrow infusion in extensive stage small-cell lung cancer. J Clin Oncol 1986; 4:1443–1454.

55. Cunningham D, Banham SW, Hutcheon AH, et al. High-Dose Cyclophosphamide and VP-16 as late dosage intensification therapy for small cell carcinoma of lung. Cancer Chemother Pharmacol 1985; 15:303–306.

56. Sculier JP, Klastersky J, Stryckmans P, et al. Late intensification in small-cell lung cancer: a phase I study of high doses of cyclophosphamide and etoposide with autologous bone marrow transplantation. J Clin Oncol 1985; 3:184–191.

57. Klastersky J, Nicaise C, Longeval E, et al. Cisplatin, adriamycin and etoposide (CAV) for remission induction of small-cell bronchogenic carcinoma: evaluation of efficacy and toxicity and pilot study of a "late intensification" with autologous bone marrow rescue. Cancer 1982; 50:652–658.

58. Cornblett M, Gregor A, Allen S, Leonard R, Smyth J. High dose melphalan as consolidation therapy for good prognosis patients with small cell carcinoma of the bronchus (SCCB). Proc ASCO 1984; 3:210.

59. Wilson C, Pickering D. Stewart S, Vallis K, Kalofonos H, Cross A, Snook D, Goldman JM, McKenzie CG, Epenetos AA. High dose chemotherapy with autologous bone marrow rescue in small cell lung cancer. In Vivo 1988; 2:331–334.

60. Humblet Y, Symann M, Bosly A, et al. Late intensification chemotherapy with autologous bone marrow transplantation in selected small-cell carcinoma of the lung: a randomized study. J Clin Oncol 1987; 5:1864–1873.

61. Stewart P, Buckner CD, Thomas ED, et al. Intensive chemoradiotherapy with autologous marrow transplantation for small cell carcinoma of the lung. Cancer Treat Rep 1983; 67:1055–1059.

62. Elias AD, Ayash L, Frei E III, Skarin AT, Hunt M, Wheeler C, Schwartz G, Mazanet R, Tepler I, Eder JP, McCauley M, Herman T, Schnipper L, Antman KH. Intensive combined modality therapy for limited stage small cell lung cancer. J Natl Cancer Inst 1993; 85:559–566.

63. Tomeczko J, Pacuszko T, Napora P, Lange A. Treatment intensification which includes high dose induction improves survival of lung carcinoma patients treated by high-dose chemotherapy with hematopoietic progenitor cell rescue but does not prevent high rate of relapses. Bone Marrow Transplant 1996; 18(suppl 1):S44–S47.

64. Brugger W, Frommhold H, Pressler K, Mertelsmann R, Kanz L. Use of high-dose etoposide/ifosfamide/carboplatin/epirubicin and peripheral blood progenitor cell transplantation in limited-disease small cell lung cancer. Semin Oncol 1995; 22(suppl 2):3–8.

65. Brugger W, Fetscher S, Hasse J, et al. Multimodality treatment including early high-dose chemotherapy with peripheral blood stem cell transplantation in limited-disease small cell lung cancer. Semin Oncol 1998; 25(suppl 2):42–48.

66. Elias A, Ibrahim J, Skarin AT, Wheeler C, McCauley M, Ayash L, Richardson P, Schnipper L, Antman KH, Frei E III. Dose intensive therapy for limited stage small cell lung cancer: long-term outcome. J Clin Oncol 1999; 17:1175–1184.

67. Farha P, Spitzer G, Valdivieso M, et al. High-dose chemotherapy and autologous

bone marrow transplantation for the treatment of small cell lung carcinoma. Cancer 1983; 52:1351–1355.

68. Marangolo M, Rosti G, Ravaioli A, et al. Small cell carcinoma of the lung (SCCL): high-dose (HD) VP-16 and autologous bone marrow transplantation (ABMT) as intensification therapy: preliminary results. Int J Cell Cloning 1985; 3:277.

69. Pignon JP, Arriagada R, Ihde DC, et al. A meta-analysis of thoracic radiotherapy for small-cell lung cancer. N Engl J Med 1992; 327:1618–1624.

70. Warde P, Payne D. Does thoracic irradiation improve survival and local control in limited-stage small-cell carcinoma of the lung? A meta-analysis. J Clin Oncol 1992; 10:890–895.

71. Perry MC, Eaton WL, Propert KJ, Ware JH, Zimmer B, Chahinian AP, Skarin A, Carey RW, Kreisman H, Faulkner C, Comis R, Green MR. Chemotherapy with or without radiation therapy in limited small-cell carcinoma of the lung. N Engl J Med 1987; 316:912–918.

72. Bunn PA, Lichter AS, Makuch RW, Cohen MH, Veach SR, Matthews MJ, Anderson AJ, Edison M, Glatstein E, Minna JD, Ihde DC. Chemotherapy alone or chemotherapy with chest radiation therapy in limited stage small cell lung cancer. Ann Intern Med 1987; 106:655–662.

73. Kies MS, Mira JG, Crowley JJ, Chen TT, Pazdur R, Grozea PN, Rivkin SE, Coltman CA, Ward JH, Livingston RB. Multimodal therapy for limited small-cell lung cancer: a randomized study of induction combination chemotherapy with or without thoracic radiation in complete responders; and with wide-field versus reduced-field radiation in partial responders: a Southwest Oncology Group study. J Clin Oncol 1987; 5: 592–600.

74. Arriagada R, Kramar A, Le Chevalier T, De Cremoux H. Competing events determining relapse-free survival in limited small-cell lung carcinoma. J Clin Oncol 1992; 10:447–451.

75. Turrisi AT, Kim K, Johnson DH, Komaki R, Sause W, Curran W, Livingston R, Wagner H, Blum R. Daily (qd) v twice-daily (bid) thoracic irradiation (TI) with concurrent cisplatin-etoposide (PE) for limited small cell lung cancer (LSCLC): preliminary results on 352 randomized eligible patients. Lung Cancer 1994; 11(suppl 1):172 (667).

76. Turrisi AT, Kim K, Blum R, et al. Twice-daily compared with once-daily thoracic radiotherapy in limited small-cell lung cancer treated concurrently with cisplatin and etoposide. N Engl J Med 1999; 340:265–271.

77. Choi NC, Herndon II JE, Rosenman J, et al. Phase I study to determine the maximum tolerated dose (MTD) of radiation in standard daily and hyperfractionated accelerated twice daily radiation schedules with concurrent chemotherapy for limited stage small cell lung cancer (Cancer and Leukemia Group B 8837). J Clin Oncol 1998; 16:3528–3536.

78. Tepler I, Cannistra SA, Frei E III, Gonin R, Anderson KC, Demetri G, Niloff J, Goodman H, Muntz H, Muto M, Sheets E, Elias AD, Mazanet R, Wheeler C, Ayash L, Schwartz G, McCauley M, Gaynes L, Harvey S, Schnipper LE, Antman KH. Use of peripheral blood progenitor cells abrogates the myelotoxicity of repetitive outpatient high-dose carboplatin and cyclophosphamide chemotherapy. J Clin Oncol 1993; 11:1583–1591.

79. Woll PJ, Lee SM, Lomax L, Hodgetts J, Stout R, Burt PA, Sims T, Kitchin R, Thatcher N. Randomised phase II study of standard versus dose-intensive ICE chemotherapy with reinfusion of haemopoietic progenitors in whole blood in small cell lung cancer (SCLC). Proc ASCO 1996; 15:333 (957).
80. Pettengell R, Woll PJ, Thatcher N, Dexter TM, Testa NG. Multicyclic, dose-intensive chemotherapy supported by sequential reinfusion of hematopoietic progenitors in whole blood. J Clin Oncol 1995; 13:148–156.
81. Perey L, Rosti G, Lange A, Pampallona S, Bosquee L, Pasini F, Humblet Y, Hamdan O, Cetto GL, Marangolo M, Leyvraz S. Sequential high-dose ICE chemotherapy with circulating progenitor cells (CPC) in small cell lung cancer: an EBMT study. Bone Marrow Transplant 1996; 18(suppl 1):S40–S43.
82. Crown J, Wasserheit C, Hakes T, et al. Rapid delivery of multiple high-dose chemotherapy courses with granulocyte colony-stimulating factor and peripheral blood-derived hematopoietic progenitor cells. J Natl Cancer Inst 1992; 84:1935–1936.
83. Gianni AM, Siena S, Bregni M, et al. Prolonged disease-free survival after high-dose sequential chemo-radiotherapy and hemopoietic autologous transplantation in poor prognosis Hodgkin's disease. Ann Oncol 1991; 2:645–653.
84. Ayash L, Elias A, Wheeler C, Reich E, Schwartz G, Mazanet R, Tepler I, Warren D, Lynch C, Gonin R, Schnipper L, Frei E III, Antman K. Double dose-intensive chemotherapy with autologous marrow and peripheral blood progenitor cell support for metastatic breast cancer: a feasibility study. J Clin Oncol 1994; 12:37–44.
85. Humblet Y, Bosquee L, Weynants P, Symann M. High-dose chemo-radiotherapy cycles for LD small cell lung cancer patients using G-CSF and blood stem cells. Bone Marrow Transplant 1996; 18(suppl 1):S36–S39.
86. Gribben JG, Freedman AS, Neuberg D, Roy DC, Blake KW, Woo SD, Brossbard ML, Rabinowe SN, Coral F, Freeman GJ, Ritz J, Nadler LM. Immunologic purging of marrow assessed by PCR before autologous bone marrow transplantation for B-cell lymphoma. N Engl J Med 1991; 325:1525–1533.
87. Brenner MK, Rill DR, Moen RC, Krance RA, Mirro J Jr, Anderson WF, Ihle JN. Gene-marking to trace origin of relapse after autologous bone-marrow transplantation. Lancet 1993; 341:85–86, and verbal communication, Stem Cell Conference, San Diego, March, 1993.
88. Brenner MK, Rill DR. Gene marking to improve the outcome of autologous bone marrow transplantation. J Hematother 1994; 3:33–36.
89. O'Shaughnessy JA, Cowan KH, Cottler-Fox M, Carter CS, Doren S, Leitman S, Wilson W, Moen R, Nienhuis AW, Dunbar CE. Autologous transplantation of retro-virally-marked CD34-positive bone marrow and peripheral blood cells in patients with multiple myeloma or breast cancer. Proc ASCO 1994; 13:296 (963).
90. Stahel RA, Mabry M, Skarin AT, Speak J, Bernal SD. Detection of bone marrow metastasis in small-cell lung cancer by monoclonal antibody. J Clin Oncol 1985; 3: 455–461.
91. Canon JL, Humblet Y, Lebacq-Verheyden AM, Manouvriez P, Bazin H, Rodhain J, Prignot J, Symann M. Immunodetection of small cell lung cancer metases in bone marrow using three monoclonal antibodies. Eur J Cancer Oncol 1988; 24:147–150.
92. Trillet V, Revel D, Combaret V, Favrot M, Loire R, Tabib A, Pages J, Jacquermet P, Bonmartin A, Mornex JF, Cordier JF, Binet R, Brune J. Bone marrow metastases

in small cell lung cancer: detection with magnetic resonance imaging and monoclonal antibodies. Br J Cancer 1989; 60:83–88.

93. Berendsen HH, De Leij L, Postmus PE, Ter Haar JG, Popperna S, The TH. Detection of small cell lung cancer metastases in bone marrow aspirates using monoclonal antibody directed against neuroendocrine differentiation antigen. J Clin Pathol 1988; 41:273–276.

94. Beiske K, Myklebust AT, Aamdal S, Langhom R, Jakobsen E, Fodstad O. Detection of bone marrow metases in small cell lung cancer patients. Am J Pathol 1992; 141: 531–538.

95. Hay FG, Ford A, Leonard RCF. Clinical applications of immunocytochemistry in the monitoring of the bone marrow in small cell lung cancer (SCLC). Int J Cancer 1988; (suppl 2):8–10.

96. Leonard RCF, Duncan LW, Hay FG. Immunocytological detection of residual marrow disease at clinical remission predicts metastatic relapse in small cell lung cancer. Cancer Res 1990; 50:6545–6548.

97. Brugger W, Bross KJ, Glatt M, Weber F, Mertelsmann R, Kanz L. Mobilization of tumor cells and hematopoietic progenitor cells into peripheral blood of patients with solid tumors. Blood 1994; 83:636–640.

98. Elias A, Li Y, Wheeler C, Richardson P, Ayash L, McCauley M, Newquist E, Cap B, Tuchin J, Webb I, Schnipper L, Frei E III, Skarin AT, Chen LB. CD34-selected peripheral blood progenitor cell (PBPC) support in high dose therapy of small cell lung cancer (SCLC): use of a novel detection method for minimal residual tumor (MRT). Proc ASCO 1996; 15:341 (991).

8

Dose Intensification of Chemotherapy in SCLC: Con

Russell F. DeVore III*

Vanderbilt–Ingram Cancer Center and Vanderbilt University School of Medicine, Nashville, Tennessee

INTRODUCTION

Small cell lung cancer (SCLC) is a chemosensitive malignancy in which high overall and complete response rates can be achieved. Despite the presence of systemic micrometastases in virtually all patients at the time of presentation (1), a proportion of patients with limited-stage disease can be cured with a combination of chemotherapy and thoracic radiotherapy (2). Therefore, SCLC is an excellent model for testing strategies to overcome drug resistance in an effort to increase long-term survival rates (3).

In preclinical tumor models, one of the simplest methods used to overcome drug resistance is dose escalation (3). Testing of dose escalation strategies in SCLC began in the late 1970s when Cohen and colleagues undertook a randomized trial in which SCLC patients were randomly assigned to receive either standard dosages of cyclophosphamide, methotrexate, and lomustine or higher-dose cyclophosphamide, lomustine, and standard-dose methotrexate (4). These investigators observed both a higher overall response rate and a prolonged survival in the high-dose-chemotherapy group. Long-term survivors were observed only

---

*Current affiliation: East Tennessee Oncology/Hematology, Knoxville, Tennessee.

among those patients given high-dose chemotherapy. By today's standards, the "high dose" regimen used by Cohen and his colleagues would be considered relatively modest. Nevertheless, this trial spawned a series of studies aimed at overcoming drug resistance through dose escalation.

A number of strategies have been employed to dose-intensify therapy in SCLC. These include high-dose induction chemotherapy, weekly chemotherapy, use of hematopoeitic growth factors, and late intensification with bone marrow rescue. To date no randomized trial has demonstrated a survival advantage to increasing dose intensity beyond that of the best conventional regimens. Increasing dose intensity in patients with extensive-stage SCLC is harmful and only increases the rate of serious toxicities. In limited-stage patients, results of randomized trials suggest that maintaining dose intensity at or near the maximally tolerated dose of a given regimen is important, but intensifying induction therapy beyond conventional doses has not been well addressed.

In this chapter the various trials investigating the importance of dose intensity in SCLC are reviewed. Emphasis is placed on randomized controlled trials and a distinction is made between results in extensive- versus limited-stage patients. An argument is made to discontinue work testing this strategy, which has been extensively studied with overwhelmingly negative results.

HIGH-DOSE INDUCTION CHEMOTHERAPY

Extensive SCLC

Several randomized trials have tested the concept of high-dose induction therapy in SCLC (Table 1) (5–10). Based on pilot data demonstrating the feasibility of high-dose induction therapy (11), the Southeastern Cancer Study Group (SECSG) undertook a prospective study in which patients with extensive-stage SCLC were randomized to receive either high-dose cyclophosphamide, doxorubicin, and vincristine (CAV) for the initial three cycles of therapy or standard doses of the same regimen (6). No dose attenuation was allowed during the initial three cycles of therapy. Patients received a mean of ≥95% of the planned dosages of cyclophosphamide and doxorubicin during the first three treatment cycles resulting in a 15% and 67% dose escalation of each drug, respectively. Although the complete remission rate was higher in the high-dose arm (22% and 12%; $p < 0.05$), overall response rates (63% and 53%) and median survival duration (29.3 weeks and 34.7 weeks) were not significantly different between the two treatment groups. Moreover, the high-dose CAV regimen was substantially more toxic with a large percentage of patients experiencing life-threatening toxicities (grade 4 neutropenia: 79% and 40%; $p < 0.05$). Virtually identical results were reported by Figueredo and colleagues in a Canadian trial (9).

TABLE 1 Randomized Trials of High-Dose Versus Conventional-Dose Induction Chemotherapy

Ref.	Regimen[a]	Patient number	Overall response	Median survival	1-Year survival
Hande (8)	cd MCDVEH	21	67%	9 months	10%[b]
	hd MCDVEH	21	74%	9 months	7%[b]
Figueredo (9)	cd CDV	51	61%	7 months[c]	—
	hd CDV	52	71%	9 months[c]	—
Johnson (6)	cd CDV	174	53%	34.7 weeks	20%
	hd CDV	124	63%	29.3 weeks	20%
Ihde (7)	cd PE	46	83%	10.7 months	48%
	hd PE	44	86%	11.4 months	45%
Arriagada (10)	cd PCDE	50[d]	54%[e]	.14 months	26%[f]
	hd PCDE	55[d]	67%[e]	.18 months	43%[f]

Methotrexate (M); cyclophosphamide (C); doxorubicin (D); vincristine (V); etoposide (E); hexamethylmelamine (H); cisplatin (P).
[a] Conventional dose = cd; high-dose = hd.
[b] Survival at 18 months.
[c] Median duration of response.
[d] All patients limited stage.
[e] Complete remission rate.
[f] Survival at 24 months.

Hong and associates randomly assigned limited- and extensive-stage SCLC patients to receive either high-dose cyclophosphamide (2000 mg/m^2) plus vincristine (CV), standard dose CAV, or standard-dose etoposide plus cyclophosphamide and vincristine (CEV) (5). A total of 353 patients were studied. In limited-stage patients the complete response rates and median survivals for dose-intensive CV, standard-dose CAV, and standard-dose CEV were 31% and 41 weeks, 42% and 55 weeks, and 38% and 58 weeks, respectively. Because the agents employed in the various regimens were not identical, factors other than dose intensity may have affected survival outcomes. Indeed, the median survival duration for all patients was superior in the standard-dose CEV arm ($p = 0.01$), suggesting that the inclusion of etoposide may have been more important to efficacy than dose intensification.

More recently, Ihde and colleagues compared "standard-dose" etoposide (80 mg/m^2/day $\times$ 3 days) plus cisplatin (80 mg/m^2/day 1) to "high-dose" etoposide (80 mg/m^2/day $\times$ 5 days) plus cisplatin (27 mg/m^2/day $\times$ 5 days) (7) in patients with extensive disease. Both regimens were administered every 21 days. The degree of myelosuppression with high-dose therapy was approximately twice that observed with the standard dose. Despite 68% higher doses and a 46% higher dose-rate intensity actually given to patients in the high-dose group, there was no difference in response rates (85% and 81%), median survival (12 months and 11 months), or 1-year survival rates (50% and 46%).

The Johnson and Ihde trials were well designed; they tested dose intensification of induction therapy with two widely used conventional regimens; and they had similar findings. Both groups were able to approximate their planned increase in dose intensity in the "high dose" treatment arms but not even a statistically insignificant trend suggesting a survival benefit was observed. It might be argued that the degree of dose intensification achieved by these investigators was not sufficient to impact clinical outcomes. Indeed, preclinical studies indicate that a survival benefit may not be observed until the dose of an active agent is increased twofold or more (3). Furthermore, in animal models the most convincing evidence for a survival benefit to dose intensification comes from models with curative potential (12). Therefore, extensive-stage SCLC may not be a good model for testing dose intensification even if a twofold increase in dose intensity can be achieved.

Limited SCLC

Efforts to exploit any biological or clinical advantage to dose intensification might better be pursued in patients with limited-stage disease. To this end Arriagada and colleagues performed a retrospective analysis of 131 consecutively treated limited-stage SCLC patients and observed a survival benefit for patients who received higher initial doses of cyclophosphamide and cisplatin (13,14).

Based on this observation, they undertook a phase III trial in which limited-stage patients were randomly assigned to receive either conventional-dose cisplatin, cyclophosphamide, etoposide, and doxorubicin alternating with thoracic radiotherapy, or the identical treatment regimen, except 20% higher doses of cyclophosphamide and cisplatin were given in the first treatment cycle only (10). The complete response rate (67% vs. 54%, $p = 0.16$) and 2-year survival (43% vs. 26%, $p = 0.02$) were superior in the dose-intensive group. These results are astounding given the minor degree to which chemotherapy doses were intensified and suggest that a twofold increase in dose intensity might not be necessary to impact survival outcomes in the clinical setting.

A more recent report by Steward and colleagues also suggests that dose intensification might effect superior survival outcomes in early-stage patients (15). These investigators enrolled patients with "good- or intermediate-prognosis" SCLC to a prospective multicenter study that involved a 2×2 factorial design, randomizing patients to conventional versus dose-intensified V-ICE chemotherapy (vincristine, ifosfamide, carboplatin, etoposide). Patients were randomly assigned to receive identical doses of all four drugs on either an every-3-week or every-4-week schedule. Therefore, dose intensification was attempted by decreasing the dosing interval rather than increasing chemotherapy doses. Both treatment groups underwent a second randomization to receive either granulocyte-macrophage colony-stimulating factor (GM-CSF) or no growth factor support. Eligibility required that patients be classified as good- or intermediate-prognosis as defined by Cerny and colleagues (16). A total of 178 of 300 patients (59%) had limited-stage disease. Although there were greater proportions of limited-stage patients and patients with more favorable prognostic scores in the dose-intensive group, these differences were not statistically significant. The addition of GM-CSF neither reduced the incidence of complications from myelosuppression, nor did it improve survival. However, patients in the 3-week-treatment arm experienced statistically superior median and 2-year survivals (443 vs. 351 days and 33% vs. 18%, respectively).

The dose-intensive patients in the Arriagada and Steward trials experienced 2-year survival rates of 43% and 33%, respectively. Although the treatment regimens used in these trials varied significantly, an indirect estimate of the relative dose intensity of the two regimens can be made by comparing the incidence of dose-limiting toxicity, that being grade IV neutropenia 59% and 65%, respectively. Turrisi and colleagues recently described the highest long-term survival rates ever observed in a multicenter phase III trial in limited-stage SCLC (2). Patients were treated with etoposide and cisplatin and concurrent thoracic radiotherapy by either a conventional once-daily or a twice-daily schedule. For the entire patient group, the 2-year survival rate was 44% and the grade IV neutropenia rate was 63%, results almost identical to those observed in the "dose-intensive" patients from the Arriagada and Steward trials. The control regimens used in the latter trials resulted in grade IV neutropenia rates of only 23% (cycle 1 only) and 49%, respectively. The dose intensity of the latter regimens might better be considered suboptimal rather than standard. Similar to the experience of Cohen and colleagues in patients with extensive-stage disease (4), the Arriagada and Steward trials demonstrated that reducing chemotherapy dose intensity below the optimum of a given induction regimen leads to inferior survival outcomes.

It is safe to conclude that dose intensification of induction therapy is of no benefit to patients with extensive-stage disease. Optimal therapy for limited-stage disease should include doses at or near the maximal tolerated doses of the induction regimen. Compromising dose intensity in these patients may negatively impact long-term survival rates. Whether a survival benefit can be derived by intensifying induction therapy beyond the maximally tolerated doses of conventional outpatient therapy is unknown at this time and is a reasonable area for continued investigation in limited-stage patients.

WEEKLY CHEMOTHERAPY

As described in the preceding section, Steward and colleagues were able to effect a significant improvement in median survival in good- or immediate-prognosis SCLC patients by decreasing the treatment interval from 4 to 3 weeks. This suggests that increasing dose intensity by more frequent dosing might be beneficial. This may be even better achieved with weekly chemotherapy using standard chemotherapy doses but alternating between myelosuppressive and nonmyelosuppressive agents. Early pilot trials testing this approach have produced very promising results leading to a number of phase III trials comparing weekly chemotherapy to conventional regimens (Table 2) (17–20). The EORTC conducted a large phase III study comparing a weekly multidrug chemotherapy regimen (doxorubicin, etoposide, cyclophosphamide, cisplatin, vindesine, vincristine, and methotrexate) to a standard chemotherapy regimen (cyclophosphamide, doxorubicin, and etoposide) administered every 3 weeks (17). Both limited- and extensive-stage patients were enrolled. Although the response rate in the weekly regimen was higher in limited-stage patients, there was no difference in overall response rate, median survival, and 2-year survival. The total relative dose intensity for the drugs common to both regimens was significantly less in the weekly chemotherapy arm due to frequent treatment delays. This study failed to directly address the question of dose intensity but suggests increasing dose intensity or dose density with weekly chemotherapy may not be possible without hematopoietic support because of excessive toxicity.

Souhami and colleagues, reporting for the Cancer Research Campaign of the United Kingdom, also found no survival benefit when they compared a weekly multidrug regimen to a standard every-3-week approach (18). In the U.K.

TABLE 2 Randomized Trials of Weekly Versus Every-Three-Week Chemotherapy

Ref.	Regimen	Patient number	Overall response (%)	Median survival	2-Year survival (%)
Sculier (17)	Weekly[a]	98	69	49 weeks	8.5
	Every 3 weeks[b]	101	62	43 weeks	7.9
Souhami (18)	Weekly[c]	221	82.3	10.8 months	11.8
	Every 3 weeks[d]	217	81.1	10.6 months	11.7
Murray (19)	CODE	110	87	0.98 years	10[e]
	CAV/EP	109	70	0.91 years	10[e]
Furuse (20)	CODE, GCSF	114	84	11.6 months	8.5
	CAV/EP	113	77	10.9 months	12

[a] Doxorubicin, etoposide, cyclophosphamide, cisplatin, vindesine, vincristine, methotrexate.
[b] Cyclophosphamide, doxorubicin, etoposide.
[c] Ifosfamide, doxorubicin alternating with cisplatin, etoposide.
[d] Cyclophosphamide, doxorubicin, vincristine alternating with cisplatin and etoposide.
[e] Progression-free survival.

trial, 438 patients with either limited disease or "good prognosis" extensive disease were randomized to receive 12 weekly cycles of ifosfamide and doxorubicin alternating weekly with cisplatin and etoposide or six cycles of CAV alternating every 3 weeks with EP. Thoracic irradiation was administered only to limited-stage patients in complete or partial response. There were no reported differences in overall response rates (82.3% and 81.1%), median survival (10.8 months and 10.6 months), or 2-year survival rates (11.8% and 11.7%). Hematological toxicity was greater in the weekly-chemotherapy arm and the ratio of intended/delivered dose intensity was greater in the standard arm.

In both the EORTC and U.K. trials the chemotherapeutic agents differed between the two treatment arms. Although the ability to deliver full intended doses was superior in the standard regimens, it was not possible to directly compare dose intensity between the regimens.

Canadian investigators reported promising results from a pilot study of a weekly regimen referred to as CODE: cisplatin (25 mg/m^2 for 9 consecutive weeks); vincristine (1 mg/m^2 weeks 1, 2, 4, 6, 8); doxorubicin (40 mg/m^2 weeks 1, 3, 5, 7, 9); and etoposide (80 mg/m^2 days 1–3, weeks 1, 3, 5, 7, 9) (21). Excluding cyclophosphamide, the CODE regimen contained the same agents and same total cumulative doses as the conventional alternating CAV/EP regimen but therapy was completed in 9 rather than 18 weeks. Thoracic and prophylactic cranial radiation therapy was also given to selected patients. These investigators were able to deliver close to full intended doses, thus achieving the goal of an approximately twofold increase in dose intensity for the four drugs common to the two regimens. A 2-year survival rate of 30% was observed, far superior to the historical rate of <5% in extensive-stage patients.

NCI Canada and SWOG collaborated on a phase III trial comparing CODE to conventional alternating CAV/EP in patients with extensive-stage SCLC (19). Greater than 70% of intended doses were delivered for both regimens. CODE patients received slightly higher cumulative doses of each of the four common agents but completed their therapy as intended in just 9 weeks rather than the 18 weeks targeted for control patients. Therefore, a twofold increase in the dose intensity of the four common agents was again achieved. Although rates of neutropenia and fever were similar, 10/110 CODE patients versus 1/109 CAV/EP patients died during chemotherapy. Response rates were higher for the CODE patients but progression-free and overall survival were not statistically different. In view of the increased mortality and a lack of survival benefit, CODE was not recommended.

In the Canadian pilot and intergroup phase III trials, CODE patients received aggressive supportive care but were not routinely treated with prophylactic colony-stimulating factor (CSF). Japanese investigators conducted a small randomized trial of CODE with or without granulocyte-colony stimulating factor (G-CSF) in patients with extensive-stage SCLC (22). Use of G-CSF resulted in increased mean total received dose intensity for all drugs, reduced neutropenia and neutropenic fever, and a significant improvement in survival. This led to a phase III trial designed almost identical to that of the NCI Canada/SWOG trial (20). A total of 227 patients with extensive-stage SCLC were randomized to receive either CODE + G-CSF or conventional alternating CAV/EP. CODE patients received G-CSF on nontreatment days. The achieved dose intensity for CODE + G-CSF was twice that of the CAV/EP regimen. The incidence of leukopenia was not different but anemia and thrombocytopenia were significantly increased in the CODE + G-CSF patients. The incidence of neutropenic fever was 18.8% versus 8.8% of patients in the CODE + G-CSF and CAV/EP arms, respectively, and 4/114 (3.5%) of CODE + G-CSF patients died from therapy-related causes. The response rate was slightly higher (77% vs. 84%) in the CODE + G-CSF arm, but there was no survival difference.

Even with a twofold increase in dose intensity and growth factor support, dose intensification with the CODE regimen yielded no survival benefit in extensive-stage patients. As demonstrated in the induction therapy trials, dose intensification with weekly therapy leads to excessive toxicity rates and no therapeutic advantages. Dose intensification has been well tested in patients with extensive-stage SCLC and no evidence for benefit has been observed.

COLONY STIMULATING FACTORS

As outlined in the preceding sections, the addition of a CSF allowed for dose intensification of the VICE and CODE regimens (15,22). Decreasing the dosing interval of VICE improved survival, but the addition of GM-CSF had no independent impact on this outcome. The initial Japanese CODE + G-CSF trial, reported by Fukuoka and colleagues, was designed to address dose intensity as the primary endpoint rather than survival. Therefore, only 63 patients were accrued, but median survival was superior for patients who received G-CSF (59 vs. 32 weeks, $p = 0.0004$). Several phase III trials have investigated the impact of CSFs on SCLC chemotherapy (Table 3) (15,22–29). The primary endpoint of most trials was the incidence of neutropenia and associated sequelae. Most were not designed to directly address the relationship between dose intensity and therapeutic outcomes. In the study described above by Steward and colleagues, dose intensity was increased by adding GM-CSF to the regimen but the addition of growth factor had no independent impact on survival (15). Likewise, when Woll and colleagues added G-CSF to the VICE regimen, they were able to increase dose intensity but the trial was not powered to accurately address survival endpoints (28). Pujol and colleagues treated 125 patients with extensive-stage SCLC with either a dose-intensive regimen containing high doses of cyclophosphamide, epidoxorubicin, etoposide, and cisplatin plus GM-CSF or the same chemotherapy at conventional doses without GM-CSF (24). Despite their attempt to improve

TABLE 3 Randomized Trials of Chemotherapy With and Without Colony-Stimulating Factors (CSF) in SCLC

Ref.	CSF	LD/ED	Attempt ↑ DI[a]	Effect on DI	Effect on toxicity	Effect on median survival
Pujol (24)	GM	ED	Yes	Decreased	Increased	Decreased
Steward (15)	GM	59% LD	Yes	Increased	None	None
Fukuoka (22)	G	ED	No	Increased	Decreased	Increased
Bunn (23)	GM	LD	No	Decreased	Increased	None
Hamm (25)	GM	Both	No	Increased	↓ Neutropenia ↑ Thrombocytopenia	None
Miles (26)	G	Both	No	None	Decreased	None
Crawford (27)	G	Both	No	NA	Decreased	None
Trillet-Lenoir (29)	G	Both	No	Increased	Decreased	None
Woll (28)	G	92% LD	Yes	Increased	Increased deaths	None

[a] An attempt was made to increase either doses or dose frequency in the CSF patients.
Dose intensity (DI); granulocyte-colony stimulating factor (G); granulocyte-macrophage-stimulating factor (GM); limited disease (LD); extensive disease (ED).

survival by increasing dose intensity with the aid of GM-CSF, these investigators reported decreased dose intensity, worse hematological toxicities, and inferior median survival (10.8 vs. 8.9 months, $p = 0.0005$) for the high-dose chemotherapy/GM-CSF-treated patients.

The Pujol data further corroborate the overwhelming evidence that attempting to intensify chemotherapy for extensive-stage patients is not beneficial, but is, in fact, harmful. However, the Arriagada and VICE data suggest dose intensification might be beneficial in limited-stage patients. Although the trial by Woll and colleagues was not designed to address a primary survival endpoint, they did demonstrate a statistically significant increase in 2-year survival (32 vs. 15%) in primarily limited-stage patients receiving dose-intensified VICE + G-CSF, even though median survival was not improved (69 vs. 65 weeks). Bunn and colleagues conducted a phase III trial in 230 limited-stage SCLC patients to determine whether GM-CSF could be used to reduce the incidence of neutropenic fever and hematological toxicities of combined chemoradiotherapy (23). All patients initially received etoposide 80 mg/m^2 and cisplatin 40 mg/m^2 days 1–3. Thoracic radiotherapy consisted of 45 Gy total delivered in 25 daily fractions of 1.8 Gy, 5 days per week, given simultaneously with the chemotherapy over the first 5 weeks. GM-CSF was dosed at 250 µg/m^2 subcutaneously twice daily on days 4–18 of each cycle of therapy. There was a statistically significant increase in the frequency and duration of life-threatening thrombocytopenia ($p < 0.001$), more nonhematological toxicity, more days of hospitalization, a higher incidence of intravenous antibiotic usage, more transfusions, and more toxic deaths in the patients receiving GM-CSF. There was no significant difference in median survival.

In summary, the addition of CSFs to chemotherapy in patients with SCLC can reduce the incidence of hematological side effects if chemotherapy is given at conventional doses. Chemotherapy dose escalation or the addition of concurrent radiotherapy to CSFs has resulted in increased toxicity and death rates in some studies. Considering the expense and inconveniences associated with the use of CSFs, the lack of benefit from dose intensification, and the intolerability of concurrent use with radiotherapy, the routine use of these agents in the management of SCLC cannot be recommended (30–32). This represents yet a third failed strategy to improve treatment outcomes with dose intensification.

LATE INTENSIFICATION CHEMOTHERAPY

Of the dose intensification strategies discussed thus far, only the CODE regimen yields a greater-than-twofold increase in dose intensity. Some type of hematopoietic stem cell support is needed to intensify therapy further. Late intensification has both scientific and clinical appeal (33,34). Because SCLC patients are often quite ill at the time of presentation they are often poor candidates for highly aggressive approaches upfront. Patients are generally in better medical condition to be considered for high-dose therapy following induction. Consolidation with high-dose therapy also allows for the prospective identification and selection of patients who are most likely to benefit—those with limited-stage disease, good performance status, and those who obtained a major remission with induction chemoradiotherapy (34). This approach has been studied by a number of investigators albeit rarely in a randomized trial. Humblet and colleagues reported the results of the only published multicenter randomized study testing late intensification chemotherapy in patients responding well to induction therapy (35). Autologous bone marrow transplantation was used to rescue patients from hematological toxicities. Of 101 patients receiving standard induction chemotherapy, 45 patients with chemotherapy-sensitive disease were randomized to receive one additional cycle of either high-dose cyclophosphamide, carmustine (BCNU), and etoposide or conventional doses of the same drugs. In this highly selected group of patients, median overall survival after induction therapy was 68 weeks for the intensified group compared to 55 weeks for the conventional therapy group, a difference that proved not to be statistically significant ($p = 0.13$).

In a large phase II study, the Southwest Oncology Group treated 58 limited-stage SCLC patients with induction chemoradiotherapy followed by high-dose cyclophosphamide (150 mg/kg) intensification and autologous bone marrow rescue (36). Only 21 patients completed the entire course of therapy, and there were seven treatment-related deaths, four of which occurred during late-intensification chemotherapy. Median survival for all patients was 11.1 months. Nine of the 21 patients receiving late intensification were alive in complete remission with a median survival of 27 months.

Dana Farber Cancer Center investigators employed high-dose consolidation chemotherapy in patients with limited-stage SCLC in partial or complete remission following conventional first-line chemotherapy (37). Patients received cumulative doses of 5625 mg/m^2 cyclophosphamide, 165 mg/m^2 cisplatin, and 480 mg/m^2 carmustine followed by thoracic and prophylactic cranial irradiation. Of the 36 patients treated in this phase II trial, 29 of whom were in complete or near-complete remission before high-dose therapy, 14 remained disease free at a median of 21 months after treatment. Actuarial 2- and 5-year disease-free survival rates were 53% and 41%, respectively. Morbidity was relatively low and most patients were able to return to full-time work. Although the results of this trial are provocative, patients were highly selected and accrued over a 9-year period. Furthermore, the median age of patients entered into this trial was 49 years, several years below the typical age of SCLC patients. There are few reports of similarly selected patients from which historical control data can be derived and compared. However, the SECSG reported a phase III trial involving a similar subset of selected patients (38). Patients with limited-stage SCLC were randomly assigned to receive either six cycles of induction chemotherapy with CAV or the same therapy with concurrent radiotherapy. Good-performance-status patients who had achieved an objective remission at the end of induction therapy were randomized to receive two cycles of consolidation etoposide and cisplatin or no further therapy. Twenty-six patients had received induction chemotherapy and radiotherapy and consolidation with etoposide and cisplatin. From the time of consolidation therapy initiation, these patients achieved a 2-year survival rate of 55%, almost identical to the results reported by the Dana Farber group.

The results with high-dose consolidation therapy in patients with SCLC have not been sufficiently promising to justify phase III testing. More compelling data are needed to generate enthusiasm for more extensive testing of this costly and toxic therapy in a disease that occurs primarily in elderly patients with significant comorbidities.

CONCLUSIONS

Dose-intensive induction therapy, weekly chemotherapy, attempts to intensify therapy with CSFs, and high-dose consolidation therapy have all failed to show a survival benefit for patients with SCLC. Intensification of therapy beyond that of conventional regimens has generally been harmful. A large body of clinical evidence indicates that further study of dose intensification strategies in extensive-stage SCLC is not justified and ethically questionable given the high rates of morbidity and mortality observed with this approach to date.

For patients with limited-stage SCLC, the available data suggest that survival is compromised when induction chemotherapy is given below the maximally tolerated doses of conventional combined-modality regimens. Intensification of induction therapy beyond this level in limited-disease patients has not been well studied and remains a legitimate area of research.

The utility of late intensification therapy for limited-stage SCLC is still not well addressed in randomized controlled studies. However, it is questionable whether pilot trials have generated sufficiently promising clinical evidence to justify phase III testing of this approach.

Based on an extensive body of clinical data, we can safely conclude that dose intensification with current agents is of no benefit and may even be harmful to patients with SCLC. Early intensification of therapy in limited-stage disease remains a legitimate area of research, but it is difficult to be optimistic given the futility of this approach in other disease settings. Unless new and significantly more active and non-cross-resistant agents are identified, substantial additional effort in this area of research is largely a waste of valuable patient resources.

REFERENCES

1. Matthews MJ, Kanhouwa S, Pickren J, Robinette D. Frequency of residual and metastatic tumor in patients undergoing curative resection for lung cancer. Cancer Chemother Rep 1973; 4(part 3):63–67.
2. Turrisi AT, Kim K, Blum R, Sause WT, Livingston RB, Komaki R, Wagner H, Aisner S, Johnson DH. Twice-daily compared with once-daily thoracic radiotherapy in limited small-cell lung cancer treated concurrently with cisplatin and etoposide. N Engl J Med 1999; 340(4):265–271.
3. Schabel FM, Griswold DP, Corbett TH, Laster R, Mayo JG, Lloyd HH. Testing therapeutic hypotheses in mice and man: observations on the therapeutic activity against advanced solid tumors of mice treated with anticancer drugs that have demonstrated or potential clinical utility for treatment of advanced solid tumors in man. In: DeVita VT, Busch H, eds. Methods in Cancer Research. Cancer Drug Development Part B. Vol. XVII. New York: Academic Press, 1979: 4–52.
4. Cohen MH, Creaven PJ, Fossieck BE, Broder LE, Selawry OS, Johnston A, Williams CL, Minna JD. Intensive chemotherapy of small cell bronchogenic carcinoma. Cancer Treat Rep 1977; 61:349–354.
5. Hong WK, Nicaise C, Lawson R, Maroun JA, Comis R, Speer J, Leudke D, Hurtubise M, Lanzotti V, Goodlow J, Rozencweig M. Etoposide combined with cyclophosphamide plus vincristine compared with doxorubicin plus cyclophosphamide plus vincristine and with high-dose cyclophosphamide plus vincristine in the treatment of small cell carcinoma of the lung: a randomized trial of the Bristol Lung Cancer Study Group. J Clin Oncol 1989; 7:450–456.
6. Johnson DH, Einhorn LH, Birch R, Vollmer R, Perez C, Krauss S, Omura G, Greco FA. A randomized comparison of high-dose versus conventional-dose cyclophosphamide, doxorubicin, and vincristine for extensive-stage small cell lung cancer: a phase III trial of the Southeastern Cancer Study Group. J Clin Oncol 1987; 5:1731–1738.
7. Ihde DC, Mulshine JL, Kramer BS, Steinberg SM, Linnoila RI, Gazdar AF, Edison M, Phelps RM, Lesar M, Phares JC, Grayson J, Minna JD, Johnson BE. Prospective randomized comparison of high-dose and standard-dose etoposide and cisplatin chemotherapy in patients with extensive-stage small-cell lung cancer. J Clin Oncol 1994; 12:2022–2034.
8. Hande KR, Oldham RK, Fer MF, Richardson RL, Greco FA. Randomized study of high-dose versus low-dose methotrexate in the treatment of extensive small cell lung cancer. Am J Med 1982; 73:413–419.
9. Figueredo AT, Hryniuk WM, Strautmanis I, Frank G, Rendell S. Co-trimoxazole prophylaxis during high-dose chemotherapy of small cell lung cancer. J Clin Oncol 1985; 3:54–64.
10. Arriagada R, Le Chevalier T, Pignon JP, Riviere A, Monnet I, Chomy P, Tuchais C, Tarayre M, Ruffie P. Initial chemotherapeutic doses and survival in patients with limited small-cell lung cancer. N Engl J Med 1993; 329(25):1848–1852.
11. Lowenbraun S, Birch R, Buchanan R, Krauss S, Durant J, Perez C, Mill W, Vollmer R, Ogden L. Combination chemotherapy in small cell lung carcinoma: a randomized study of two intensive regimens. Cancer 1984; 54:2344–2350.

12. Murray N. Importance of dose and dose intensity in the treatment of small-cell lung cancer. Cancer Chemother Pharmacol 1997; 40 (suppl):S58–S63.

13. Arriagada R, de The H, Le Chevalier T, Thomas F, Ruffie P, de Cremoux H, Martin M, Duroux P, Dewar J, Sancho-Garnier H. Limited small cell lung cancer: possible prognostic impact of initial chemotherapy doses. Bull Cancer 1989; 76(6):604–615.

14. De Vathaire F, de The H. Dose intensity of initial chemotherapy may have an impact on survival in limited small cell lung carcinoma. Lung Cancer 1993; 8:301–308.

15. Steward WP, von Pawel J, Gatzemeier U, Woll P, Thatcher N, Koschel G, Clancy L, Verweij J, de Wit R, Pfeifer W, Fennelly J, von Eiff M, Frisch J. Effects of granulocyte-macrophage colony-stimulating factor and dose intensification of V-ICE chemotherapy in small-cell lung cancer: a prospective randomized study of 300 patients. J Clin Oncol 1998; 16(2):642–650.

16. Cerny T, Anderson H, Bramwell V, Thatcher N. Pretreatment prognostic factors and scoring system in 407 small-cell lung cancer patients. Int J Cancer 1987; 89(February):146–149.

17. Sculier JP, Paesmans M, Bureau G, Dabouis G, Libert P, Vandermoten G, Van Cutsem O, Berchier MC, Ries F, Michel J, Sergysels R, Mommen P, Klastersky J. Multiple drug weekly chemotherapy versus combination regimen in small cell lung cancer: a phase III randomized study conducted by the European Lung Cancer Working Party. J Clin Oncol 1993; 11:1858–1865.

18. Souhami RL, Rudd R, Ruiz de Elvira M-C, James L, Gower N, Harper PG, Tobias JS, Partridge MR, Davison AG, Trask C, Spiro SG. Randomized trial comparing weekly versus 3-week chemotherapy in small cell lung cancer: a Cancer Research Campaign trial. J Clin Oncol 1994; 12:1806–1813.

19. Murray N, Shepherd F, James K, Zee B, Lantgleben A, Kraut M, Bearden J, Goodwin JW, Grafton C, Turrisi A, Walde D, Croft H, Osoba D, Ottaway J, Gandara D. A randomized study of CODE versus alternating CAV/EP for extensive stage small cell lung cancer: an intergroup study of the National Cancer Institute of Canada Clinical Trials Group and the Southwest Oncology Group. J Clin Oncol 1999; 17:2300–2308.

20. Furuse K, Fukuoka M, Nishiwaki Y, Kurita Y, Watanabe K, Noda K, Ariyoshi Y, Tamura T, Saijo N. Phase III study of intensive weekly chemotherapy with recombinant human granulocyte colony-stimulating factor versus standard chemotherapy in extensive-disease small-cell lung cancer. The Japan Clinical Oncology Group. J Clin Oncol 1998; 16(6):2126–2132.

21. Murray N, Shah A, Osoba D, Page R, Karsai H, Grafton C, Goddard K, Fairley R, Voss N. Intensive weekly chemotherapy for the treatment of extensive-stage small cell lung cancer. J Clin Oncol 1991; 9:1632–1638.

22. Fukuoka M, Masuda N, Negoro S, Matsui K, Yana T, Kudoh S, Kusunoki Y, Takada M, Kawahara M, Ogawara M, Kodama N, Kubota K, Furuse K. CODE chemotherapy with and without granulocyte colony-stimulating factor in small-cell lung cancer. Br J Cancer 1997; 75(2):306–309.

23. Bunn PA, Jr., Crowley J, Kelly K, Hazuka MB, Beasley K, Upchurch C, Livingston R. Chemoradiotherapy with or without granulocyte-macrophage colony-stimulating factor in the treatment of limited-stage small-cell lung cancer: a prospective phase

III randomized study of the Southwest Oncology Group. J Clin Oncol 1995; 13(7): 1632–1641.

24. Pujol JL, Douillard JY, Riviere A, Quoix E, Lagrange JL, Berthaud P, Bardonnet-Comte M, Polin V, Gautier V, Milleron B, Chomy F, Chomy P, Spaeth D, Le Chevalier T. Dose-intensity of a four-drug chemotherapy regimen with or without recombinant human granulocyte-macrophage colony-stimulating factor in extensive-stage small-cell lung cancer: a multicenter randomized phase III study. J Clin Oncol 1997; 15(5):2082–2089.

25. Hamm J, Cuffie C, Oken M, Risher R, Shepherd F, Kaiser G. Dose-ranging study of recombinant human granulocyte-macrophage colony-stimulating factor in small-cell lung carcinoma. J Clin Oncol 1994; 12:2667–2676.

26. Miles DW, Fogarty O, Ash CM, Rudd RM, Trask CW, Spiro SG, Gregory WM, Ledermann JA, Souhami RL, Harper PG. Received dose-intensity: a randomized trial of weekly chemotherapy with and without granulocyte colony-stimulating factor in small-cell lung cancer. J Clin Oncol 1994; 12(1):77–82.

27. Crawford J, Ozer H, Stoller R, Johnson D, Lyman G, Tabbara I, Kris M, Grous J, Picozzi V, Rausch G, Smith R, Gradishar W, Yahanda A, Vincent M, Stewart M, Glaspy J. Reduction by granulocyte colony-stimulating factor of fever and neutropenia induced by chemotherapy in patients with small cell lung cancer. N Engl J Med 1991; 325:164–170.

28. Woll PJ, Hodgetts J, Lomax L, Bildet F, Cour-Chabernaud V, Thatcher N. Can cytotoxic dose-intensity be increased by using granulocyte colony-stimulating factor? A randomized controlled trial of lenograstim in small-cell lung cancer. J Clin Oncol 1995; 13(3):652–659.

29. Trillet-Lenoir GJ, Manegold C, Von Pawel J, Gatzemeier U, Lebeau B, Depierre A, Johnson P, Decoster G, Tomita D, Ewen C. Recombinant granulocyte colony stimulating factor reduces the infectious complications of cytotoxic chemotherapy. Eur Cancer 1993; 29A:319–324.

30. Nichols CR, Fox EP, Roth BJ, Williams SD, Loehrer PJ, Einhom LH. Incidence of neutropenic fever in patients treated with standard-dose combination chemotherapy for small-cell lung cancer and the cost impact of treatment with granulocyte colony-stimulating factor. J Clin Oncol 1994; 12(6):1245–1250.

31. Chouaid C, Fuhrman C, Monnet I, Housset B. Routine use of granulocyte colony-stimulating factor is not cost-effective and does not increase patient comfort in the treatment of small-cell lung cancer: an analysis using a Markov model. J Clin Oncol 1998; 16(August):2700–2707.

32. Messori A, Tnendi E. G-CSF for the prophylaxis of neutropenic fever in patients with small cell lung cancer receiving myelosuppressive antineoplastic chemotherapy: meta-analysis and pharmacoeconomic evaluation. J Clin Pharm Ther 1996; 21(April):57–63.

33. Norton L, Simon R. Tumor size, sensitivity to therapy, and design of treatment schedules. Cancer Treat Rep 1977; 61:1307–1317.

34. Elias A. Dose-intensive therapy in lung cancer. In: Armitage JAK, ed. High-Dose Cancer Therapy. Baltimore: Williams & Wilkins, 1995:824–846.

35. Humblet Y, Symann M, Bosly A, Delaunois L, Francis C, Machiels J, Beauduin M, Doyen C, Weynants P, Longueville J, Prignot J. Late intensification chemotherapy

with autologous bone marrow transplantation in selected small cell carcinoma of the lung: a randomized study. J Clin Oncol 1987; 5:1864–1873.

36. Goodman GE, Crowley J, Livingston RB, Rivkin SE, Albain K, McCulloch JH. Treatment of limited small cell lung cancer with concurrent etoposide/cisplatin and radiotherapy followed by intensification with high-dose cyclophosphamide: a Southwest Oncology Group study. J Clin Oncol 1991; 9:453–457.

37. Elias A, Skarin A, Wheeler C, McCauley M, Ayash L, Richardson P, Schnipper L, Antman K, Frei E. Dose-intensive therapy for limited-stage small-cell lung cancer: Long-term outcome. J Clin Oncol 1999; 17(April):1175–1184.

38. Johnson DH, Bass D, Einhorn LH, Crawford J, Perez CA, Bartolucci A, Omura GA, Greco FA. Combination chemotherapy with or without thoracic radiotherapy in limited-stage small-cell lung cancer: a randomized trial of the Southeastern Cancer Study Group. J Clin Oncol 1993; 11(7):1223–1229.

9

The Role of Surgery in SCLC

Frances A. Shepherd
University of Toronto and Princess Margaret Hospital, Toronto, Ontario, Canada

HISTORICAL PERSPECTIVE

Twenty to twenty-five percent of all primary bronchogenic carcinomas are of the small cell subtype. However, since dissemination to regional lymph nodes and/ or distant metastatic sites can be identified in more than 90% of patients at the time of initial presentation (1), these tumors represent less than 5% of cases in most surgical series. Furthermore, in the patients with apparently "limited"-stage or operable tumors, widespread micrometastic disease is likely present, and these subclinical deposits have the potential to proliferate if only local therapeutic modalities, such as surgery or radiotherapy, are employed. This explains why almost all surgical series from the prechemotherapy era reported 5-year survival rates approaching zero for patients with small cell carcinoma (2,3).

To assess the role of surgery in the treatment of small cell lung cancer, a prospective randomized trial was mounted by the Medical Research Council of Great Britain (4,5). Seventy-one patients were randomized prospectively to undergo surgery, and 73 to receive thoracic irradiation (30 Gy or more over 20–40 days). The median survivals for patients in the surgical and radiotherapy arms were 199 and 300 days, respectively (Figure 1). At 5 years, one surgical and three radiotherapy patients were alive ($p = 0.04$), and at 10 years, only the three patients in the radiotherapy arm remained alive. It was concluded from this study

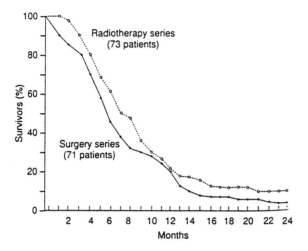

FIGURE 1   Survival in the two treatment series (all patients). (From Ref. 4.)

that radical radiotherapy was preferable to surgery, but that neither of the treatment policies was really effective. The investigators stated that it would be improbable that any advance in therapy could exert a significant effect on the death rate from this disease in the absence of successful smoking prevention programs. How true these words are, even today!

The results of this study led to trials of preoperative radiotherapy followed by surgery for patients with small cell lung cancer. Several prospective phase II trials showed that it was possible to combine these two local treatment modalities safely, but few patients achieved long-term survival (6–8).

The observation in the 1970s that patients with small cell lung cancer were dying from systemic metastases led to the hypothesis that chemotherapy might add to the effects of local radiotherapy. Bergsagel et al. from the Princess Margaret Hospital were the first to show a modest survival advantage with the addition of single-agent, low-dose cyclophosphamide (9). The British Medical Research Council Lung Cancer Working Party also showed that adding low-dose cyclophosphamide and 1-(2-chloroethyl)-3 cyclohexyl-1-nitrosourea (CCNU) to radiotherapy resulted in a significant prolongation of progression-free, but not overall, survival (10).

At the same time, other investigators were applying the same adjuvant-chemotherapy principles to surgical patients. In 1977, Shields reviewed the results of four Veterans Administration Surgical Adjuvant Group (VASOG) adjuvant chemotherapy studies, and undertook a separate analysis of the 148 patients (47%) in those trials who had small cell lung cancer (11). No survival advantage was seen for the patients in the chemotherapy arms of either of the trials that evaluated single-agent nitrogen mustard or single-agent cyclophosphamide. A small survival advantage was seen for patients in the chemotherapy arm of a three-arm trial in which patients were randomized to receive prolonged intermittent courses of CCNU and hydroxyurea or no further therapy (Figure 2).

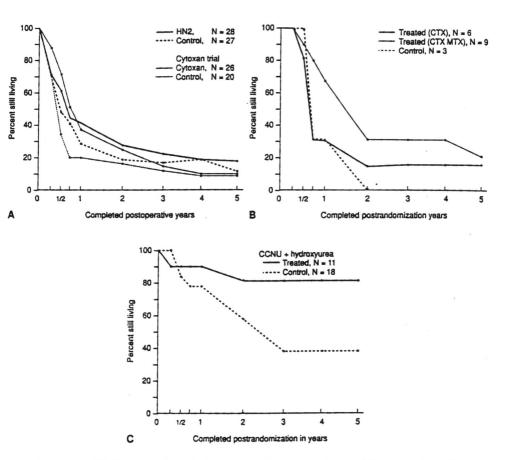

FIGURE 2   (A) Survival of treated and control patients with undifferentiated small cell carcinoma in the nitrogen mustard (HN$_2$) and cyclophosphamide (Cytoxan) adjuvant chemotherapy VASOG lung trials. (B) Survival of treated and control patients with undifferentiated small cell carcinoma in the prolonged intermittent cyclophospharide (Cytoxan, CTX) and methotrexate (MTX) adjuvant chemotherapy VASOG lung trials. (C) Survival of treated and control patients with undifferentiated small cell carcinoma in the CCNU and hydroxyurea adjuvant chemotherapy VASOG lung trials. (From Ref. 12.)

Shields and his colleagues also made other important observations from their analysis of the small cell patients in the VASOG trials (12). They demonstrated the importance of tumor, node, metastasis (TNM) staging, which has long been recognized to have prognostic significance for non–small cell lung cancer. Sixty percent of patients with $T_1 N_0 M_0$ tumors were alive at 5 years, whereas there were almost no 5-year survivors among the patients who presented either with T_{2-3} tumors or with mediastinal lymph node involvement (Figure 3). Patients with small stage II tumors had an intermediate 5-year survival of approximately 30%.

These observations suggested that there could be a small subpopulation of patients with small cell lung cancer for whom it might be appropriate to consider a surgical approach. In a retrospective review of 40 patients with small cell lung cancer who underwent potentially curative resection between 1959 and 1972, Shore and Paneth reported an overall 5-year survival rate of 25%. Four of 10 patients (40%) without nodal involvement achieved long-term survival compared to nine of 26 patients (25%) who had hilar or mediastinal nodal involvement (13).

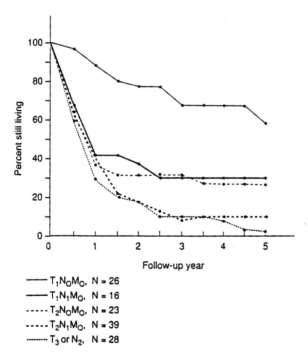

FIGURE 3 Survival, computed by the life table method, from postoperative day 30 (early trials) or from randomization (recent trials) by TNM classification for patients with undifferentiated small cell carcinoma who had undergone a "curative" resection in the VASOG lung trials. (From Ref. 12.)

Small cell lung cancer usually presents with a central mass associated with hilar and mediastinal adenopathy. Lennox et al. observed that patients who had large proximal tumors and who required a pneumonectomy were less likely to achieve long-term survival. The 2- and 5-year survival rates for patients who required only a lobectomy were 32% and 18%, respectively, compared to 14.4% and 7.2% for pneumonectomy patients (14). It is unusual for small cell lung cancer to present as a solitary pulmonary nodule. In the VASOG review of solitary pulmonary nodules, only 15 patients (4%) were found to have small cell pathology, and 11 were able to undergo surgery (15). One-, 5-, and 10-year survival rates for those 11 patients were 63.6%, 36.4%, and 18.2%, respectively. Since most of these patients underwent surgery before the chemotherapy era, it may be assumed that approximately one-third were cured by their surgery alone as measured by survival at the 5-year mark.

From this historical review it is clear that local treatment, whether surgery, or radiation, or both, is inadequate therapy for small cell lung cancer. If surgery is to play a role, it must be in the context of a combined-modality treatment program with systemic combination chemotherapy.

RATIONALE FOR SURGERY

Improved Control at the Primary Site

Response rates of 80% or more are achieved with current chemotherapy combinations for small cell lung cancer, and complete clinical response is seen in approximately 50% of patients with limited-stage disease (16). However, most patients relapse shortly after discontinuing treatment, and the 2-year survival rate is 20% or less in most series. For patients with limited disease, the most frequent site of failure is the primary tumor and the hilar or mediastinal lymph nodes. In total, up to 50% of patients fail at the primary site, and for half of those patients, the primary site may be the *only* area of failure. Similar results have been found at autopsy. In a review by Elliott et al., residual tumor was identified at autopsy in the primary site in 64%, and in the hilar and mediastinal lymph nodes in 53% of patients with limited disease who had at some time achieved a complete clinical response (17).

Two meta-analyses of thoracic radiotherapy for small cell lung cancer have been published (18,19). The survival data for almost 2000 patients in 16 trials were available, and data on local control rates were available for nine studies. Both meta-analyses showed that thoracic irradiation resulted in a reduction in local relapse rate from 47.9% to 23.3% ($p < 0.0001$) (18). They also demonstrated a small but significant survival benefit for patients who received radiotherapy (18,19).

Based on the results of these meta-analyses, the standard therapy for patients with limited small cell lung cancer now consists of combination chemotherapy and thoracic irradiation with or without prophylactic cranial irradiation. Median survival longer than 20 months and 5-year survival rates of approximately 20% have been reported (16,20). However, even the most successful combined-modality treatment programs report isolated initial relapse at the primary site in 20–25% of patients, and a cumulative risk of recurring locally of 50% (20).

This high local failure rate led several investigators to question whether surgical resection would result in improved local control. They postulated that control of bulk disease in the chest by surgery and eradication of low-volume micrometastatic disease by systemic chemotherapy would result in an increased cure rate. Small studies from several centers suggested that this might, indeed, be the case. The University of Toronto Lung Oncology Group reported only two local recurrences in 35 patients treated with combined-modality therapy that included surgical resection (21). Similar results were reported by Comis et al., who observed no local recurrences in 16 patients who underwent adjuvant surgical resection after induction chemotherapy (22).

Mixed Histology Tumors

In approximately 5–10% of cases, small cell lung cancer is found in combination with other histologies such as adenocarcinoma or squamous cell carcinoma (23). Investigators for the Eastern Cooperative Oncology Group reported that mixed-histology tumors were more likely to present as peripheral lesions on chest x-ray, although they found that all other clinical characteristics were similar to those of the pure small cell lung cancer patients (24). Surgical series of small cell lung cancer report higher percentages of mixed histological tumors. The University of Toronto Lung Oncology Group reported mixed histology in 14 of 79 patients (17.7%) who underwent initial surgery followed by adjuvant chemotherapy, and in three of 40 patients (7.5%) who had surgical resections after induction chemotherapy (25).

Since non–small cell lung cancers are relatively insensitive to chemotherapy, they are not likely to be controlled by systemic treatment. Thus, it may be appropriate to consider a combined-modality treatment program for patients with mixed-histology tumors if they meet standard surgical criteria and have no evidence of extrathoracic spread.

Late Recurrence After Successful Treatment of Small Cell Lung Cancer

Several reviews have now suggested that long-term survivors of small cell lung cancer are at high risk of developing second primary tumors, in particular second primary lung cancers (26–30). Although the patient population at risk for these second tumors is low because of the low cure rate for small cell lung cancer, clinicians seeing patients in follow-up must be aware that a new lesion on chest x-ray may not represent relapse, but may be a new tumor of different histology.

Such patients should be investigated as any other patient who is presenting with a lung mass for the first time. Histological or cytological confirmation of malignancy should be obtained, and if non–small cell lung cancer pathology is found, further workup should be directed at determining operability since surgical resection has the potential to be curative for some patients.

ADJUVANT CHEMOTHERAPY FOLLOWING SURGICAL RESECTION

The favorable results reported in Shields's review of the VASOG trials led several investigators to administer combination chemotherapy to all patients following complete resection of small cell lung cancer. A summary of 11 such trials is shown in Table 1 (12,31–42). All of the studies were retrospective reviews and suffer from the inherent weaknesses of any retrospective assessment of a treatment policy.

Frequently surgery was undertaken for patients in these series because a preoperative diagnosis of small cell lung cancer had not been made. For some, it had not been possible to obtain adequate tissue for any malignant diagnosis, and for others a preoperative diagnosis of non–small cell lung cancer had been made. Some of those patients were found subsequently to have mixed-histology tumors, whereas others had pure small cell tumors that had been incorrectly diagnosed preoperatively. Maassen and Greschuchna (36) reported that only 18 of 24 patients had a correct histological diagnosis of small cell lung cancer preoperatively. Similarly, the University of Toronto Group (37) found that a correct preoperative diagnosis of small cell cancer was found in only 18 of 63 patients. Postoperatively small cell lung cancer was seen in 54 patients and mixed-histology tumors in nine.

Most of the series in Table 1 included patients seen over a 10-or-more-year period, and frequently, multiple-chemotherapy protocols were employed. However, with the exception of the early trials reported by Shields et al. (12) and Hayata et al. (31), all patients were treated with combinations of drugs that would be considered adequate even today. The duration of chemotherapy treatment was also variable, and ranged from a single course of postoperative therapy, to multiple courses for up to 18 months. Most groups administered approximately six cycles of treatment.

In addition to postoperative chemotherapy, some centers also administered thoracic radiotherapy as well as prophylactic cranial irradiation. In view of the variability in radiation treatment, and incomplete reporting in several series, no conclusions can be drawn concerning the advisability of trimodality therapy.

Because so few patients with small cell lung cancer are surgical candidates, the TNM staging system is not generally applied to this subtype of lung cancer, and instead, patients are classified simply as having limited or extensive disease. The patients in the reviews summarized in Table 1 differ from limited-stage small

TABLE 1 Survival by Pathological Stage for Patients Treated with Adjuvant Chemotherapy After Surgery for Small Cell Lung Cancer

Author	Number of patients		Stage			Total
			I	II	III	
Hayata, 1978 (31)	Number		27	6	39	72
	Survival		26%	17%	0%	11% (5 yr)
Shields, 1982 (12)	Number		49	55	28	132
	Survival		51%	20%	3%	28% (5 yr)
Meyer, 1983, 1984 (32,33)	Number		6	4	10	30
	Survival		>50%	50%	0	? (5 yr)
Wada, 1995 (34)	Number		5	5	7	17
	Survival		37%[a]	—	33%	32%
Osterlind, 1986 (35)	Number		18	8	10	36
	Survival		22%	?	?	25% (3.5 yr)
Maassen, 1986 (36)	Number		41	19	64	124
	Survival		34%	21%	11%	20% (3 yr)
Shepherd, 1988 (37)	Number		19	24	20	63
	Survival		48%	24%	24%	31% (5 yr)
Karrer, 1990, 1991 (38,39)	Number		63	54	40	157
	Survival		61%	35%	35%	? (4 yr)
Macchiarini, 1991 (40)	Number		26	—	15 (T_3N_0)	42
	Survival		52%	—	13%	36% (5 yr)
Hara, 1991 (41)	Number		13	10	14	37
	Survival		64%	42%	10.7%	? (5 yr)
Davis, 1993 (42)	Number		11	16	5	32
	Survival		50%	35%	21%	36% (5 yr)

[a] Stage I and II combined.

cell lung cancer patients overall in that they all underwent pretreatment surgical resection, and therefore detailed pathological staging is available. The results show clearly that the TNM staging system is highly prognostic for patients with limited small cell lung cancer. In every study, the best survival was achieved by patients who had *pathological* stage I tumors, and the poorest survival was seen for patients with *pathological* stage III tumors (Figures 4 and 5) (38,39). For stage I patients, survival ranged from 22% at 3.5 years in the Danish series (35) to 61% at 4 years in the International Society of Chemotherapy LCSG. On average, it would appear that approximately 50% of patients with pathological stage I small cell lung cancer may be cured with a combined-modality approach that includes surgical resection and adjuvant combination chemotherapy. In the early trials, virtually no patients with stage III tumors achieved long-term survival. In the later reviews in which more aggressive combination chemotherapy regimens were employed, long-term survival ranged from 11% (36,43) to 35% (38,39). In all series, the survival of stage II patients was intermediate between that of patients with stages I and III. In fact, stage for stage, the survival rates are very similar to those seen after surgical resection of non–small cell lung cancer.

All of the studies that employed intensive combination chemotherapy reported survival rates that appear to be superior to the survival rates seen in patients

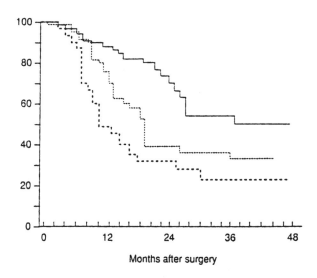

FIGURE 4 Life table survival curves for small cell lung cancer patients according to lymph node involvement. Patients with stage pT, N_0, M_0 disease (solid line), n = 63; pT, N_1, M_0 (dotted line), n = 51: pT, N_2, M_0 (dashed line), n = 32. (From Ref. 39.)

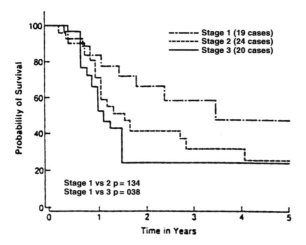

FIGURE 5 A comparison of survival by stage for patients treated with adjuvant chemotherapy after surgical resection for small cell lung cancer. (From Ref. 37.)

following surgery without adjuvant chemotherapy. Since it is likely that the improved survival is attributable to the postoperative chemotherapy treatment and not to improvements in surgical techniques or supportive care, it seems appropriate to recommend that chemotherapy be given to all patients who have undergone resection for limited small cell lung cancer. The short-term toxicity of such treatment is usually quite manageable and reversible, and the long-term toxicity is minimal. The Toronto Group recommend no more than six treatment cycles (37), since survival does not seem to be superior for patients in the retrospective studies who received 12–18 months of postoperative treatment (34,35). Whether fewer than six cycles may also be adequate is unknown. In the study reported by Hara et al. (41), 11 patients treated before 1981 received only one postoperative course of combination chemotherapy, and 26 patients treated from 1982 to 1989 received two courses followed by consolidation radiotherapy. Although the 5-year survival rates for patients with stage I and II tumors were excellent, only 10.7% of patients with stage III tumors were alive at 5 years. These results appear to be somewhat poorer than those achieved by other groups who administered a more prolonged course of adjuvant chemotherapy, although firm conclusions cannot be drawn from these retrospective analyses. Littlewood et al. (44) treated two young patients by pneumonectomy followed by a single course of very-high-dose chemotherapy and autologous bone marrow transplantation. Both patients relapsed, 118 and 80 weeks after treatment. It would appear, therefore, that a brief course (maximum six treatment cycles) of standard-dose combination chemotherapy should be the treatment of choice for patients.

It is not possible to state with certainty whether it is necessary to administer adjuvant chemotherapy to all patients. Shah et al. (45) reported 43.3% *actual* 5-year survival for 28 patients who underwent complete surgical resection without postoperative chemotherapy. More than half the patients in this study had peripheral tumors, and their survival was better than that of the patients who had central tumors. However, peripheral stage I small cell lung cancer is uncommon, as shown by the VASOG study of solitary pulmonary nodules in which only 15 of 309 patients were found to have small cell cancer (15). Their 5-year and 10-year survivals were 36.4% and 18.2%, respectively. The details of postoperative therapy, if any, for these patients were not provided, but it is likely that they did not receive aggressive combination chemotherapy. The 5-year survival rate is less than that reported by Shah et al. (45), and one can only speculate whether superior survival might have been achieved with the addition of combination chemotherapy.

It is not, on the other hand, possible to draw firm conclusions concerning the contribution of the *surgery* to the overall survival of these patients. It must be remembered that these surgical series included only a select subgroup with limited disease from which patients with adverse prognostic factors, such as supraclavicular adenopathy, bulky primary tumors with superior vena caval obstruction, and/or pleural effusions, were specifically excluded.

Surgery, if it does play a role in the treatment of small cell lung cancer, will do so by improving control at the primary site. Relapse patterns were reported in only seven of the trials reviewed (32,37,40–44), but the results from those studies suggest that surgery did, indeed, contribute to local control, since isolated local relapse was seen in only eight of the 201 patients in those studies (Table 2). It is still possible, however, that this high rate of local control was due only

TABLE 2 Pattern of Relapse for Patients with Small Cell Lung Cancer Treated with Surgery Followed by Adjuvant Chemotherapy

		No. of patients with relapse		
Investigators	No. of patients	Local only	Distant only	Both
Meyer, 1983 (32)	10	—	1	—
Friess, 1985 (43)	15	1	5	1
Littlewood, 1987 (44)	2	1	1	—
Shepherd, 1988 (37)	63	2	26	5
Macchiarini, 1991 (40)	42	2	24	—
Hara, 1991 (41)	37	2	?	—
Davis, 1993 (42)	32	—	15	2
Total	201	8	72	8

to the fact that the patients in these series had less locally advanced tumors and that the local control rate might have been equivalent with a combination of systemic chemotherapy and thoracic irradiation.

PROSPECTIVE TRIALS OF INDUCTION CHEMOTHERAPY FOLLOWED BY SURGICAL RESECTION FOR SMALL CELL LUNG CANCER

Phase II Trials

The encouraging results achieved with initial surgery followed by adjuvant chemotherapy led several groups to undertake prospective studies of systemic chemotherapy *followed by* surgery for certain patients with limited small cell lung cancer. The results of nine prospective phase II trials are summarized in Table 3 (46–54).

In all studies, patients received multiple courses of combination chemotherapy that included agents considered, even today, to be active against small cell lung cancer (cyclophosphamide, doxorubicin, vincristine, etoposide, and cisplatin). The number of preoperative chemotherapy courses ranged from two to six, and the overall response rate was greater than 88% in all studies except that of Baker et al. (49) in which only two preoperative courses of chemotherapy were given. This perhaps suggests that a longer course of induction chemotherapy is advisable, although in the small study reported by Benfield et al. (51) 88% of patients responded to treatment, and 100% were able to undergo complete surgical resection after only two courses of chemotherapy.

Not all responding patients in this series were eligible for thoracotomy after chemotherapy. On average, approximately 60% of patients were considered to have responded adequately enough for surgical exploration, and of those, more than 80% could be resected completely. When calculated from the total number of patients who entered the studies, however, the overall complete surgical resection rate was only approximately 50%. Not all studies reported surgical toxicity, but it does not appear that the postoperative death rate or complication rate was significantly increased by the preoperative chemotherapy. Only three postoperative deaths were reported (50,52,54), all in patients who had required a complete pneumonectomy. Other postoperative complications included infection, bronchopleural fistula formation, and reversible supraventricular tachycardias.

As would be expected, the complete pathological response rate was considerably lower than the clinical response rate. The rate ranged from 4% (50) to 37% (48) and on average was approximately 10%. It is of interest that this complete pathological response rate is very similar to that which has been reported in studies of induction chemotherapy followed by surgery for patients with locally advanced (stage IIIA or IIIB) non–small cell lung cancer (58).

TABLE 3 Prospective Phase II Trials of Induction Chemotherapy Followed by Surgery for Limited Small Cell Lung Cancer

Investigators	No. of patients	Clinical stage			Chemotherapy	Response CR/PR (ORR%)	Surgery: thoracotomy /CSR (%)	Complete pathological response (%)
		I	II	III				
Prager, 1984 (46)	39	2	12	25	CAVE × 2–4	13/21 (88)	11/8 (21)	2 (5)
Williams, 1987 (47)	38	—	—	—	CAE × 3	5/26 (82)	25/21 (55)	4 (11)
Johnson, 1987 (48)	24	3	7	14	CAV × 6 ± EP	? (100)	23/15 (62)	9 (37)
Baker, 1987 (49)	37	—	—	—	CAE × 2	1/19 (54)	20/20 (54)	2 (5)
Shepherd, 1989 (50)	72	21	16	35	CAV × 6 ± EP	27/30 (80)	38/33 (36)	3 (4)
Benfield, 1989 (51)	8	—	5	3	CAEV × 2	5/2 (88)	8/8 (100)	0
Zatopek, 1991 (52)	25	10	1	24	COPE × 3	10/14 (96)	14/10 (40)	5 (20)
Hara, 1991 (53)	17	4	6	7	Various	4/10 (82)	17/17 (100)	?
Eberhardt, 1997 (54)	46	6	2	38	EP	15/28 (94)	32/23 (50)	11 (24)

CR, complete response; PR, partial response; ORR, overall response rate; CSR, complete surgical resection; V, vincristine; E, etoposide; O, vincristine; P, cisplatin; C, cyclophosphamide; A, doxorubicin.

All investigators reported that survival was strongly dependent on TNM stage (Figure 6). Patients with stage I (T_{1-2} N_0) tumors had the best prognosis with 5-year survival rates that approached 70% for completely resected patients. Stage II and III patients fared less well, but all series reported a small number of patients with stage IIIA tumors (N_2) who achieved long-term survival and appeared to be cured by their combined-modality treatment program. The median survival for the entire group of patients who entered the trials (including those who did not proceed to thoracotomy) was reported for only six studies, and ranged from 13 to 33 months (47,48,50–52,54). Several authors reported the highest cure rate for patients who required only a lobectomy (47,54), although this was not confirmed by all authors (46,48). Almost no long-term survival was seen in patients who had unresectable tumors at the time of thoracotomy. Patients who achieved a complete pathological response and who had no viable tumor identified at thoracotomy had the best survival. Williams et al. (47) reported that all patients who had pathological complete response (five) were cured of their tumors compared to only 20% of patients who were operable but had gross or microscopic evidence of residual cancer.

Local relapse rates ranged from 0% (46) to 40% of completely resected patients (49). Most series reported local failure rates that ranged from 10 to 20% for patients who were able to undergo successful resection (Table 4) (46–48,50–53,55,56,59). Local control was found to correlate with the degree of response to chemotherapy and the completeness of the surgical resection. If the 15% of

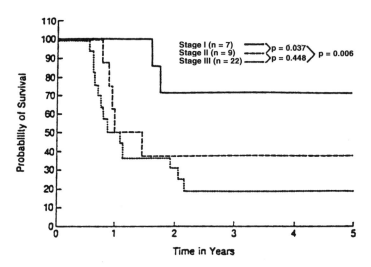

FIGURE 6 Comparison of survival by pathological stage for 38 patients with small cell lung cancer treated with adjuvant surgical therapy after chemotherapy. (From Ref. 50.)

TABLE 4   Pattern of Relapse for Patients with Small Cell Lung Cancer Treated
with Induction Chemotherapy Followed by Surgery[a]

Investigators	Thoracotomy/ CSR	Relapse pattern			
		None	Local only	Distant only	Both
Prager, 1984 (46)	11/8	4	—	4	—
Williams, 1987 (47)	25/21	12	3	6	—
Johnson, 1987 (48)	23/15	2	3	7	3
Shepherd, 1989 (50)	38/33	10	3	20	—
Benfield, 1989 (51)	8/8	2	—	6	0
Zatopek, 1991 (52)	14/10	5	—	5	—
Hara, 1991 (53)	17/17	10	3	7	—
Yamada, 1991 (55)	20/18	13	3	7	—
Muller, 1992 (56)	48/45	26	4	15	—
Total	204/175	106	19	70	6

[a] Excluding patients who did not have complete surgical resection (CSR) at time of thoracotomy.

patients who had unresectable tumors are added to those who relapsed locally, the real local failure rate rises to over 25% of the surgical patients.

These phase II trials led to observations that were important in the design of subsequent randomized trials of surgery for limited small cell lung cancer (57). They showed that combined-modality treatment was feasible and that the preoperative administration of chemotherapy did not result in excessive postoperative morbidity or mortality. It was recognized by all investigators that the favorable survival achieved in these trials might be due to patient selection. The Toronto group emphasized the importance of selection bias after their review of all limited-stage small cell lung cancer patients treated at their institutions over a 10-year period (58). They reported a significant survival advantage for patients who had no clinical evidence of mediastinal node involvement or pleural effusion. This group, which would be typical of patients who might be considered for surgery protocols, had a 20% cure rate with standard chemotherapy and radiation alone, compared to no long-term survival for patients with more advanced tumors.

Randomized Trials

In an attempt to determine whether the addition of surgery to combination chemotherapy and radiotherapy could prolong survival and improve the cure rate for patients with limited small cell lung cancer, the LCSG initiated a prospective randomized trial of adjuvant surgical resection in 1983 (59). Most patients with limited-stage tumors were eligible for this trial, even those with clinically evident mediastinal lymph node involvement. Induction chemotherapy initially consisted of cyclophosphamide, doxorubicin, vincristine, and etoposide but was changed to cyclophosphamide, doxorubicin, and vincristine alone in the later phase. In the absence of toxicity or progressive disease, patients received five preoperative cycles of chemotherapy. They were then restaged and medically assessed to determine their suitability for thoracotomy. At that point, eligible patients were randomized to receive either surgical resection followed by radiotherapy to the chest and prophylactic cranial irradiation or the same radiotherapy alone. A total of 340 patients entered the trial. Although the clinical response rate to chemotherapy was 68% (28% CR, 37% PR), only 144 (42%) of patients were randomized, 68 to receive surgery and radiotherapy, and 76 to receive radiotherapy alone. Of the 68 patients who were randomized to surgery, six did not undergo thoracotomy, but eight patients in the nonsurgical arm had off-study surgery, so a total of 70 thoracotomies were performed. Fifty-eight patients had some resection of tumor (83%) but only 54 had a pathological complete resection (77%). A complete pathological response was documented for 18% of patients who underwent surgery. Non–small cell pathology was found in 11% of patients. All randomized patients received radiotherapy to the chest, 50 Gy delivered over 5 weeks, and prophylactic cranial irradiation, 30 Gy over 3 weeks.

The median survival from enrollment for all patients was 14 months, and for the randomized patients it was 18 months, with no difference seen between the groups in either median survival or long-term survival (Figure 7). Because only half of the randomized patients in this study underwent surgical resection, it is not possible to compare survival based on pathological stage or TNM subgroup. The Toronto group were the first to draw attention to the discrepancy between clinical staging and pathological staging for patients with small cell lung cancer (25,50); they showed that clinical staging could not identify subgroups of patients with different prognoses (Figure 8). Similar results were found in the LCSG study in which patients were staged very carefully at the time of surgery. Clinical and surgical TNM stages after chemotherapy were the same in only 20 patients (29%) and most frequently patients moved into a more advanced stage (59). For the surgical group, no difference in *resectability* was identified for patients in any T or N subgroup although there seemed to be a trend toward unresectability for patients with T_3 tumors ($p = 0.08$). All pathological T and N subsets in the surgical patients had similar survival.

Why was survival not improved by surgery, and how should the results of this LCSG trial be interpreted? The survival curves shown in Figure 9 were generated on an ''intent to treat'' basis, which is, of course, mandatory for any prospective randomized trial. It should be noted, though, that 10% of the patients did not receive protocol-specified therapy. Six patients randomized to surgery declined operation, and of perhaps even greater significance, eight patients in the nonsurgi-

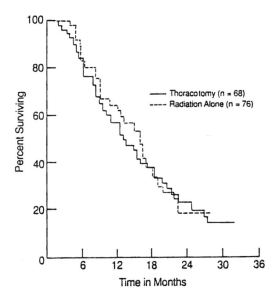

FIGURE 7   A comparison of survival for patients randomized to thoracotomy and radiation or radiation alone. (From Ref. 62.)

cal arm underwent thoracotomy and surgical resection. In such a small study, a 10% protocol violation of this nature may have masked a small, but significant, survival advantage between the treatment arms.

The next question to be asked is why complete surgical resection was possible for only three-quarters of the patients subjected to thoracotomy. Although the combination of cyclophosphamide, doxorubicin, and vincristine was considered standard therapy at the time, a disappointingly low response rate of only 65% was seen in this study. With newer regimens that incorporate etoposide and cisplatin and concurrent radiotherapy administered early in the course of the disease, response rates of 90% or more are standard (16,20). One might speculate, therefore, that a more complete response to chemotherapy might have resulted in a higher complete surgical resection rate.

Seventeen percent of patients underwent "open and closed" procedures with no attempt at surgical resection. For some patients the residual tumor was clearly unresectable at the time of thoracotomy. For other patients, though, the decision not to proceed to resection was based on scar tissue formation at the area of the primary tumor and in the mediastinum. Response to chemotherapy is often accompanied by an intense local scirrhous reaction, which makes surgical resection more difficult. Tumors that may appear initially unresectable because of fibrosis may, in fact, be resected safely with careful dissection of the tumor

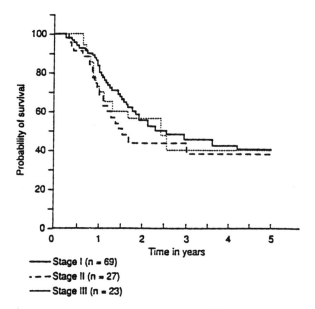

FIGURE 8 A comparison of survival by pretreatment clinical stage for 119 patients who underwent surgery for limited small cell lung cancer. (From Ref. 25.)

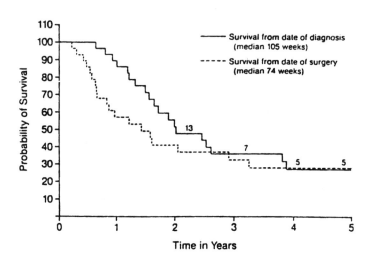

FIGURE 9 Survival of 28 patients who underwent salvage operations for small cell lung cancer. (From Ref. 60.)

bed and mediastinum. Because this was an international multi-institutional study, any individual surgeon operated on only a few patients. It is possible that had this been a larger study, the overall resectability rate might have been higher. This is suggested by the observation that the resectability rate was higher for LCSG surgeons than it was in other centers that joined the trial at a later date. This may have been due to their greater experience in operating on both small cell and non–small cell patients after induction chemotherapy.

Finally, patient selection undoubtedly played a large role in the ultimate results of this trial. All patients with limited disease were eligible to enter this study, with the exception of those who had supraclavicular lymph node involvement or pleural or pericardial effusions. Therefore, the majority of patients had stage III tumors. It has long been recognized that surgery has a limited role in the management of stage III patients with non–small cell lung cancer, and this trial suggests that the same is true for patients with small cell lung cancer. Since many, if not most, patients with limited small cell lung cancer have mediastinal node involvement (often bulky) at the time of initial diagnosis, it is clear that surgical resection will have very little role to play for the majority of patients with this disease. Nonetheless, it still remains possible that patients with early-stage disease (T_{1-2} N_0, and perhaps nonbulky stage II) may benefit from a combined-modality approach that includes surgery. Because so few patients fall into this subgroup (likely less than 10%) it will probably never be possible to undertake a prospective randomized trial to prove or disprove that surgery is appropriate in this setting.

SALVAGE SURGERY FOR PATIENTS WITH SMALL CELL LUNG CANCER

There are few treatment options for patients with small cell cancer who fail to respond to initial therapy, or who relapse after a primary response. Typically, only brief periods of palliation or prolongation of survival are achieved with second-line chemotherapy or radiation. This has led some investigators to evaluate whether surgery might be useful as salvage therapy for certain patients with limited small cell lung cancer.

Yamada et al. (55) operated on nine patients, two who had failed to respond to chemotherapy, six who had achieved partial response, and one complete responder. Four patients achieved long-term disease-free survival, which ranged from 3 to 11+ years. The Toronto group performed salvage operations on 28 patients, only 18 of whom were found on pathological examinations to have pure small cell tumors (60). Overall median survival of the 28 patients was 105 weeks, but only two pure small cell patients survived beyond 5 years (Figure 9). In view of these results, surgery cannot be recommended for patients with pure small cell tumors who fail to respond or who relapse after initial standard therapy.

Mixed-histology tumors are reported more frequently in surgical series (25,61). In the series of salvage operations reported by the Toronto group (60) 10 patients had mixed-histology or non–small cell tumors, and their median survival was 108 weeks. Four of the 10 patients (three stage I) achieved long-term survival after operation. Because a small number of patients with tumors of mixed histological type may be cured by surgical treatment, consideration should be given to a second biopsy for patients who have *localized* resistant small cell lung cancer.

Several authors have now reported that long-term survivors of small cell lung cancer are at increased risk of developing second primary tumors (26–30). In fact, a long-term survivor is more likely to have a second primary malignancy than a relapse of small cell lung cancer, and many of these tumors arise in the lung. In the University of Toronto series, eight patients underwent surgical resection at the time of "relapse" following a long disease-free interval after initial treatment for small cell lung cancer. Two were found to have non–small cell tumors, and both achieved long-term survival after surgery. It is recommended, therefore, that a biopsy should be undertaken for long-term survivors of small cell lung cancer who develop a new lung lesion. If non–small cell pathology is documented, the patient should be staged completely, and surgery should be considered if the standard medical and surgical criteria for resection that would be applied to all patients with non–small cell tumors are met.

SUMMARY

It has now been shown that combined-modality therapy with surgery and chemotherapy is feasible, the toxicity is manageable, and the postoperative morbidity and mortality rates acceptable. Patient selection is important and the results of the LCSG trial indicate that surgical resection will not benefit the majority of patients with limited small cell lung cancer. The chances of long-term survival and cure are strongly correlated with pathological TNM subgroup, and the results suggest that consideration of surgery for patients with small cell lung cancer should be limited to those with stage I and perhaps some stage II patients. Therefore, before surgery is undertaken, patients should undergo full staging of the mediastinum including mediastinoscopy.

Surgery may be considered for patients with $T_{1-2} N_0$ small cell tumors, and whether it is offered as the initial treatment or after induction chemotherapy does not seem to be important, as shown by Wada et al. (34) and the University of Toronto group (28).

If a small cell tumor is identified unexpectedly at the time of thoracotomy, complete resection and mediastinal lymph node resection should be undertaken if possible. Chemotherapy should be administered postoperatively to all patients, even those with pathological stage I tumors.

Surgery likely has very little role to play for most stage II patients and virtually no role for patients with stage III tumors. Even though chemotherapy can result in dramatic shrinkage of bulky mediastinal tumors, the addition of surgical resection does not contribute significantly to long-term survival for the majority of patients as shown conclusively by the LCSG trial.

The final group of patients who may benefit from surgical resection are those with combined small cell and non–small cell tumors. If a mixed-histology cancer is identified at diagnosis, the initial treatment should be with chemotherapy to control the small cell component of the disease, and surgery should be considered for the non–small cell component. For patients who demonstrate an unexpectedly poor response to chemotherapy, and for patients who experience localized late relapse after treatment for pure small cell tumors, a repeat biopsy should be performed. Surgery may be considered if non–small cell pathology is confirmed.

REFERENCES

1. Hansen HH, Dombernowsky P, Hirsch FR. Staging procedures and prognostic features in small cell anaplastic bronchogenic carcinoma. Semin Oncol 1978; 5:280–287.
2. Martini N, Wittes RE, Hilaris BS, et al. Oat cell carcinoma of the lung. Clin Boll 1975; 5:144–148.
3. Mountain C. Clinical biology of small cell carcinoma: relationship to surgical therapy. Semin Oncol 1978; 5:272–279.
4. Working-party on the evaluation of different methods of therapy in carcinoma of the bronchus comparative trial of surgery and radiotherapy for the primary treatment of small cell, or oat-cell carcinoma of the bronchus. Lancet 1966; 2:979–986.
5. Fox W, Scadding JG. Medical Research Council comparative trial of surgery and radiotherapy for primary treatment of small cell or oat-cell carcinoma of the bronchus. Ten-year follow-up. Lancet 1973; 2:63–65.
6. Bates M, Levison V, Hurt R, Sutton M. Treatment of oat-cell carcinoma of bronchus by pre-operative radiotherapy and surgery. Lancet 1975; 1:1134–1135.
7. Levison V. Pre-operative radiotherapy and surgery in the treatment of oat-cell carcinoma of the bronchus. Clin Radiol 1980; 31:345–348.
8. Sherman DM, Neptune W, Weichselbaum R, Order SE, Piro AJ. An aggressive approach to marginally resectable lung cancer. Cancer 1978; 41:2040–2045.
9. Bergsagel DE, Jenkin RDT, Pringle JF. Lung cancer: Clinical trial of radiotherapy alone versus radiotherapy plus cyclophosphamide. Cancer 1972; 30:321.
10. Medical Research Council Lung Working Party. Radiotherapy alone or with chemotherapy in the treatment of small cell carcinoma of the lung. Br J Cancer 1979; 40:1–10.
11. Shields TW, Humphrey EW, Eastridge CE, Keehn RJ. Adjuvant cancer chemotherapy after resection of carcinoma of the lung. Cancer 1977; 40:2057–2062.
12. Shields TW, Higgins GA, Matthews MG, Keehn RJ. Surgical resection in the management of small cell carcinoma of the lung. J Thorac Cardiovasc Surg 1982; 84:481–488.

13. Shore DF, Paneth M. Survival after resection of small cell carcinoma of the bronchus. Thorax 1987; 35:819–822.
14. Lennox SC, Flavell G, Pollock DJ, Thompson VC, Wilkins JL. Results of resection for oat-cell carcinoma of the lung. Lancet 1968; 2:925–927.
15. Higgins GS, Shields TW, Keehn RJ. The solidary pulmonary nodule. Ten-year follow-up of Veteran's Administration–Armed Forces Co-operative study. Arch Surg 1975; 110:570–575.
16. Shepherd FA, The role of chemotherapy in the treatment of small cell lung cancer. Chest Surg Clin North Am 1997; 7:113–133.
17. Elliott JA, Osterlind K, Hirsch FR, Hansen HH. Metastatic patterns in small cell lung cancer: correlation of autopsy findings with clinical parameters in 537 patients. J Clin Oncol 1987; 5:246–254.
18. Warde P, Payne D. Does thoracic irradiation improve survival and local control in limited-stage small cell carcinoma of the lung? A meta-analysis. J Clin Oncol 1992; 10:890–895.
19. Pingnon J-P, Arriagada R, Ihde D, Johnson DH, Perry MC, et al. A meta-analysis of thoracic radiotherapy for small cell lung cancer. N Engl J Med 1992; 327:1618–1624.
20. Murray N, Coy P, Pater J, Hodson I, Arnold A, et al. Importance of timing for thoracic irradiation in the combined modality treatment of limited-stage small cell lung cancer. J Clin Oncol 1993; 11:336–344.
21. Shepherd FA, Ginsberg RJ, Evans WK, Feld R, Cooper JD, et al. Reduction in local recurrence and improved survival in surgically treated patients with small cell lung cancer. J Thorac-Cardiovasc Surg 1983; 86:498–504.
22. Comis R, Meyer J, Ginsberg S, et al. The impact of TNM stage on results with chemotherapy and adjuvant surgery in small cell lung cancer. Proc Am Soc Clin Oncol 1984; 3:226 (abstr C-884)
23. Hirsch FR, Osterlind K, Hansen H. The prognostic significance of histopathologic subtyping of small cell carcinoma of the lung according to the classification of the World Health Organization. Cancer 1983; 52:2144–2150.
24. Magnum MD, Greco FA, Hainsworth JD, Hande KR, Johnson DH. Combined small cell and non–small cell lung cancer. J Clin Oncol 1989; 7:607–612.
25. Shepherd FA, Ginsberg RJ, Feld R, Evans WK, Johansen E. Surgical treatment for limited small cell lung cancer. J Thorac Cardiovasc Surg 1991; 101:385–393.
26. Heyne KH, Lippman SM, Lee JJ, Lee JS, Hong WK. The incidence of second primary tumors in long-term survivors of small cell lung cancer. J Clin Oncol 1992; 10:1519–1524.
27. Tucker MA, Murray N, Shaw EG, Shepherd FA, et al. Second cancers related to smoking and treatment for small cell lung cancer. J Natl Cancer Inst 1997; 89(23): 1782–1788.
28. Sagman U, Lishner M, Maki E, Shepherd F, Haddad R, et al. Second primary malignancies following diagnosis of small cell lung cancer. J Clin Oncol 1992; 10:1525–1533.
29. Ihde DC, Tucker MA. Second primary malignancies in small cell lung cancer: a major consequence of modest success. J Clin Oncol 1992; 10:1511–1513.
30. Osterlind K, Hansen HH, Hansen M, et al. Mortality and morbidity in long-term

surviving patients treated with chemotherapy with or without irradiation for small cell lung cancer. J Clin Oncol 1986; 4:1044–1052.

31. Hayata Y, Funatsu H, Suemasu K, Yoneyama T, Hashimoto K, Doi O, Ohota M. Surgical indications for small cell carcinoma of the lung. Jpn J Clin Oncol 1978; 8:93–100.

32. Meyer J, Comis RL, Ginsberg SJ, Burke WA, Ikins PM, DiFino S, et al. The prospect of disease control by surgery combined with chemotherapy in stage I and stage II small cell carcinoma of the lung. Ann Thorac Surg 1983; 36:37–43.

33. Meyer JA, Gullo JJ, Ikins PM, Comis RL, Burke WA, DiFino SM, Parker FB. Adverse prognostic effect of N_2 disease in treated small cell carcinoma of the lung. J Thorac Cardiovasc Surg 1984; 88:495–501.

34. Wada H, Yokomise H, Tanaka F et al. Surgical treatment of small cell carcinoma of the lung: advantage of preoperative chemotherapy. Lung Cancer 1995; 13:45–56.

35. Osterlind K, Hansen M, Hansen HH, Dombernowsky P. Influence of surgical resection prior to chemotherapy on the long-term results in small cell lung cancer. A study of 150 operable patients. Eur J Cancer Clin Oncol 1986; 22:589–593.

36. Maassen W, Greschuchna D. Small cell carcinoma of the lung—to operate or not? Surgical experience and results. Thorac Cardiovasc Surg 1986; 34:71–76.

37. Shepherd FA, Evans WK, Feld R, Young V, Patterson GA, Ginsberg R, Johansen E. Adjuvant chemotherapy following surgical resection for small cell carcinoma of the lung. J Clin Oncol 1988; 6:832–838.

38. Karrer K, Denck H, Karnicka-Mlodkowska H, Drings P, Salzer GM, et al. The importance of surgery as the first step in multimodality treatment of small cell bronchial carcinoma. Int J Clin Pharm Res 1990; 10:257–263.

39. Ulsperger E, Karrer K, Denck H, ISC-Lung Cancer Study Group. Multi-modality treatment for small cell bronchial carcinoma. Eur J Cardio-Thorac Surg 1991; 5: 306–310.

40. Macchiarini P, Hardin M, Basolo F, Bruno J, Chella A, Angeletti CA. Surgery plus adjuvant chemotherapy for $T_{1-3}N_0M_0$ small cell lung cancer. Am J Clin Oncol 1991; 14:218–224.

41. Hara N, Ichinose Y, Kuda T, Asoh H, Yano T, Kawasaki M, Ohta M. Long-term survivors in resected and non-resected small cell lung cancer. Oncology 1991; 48: 441–447.

42. Davis S, Crino L, Tonato M, Darwish S, Pelicci PG, Grignani F. A prospective analysis of chemotherapy following surgical resection of clinical stage I-II small cell lung cancer. Am J Clin Oncol 1993; 16:93–95.

43. Friess GG, McCracken JD, Troxell ML, Pazdur R, Coltman CA, Eyre HG. Effects of initial resection of small cell carcinoma of the lung: a review of Southwest Oncology Group study 7628. J Clin Oncol 1985; 3:964–968.

44. Littlewood TH, Smith AP, Bentley DP. Treatment of small cell lung cancer by pneumonectomy and single course high dose chemotherapy. Thorax 1987; 42:315–316.

45. Shah SS, Thompson J, Goldstraw P. Results of operation without adjuvant therapy in the treatment of small cell lung cancer. Ann Thorac Surg 1992; 54:498–501.

46. Prager RL, Foster JM, Hainsworth JD, Hande KR, Johnson DH, Wolff SN, Greco FA, Bender HW. The feasibility of adjuvant surgery in limited-stage small cell carcinoma: a prospective evaluation. Ann Thorac Surg 1984; 38:622–627.

47. Williams CJ, McMillan I, Lea R, Mead DJ, Thompson J, Sweetenham J, Herbert A, et al. Surgery after initial chemotherapy for localized small cell carcinoma of the lung. J Clin Oncol 1987; 5:1579–1588.
48. Johnson DH, Einhorn LH, Mandelbaum I, Williams SD, Greco FA. Post chemotherapy resection of residual tumor in limited stage small cell lung cancer. Chest 1987; 92:241–246.
49. Baker RR, Ettinger DS, Ruckdeschel JD, Eggleston JC, McKneally MF, Abeloff MD, Woll J, Adelstein DJ. The role of surgery in the management of selected patients with small cell carcinoma of the lung. J Clin Oncol 1987; 5:697–702.
50. Shepherd FA, Ginsberg RJ, Patterson GA, Evans WK, Feld R. A prospective study of adjuvant surgical resection after chemotherapy for limited small cell lung cancer. J Thorac Cardiovasc Surg 1989; 97:177–186.
51. Benfield GFA, Matthews HR, Watson DCT, Colling FJ, Cullen MH. Chemotherapy plus adjuvant surgery for local small cell lung cancer. Eur J Surg Oncol 1989; 15: 341–344.
52. Zatopek N, Holoye P, Ellerbroek NA, Hong WK, Roth JA, Ryan B, Komaki R, et al. Resectability of small cell lung cancer following induction chemotherapy in patients with limited disease (stage II–IIIb). Am J Clin Oncol 1991; 14:427–432.
53. Hara N, Ohta M, Ichinose Y, Motohiro A, Kuda T, Asoh H, Kawasaki M. Influence of surgical resection before and after chemotherapy on survival in small cell lung cancer. J Surg Oncol 1991; 47:53–61.
54. Eberhardt W, Wilke H, Stamatis G, et al. Preliminary results of a stage oriented multimodality treatment including surgery for selected subgroups of limited disease small cell lung cancer. Lung Cancer 1997; 18(suppl 1):61 (abstr 235).
55. Yamada K, Saijo N, Kojima A, Ohe Y, Tamura T, Sasaki Y, Euguchi K, et al. A retrospective analysis of patients receiving surgery after chemotherapy for small cell lung cancer. Jpn J Clin Oncol 1991; 21:39–46.
56. Muller LC, Salzer GM, Huber H, Prior C, Ebner I, Frommhold H, Prauer H-W. Multimodal therapy of small cell lung cancer in TNM stages I–IIIa. Ann Thorac Surg 1992; 54:493–497.
57. Shepherd FA. Induction chemotherapy for locally advanced non–small cell lung cancer. Ann Thorac Surg 1993; 55:1585–1592.
58. Shepherd FA, Ginsberg RJ, Haddad R, et al. Importance of clinical staging in limited small cell lung cancer: a valuable system to separate prognostic subgroups. J Clin Oncol 1993; 8:1592–1597.
59. Lad T, Piantadosi S, Thomas P, Payne D, Ruckdeschel J, Giaccone G. A prospective randomized trial to determine the benefit of surgical resection of residual disease following response of small cell lung cancer to combination chemotherapy. Chest 1994; (suppl 6):3205–3235.
60. Shepherd FA, Ginsberg RJ, Patterson GA, Feld R, Goss PE, Pearson FG, Todd TJR, et al. Is there ever a role for salvage operations in limited small cell lung cancer? J Thorac Cardiovasc Surg 1991; 101:196–200.
61. Mangum MD, Greco FA, Hainsworth JD, Hande KR, Johnson DH. Combined small cell and non–small cell lung cancer. J Clin Oncol 1989; 7:607–612.
62. Shields TW, ed. General Thoracic Surgery, 4th edition. Baltimore: Williams & Wilkins, 1994.

10

Adjuvant Therapy for Resected Stages II and IIIA NSCLC: Pro

Ritsuko Komaki

University of Texas M.D. Anderson Cancer Center, Houston, Texas

INTRODUCTION

The role of adjuvant radiation therapy for completely resected non–small cell lung cancer (NSCLC) remains controversial. This is due to differences in the behavior of tumors and the extent of metastasis depending on the histology, adequacy of staging, and extent of surgery. These variations make it difficult to compare the results of local control, survival, and failure patterns. Nevertheless, in certain circumstances, radiation therapy does have a distinct role in the adjuvant treatment of selected patients with NSCLC.

Much of the published data includes outdated staging workup (without imaging of the brain, CT of the chest and upper abdomen), as well as suboptimal radiation therapy equipment (e.g., Co-60 or low-energy Linac accelerators), without postoperative CT planning. Without reviewing isodose curves, suboptimal doses delivered to the target volume may cause sublethal damage on malignant cells leading to tumor recurrence and/or excessive doses to the normal surrounding tissue, such as the lung, heart, esophagus, or spinal cord, possibly contributing to intercurrent death. Evaluating the benefit of adjuvant treatment requires long follow-up. There is little published data to date with adequate follow-

up after thorough staging workup, modern surgical techniques, advanced radiotherapy with CT-based planning, and/or 3-D conformal techniques, as well as
efficacious chemotherapeutic agents, in carefully selected patients who require
postoperative adjuvant treatment.

RATIONALE FOR ADJUVANT RADIATION THERAPY
FOR NSCLC

Surgery and radiation therapy (RT) can eradicate cancer cells if the cancer is
localized and patients can tolerate aggressive treatment. However, since patients
with lung cancer usually have a smoking history with compromised cardiopulmonary function, radical cancer surgery is not feasible for many patients. Adjuvant
RT instead of reoperation is a reasonable treatment choice for these patients who
have microscopic residual tumor in the form of positive margins or positive
lymph nodes after surgery.

In theory, hypoxic conditions exist in large epithelial tumors, making RT
less effective in patients with these tumors (1). However, as surgery can remove
hypoxic cells, the remaining microscopic cancer cells are potentially better oxygenated, and these can be eradicated by adjuvant radiation therapy. A more detailed explanation of the role of hypoxia in lung cancer is provided in another
chapter. In addition, as long as the volume and fractionation are reasonable, adjuvant RT for epithelial tumors is relatively free of serious side effects. This combination of factors makes adjuvant RT a reasonable choice in patients with possible
residual tumor.

FAILURE PATTERNS AFTER SURGERY

Approximately one-third of patients with NSCLC undergo surgery, and only one-
quarter of these patients are completely resected (with negative lymph nodes)
and do not require adjuvant treatment. The rest are candidates for adjuvant treatment due to positive margins, hilar lymph node involvement (stage II), or mediastinal nodal involvement (N_2, stage IIIA disease), according to the recent staging
system (2). Patients with mediastinal lymph node involvement (N_2) have a 5-
year survival rate of 15–30% (3,4). Patients with stage II disease (hilar or peribronchial nodal involvement) have a 5-year survival rate of 30–60% (5,6). Most
recurrences following curative complete resections are distant metastases. Adjuvant radiation therapy to the hilar or mediastinal lymph nodes has not, however,
led to an improvement in overall survival, according to the Lung Cancer Study
Group (LCSG) trial, although locoregional control was significantly improved
by postoperative RT compared with surgery alone (7).

There are no published clinical trials or retrospective studies, except for some
limited autopsy-based studies, documenting the cause of death. This stems from the

TABLE 1 Pattern of Failure After Surgery for Lung Cancer

Investigators	Tumor stage	No. of patients	Pattern of failure (%)	
			Local	Distant
Kotlyarov and Rukosuyev, 1991 (15)	All	542	12	18
Martini and Beattie, 1977 (10)	$T_{1-2}N_0$	110	0	18
Immerman et al., 1981 (13)	$T_{1-2}N_0$	77	12	27
	$T_{1-2}N_1$	22	41	23
Pairolero et al., 1984 (11)	T_1N_0	170	6	15
	T_2N_0	158	6	23
	T_1N_1	18	28	39
Feld et al., 1984 (12)	T_1N_0	162	9	17
	T_1N_1	32	9	22
	T_2N_0	196	11	30
Lung Cancer Study Group, 1986 (7)	N_{1-2}	108	20	30
Ludwig Lung Cancer Study Group, 1987 (14)	$T_{1-2}N_{0-1}$	1012	17	22
Medical Research Council, 1996 (25)	$T_{1-2}N_{1-2}$	154	47	67
The Groupe d'Etude et de Traitemant des Cancers Bronchiques, 1999 (24)	$T_{1-3}N_{0-2}$	355	28	26

fact that meticulous workup to detect all possible sites of recurrence after surgical resection for NSCLC is not routinely done at the time of follow-up. Instead, physicians tend to document only the first site of failure on the basis of obvious changes in radiological images or in symptoms or signs of the recurrence.

A further difficulty in assessing the patterns of failure in patients with resected NSCLC is that autopsies are done on few patients. Matthews and colleagues in 1973 reported the autopsy findings in 202 patients who died within 30 days after a curative resection of lung cancer. Interestingly, 22 of 24 patients who had residual cancer within the thorax had squamous cell carcinoma. This suggests that failure in the thorax occurs more frequently in patients with squamous cell carcinoma than in those with adenocarcinoma (8). In a series of 227 patients who underwent surgery for lung cancer, Rasmussen (9) reported autopsy data for 64 patients who died at least 2 months after surgery. Fifty-four (84%) of the 64 had residual cancer in the thorax. Twenty-three of the 57 patients with N_2 disease had autopsies, and residual cancer was found in the thorax in 20 (87%).

Several clinical studies (7,10–15) have analyzed the failure patterns after surgery in patients who did not receive adjuvant treatment for lung cancer; the findings are summarized in Table 1. According to these series, distant metastases appear to be a problem in most patients, although these were not autopsy series and these patients were not evaluated by computed tomography (CT) of the chest to investigate locoregional recurrence. The local recurrence rate reported was likely lower than reality because it is difficult to detect minimal or asymptomatic local recurrence on routine follow-up chest x-ray studies. When the patient develops symptoms or signs of locoregional recurrences, the disease is usually too advanced to be controlled. On the other hand, the incidence of distant metastases has likely been overestimated. Locoregional failure is not an uncommon event, and the risk of such failure appears to be related to the nodal status (7,10–12,14,15). Indeed, many studies do not report locoregional recurrences when patients die of distant metastases.

EFFICACY OF SALVAGE TREATMENT FOR LOCOREGIONAL RECURRENCE

If the salvage treatment for locoregional recurrence were efficacious, adjuvant treatment would not be a critical issue. However, to date, no efficacious salvage treatment exists for locoregional recurrence in the chest, whether additional surgery or a curative type of RT (with or without chemotherapy) has been attempted. Some authors have, however, reported that RT can be efficacious in controlling local recurrence after curative resection for lung cancer (16–18). The 2-year survival rate reported by these authors ranged from 5% to 28%. Most patients, however, had progression in the locoregional areas as the first site of failure after radiation therapy. Their cause of death after RT was locoregional progression, although no attempt was made to detect distant metastases (DM) at the time of death, if they were asymptomatic from DM. Patients with recurrences at the bronchial resection site had a better outcome, with a 2-year survival rate of 50% compared with patients with locoregional recurrence in the hilar or mediastinal nodal area.

PROSPECTIVE RANDOMIZED CLINICAL TRIALS

Adjuvant Radiotherapy

Table 2 compares the patient data reported for seven prospective randomized trials of postoperative RT versus observation (7,19–24). The majority of these studies were conducted in the pre-CT era, and many patients were treated with cobalt 60 or orthovoltage therapy.

Paterson and Russell (19) studied the efficacy of postoperative RT after pneumonectomy in 202 patients with or without lymph node involvement. After the pneumonectomy, patients were randomized to receive either 45 Gy in 4 weeks versus observation. The authors did not stratify patients by the tumor stage, nodal stage, or histological type. They also included node-negative patients treated by cobalt 60 or orthovoltage using large fields that encompassed a portion of the heart and the opposite side of the lung. Their 3-year survival rates were 36% without postoperative RT versus 33% with RT.

In the trial conducted by Bangma, patients were alternately (rather than prospectively) randomized to receive either postoperative RT or observation alone. All patients had early-stage cancer, and two-thirds had negative lymph nodes. Survival in patients who received postoperative RT (45 Gy over 5 weeks) was not statistically different from survival in the observation-alone group (20).

In 1979, Israel et al. (21) published interim results of the trial conducted by the European Organization for Research and Treatment of Cancer (EORTC). This trial included two arms in which patients were consecutively randomized to receive either adjuvant local treatment or systemic treatment. This trial included only patients with squamous cell carcinoma with or without postoperative thoracic RT (total dose of 45 Gy over 4.5 weeks to the mediastinum). After the completion of thoracic RT, patients were randomized to undergo observation or to receive one of the following systemic treatments: chemotherapy, such as cyclophosphamide, methotrexate, and lomustine; immunotherapy, such as bacille Calmette Guérin; or chemotherapy and immunotherapy together. The 1979 interim analysis showed that patients receiving adjuvant chemotherapy had a significantly lower survival than those in the immunotherapy or observation groups. Although postoperative RT did not improve survival, it did reduce locoregional relapses, especially in patients with nodal involvement. Specifically 12 of the 104 patients (11.5%) who received postoperative RT developed local relapse compared with 26 of 126 patients (20.6%) who had surgery alone.

TABLE 2 Postoperative Radiotherapy for Lung Cancer: Prospective Randomized Trials

Investigators	Radiation dose	Equipment	No. of patients	Pathology	Surgery	Patient selection	Survival
Paterson and Russell, 1962 (19)	45 Gy/4 wk	Ortho	202	All	Pneumo	N_0, N+	NI
Bangma, 1972 (20)	45 Gy/4 wk	Co-60	73	All	All	N_0, N+	NI
Israel et al., 1979 (21)	45 Gy/4.5 wk	Co-60	392	Sq	All	N_0, N+	NI
van Houtte et al., 1980 (22)	60 Gy/6 wk	Co-60	224	All	All	N_0	NI
Lung Cancer Study Group, 1986 (7)	50 Gy/5 wk	Co-60	230	Sq	All	N+	LCI
MRC, 1996 (25)	40 Gy/3 wk	Co-60/LA	308	NSC	All	N+	LCI
GETCB, 1999 (24)	60 Gy/6 wk	Co-60/LA	728	All	All	N_0, N+	NI

NSC: non–small cell; Sq: squamous cell; NI: no improvement; LCI: local control improved; MRC: Medical Research Council Lung Working Party; GETCB: Groupe d'Etude et de Traitemant des Cancers Bronchiques; Ortho: orthovoltage; LA: linear accelerator.

Van Houtte and colleagues conducted a randomized study in patients without lymph node metastasis (N_0) who had T_1, T_2, or T_3 lesions and underwent complete surgical resection of the primary tumor. Postoperative RT was associated with a slight decrease in the rate of locoregional recurrence within the irradiated field from 18% to 13%. Survival, however, was inferior in the patients who received postoperative RT, especially those patients who had a pneumonectomy. There was also a high rate of radiation-induced late effects, such as cardiac toxicity. This adverse effect appeared to be related to use of a cobalt 60 unit that delivered 60 Gy in 6 weeks employing a three-field technique, without correction for lung inhomogeneity. Very large fields were also used to irradiate mediastinal nodes, including a large portion of the heart. A further problem was that there was no CT-based treatment planning capability available at that time (22).

The LCSG conducted a randomized study to evaluate postoperative radiation therapy in patients with completely resected stage II and stage IIIA squamous cell carcinoma of the lung. Patients were randomized after complete resection to an observation-only group or a RT group that received a total tumor dose of 50 Gy in 5 weeks (7). Only patients with squamous cell carcinoma who had disease in either the hilar lymph nodes (N_1) or the mediastinal lymph nodes (N_2) were included in the study. Patients received 50 Gy in 5 weeks using a cobalt 60 unit or a Linac accelerator. Although there was no difference in overall survival between the two groups, the patients who received postoperative RT had a significant reduction in the incidence of local recurrence (1%) compared with those who were observed postoperatively (19%) ($p = 0.05$). The reduction in the incidence of locoregional recurrence was especially pronounced in patients with N_2 disease.

The British Medical Research Council (MRC) (25) conducted a randomized study in 308 patients with pathologically staged T_1 or T_2 NSCLC who had positive hilar or mediastinal lymph nodes. They were randomized either to undergo observation or to receive a total dose of postoperative RT to 40 Gy in 3 weeks using a cobalt 60 or low-energy linear accelerator. Postoperative RT was associated with improved locoregional recurrence-free survival in a subset group (106 patients) with T_2N_2 NSCLC. The 2-year survival rate in the group was 46% as compared with 27% in the observation group. However, there was no significant difference in overall survival rate between the two groups. The most significant difference between the observation and postoperative RT groups was in the incidence of distant metastases. There was a highly significant increase in the incidence of bone metastases in N_2 patients in the observation group over the 3–4 years following treatment. There was no significant difference in the incidence of local recurrence among the patients with pathological N_1 disease with or without postoperative RT.

A prospective multicenter randomized trial assessed the value of postoperative RT after complete tumor resection in patients with NSCLC in Europe (24).

There were 728 patients with NSCLC (221 stage I, 180 stage II, and 327 stage III) in the study, and they were randomized to receive either postoperative RT or observation only. There were 303 patients who had a pneumonectomy and 425 patients who were treated by lobectomy. Patients were assigned to a study group within 1 month of complete resection, although it is not clear exactly when the RT was initiated. The RT was administered by cobalt 60 or higher energy for a total dose of 60 Gy over 6 weeks. The total dose was prescribed at the isocenter, without inhomogeneity calculation. The daily fraction was also higher than the usual fraction size (1.8–2.0 Gy per fraction) at 2.5 Gy per fraction, when a high-energy photon source (of more than 10 MV) was used. The first 40 Gy in the initial 4 weeks encompassed the bronchial stump, ipsilateral hilum, upper and middle mediastinum, and supraclavicular area. This was followed by 20 Gy in 2 weeks delivered by lateral or oblique fields to avoid the spinal cord. Computer dosimetry was recommended but not required. At the conclusion of the study period, 218 of 355 patients (61%) in the observation group and 262 of the 373 patients (70%) in the postoperative RT group had died. The 5-year overall survival was 43% in the observation group and 30% in the RT group ($p = 0.002$). This result was not altered following adjustment for potential prognostic factors. The excessive mortality rate in the postoperative RT group was due to excess of intercurrent deaths owing to a high incidence of intercurrent cardiac or respiratory complications, which accounted for 31% of the deaths in the RT group and 8% of the deaths in the observation group over 5 years ($p = 0.0001$). This study suggests that unnecessary and technically limited RT can cause treatment-related deaths rather than conferring any benefit. More than half of the patients did not need any postoperative RT since they had undergone resection and had stage I or II disease.

Adjuvant Radiotherapy With or Without Chemotherapy

One randomized trial (26) from the LCSG evaluated adjuvant therapy in patients with incompletely resected stage II or III NSCLC of all histological types. Incomplete resection was defined by the finding of either disease in the highest resected mediastinal node or positive surgical margins. A total of 172 patients were randomized to undergo either postoperative thoracic RT (40 Gy in a split course) or cyclophosphamide (Cytovan), doxorubicin (Adriamycin), and cisplatin (CAP) chemotherapy plus RT. CAP was administered every 4 weeks for six courses. Chemotherapy improved the median survival from 13 months to 20 months and improved the median time to recurrence from 8 months to 14 months. Also, the survival rate at 1 year improved by 14%, from 54% to 68%, in the adjuvant chemotherapy/RT group. Although the differences in median and 1-year overall survivals were not statistically significant, death due to cancer in the first postoperative year was significantly less in the group that received the combination of chemotherapy and RT ($p = 0.02$) (26).

In Intergroup Study 0015 (RTOG 91-05), patients with resected stage II (N_1) and stage III (N_2) NSCLC were randomized to receive postoperative RT alone or concurrent RT and chemotherapy. In this study, 488 patients were randomized between April 1991 and February 1997. Chemotherapy consisted of four cycles of cisplatin (60 mg/m^2/day 1) and etoposide (VP-16, 120 mg/m^2/day 1–3), and RT was delivered to a total dose of 50.4 Gy in 28 fractions (in a daily dose of 1.8 Gy). Patients were stratified by weight loss, histological type, nodal biopsy technique, and stage (N_1 vs. N_2). A total of 351 patients were eligible for analysis at a median follow-up of 37 months. A total of 121 of the 183 (66%) patients in the combination therapy group received four cycles of chemotherapy, while 139 of the 183 patients (76%) in the RT group received the planned RT. Treatment-associated mortality was 2.2% in the chemotherapy/RT arm and 2.4% in the RT arm. The median survival in the RT arm was 41.1 months, and it was 38.6 months in the chemotherapy/RT arm ($p = 0.99$). Analysis of the stratified subgroups showed no statistically significant advantage for either treatment arm. The conclusion was that adjuvant chemotherapy in combination with RT does not prolong survival in patients with completely resected stage II or III NSCLC over that in patients treated with RT alone (27).

RETROSPECTIVE STUDIES AND META-ANALYSIS

Retrospective studies have shown some benefit from postoperative RT in selected groups of patients. For example, postoperative RT proved beneficial in patients with locoregionally advanced disease (T_3, N_1, N_2, or N_3) from the standpoint of survival and locoregional control (Table 3). None of the studies listed demonstrated any significant benefit from postoperative RT (28,29) for patients who underwent complete resection of an early-stage tumor without positive lymph nodes (T_1 or T_2, N_0).

In retrospective comparisons of outcome in patients treated with surgery alone versus postoperative RT, Green and Kern (16), Ennuyer (28), and Chung et al. (30) observed a trend toward improvement in the 5-year survival rate in patients treated with postoperative RT. Green (29), Choi (32), and Sawyer (31), and their colleagues, reported a benefit from postoperative RT in patients with adenocarcinoma, suggesting that locoregional adjuvant treatment improves survival. The findings from these studies contrast to those from a more recent meta-analysis conducted by PORT (33) in which adjuvant RT was associated with a decrement in survival. From the retrospective studies, it appears that mostly patients with T_3 disease or positive lymph nodes benefited from postoperative RT. One of many drawbacks to the PORT meta-analysis is that it included mostly early stage and N_0 patients (7,10,13,14,16,28,30–32,34–40).

Table 4 summarizes survival data reported in the literature for patients with more locally advanced disease (T_3 disease and positive lymph nodes) and shows a wide range in survival depending on the treatment (surgery alone vs. postopera-

TABLE 3 Postoperative Radiotherapy for Locally Advanced Lung Cancer (T_3, N+): Results of Uncontrolled Studies

Investigators	Dose (Gy)	Pathology	Surgery		Postoperative radiation therapy		Survival
			No. pts.	Survival (%)	No. pts.	Survival (%)	@ year #
Ennuyer, 1963 (28)	60–65	Sq	42	26	37	40	2
Martini and Beattie, 1977 (10)	40–45	Sq			25	44	3
Green and Kern, 1978 (16)	50–60	All	30	3	66	35	5
Chung et al., 1982 (30)	46	All	29	9	38	39	3
Kirsh and Sloan, 1982 (34)	50–55	All	20	0	105	24	5
Astudillo and Conill, 1990 (37)	45–50	All	60	12	86	19	5
Durci et al., 1991 (38)	50–60	All	41	25	48	30	5
Reinfuss et al., 1993 (39)	50–60	All			37	38	5
Emami et al., 1997 (40)	50–60	Sq			62	29	5
Sawyer et al., 1997 (31)[a]	45–55	All	35	4	27	37	4

Sq: squamous cell.
[a] High-risk group for recurrence.

TABLE 4 Postoperative Radiation Therapy for Lung Cancer: Locoregional Relapses (T$_3$, N+)

Investigators	Surgery		Postoperative radiation therapy	
	No. pts.	Local relapse (%)	No. pts.	Local relapse (%)
Choi et al., 1980 (32)	32	53	41	31
Immerman et al., 1981 (13)	22	41		
Chung et al., 1982 (30)	29	48	38	8
Iascone et al., 1986 (35)	59	20		
Lung Cancer Study Group, 1986 (7)	108	20	102	1
Ludwig Lung Cancer Study, 1987 (14)	253	30		
Herskovic et al., 1988 (36)			64	19
Astudillo and Conill, 1990 (37)	60	12	71	19
Durci et al., 1991 (38)	41	36	38	45
Emami et al., 1997 (40)			150	20
Sawyer et al., 1997 (31)	136	LR 37 IM 58 HR 100	88	LR 20 IM 15 HR 11

LR: low risk; IM: intermediate risk; HR: high risk.

tive RT), histology, and the series. For example, Choi et al. (32) reported that postoperative RT was associated with a significant increase in survival in patients with adenocarcinoma, but not squamous cell carcinoma. In their 29 patients with squamous cell carcinoma who had positive lymph nodes but did not receive postoperative RT, the 5-year survival rate was 33%, identical to the survival rate in 46 patients with squamous cell carcinoma and positive mediastinal lymph nodes treated with postoperative RT. However, the 5-year survival rate in the 21 patients with adenocarcinoma treated with surgery alone was 8%, versus 43% in the 40 patients with adenocarcinoma treated with postoperative RT, with doses ranging from 40 to 56 Gy (32). Martini et al. (41) also suggested that postoperative RT was more beneficial for patients with positive regional lymph nodes who had adenocarcinoma than in those with positive nodes who had squamous cell carcinoma.

The average local relapse rate for the 11 studies summarized in Table 4 was 30% (ranging from 12% to 53%) in patients who underwent surgery alone (7,13,14,30–32,35–38) and 12% (ranging from 1% to 31%) in those who received postoperative RT (7,13,14,30–32,35–38,40). The key question as to whether local control will translate into an improvement in survival remains controversial. It is critical to assess biomarkers and underlying risk factors in such patients to determine which patients will potentially benefit most from postoperative RT (10,16,28,30,32,34,37–39,42,43).

Despite these findings, a recent meta-analysis of nine randomized trials from the same group revealed a significant survival decrement in patients who received postoperative RT (33). However, this meta-analysis included node-negative patients in whom postoperative radiation is not indicated. Indeed, the use of postoperative RT in such node-negative patients adversely affected survival, especially when cobalt 60 teletherapy was utilized with large fields (22). Few, if any, contemporary clinical investigators would now prescribe RT for such patients with negative nodes. Another problem in interpreting the findings from some of the trials included in this meta-analysis is that, in the absence of CT of the chest, it would have been difficult to localize the positive nodal area in the mediastinum or hilar region, in patients status postpneumonectomy. In addition, anterior/posterior rectangular fields with cobalt 60 were often employed, leading to potential "hot spots" over the spinal cord and esophagus, as well as the anterior portion of the heart (Figure 1A). Indeed, cobalt 60 is no longer considered an acceptable modality for the treatment of patients with thoracic malignancies due to the inhomogeneous dose distribution compared to higher-energy linear accelerators (Linac) (Figure 1B). This meta-analysis also incorporated patients who were treated in the 1960s when adequate staging was not done (33). Without adequate staging, including CT of the chest and upper abdomen, CT or MRI of the brain, and bone scan, it is difficult to evaluate the efficacy of local control from the standpoint of survival. It is often difficult to ascertain the exact cause of death in a meta-analysis, owing to inconsistency in the reporting or analysis of the data.

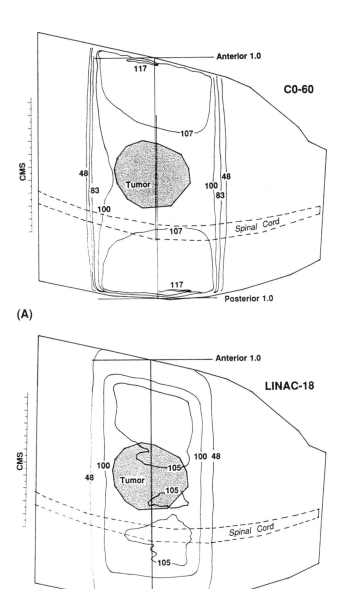

FIGURE 1 (A) Sagittal section of the thorax showing isodose curves from AP/PA fields delivered by cobalt 60. The target volume was not encompassed by the maximum dose curve, and the patient received a 7% higher dose to the heart and spinal cord compared with the dose to the target volume (tumor). (B) Sagittal section of the thorax shown by AP/PA fields delivered by 18-MV photons, which did not cause as much of the inhomogeneous dose distribution as seen for cobalt-60 treatment. A higher dose to the heart and spinal cord was avoided by using 18-MV photons.

The timing of the postoperative RT is also an important factor that impacts on local control and survival in patients with epithelial carcinoma. For example, if RT is not initiated within approximately 6 weeks of surgery in patients with positive lymph nodes, local control and survival may be reduced, according to the results from a study of patients with head and neck cancer (44). Observations in breast cancer patients have also shown that local control is an important factor influencing survival once systemic treatment improves. In breast cancer, the role of RT after mastectomy has been evaluated in several randomized trials, and these have shown there is a significant reduction in locoregional recurrences with postoperative RT. Once adequate adjuvant chemotherapy became available, the role of postoperative RT became more important in the control of locoregional disease, which ultimately influenced overall survival (45,46).

TECHNICAL CONSIDERATIONS OF POSTOPERATIVE RT

Equipment and Target Volume

It is very important to utilize adequate treatment equipment for postoperative RT to avoid the inhomogeneous dose distribution and large penumbra associated with the use of orthovoltage or cobalt units, compared to high-energy linear accelerators.

For example, in some patients treated on the trial conducted by the Medical Research Council (MRC), the RT technique was suboptimal owing to the use of a midline block, resulting in suboptimal dose to the mediastinum. A further drawback in the randomized or retrospective studies listed in Tables 1 and 2 was that none utilized planning CT to identify the shift of the mediastinum postoperatively to ensure delivery of an adequate dose to the mediastinal lymph nodes or ipsilateral hilar lymph nodes. At the same time, an overdose of radiation may have been delivered to the heart and residual lungs.

Figure 1A shows the sagittal section of the thorax and the isodose curve in the anteroposterior/posteroanterior (AP/PA) fields given by cobalt 60. The target volume was not encompassed by the high-dose area, and the patient received a 7% higher dose to the heart and spinal cord compared to the dose to the target volume. Higher-energy sources (Figure 1B) do not cause this inhomogeneous dose distribution or the delivery of higher doses to the heart and spinal cord. The difference between the maximum dose and target volume becomes more significant when parallel opposed oblique or lateral fields are used because of the distance from the surface of the skin to the target volume, which is at midline.

Philips et al. (47) reviewed the efficacy and toxicity of postoperative RT using cobalt 60 versus linear accelerator in patients who had undergone a pneumonectomy. Fifty-one patients were treated with 60 and 25 patients by a linear accelerator. Twenty-seven patients who had T_1, T_2, or T_3 disease without any positive lymph nodes did not receive any postoperative RT, and these 27 patients were used as the control group. Twenty of 51 patients who were treated by cobalt 60 had positive lymph nodes and 17 of 25 who were treated by the linear accelerator had positive lymph nodes. The 5-year survival rate in patients treated with cobalt 60 was significantly lower at 8% compared to 30% in those treated by a linear accelerator. The 5-year survival rate in the control group was 31%. Those patients who were treated with cobalt 60 developed more cases of respiratory insufficiency and cardiac complications, with a 12% rate of lethal complications due to treatment compared to only a 4% incidence of lethal complications in patients treated by the linear accelerator. However, the incidence of distant metastases was higher in those patients treated by the linear accelerator than in those treated with cobalt 60. The authors concluded that poor treatment led to treatment-related deaths and that locoregional control did not confer a survival benefit (47).

Figure 2 shows the shift of the mediastinum after pneumonectomy creating a 1.5-cm margin lateral to the vertebral body on the opposite side, leading to

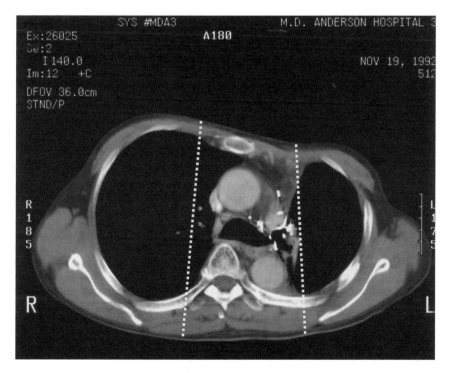

FIGURE 2 The mediastinum shifted after pneumonectomy, placing a 1.5-cm margin lateral to the vertebral body on the opposite side and causing the inclusion of a fairly large amount of the opposite side of the lung.

inclusion of a fairly large volume of the opposite lung. Because of the shift of the mediastinum after left pneumonectomy, an AP/PA field delivered by cobalt may cause more severe cardiac damage in those patients who already have borderline cardiovascular problems (Figure 2). When the AP/PA field was set up without a computerized plan, the right hilum and a portion of the mediastinum were partially missed from the RT ports, owing to the shift of the mediastinum after bilobectomy on the right side (Figure 3, A and B). This problem could be corrected by a computerized system (Figure 4, A and B).

CT-based treatment planning, the linear accelerator with tissue inhomogeneity correction, and three-dimensional conformal treatment planning are helpful tools to define the target volume and avoid radiation to the surrounding normal tissue (22,47). However, the CT scan for the treatment plan must be performed with the patient in the treatment position. The formulation of an optimal treatment plan to define the target volume and avoid critical structures is essential, especially in patients who have had a pneumonectomy or bilobectomy (Figure 4, A and B), which limits lung capacity and compromises cardiac function (48). At the same time, while tighter margins are necessary for these patients, it is essential not to miss the target volume due to respiratory motion or movement of the heart and aorta.

The target volume for postoperative RT needs to include the bronchial resection line, the ipsilateral hilum, and the mediastinum usually 5 cm below the carina and supraclavicular fossa if the lesion is in the upper lobe. We place the lower border 3 cm below the carina if there were no involved subcarinal nodes and the patient is receiving concurrent chemotherapy and RT. More recently, the contralateral hilum and supraclavicular regions are not routinely treated. If the primary tumor was in the lower lobe and the patient has positive mediastinal lymph nodes, the lower mediastinum, ipsilateral hilum, and an area several centimeters above the carina in the mediastinum are typically irradiated. The arrangement of the beam for postoperative RT has been well documented by Emami et

---

FIGURE 3   (A) When the AP/PA field was configured without a computerized plan postoperatively, the right hilum and a portion of the mediastinum were missed from the radiation therapy ports due to the shift of the mediastinum after right middle and lower lobectomy. This is shown by a horizontal line in the circle, which was the center. This was corrected by a computerized system, and the new center became the cross in the middle of the circle, marked to cover the right hilum and mediastinum adequately and to avoid the medial portion of the left lung. The black outline shows 4500 cGy, which was set up by AP/PA fields without a CT plan. The white outline shows a 5000-cGy isodose curve that is missing the right hilum. (B) Coronal section of the isodose curve without a CT plan. The margin is too tight around the right hilum.

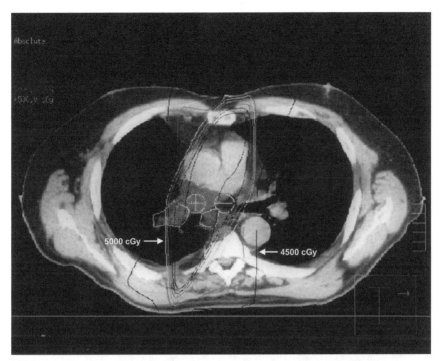

(A)

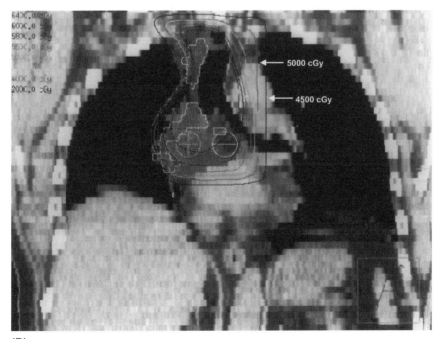

(B)

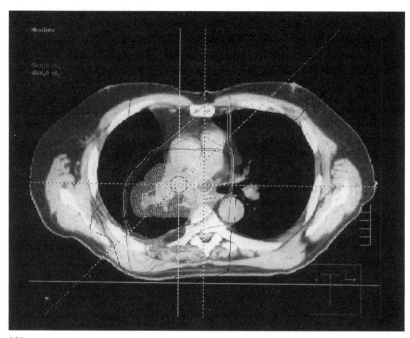

(A)

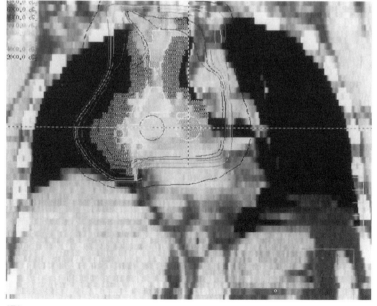

(B)

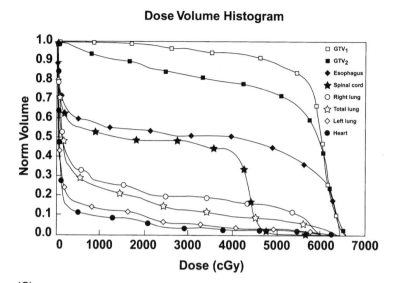

(C)

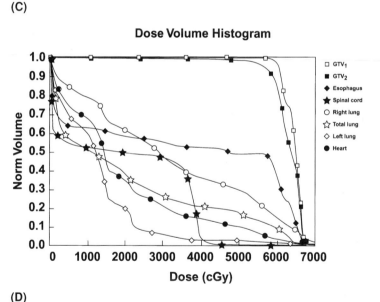

(D)

FIGURE 4   (A) Axial section of the CT plan. The white circle is the old central axis, the black circle is the new central axis, and the shaded gray part indicates motion, which was recognized. The motion of the hilum depended on breathing and pulsation of the heart. (B) Coronal section showing inclusion of the same margin and the shaded area representing respiration and motion of the heart. The white circle is the old isocenter, and the black circle is the new isocenter. (C) Dose-volume histogram without planning CT. (D) Dose-volume histogram with planning CT and with an inhomogeneity correction.

al. (40). No longer are the generous treatment fields of the past utilized, which included the bilateral hilum and bilateral upper, mid-, and lower portions of the mediastinum (32,42).

Optimal Postoperative RT Dose

The optimal radiation dose to be prescribed after complete resection to control microscopic residual tumor has not been well defined, but is currently between 50 Gy and 60 Gy for conventional RT (delivered in fractions of 1.8–2 Gy). Emami et al. (40) recommend 60 Gy for positive margins and 50 Gy for subclinical nodal disease. This was confirmed by the LCSG, which administered 50 Gy over 5 weeks postoperatively with a local recurrence rate of 1%. According to Emami's data, local control was achieved in 75% of patients with positive margins given 50–60 Gy and there was no difference in the local control rate associated with doses in this range. However, locoregional control was achieved in only 45% of the patients who received less than 50 Gy. There was improvement in the survival rate in patients with positive margins who received 60 Gy or higher, compared with the rate in patients given lower doses. Emami and colleagues also emphasized the importance of adequate portal coverage for achieving local control. As long as the portal and target volumes were adequately covered, there was no significant difference in the local control with doses between 50 and 60 Gy. However, there was a significant decrease in the local control rate in patients who received <50 Gy or those given ≥60 Gy if the portal did not adequately cover the target volume. Emami et al. recommend 50 Gy for microscopic residual disease, 60 Gy for positive margins, and 70 Gy for macroscopic residual disease (2 Gy/fraction) to 90% of the dose line. Adequate coverage was also associated with significant improvement in the actuarial survival rate compared with the rate in patients who received inadequate coverage regardless of the dose level (i.e., <50 Gy, 50–60 Gy, >60 Gy). A study by Choi and colleagues (32) showed that all patients with local relapse had received a dose of <50 Gy.

COMPLICATIONS RELATED TO POSTOPERATIVE RT

Clinical and experimental studies have shown that the total dose and fraction size of the RT are associated with pericardial and myocardial complications (49). According to the GETCB study, intercurrent death was related to the fraction size of radiation therapy (24). Seven percent of the patients in their study died of intercurrent disease in the control group. However, of those who received RT, 16% of the patients who received less than 2 Gy per fraction, 18% of patients who received 2 Gy per fraction, and 26% of patients who received more than 2 Gy per fraction died of intercurrent disease. These authors did not, however, find any correlation between the intercurrent death rate and the total tumor dose (24).

An increased rate of intercurrent deaths in patients who received RT was documented in the van Houtte trial (22) and also by the LCSG (7). According to the LCSG, 14 intercurrent deaths (14%) occurred in the RT group, compared with seven (7%) in the control group. These intercurrent deaths were mainly due to cardiovascular failure and infections. It is important to recognize this potential complication in patients at high risk of cardiovascular disease prior to the initiation of postoperative RT. Usually acute toxicity during RT does not predict for intercurrent death or late effects.

Radiation Effects on the Lung

The pulmonary effects of irradiation depend on an interplay of host and treatment factors, especially the volume of the radiated lung, the site of the irradiated lung, the total dose and fraction schedule, and the different chemotherapeutic regimens. Rubin (50) noted that when the whole lung is irradiated, there is a steep upward dose-response curve at a threshold of 7 Gy and a rapid rise to a cell lethality of 80% due to pulmonary toxicity at 11 Gy (Figure 5). No pneumonitis was manifest when ≥20 Gy was delivered to <22% of the lung volume. However, there is a steep increase in the extent of radiation pneumonitis if 20 Gy is given to >40% of the total lung, and this was observed to cause 23% of the cases of grade 3 (severe) to 5 (lethal) pneumonitis, as calculated by dose-volume histograms (51). The late or fibrotic changes may begin to occur at 3–6 months and are characterized by sclerosis of the alveolar wall and damage to small blood vessels, replacement of alveolar spaces by fibrotic tissue, and functional loss. Interstitial fibrosis, pleural thickening, and increased lung density are seen on radiographs with gradual volume loss (52). Patients are usually not symptomatic, however, even with fibrotic changes on the CT scan, because the volume of the sclerotic area is less than 20% and because the patient's pretreatment condition obscures the development of subsequent symptoms. To prevent pneumonitis and other pulmonary complications, it is important to assess a dose-volume histogram to reduce lung volume irradiated by ≥20 Gy to <40% (Figure 5). Of further concern is the well-known fact that certain types of chemotherapy such as bleomycin, actinomycin D, cyclophosphamide, methotrexate, BCNU, and possibly CPT-11 and paclitaxel (Taxol) have pulmonary toxicities that may increase pulmonary injury, especially when they are administered concurrently with radiation therapy (50,52–55).

Radiation Effects on the Heart

The cardiac effects of radiation have been best studied in patients who received RT for Hodgkin's disease, breast cancer, or lung cancer. For example, a radiation effect on the coronary vessels (56–58) and myocardium (59,60) has been reported, although these were not solely due to radiation. Usually the cardiac tolerance dose is 40 Gy in 4–5 weeks when the entire heart is irradiated. Among

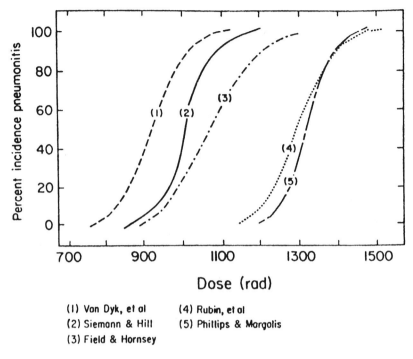

(1) Van Dyk, et al   (4) Rubin, et al
(2) Siemann & Hill   (5) Phillips & Margolis
(3) Field & Hornsey

FIGURE 5   Incidence of pneumonitis correlated with dose of radiation. (From Ref. 50.)

patients who received a total dose of 40 Gy in 4–5 weeks to the entire heart, 4–7% developed symptoms of radiation pericarditis (61–63). Symptomatic pericarditis typically develops within 12–24 months of the completion of radiation therapy (64), and the manifestations are usually chest pain, fever, friction rub, and pericardial effusion. Coronary occlusion is only manifest many years later.

A total radiation dose of 35 Gy to the heart reduced the ventricular ejection fraction in more than one-half of irradiated patients (65). This was mainly subclinical, however, in those patients with Hodgkin's disease who received radiation to the mediastinum. None of the patients who received this amount of radiation to the heart presented with congestive heart failure or constrictive pericarditis. Electrocardiographic changes have been observed, as well as transient and clinically silent perimyocarditis following cardiac radiation in breast cancer patients receiving internal mammary radiation on the left side (66). Not surprisingly, there were reports of deaths due to cardiac disease in node-negative patients who received 60 Gy using cobalt 60 in the study conducted by van Houtte and Dautzenberg (22,24). With careful CT-based planning, however, it should now be possible to minimize radiation to the heart so that less than 30% of the cardiac volume receives a dose of 50 Gy or higher (67,68).

Radiation Effects on the Esophagus

The effects of radiation on the esophagus may either be acute (e.g., esophagitis during radiation therapy to the mediastinum) or chronic (e.g., stricture of the esophagus months after radiation therapy). The germinal layer of the epithelium is most sensitive to radiation, especially if chemotherapy is given concurrently as a sensitizer for radiation. Acute esophagitis causes dysphagia usually around 2 weeks after the initiation of radiation therapy (at a dose of ~20 Gy or higher). It is very difficult, however, to avoid acute esophagitis when patients require mediastinal RT. However, an esophageal stricture may be avoided by reducing the length of the irradiated area and limiting the total esophageal dose to less than 60 Gy. There have been reports of severe stricture in less than 5% of patients given a total dose of 60–70 Gy of radiation to the esophagus (69). If less than 10 cm of the esophagus is irradiated and the total radiation dose is 50 Gy in 5 weeks, the risk of an esophageal stricture is less than 2% (70). Many chemotherapeutic agents are known to augment the radiation effect on the esophagus, especially doxorubicin (71–73), cyclophosphamide (50), bleomycin (74), fluorouracil and dactinomycin (75), and etoposide (76).

At present, we are conducting a randomized study of radioprotectors in patients (WR-2721) for unresectable NSCLC who are being treated with concurrent chemotherapy and radiation therapy. Similarly, the Radiation Therapy Oncology Group has a randomized trial to determine if amifostine (WR-2721) can reduce esophagitis from intensive chemoradiation in locally advanced NSCLC (RTOG 98-01). WR-2721 has been shown to protect normal tissue from radiation chemotherapy effects (77,78).

Radiation Effects on the Spinal Cord

A transient radiation myelopathy may be seen weeks to months following RT to the cervical or upper thoracic spinal cord. Lhermitte's sign of electrical paresthesias is the only clinical feature of this subacute effect, which does not translate into a higher risk of developing myelopathy. Affected patients experience electric-like shocks that radiate down the extremities, especially the buttocks and legs, on ventral flexion of the neck. This is most likely to be the result of transient demyelination of the spinal cord (79). This transient myelopathy has been noted in 3–15% of patients who receive RT to the thoracic spinal cord (80,81).

Late radiation effects on the spinal cord include a progressive radiation myelopathy, often presenting with clumsiness and weakness of the legs. A common early finding is the Brown-Séquard syndrome. The onset of the myelopathy is around 6 months or longer after the completion of RT, and symptoms may begin 3 or more years after treatment. Permanent spinal cord damage from RT is rare if the total dose is limited to less than 50 Gy in 5 weeks with standard fractionation such as less than 2 Gy per fraction. The fraction size to the spinal cord is an important factor related to permanent radiation myelitis (82). This damage to the spinal cord can be avoided by using careful CT-based treatment planning and by fractionating the radiation therapy.

Effects on Peripheral Nerves

When postoperative RT is given to the apex of the thorax in patients with positive margins or positive lymph nodes, there is always a concern regarding damage to the brachial plexus. However, peripheral nerves have a relatively high tolerance to ionizing radiation, and the incidence of damage to the peripheral nerves from the RT itself is rare. There are no recognized acute or subacute effects, and damage to peripheral nerves from radiation is manifested late, usually a few years or more after RT. Stoll and Andrews (83) reported the symptoms and signs related to brachial plexus damage among patients who received radiation to the supraclavicular area with 4-MV photons. However, patients with involvement of the brachial plexus by supraclavicular lymph nodes were not consistently excluded. Thomas and Colby (84) observed injury in only 1.2% (14/1202 patients) of those treated to supraclavicular area by RT. Stoll and Andrews reported that radiation-induced brachial plexus lesions were correlated with the dose-time-fraction size, as well as with the volume included within the radiation fields. They also suggested that the equipment that caused an inhomogeneous dose distribution, such as low-energy kilovoltage equipment, would more likely cause brachial plexus damage.

DISCUSSION AND RECOMMENDATION

Postoperative RT for Resected N_2 (Stage IIIA) NSCLC

It is obvious that survival is significantly lower in patients with positive mediastinal lymph nodes. This is borne out by findings such as those reported by Wilkins et al. (85), who reported 5-year survival rates of 42% in patients without mediastinal lymph node involvement compared with only 16% in patients with positive mediastinal lymph nodes. Mountain (86) also pointed out a significant reduction in the 5-year survival rate when there was mediastinal lymph node involvement. However, the preoperative staging in these studies was not uniform. For example, it did not include CT scan of the chest and upper abdomen, MRI of the brain, bone scan, etc., since these studies were performed before CT was applied to all lung cancer patients. A further difficulty in interpreting the results of some of the studies is that gross N_2 disease versus microscopic residual N_2 disease was not documented. A further consideration is that the nodal level determines a different outcome, according to Naruke et al. (87) and Pearson et al. (88). A number of retrospective studies have been interpreted to show that postoperative RT is beneficial to patients with mediastinal lymph node involvement (29,30,32,34,89). However, these retrospective studies usually had a fairly small sample size, and comparisons were made with historical controls or with controls in other studies conducted by different investigators.

Nevertheless, it cannot be ignored that an improvement in local control was found in most of the randomized studies in patients with N_2 disease. As well, local control will only become more important for improvement in survival once an efficacious systemic treatment is developed (54). A major problem in interpreting the cited studies is that many patients died of intercurrent disease stemming from inadequate planning and treatment equipment as well as inadequate staging, making it difficult to assess the true value of postoperative RT in these patients. Among patients with N_2 NSCLC, squamous cell carcinoma will more likely recur locally and postoperative RT will reduce local recurrence without influencing survival, compared with adenocarcinoma in which postoperative RT might reduce the risk of local recurrence, as well as improve survival (29,30,32).

Sawyer et al. (31) analyzed 224 patients who had N_2 NSCLC and underwent surgery and postoperative RT. Eighty-eight of the 224 patients had at least one positive mediastinal lymph node and received postoperative RT (50.4 Gy in 5.5 weeks). These investigators separated patients into three groups: a low-risk group with no nodal involvement, N_1 nodal involvement, T_1 or T_2 disease, and discordant T_{3-4} lesions without superior or inferior mediastinal lymph node involvement; an intermediate-risk group with negative N_1 nodes and discordant T_{3-4} lesions with superior or inferior mediastinal lymph node involvement or positive N_1 lymph nodes with superior or inferior mediastinal lymph node involvement; and a high-risk group with superior and inferior mediastinal lymph node involvement. According to their analysis, those patients in the high-risk group had a significant benefit from the adjuvant postoperative RT in terms of freedom from local recurrence and survival. This was also the case for patients of intermediate risk, although the benefit from RT was moderate. There was no improvement with regard to freedom from local recurrence or survival among those patients who were in the low-risk group. Sawyer et al. therefore advocated that patient selection is important to identify those patients with N_2 disease who benefit from postoperative RT.

Postoperative RT in Resected T_3, N_0, M_0 (New Staging System Stage IIB) Disease Involving the Chest Wall

Patients with resected T_3 tumors involving the chest wall, such as the parietal pleura, intercostal muscle, and ribs, need postoperative RT (90). However, Piehler and colleagues (91) made contrasting observations in 93 patients operated on from 1960 through 1980 for lung cancer invading the chest wall. Sixty-six had complete en bloc resection, and of those, 31 had T_3N_0 NSCLC. Sixteen of these 31 patients received postoperative RT; their actuarial survival at 5 years was the same as for those who did not receive postoperative RT (53.3% vs. 54.4%). Patterson and colleagues (92) reported on 35 patients treated between 1969 and 1981, 83% of whom had en bloc resection. Twenty-one patients with $T_3N_0M_0$ disease had a complete resection. Unlike the findings in Piehler and associates' study, seven of their nine patients (78%) who received postoperative RT were alive at 5 years compared with only three of the 14 (21%) who received no postoperative RT. None of the 13 patients who received postoperative RT had a recurrence locally, while six of the 22 (27%) who did not receive postoperative RT failed locally.

However, the role of postoperative RT in patients with $T_3N_0M_0$ NSCLC whose tumor has been completely resected has been controversial. This has been compounded by the fact that there has not been any randomized study to compare postoperative RT with no postoperative RT for completely resected $T_3N_0M_0$ NSCLC. In the study of Gould et al. (93), 92 patients underwent complete resection for $T_3N_0M_0$ NSCLC. They reviewed prognostic factors, including histological type, tumor size, location, grade, patient age, adjuvant RT, and type of surgical procedure. The actuarial local control rate at 4 years in their patients was 94%, with or without additional postoperative RT.

Superior sulcus tumors are a special consideration with regard to postoperative RT as there is typically not an adequate margin, even if patients had a complete resection. The majority of patients will have microscopic residual tumor without any preoperative RT. Whether resectable $T_3N_0M_0$ superior sulcus tumors need to be treated with RT preoperatively or postoperatively has been controversial. Recently, the effectiveness of preoperative versus postoperative RT for superior sulcus tumors was analyzed, but there was no significant difference in the outcome of the patients (Komaki, unpublished observations). In stage IIB (T_3N_0) or stage IIIA patients with the superior sulcus tumors, the 2-year survival rate was 46.5% compared with 20.6% in stage IIIB patients with superior sulcus tumors (94).

Postoperative RT for T_{1-2}, N_{0-1} NSCLC

Patients with squamous cell carcinoma and completely resected stage I–II disease should have less of a survival benefit from postoperative RT according to retrospective studies (16,34,95). For example, in a study of 134 patients with N_1 squamous cell carcinoma, the LCSG (7) showed a significant improvement in the local control rate in those who received postoperative RT compared with those who received surgery alone, but there was no significant improvement in overall survival.

According to our analysis of patients with pathologically confirmed N_1 squamous cell carcinoma who underwent complete resection, patients did extremely well without any adjuvant treatment (96,97). The original study included 173 patients who had complete resection of their NSCLC that was clinically graded as N_0. However, at surgery, patients were found to have hilar lymph node involvement. There were 86 patients with squamous cell carcinoma and 73 patients with adenocarcinoma; the other histological types were large cell or unclassified. The 5-year survival rate in patients with squamous cell carcinoma was 43% compared with 21% in the non–squamous cell cases ($p = 0.03$). A further finding was that the apoptosis and mitosis indices in the squamous cell group predicted a significantly better survival (96). When other prognostic biomarkers were studied (S + G2M, p53 status, Ki-67, DNA index) in addition to the apoptosis and mitosis indices, apoptosis and Ki-67 proved to be significant prognostic factors in squamous cell carcinoma for less distant metastasis and better overall survival. Multivariate analysis showed that the DNA index and Ki-67 status were significant predictors. In patients with non–squamous cell carcinoma of the lung, only the mitotic index was a significant predictor of overall survival (97).

Postoperative RT and Chemotherapy

Although the recent Intergroup Study showed no benefit to the addition of cisplatin and etoposide to postoperative radiation, the Radiation Therapy Oncology Group (RTOG) and other groups have decided to test newer systemic agents such as carboplatin and paclitaxel (98). In a recent Eastern Cooperative Oncology Group (ECOG) study of multiple cisplatin analogs in combinations, initial therapy with carboplatin and paclitaxel produced the best long-term survival, with a p value of ≤ 0.001 (99). Several studies (100–104) have indicated that paclitaxel is an active chemotherapeutic agent for NSCLC and that chemoradiation therapy with paclitaxel and carboplatin is well tolerated in patients with inoperable, locally advanced NSCLC. This approach was thus adapted to the adjuvant setting in patients who do not have bulky disease, i.e., in a setting where cure rates may be substantially enhanced. In the RTOG 97-05 phase III study (98), adjuvant therapy with paclitaxel, carboplatin, and concurrent thoracic RT was evaluated in patients with completely resected stage II and IIIA NSCLC. A total of 93 patients were entered, and toxicity data were available for 62 patients. Overall, the treatment regimen was reasonably well tolerated, with only one patient death secondary to sepsis and grade IV respiratory toxicity after completion of four cycles of chemotherapy. There was one grade IV esophagitis after two cycles of chemotherapy. Overall, there was a 16% rate of grade III/IV acute esophagitis and two late grade III toxicities. While waiting for mature data from RTOG 97-05, RTOG would like to build on this experience by exploring a promising approach that could be added to this regimen without risking increased toxicity. The adjuvant approach selected for this study is active immunotherapy with vaccines directed against tumor-associated antigens. These antigens are seen as self-antigens by the immune system and thus the patient is typically immunologically tolerant to them.

CONCLUSIONS

Postoperative RT will be more effective once more efficacious systemic treatment and better prognostic predictors become available. Further advances will come with improvements in CT-based planning and equipment and once we are better able to determine the volume to be irradiated, dose-time-fractionation schedule, and total dose. The role of postoperative chemotherapy will also need to be reinvestigated as better sensitizers to radiation and better systemic agents become available.

REFERENCES

1. Hall EJ. Radiobiology for Radiologist, 4th edition. Philadelphia: Lippincott, 1994: 141–145.
2. Mountain CF, Dresler CM. Regional lymph node classification for lung cancer staging. Chest 1997:1718–1723.
3. Pearson FG. Management of stage III disease: mediastinal adenopathy—the N_2 lesion. In: Delarue NC, Eschapasse H, eds. International Trends in General Thoracic Surgery, Vol 1, Lung Cancer. Philadelphia: WB Saunders, 1985:104–107.
4. Martini N, Flehinger BJ, Bains MS, McCormack P. Alternate approaches to the management of mediastinal adenopathy. In: Delarue NC, Eschapasse H, eds. International Trends in General Thoracic Surgery, Vol. I, Lung Cancer. Philadelphia: WB Saunders, 1985:108–120.
5. Martini N, Flehinger BJ, Nagasaki F, Hart B. Prognostic significance of N_1 disease in carcinoma of the lung. J Thorac Cardiovasc Surg 1983; 86:646–653.
6. Ferguson M, Little AG, Golomb HM, Hoffman PC, DeMeester TR, Beveridge R, Skinner DB. The role of adjuvant therapy after resection of $T_1N_0M_0$ and $T_2N_0M_0$ nonsmall cell lung cancer. J Thorac Cardiovasc Surg 1986; 99:344–349.
7. Lung Cancer Study Group. Effects of postoperative mediastinal radiation on completely resected stage II and stage III epidermoid cancer of the lung. N Engl J Med 1986; 315:1377–1381.
8. Matthews MJ, Kanhouwa S, Pickren J, Robinette D. Frequency of residual and metastatic tumor in patients undergoing curative surgical resection for lung cancer. Cancer Chemother Rep 1973; 4:63–67.

9. Rasmussen PS. The incidence of local recurrence and distant metastases in surgically treated cases of lung cancer. Acta Pathol Microbiol Scand 1964; 62:145–150.

10. Martini N, Beattie EJ Jr. Results of surgical treatment in stage I lung cancer. J Thorac Cardiovasc Surg 1977; 74:499–505.

11. Pairolero PC, Williams DE, Bergstrahl EJ, Piehler JM, Bernatz PE, Payne WS. Postsurgical stage I bronchogenic carcinoma: morbid implications of recurrent disease. Ann Thorac Surg 1984; 38:331–338.

12. Feld R, Rubenstein LV, Weisenberger TH. The Lung Cancer Study Group: sites of recurrence in resected stage I nonsmall cell cancer: a guide for future studies. J Clin Oncol 1984; 2:1352–1357.

13. Immerman SC, Vanecko RM, Fry WA, Head LR, Shields TW. Site of recurrence in patients with stages I and II nonsmall cell carcinoma of the lung. Ann Thorac Surg 1981; 32:23–27.

14. Ludwig Lung Cancer Study Group. Patterns of failure in patients with resected stage I and II nonsmall cell carcinoma of the lung. Ann Surg 1987; 205:67–71.

15. Kotlyarov EV, Rukosuyev AA. Long-term results and patterns of disease recurrence after radical operations for lung cancer. J Thorac Cardiovasc Surg 1991; 102: 24–28.

16. Green N, Kern W. The clinical course and treatment results of patients with postresection locally recurrent lung cancer. Cancer 1978; 42:2478–2482.

17. Kopelson G, Choi N. Radiation therapy for postoperative loco-regionally recurrent lung cancer. Int J Radiat Oncol Biol Phys 1980; 6:1503–1506.

18. Curran WJ, Herbert SH, Stafford PM, Sandler HM, Rosenthal SA, McKenna WG, Hughes E, Dougherty MJ, Keller S. Should patients with postresection locoregional recurrence of lung cancer receive aggressive therapy? Int J Radiat Oncol Biol Phys 1992; 24:25–30.

19. Paterson R, Russell MH. Clinical trial in malignant disease. IV. Lung cancer. Value of postoperative radiotherapy. Clin Radiol 1962; 13:141–144.

20. Bangma PJ. Postoperative radiotherapy. In: Deeley TJ, ed. Carcinoma of the Bronchus: Modern Radiotherapy. New York: Appleton-Century-Crofts, 1972:163–170.

21. Israel L, Bonadonna G, Sylvester R. Controlled study with adjuvant radiotherapy, chemotherapy, immunotherapy and chemoimmunotherapy in operable squamous cell carcinoma of the lung. In: Muggia FM, Rozencweig M, eds. Lung Cancer: Progress in Therapeutic Research. New York: Raven Press, 1979:443–452.

22. van Houtte P, Rocmans P, Smets P, Goffin J-C, Lustman-Marechal J, Vanderhoeft P, Henry J. Postoperative radiation therapy in lung cancer: a controlled trial after resection of curative design. Int J Radiat Oncol Biol Phys 1980; 6:983–986.

23. Bleehen NM, British Medical Research Council Lung Cancer Working Party. Randomized trial of surgical resection with or without post-operative radiotherapy (RT) in nonsmall cell lung cancer NSCLC. Lung Cancer 1994; 11(suppl 1):148.

24. Dautzenberg B, Arriagada R, Chammard AB, Jarema A, Mezzetti M, Mattson K, Lagrange JL, Le Pechoux C, Lebeau B, Chastang C. A controlled study of postoperative radiotherapy for patients with completely resected nonsmall cell lung carcinoma. Cancer 1999; 86:265–273.

25. Medical Research Council Lung Cancer Working Party. The role of postoperative

radiotherapy in nonsmall cell lung cancer: a multicentre randomised trial in patients with pathologically staged $T_1–T_2$, $N_1–N_2$, M_0 disease. Br J Cancer 1996; 74:632–639.

26. Holmes EG, Gail M for the LCSG. Surgical adjuvant therapy for stage II and III adenocarcinoma and large cell undifferentiated carcinoma. J Clin Oncol 1986; 4: 710–715.

27. Keller SM, Adak S, Wagner H, Herskovic A, Bruke JB, Perry MC, Livingston RB, Johnson DH. Prospective randomized trial of postoperative adjuvant therapy in patients with completely resected stages II and IIa non-small cell lung cancer: an intergroup trial (E3590). Proc Am Soc Clin Oncol 1999; 18:465a.

28. Ennuyer A. L'irradiation du mediastin apras pneumectomie pour cancer bronchique. Poumon Coeur 1963; 9:1093–1098.

29. Green N, Kurohara SS, George FW. Postresection irradiation for primary lung cancer. Radiology 1975; 116:405–407.

30. Chung CK, Stryker JA, O'Neil M, DeMuth WE Jr. Evaluation of adjuvant postoperative radiotherapy for lung cancer. Int J Radiat Oncol Biol Phys 1982; 8:1877–1880.

31. Sawyer TE, Bonner JA, Gould PM, Foote RL, Deschamps C, Trastek VF, Pairolero PC, Allen MS, Lange CM, Li H. Effectiveness of postoperative irradiation in stage IIIA non–small cell lung cancer according to regression tree analyses of recurrence risks. Ann Thorac Surg 1997; 64:1402–1408.

32. Choi NC, Grillo HC, Gardiello M, Scannell JG, Wilkins EW Jr. Basis for new strategies in postoperative radiotherapy of bronchogenic carcinoma. Int J Radiat Oncol Biol Phys 1980; 6:31–35.

33. PORT Meta-analysis Trialists Group. Postoperative radiotherapy in nonsmall cell lung cancer: systematic review and meta-analysis of individual patient data from nine randomised controlled trials. Lancet 1998; 352:257–263.

34. Kirsh M, Sloan H. Mediastinal metastases in bronchogenic carcinoma: influence of postoperative irradiation, cell types and location. Ann Thorac Surg 1982; 33: 459–463.

35. Iascone C, DeMeester TR, Albertucci M, Little AG, Golomb HM. Local recurrence after resectable non-oat cell carcinoma of the lung. A warning against conservative treatment for N_0 and N_1 disease. Cancer 1986; 57:471–476.

36. Herskovic A, Bauer M, Seydel HG, Yesner R, Doggett RLS, Perez CA, Durbin LM, Zinninger M. Post-operative thoracic irradiation with or without levamisole in non–small cell lung cancer: results of a radiation therapy oncologic group study. Int J Radiat Oncol Biol Phys 1988; 14:37–42.

37. Astudillo J, Conill C. Role of postoperative radiation therapy in stage IIIA nonsmall cell lung cancer. Ann Thorac Surg 1990; 50:618–623.

38. Durci ML, Komaki R, Oswald MJ, Mountain CF. Comparison of surgery and radiation therapy for nonsmall cell carcinoma of the lung with mediastinal metastasis. Int J Radiat Oncol Biol Phys 1991; 21:629–636.

39. Reinfuss M, Glinski B, Mitus J, Kowalska T, Rzepecki W. Radiotherapie postoperatoire des cancers bronchopulmonaires non petites cellules. A propos de 75 cas. Bull Cancer Radiother 1993; 80:163–167.

40. Emami B, Kaiser L, Simpson J, Shapiro S, Roper C, Lockett MA. Postoperative

radiation therapy in non–small cell lung cancer. Am J Clin Oncol 1997; 20:441–448.

41. Martini H, Flehinger BJ, Zaman M, Beattie, Jr, EJ. Prospective study of 445 lung carcinomas with mediastinal lymph node metastases. J Thorac Cardiovasc Surg 1980; 80:390–399.

42. Emami B, Kim T, Roper C, Simpson JR, Pilepich MV, Hederman MA. Postoperative radiation therapy in the management of lung cancer. Radiology 1987; 164:251–253.

43. van Houtte PJ. Personal communication.

44. Marcus RB Jr, Million RR, Cassisi NJ. Postoperative irradiation for squamous cell carcinomas of the head and neck: analysis of time-dose factors related to control above the clavicles. Int J Radiat Oncol Biol Phys 1979; 5:1943–1949.

45. Overgaard M, Hansen PS, Overgaard J, Rose C, Andersson M, Bach F, Kjaer M, Gadsberg CC, Mouridsen HT, Jensen M-B, Zedeler K. Postoperative radiotherapy in high-risk premenopausal women with breast cancer who receive adjuvant chemotherapy. N Engl J Med 337; 949–955, 1997.

46. Early Breast Cancer Trialists' Collaborative Group. Effects of radiotherapy and surgery in early breast cancer: an overview of the randomized trials. N Engl J Med 1995; 333:1444–1455.

47. Philips P, Rocmans P, Vanderhoeft P, van Houtte P. Postoperative radiotherapy after pneumonectomy: impact of modern treatment facilities. Int J Radiat Oncol Biol Phys 1993; 27:525–529.

48. Rosenzweig KE, Hanley J, Mychalczak B, Raben A, Fuks Z, Mageras G, Mah D, Ling CC, Burman C, Kutcher G, Ginsberg R, Rusch V, Downey R, Bains M, Kris M, Leibel S. Final report of the 70.2 and 75.6 Gy dose levels of a phase I dose escalation study using three dimensional conformal radiotherapy in the treatment of inoperable lung cancer. Proc Am Soc Ther Radiat Oncol 1998; 42:165.

49. Stewart JR, Fajardo LF, Gilette SM, Constine LS. Radiation injury to the heart. Int J Radiat Oncol Biol Phys 1995; 31:1205–1211.

50. Rubin P. The Franz Buschke Lecture: Late effects of chemotherapy and radiation therapy: a new hypothesis. Int J Radiat Oncol Biol Phys 1984; 10:5–34.

51. Graham MV, Purdy JA, Emami B, Harms W, Bosch W, Lockett MA, Perez CA. Clinical dose-volume histogram analysis for pneumonitis after 3D treatment for non–small cell lung cancer (NSCLC). Int J Radiat Oncol Biol Phys 1999; 45:323–329.

52. Travis EL, Komaki R. Treatment-related lung damage. In: Pass HI, Mitchell JB, Johnson DH, Turrisi AT, eds. Lung Cancer: Principles and Practice. Philadelphia: Lippincott-Raven, 1996:285–301.

53. Phillips TL, Margolis L. Radiation pathology and the clinical response of lung and esophagus. In: Vaeth JM, ed. Frontiers of Radiation Therapy and Oncology, vol 6, Radiation Effects and Tolerance, Normal Tissue, Baltimore: University Park Press, 1972:254–273.

54. Wara WM, Phillips TL, Margolis LW, Smith V. Radiation pneumonitis: a new approach to the derivation of time-dose factors. Cancer 1973; 32:547–552.

55. Einhorn L, Krause M, Hornback N, Furnas B. Enhanced pulmonary toxicity with bleomycin and radiotherapy in oat cell lung cancer. Cancer 1976; 37:2414–2416.

56. Dollinger MR, Lavine DM, Foye LV, Jr.: Myocardial infarction due to postirradiation fibrosis of the coronary arteries: case of successfully treated Hodgkin's disease with lower esophageal involvement. JAMA 1966; 195:316–319.
57. McReynolds RA, Gold GL, Roberts WC. Coronary heart disease after mediastinal irradiation for Hodgkin's disease. Am J Med 1976; 60:39–45.
58. Brosius FC, Waller BF, Roberts WC. Radiation heart disease: analysis of 16 young (aged 15–33 years) necropsy patients who received over 3500 rads to the heart. Am J Med 1981; 70:519–530.
59. Ruckdeschel JC, Chang P, Martin RG, Byhardt RW, O'Connell MJ, Sutherland JC, Wiernik PH. Radiation-related pericardial effusions in patients with Hodgkin's disease. Medicine 1975; 54:245–259.
60. Kaplan HS. Hodgkin's Disease. Cambridge: Harvard University Press, 1980.
61. Cohn KJE, Stewart JR, Fajardo LF, Hancock EW. Heart disease following radiation. Medicine 1967; 46:281–285.
62. Stewart JR, Fajardo LF. Radiation-induced heart disease. Radiol Clin North Am 1971; 9:511–531.
63. Dana M, Colombel P, Bayle-Weisgerber G, Tiellet F, Desperez-Curely JP, Bernard J, Chotin G. Pericarditis after wide field mediastinal irradiation for Hodgkin's disease. J Radiol Electrol Med Nucl 1978; 59:335–341.
64. Byhardt RW, Brace K, Ruckdeschel JC, Chang P, Martin RG, Wiernik PH. Dose and treatment factors in radiation related pericardial effusion associated with a mantle technique for Hodgkin's disease. Cancer 1975; 35:795–802.
65. Gomez GA, Park JJ, Panahon AM, Parthasarathy KL, Pearce J, Reese P, Bakshi S, Henderson ES. Heart size and function after radiation therapy to the mediastinum in patients with Hodgkin's disease. Cancer Treat Rep 1983; 67:1099–1103.
66. Wehr M, Rosskopf BG, Pittner PM, Schwenk D, Prignitz R. The effect of radiation therapy on the heart in patients with left-sided mammary carcinoma. In Proceedings of the International Association for Breast Cancer Research, March 20–24, 1983, Denver, CO.
67. Applefeld MM, Cole JF, Pollock SH, Sutton FJ, Slawson RG, Singleton RT, Wiernik PN. The late appearance of chronic pericardial disease in patients treated by radiation therapy for Hodgkin's disease. Ann Intern Med 1981; 94:338–341.
68. Mill WB, Baglan RJ, Kurichety P, Prasad S, Lee JY, Moller R. Symptomatic radiation induced pericarditis in Hodgkin's disease. Int J Radiat Oncol Biol Phys 1984; 10:2061–2065.
69. Roswit B. Complications of radiation therapy: the alimentary tract. Semin Roentgenol 1974; 9:51–63.
70. Morichau-Beauchant M, Touchard G, Battandier D, Maire P, Fontanel JP, Daban A, Babin P, Matuchansky C. Chronic radiation-induced esophagitis after treatment of oropharyngeal cancer: a little known anatomo-clinical entity. Gastroenterol Clin Biol 1983; 7:843–850.
71. Greco FA, Brereton HD, Kent CH, Zimbler H, Merrill J, Johnson RE. Adriamycin and enhanced radiation reaction in normal esophagus and skin. Ann Intern Med 1976; 85:294–298.
72. Chabora BM, Hopfan S, Wittes R. Esophageal complications in the treatment of

oat cell carcinoma with combined irradiation and chemotherapy. Radiology 1977; 123:185–187.

73. Schenken LL, Burholt DR, Kovacs CJ. Adriamycin, radiation combination: drug induced delayed gastro-intestinal radiosensitivity. Int J Radiat Oncol Biol Phys 1979; 5:1265–1269.

74. Soreide O, Janssen CW, Kvam G, Hartveit F. Aorto-oesophageal fistula complicating carcinoma of the oesophagus. Scand J Thorac Cardiovasc Surg 1976; 10:79–84.

75. Philips TL, Fu KK. Quantification of combined radiation therapy and chemotherapy effects on critical normal tissues. Cancer 1976; 37:1186–1200.

76. Giever RJ, Heuskinveld RS, Manning MR, Bowden GT. Enhanced radiation reaction following combination chemotherapy for small cell carcinoma of the lung, possibly secondary to VP16-213. Int J Radiat Oncol Biol Phys 1982; 8:921–923.

77. Milas L, Hunter N, Stephens LC, Peters LJ. Inhibition of radiation carcinogenesis in mice by S-2-(3-aminopropylamino)-ethylphosphorothioic acid. Cancer Res 1992; 44:5567–5569.

78. Tannehill SP, Mehta MP, Larson M, Storer B, Pellet J, Kinsella T, Schiller JH. Effect of amifostine on toxicities associated with sequential chemotherapy and radiation therapy for unresectable non-small-cell lung cancer: results of a phase II trial. J Clin Oncol 1997; 15:2850–2857.

79. Jones A. Transient radiation myelopathy (with reference to Lhermitte's sign of electrical paresthesia). Br J Radiol 1964; 37:727–744.

80. Hutchinson G. Survival and complications of radiation therapy following involved and extended field therapy of Hodgkin's disease, stages I and II. Cancer 1976; 38: 288–305.

81. Carmel RH, Kaplan HS. Mantle irradiation in Hodgkin's disease. Cancer 1976; 37: 2813–2826.

82. Wollin M, Kagan AR. Modification of biological dose to normal tissue by daily fractionation. Acta Radiol Ther 1976; 15:481–492.

83. Stoll BA, Andrews JT. Radiation-induced peripheral neuropathy. Br Med J 1966; 1:834–839.

84. Thomas JE, Colby MY. Radiation-induced or metastatic brachial plexopathy? A diagnostic dilemma. JAMA 1972; 222:1392–1395.

85. Wilkins EW, Scannell JG, Craver JG. Four decades of experience with resection for bronchogenic carcinoma in Massachusetts General Hospital. J Thorac Cardiovasc Surg 1978; 76:364–368.

86. Mountain CF. A new international staging system for lung cancer. Chest 1986; 89: 2255–2335.

87. Naruke T, Suemasu K, Ishikawa S. Lymph node mapping and curability at various levels of metastasis in resected lung cancer. J Thorac Cardiovasc Surg 1978; 76: 832–839.

88. Pearson FG, De Larue NC, Ilves R, Todd, TRJ, Cooper JD. Significance of positive superior mediastinal nodes identified at mediastinoscopy in patients with resectable cancer of the lung. J Thorac Cardiovasc Surg 1982; 83:1–11.

89. Newman SB, Demeester TR, Golomb HM, Hoffman PC, Little AG, Raghaven V.

Treatment of modified stage II (T_1 N_1 M_0, T_2 N_1 M_0) non–small cell bronchogenic carcinoma. J Thorac Cardiovasc Surg 1983; 86:180–185.

90. Grillo HC. In: DeLarue NC, Eschapasse H, eds. International Trends in General Thoracic Surgery, vol 1, Lung Cancer. Philadelphia: WB Saunders, 1985:134–138.

91. Piehler JM, Weiland LH, Offard KP, Payne WS, Bernatz PE. Bronchogenic carcinoma with chest wall invasion: factors reflecting survival following en bloc resection. Ann Thorac Surg 1982; 34:684–691.

92. Patterson GA, Ilves R, Ginsberg RJ, Cooper JD, Todd TRJ, Pearson FG. The value of adjuvant radiotherapy in pulmonary and chest wall resection for bronchogenic carcinoma. Ann Thorac Surg 1982; 34:692–697.

93. Gould PM, Bonner JA, Sawyer TE, Deschamps C, Lange CM, Li H. Patterns of failure and overall survival in patients with completely resected T_3 N_0 M_0 non–small cell lung cancer. Int J Radiat Oncol Biol Phys 1999; 45:91–95.

94. Komaki R, Mountain CF, Holbert JM, Garden AS, Shallenberger R, Cox JD, Maor MH, Guinee VF, Samuels B. Superior sulcus tumors: treatment selection and results for 85 patients without metastasis (M_0) at presentation. Int J Radiat Oncol Biol Phys 1990; 19:31–36.

95. Chang AY, Kim K, Glick J Anderson T, Karp D, Johnson D. Phase II study of taxol, merbarone and piroxantrone in stage IV nonsmall cell lung cancer: the Eastern Cooperative Oncology Group results. J Natl Cancer Inst 1993; 85:388–394.

96. Komaki R, Fujii T, Perkins P, Ro JY, Allen PK, Mason KA, Mountain CF, Milas L. Apoptosis and mytosis as prognostic factors in pathologically staged N_1 non–small cell lung cancer. Int J Radiat Oncol Biol Phys 1996; 36:601–605.

97. Komaki R, Milas L, Ro JY, Fujii T, Perkin P, Allen P, Sikes CR, Mountain CF, Ordonez NG. Prognostic biomarker study in pathologically staged N_1 non–small cell lung cancer. Int J Radiat Oncol Biol Phys 1998; 40:787–796.

98. Ettinger. Personal communication.

99. Bonomi P, Finkelstein D, Ruckdeschel J, Blum RH, Green MD, Mason B, Hahn R, Tormey DC, Harris J, Comis R, Glick J. Combination chemotherapy versus single agents followed by combination chemotherapy in stage IV nonsmall cell lung cancer, a study of the Eastern Cooperative Oncology Group. J Clin Oncol 1989; 7:1602–1613.

100. Murphy WK, Fosella FV, Winn RJ, Shin DM, Hynes HE, Gross HM, Davilla E, Leimert J, Dhingra H, Raber MN, Krakoff IH, Hong WK. Phase II study of taxol in patients with untreated advanced nonsmall cell lung cancer. J Natl Cancer Inst 1993; 85:384–388.

101. Langer CJ, Leighton JC, Comis RL, O'Dwyer PJ, McAleer CA, Bonjo CA, Engstrom PF, Litwin S, Ozols RF. Paclitaxel and carboplatin in combination in the treatment of advanced nonsmall cell lung cancer: phase II toxocity, response and survival analysis. J Clin Oncol 1995; 13:1860–1870.

102. Langer CJ, Movsas B, Hudes R, Schol J, Keenan E, Kilpatrick D, Yeung C, Curran W. Induction paclitaxel and carboplatin followed by concurrent chemoradiotherapy in patients with unresectable locally advanced nonsmall cell lung carcinoma: report of Fox Chase Cancer Center study 94-001. Semin Oncol 1997; 24: S12–S89.

103. Belani CP, Aisner J, Day R, Ramanathan R, Jett J, Capozzoli MJ, Bahri S, Hiponia D. Weekly paclitaxel and carboplatin with simultaneous thoracic radiotherapy for locally advanced nonsmall cell lung cancer: three-year followup. Proc Am Soc Clin Oncol 1997; 16:448a.

104. Choy H, Akerley W, Safran H, Graziano S, Chung C, Williams T, Cole B, Kennedy T. Multiinstitutional phase II trial of paclitaxel, carboplatin, and concurrent radiation therapy for locally advanced nonsmall cell lung cancer. J Clin Oncol 1998; 16:3316–3322.

11

Adjuvant Therapy for Resected Stages II and IIIA NSCLC: Con

Steven M. Keller*

Beth Israel Medical Center, New York, New York, and
Albert Einstein College of Medicine, Bronx, New York

Zvi Small

Albert Einstein College of Medicine, Bronx, New York

INTRODUCTION

Following resection of pathological stages II and IIIA non–small cell lung cancer (NSCLC), 5-year survival approximates 40% and 20%, respectively (1–4). Recurrent disease presumably originates in deposits of intrathoracic and extrathoracic micrometastatic tumor foci that were present at the time of surgery. Theoretically, the minimal residual disease present following surgery should be much less likely to harbor treatment-resistant cells and would, therefore, represent an optimal scenario for the administration of curative local and systemic therapies. Unfortunately, unlike breast cancer, adjuvant therapy has not proved successful in improving patient survival.

Numerous phase II and phase III adjuvant therapy trials utilizing thoracic

---

*Current affiliation: Montefiore Medical Center, Bronx, New York.

radiotherapy and/or systemic chemotherapy have been reported. The biases associated with phase II trials are well known. Though the results of these nonrandomized trials are frequently intriguing and may form the basis for future phase III trials, they cannot be employed to determine patient care standards. Therefore, only the results of phase III trials will be analyzed. Furthermore, though "neoadjuvant" trials have been designed with substantial adjuvant therapy components, the preoperative therapy confounds the interpretation of the specific contribution of the adjuvant therapy. These trials will also not be included in this discussion.

PHASE III TRIALS

Three adjuvant phase III trials of patients with stage II and III NSCLC have been reported by the former Lung Cancer Study Group (LCSG) (5–7). CAP chemotherapy (cyclophosphamide 400 mg/m^2, adriamycin 40 mg/m^2, cisplatin 40 mg/m^2) administered in six 1-month cycles was compared to a control arm of intrapleural BCG (single injection within 14 days of surgery) and levamisole 2.5 mg/kg orally daily $\times$ 3 days every other week for 18 months in 57 patients with either adenocarcinoma or large cell undifferentiated T_2N_1 NSCLC (LCSG #772) (5). An additional 73 patients had stage III disease. When both stages were analyzed together, a 7-month median survival advantage (15 months vs. 22 months, $p < .05$) was identified in those patients who received chemotherapy. Though no stage-specific analysis was presented, the authors stated that adjustment for stage did not affect statistical significance. The results of this study were not widely accepted because the survival of patients in the treatment arm approximated that of untreated patients from previous trials, while the survival of patients in the control arm was worse than expected. The poor survival of the patients randomized to the immunotherapy arm was attributed by some to an (unproven) detrimental effect of levamisol. Moreover, long-term survival data were not reported; so it was never clear if the differences observed in median survival were sustained over time.

In a second study (LCSG #773), 210 patients with resected stages II or III squamous NSCLC received either radiotherapy (5000 cGy, 180–200 cGy daily fractions) or no further treatment (6). 136 patients had T_2N_1 disease. Among the remaining 74 patients, 44 were stage IIIA by virtue of metastases to the N_2 lymph nodes. Once again, the two stages were analyzed together. Though the median survival of patients in the control and treatment arms was 33 months and 20 months, respectively, the survival curves largely overlapped and no significant difference was found ($p = 0.618$). Subgroup analysis reportedly showed no effect of stage on the result. Radiotherapy significantly decreased local recurrence and although radiation reduced overall recurrence in patients with N_2 disease, survival was not affected.

The third LCSG study (#791) compared split-course radiotherapy (400 cGy $\times$ 5 days repeated after a 3-week rest) and CAP chemotherapy (cyclophosphamide 400 mg/m^2, adriamycin 40 mg/m^2, cisplatin 40 mg/m^2) to radiotherapy alone in 164 patients (7). Three patients were stage I, 10 were stage II, and 151 were stage III. Among the latter group, 119 had N$_2$ disease. Though the time to recurrence was significantly greater in the treatment arm than in the control arm ($p = .004$, median 14 months vs. 8 months), the time to death was not significantly different ($p = .133$). The apparent biological effect did not translate into improved survival, although the study may have been underpowered to detect a significant survival difference. Subset analysis demonstrated a slight advantage for those patients with N$_2$ disease who received both radiation and chemotherapy.

A recent phase III trial by a French cooperative group compared radiotherapy (6000 cGy) alone to three cycles of chemotherapy (cycles 1 and 3: doxorubicin 40 mg/m^2, vincristine 1.2 mg/m^2, cisplatin 75 mg/m^2, lomustine 80 mg on days 3 and 4; cycle 2: vincristine 1.2 mg/m^2, cisplatin 75 mg/m^2, cyclophosphamide 600 mg/m^2 day 1) followed by radiotherapy (RT) in 267 patients with resected NSCLC (8). Eight patients had stage I disease, 70 stage II, and 189 stage III. N$_2$ disease was present in 137 of the stage III patients. No disease-free or overall survival differences were detected ($p = .68$). Median survival in the RT group was 15.4 months; it was 14.9 months in the combined arm. Though analysis by stage was not performed, subset analysis of the 137 patients with N$_2$ disease revealed a significant improvement in disease-free survival ($p = .002$) and a decrease in the number of deaths in the combined treatment arm when compared to the radiotherapy only arm ($p = .003$). This was attributed to a decrease in the number of metastatic occurrences. However, patients with N$_0$ and N$_1$ disease who received both radiotherapy and chemotherapy actually had a statistically significant poorer survival than those patients who received radiotherapy alone ($p = .03$). Once again, though some biological effect may have been present, convincing survival benefit was lacking.

Three phase III trials from Japan have appeared in the English language literature (9–11). In a study coordinated by the National Kyushu Cancer Center (9), 209 patients with completely resected stage IIIA NSCLC were randomized to either observation or three cycles of monthly vindesine (3 mg/m^2, days 1 and 8) and cisplatin (80 mg/m^2 day 1). A total of 119 of the 181 eligible patients had N$_2$ disease. Neither the disease-free interval nor the overall survival was different between the two groups.

The remaining two Japanese trials incorporated long-term therapy with uracil and futrafur, a unique chemotherapy combination not yet investigated in patients with NSCLC in the United States and Europe. Futrafur (tegafur, FT) is an orally administered fluorourcil derivative that is converted in vivo to 5-FU. Degradation of the 5-FU is inhibited by the concomitant administration of uracil.

The combination is known as UFT. The results of these trials are difficult to interpret because of the vagaries of the staging systems utilized and the manner in which the data were analyzed.

Wada et al. reported the results of a three-arm adjuvant chemotherapy trial for the West Japan Study Group for Lung Cancer Surgery (10). A total of 323 patients with NSCLC were randomized to either surgery alone, surgery + UFT (400 mg daily $\times$ 1 year) or surgery + cisplatin (50 mg/m^2 $\times$ 1) and vindesine (2–3 mg/kg $\times$ 3 at 2-week intervals) followed by UFT (400 mg daily $\times$ 1 year). The majority of patients ($n = 210$) had stage I disease, while 36 patients had stage II disease and 55 had stage IIIA disease. The 5-year survival for those patients who received cisplatin-vindesine-UFT, UFT alone, or no postoperative treatment was 60.6%, 64.1%, and 49.0%, respectively. The differences among the three groups approached statistical significance (log-rank $p = .053$, Wilcoxon $p = .044$). The difference between the UFT group and the control arm was statistically significant, though the difference between the cisplatin-vindesine-UFT arm and the no-treatment arm approached, but did not reach, significance. Unfortunately, analysis by stage was not presented, so it remains unknown whether these findings hold for patients with stages II and IIIA NSCLC.

The Study Group of Adjuvant Chemotherapy for Lung Cancer from Chuba, Japan conducted a two-arm trial in which 383 patients with resected NSCLC were randomized to either surgery alone or surgery + cisplatin 66 mg/m^2 $\times$ 1, adriamycin 26 mg/m^2 $\times$ 1, and oral UFT 8 mg/kg/day $\times$ 6 months (11). 29 patients had stage II disease and 78 patients were stage III, the remainder were pathological stage I. When all 309 eligible patients were analyzed by treatment arm, no significant difference in survival was apparent. The authors noted, however, that there existed a statistically significant greater number of patients with nodal metastases in the treatment arm. They consequently reanalyzed the data using Cox's proportional hazard model to adjust for this imbalance and found a significant improvement in survival for the patients treated with chemotherapy ($p = .044$). However, the authors later stated that this apparent survival advantage was limited to node-negative patients and was not present for those patients with nodal metastases. In fact, survival was actually worse for those patients with N$_2$ disease who were treated with chemotherapy.

A phase III adjuvant radiotherapy trial was recently reported by Mayer et al. from Austria (12). A total of 155 patients with NSCLC who had undergone complete resection and mediastinal lymph node dissection were randomized to either no further treatment or radiotherapy (50–56 Gy in 2-Gy daily fractions, 5 $\times$/week). The 116 patients with N$_1$ or N$_2$ disease received the higher dose. No significant difference was present between the two arms or among the nodal subgroups. Local recurrence, however, was significantly decreased in those patients who had received radiotherapy.

The Eastern Cooperative Oncology Group conducted a randomized, prospective phase III trial of adjuvant therapy in patients with resected stages II and IIIA NSCLC (13). The objectives of the study were to determine if concomitant chemoradiotherapy was superior to radiotherapy alone in prolonging survival and preventing local tumor recurrence. A total of 488 patients who had undergone complete resection of the primary tumor and a thorough mediastinal lymph node sampling or dissection were randomized between April 1991 and February 1997 to receive either four cycles of cisplatin (60 mg/m^2, day 1) and VP-16 (120 mg/ m^2, days 1–3) administered concurrently with RT (5040 cGy in 28 daily 180-cGy fractions) or RT alone. Patients were stratified by weight loss (<5% vs. >5%), histology (squamous vs. other), nodal biopsy technique (sampling vs. complete lymph node dissection), and stage (II vs. IIIA). A total of 351 patients were eligible for analysis with a median follow-up of 37 months; 121/183 (66%) of patients in the chemoradiotherapy arm received all four cycles of chemotherapy, while 139 (76%) received the planned radiotherapy, and 83% (139/168) of patients in the radiotherapy-only arm received the requisite radiotherapy. Grades 3 or 4 toxicity consisting largely of leukopenia and esophagitis occurred in 8.8% and 1.3% of patients who received radiotherapy alone, and 25% and 65% of patients who received chemoradiotherapy. Treatment-associated mortality was 2.2% in the chemoradiotherapy arm and 2.4% in the radiotherapy arm. Median survival in the radiotherapy arm was 41.1 months and 38.6 months in the combined-modality arm ($p = .99$). Analysis of the stratified subgroups showed no statistically significant survival advantage for either treatment arm. Similarly, comparison of the eligible and ineligible patients revealed no survival difference.

META-ANALYSIS

The previously summarized adjuvant phase III trials are those that employed modern treatment modalities and contained sufficient data regarding TNM staging, drug administration, and radiotherapy techniques to permit accurate analysis. Though the trials required the participation of multiple investigators and numerous years to reach their accrual goals, each individual study contained insufficient numbers of patients to permit detection of fine differences between the treatment arms. In an effort to overcome this problem, which is common to most areas of clinical research, the statistical methods of meta-analysis were applied. Appropriate trials were identified via literature searches and personal communication with experts in the subject of interest. Data from disparate studies were collected, updated, and collated. The resulting large number of patients permits a greater statistical power to identify small differences among treatment groups. Though meta-analysis has achieved recent popularity and widespread utilization, not all statisticians are convinced of its accuracy or utility (14,15). Indeed, it is our opinion that the subtleties of clinical trials render the conclusions of meta-analyses suspect. With these caveats stated, the published meta-analyses of adjuvant chemotherapy and radiotherapy can be reviewed.

The Non–Small Cell Lung Cancer Collaborative Group published a meta-analysis of chemotherapy trials that were conducted between 1965 and 1991 (16). Among the 52 randomized studies containing 9387 patients with the requisite details regarding staging, treatment, and survival were 14 adjuvant therapy trials containing 4357 patients who were randomized to postoperative chemotherapy or observation, and seven studies containing 807 patients who received either adjuvant radiotherapy or combination chemoradiotherapy. The 14 adjuvant-chemotherapy trials were further divided into three groups: five containing alkylating agents (2145 patients), eight containing cisplatin (1394 patients), and four containing other drugs, principally tegafur or UFT (918 patients). (Note: some of the publications contained the results of more than one chemotherapy trial and are counted twice.)

The utilization of alkylating agents proved detrimental to survival, causing a 15% increased risk of death and decreasing survival at 2 and 5 years by 4% and 5%, respectively ($p = .005$). However, the cisplatin-containing regimens proved beneficial, producing a 13% decrease in the risk of death and improving survival at 2 and 5 years by 3% and 5%, respectively. This improved survival approached, but did not reach, statistical significance ($p = .08$). The trials containing ''other'' drugs demonstrated no significant survival difference between the study arms ($p = .30$). Six of the seven trials comparing adjuvant radiotherapy to chemoradiotherapy employed a cisplatin-containing regimen. Analysis demonstrated a 6% reduction in the risk of death favoring combined chemoradiotherapy, though the 2% improved survival at 2 and 5 years was not statistically significant ($p = .46$). The authors stated that analysis of each chemotherapy group by stage failed to identify a subgroup that either sustained a greater benefit or was more adversely affected by treatment.

The PORT Meta-analysis Trialists Group recently reported their meta-analysis of nine adjuvant trials containing 2128 patients with resected stages I–IIIa NSCLC who were randomized to either radiotherapy or no further treatment (17). Postoperative radiotherapy was associated with a 21% relative increase in the risk of death and 7% decrease in 2-year survival (55% vs. 48%, $p = .001$). Local and distant recurrence-free survival were also adversely affected by radiotherapy ($p = .005$, $p = .007$, respectively). Similarly, analysis of overall recurrence-free survival demonstrated a 13% relative increase in the risk of recurrence or death and a 4% reduction in the 2-year recurrence-free survival (46% vs. 50%, $p = .018$). Subgroup analysis by stage revealed that the greatest adverse effect of postoperative radiotherapy occurred in patients with stage I disease. A less unfavorable effect was demonstrated in patients with stage II disease, and neither a beneficial nor a detrimental effect was seen in patients with stage III disease.

TABLE 1   ECOG 3590 Morbidity

	RT $n = 230$ Grade		RT + chemo $n = 232$ Grade	
	3	4	3	4
Leukopenia	<1%		41%	38%
Granulocytopenia		1%	14%	60%
Thrombocytopenia			13%	5%
Anemia		<1%	13%	1%
Nausea	1%		20%	
Emesis	<1%		10%	5%
Esophagitis	1%		14%	3%

MORBIDITY AND MORTALITY

The extent and severity of adjuvant-therapy-induced morbidity and mortality are difficult to assess owing to a lack of uniform definitions and reporting. The LCSG documented only one death among the 543 patients entered in the three adjuvant trials previously cited (5–7). The majority of hematological, gastrointestinal, and pulmonary toxicities were grade 3 or less. As expected, the morbidity for those patients who received combined treatment was greater than for those who received radiotherapy alone. The Japanese reported similar data, with no treatment-related deaths among the 837 patients included in the three adjuvant-therapy trials (9–11).

However, Dautzenberg et al. reported 17 (6.4%) treatment-related deaths among the 267 patients in the French trial (five in the radiotherapy arm and 12 in the radio/chemotherapy arm) (8). Three patients in the radiotherapy arm and two patients in the combined arm developed bronchopleural fistula. In addition, grade 3–4 hematological toxicity was present in 6% of patients, gastrointestinal in 8%, and other organ systems in 2%.

Keller et al. (13) documented seven deaths (1.4%) among the 488 patients registered in the ECOG trial (Table 1). Treatment morbidity was, as expected, worse in the combined-treatment arm. Grade 4 granulocytopenia and leukopenia occurred in 60% and 38% of patients, respectively.

ADJUVANT THERAPY—WHY IS IT NOT MORE SUCCESSFUL?

Radiation and chemotherapy have been utilized both individually and in combination as adjuvant treatments following complete resection of NSCLC. These cyto-

TABLE 2 Administration of Chemotherapy

Trial	Planned cycles	% of patients who received the planned cycles
LCSG 772 (5)	6	58%[a]
LCSG 791 (7)	6	51%
Ohta (9)	3	41%
Wada (10)	1[c]	75%[d]
SGACLC (11)	1[b]	85%
Dautzenberg (8)	3	76%
Keller (13)	4	66%

[a] Average cumulative dose of all patients randomized to receive chemotherapy.
[b] One initial dose followed by daily oral drug for 6 months (see text).
[c] One initial dose followed by daily oral drug for 1 year (see text).
[d] All patients received the initial chemotherapy dose. This figure represents the percentage of planned daily drug actually received.

toxic modalities are thought to be most effective with small numbers of rapidly dividing cells. Yet, despite the presence of only micrometastatic disease following complete resection of the primary tumor, and laboratory evidence that documents the entry of those micrometastases into a growth phase following resection of the primary tumor (18,19), adjuvant therapy has proven ineffective. Other theoretical considerations regarding the timing of treatment in relation to operation, the number of drugs, and their mechanisms of action, as well as the order in which the two modalities are administered, have also not yet proven clinically relevant (20,21).

Practical aspects of adjuvant-therapy administration have, however, proved significant. Following surgery, many of the patients are unable to receive all the planned chemotherapy cycles (Table 2). Concomitant chemotherapy and radiotherapy compounds this problem.

CURRENT TRENDS

Though adjuvant therapy for resected stages II and IIIA NSCLC has proved disappointing, new studies with different drugs and dosage schedules are being investigated. Following operation, patients with N_1 (stage II) disease are eligible for participation in the National Cancer Center of Canada adjuvant trial NCIC BR.10. Patients are randomized to either observation or chemotherapy (four cycles of monthly cisplatin and weekly vinorelbine). The principal clinical objectives of the trial are: (1) to compare the duration of overall survival between completely resected patients who have received either adjuvant chemotherapy or

TABLE 3 Current Adjuvant Therapy Trials[a]

Group	Protocol number	Therapy	Accrual goal	Eligibility
NCIC[b]	BR10	CT/observation	600	$T_2N_0, T_{1-2}N_1$
CALGB[f]	9633	CT/observation	504	T_2N_0
CALGB[f]	9734	CT/CT + RT	480	Stage IIIA
EU[e]	94043	CT/observation	1840	Stages I–IIIA
EU[e]	96010	CT/observation	3300	Stages I–IIIA
EU[e]	97010	CT/observation	750	Stages I–IIIA
EORTC[c]	08861	RT/observation	106	Stage II–III
GETCB[d]	04CB86	RT/observation	189	Stage I–III
GETCB[d]	05CB88	RT/observation	539	Stage I–III

[a] See text for details.
[b] National Cancer Institute of Canada.
[c] European Organization for Research and Treatment of Cancer.
[d] Groupe d'Etude et de Traitement des Cancers Bronchiques.
[e] European Union.
[f] Cancer and Leukemia Group B.

observation alone and (2) to measure and compare health-related quality of life in both treatment arms throughout the study period. Accrual of the 600 necessary patients is underway and is expected to require 5.5 years. A CALGB trial, limited to stage IB patients, uses a similar approach in resected patients, comparing four cycles of adjuvant carboplatin-paclitaxel to observation. In another CALGB trial, patients with resected stage IIIa disease are randomized to chemotherapy (carboplatin/paclitaxel) versus chemotherapy (same agents) followed by mediastinal radiation.

A number of European adjuvant therapy trials include patients with stages I–IIIA NSCLC (Table 3). Following resection of stages I–IIIA NSCLC, the European Union is randomizing 1840 patients to receive either chemotherapy consisting of mitomycin, vindesine, and cisplatin or no further therapy (EU 94043). Radiotherapy may be administered at the discretion of each institution. If employed, it will be given in both study arms. In another study with similar stages (EU 96010), 3300 patients will be randomized to receive three cycles of chemotherapy consisting of cisplatin and either a vinca alkaloid or etoposide or no further therapy. Individual institutions have the option to administer sequential radiotherapy. Finally, 750 patients with resected stages I–IIIA will be randomized to receive three cycles of cisplatin and etoposide or no further treatment (EU 97010). Radiation may be administered at the discretion of the treating physician. Three additional trials evaluating adjuvant radiotherapy have been completed, but not yet reported (17).

The introduction of new chemotherapeutic agents with increased effectiveness has raised the hope of prolongation of life in patients with NSCLC. The decreased toxicity associated with these drugs has permitted their use after surgery with little or no increase in surgical morbidity or mortality. In addition, improvements in radiotherapy techniques have enabled more accurate and less toxic administration following operation. To conclusively demonstrate the role of adjuvant therapy, patients should be encouraged to participate in controlled, randomized prospective trials.

REFERENCES

1. Martini N, Burt ME, Bains MS, McCormack PM, Rusch VW, Ginsberg RJ. Survival after resection of stage II non–small cell lung cancer. Ann Thorac Surg 1992; 54: 460–466.
2. Yano T, Yokoyama H, Inoue T, Asoh H, Tayama K, Ichinose Y. Surgical results and prognostic factors of pathologic N_1 disease in non–small-cell carcinoma of the lung. J Thorac Cardiovasc Surg 1994; 107:1398–1402.
3. Goldstraw P, Mannam GC, Kaplan DK, Michail P. Surgical management of non–small cell lung cancer with ipsilateral mediastinal node metastases (N_2 disease). J Thorac Cardiovasc Surg 1994; 107:19–28.
4. Dalton R, Keller S. Survival following resection of clinically occult N_2 non small cell lung cancer. J Cardiovasc Surg 1994; 35(suppl. 1 to no. 60):13–17.
5. Holmes EC, Gail M, The Lung Cancer Study Group. Surgical adjuvant therapy for stage II and stage III adenocarcinoma and large-cell undifferentiated carcinoma. J Clin Oncol 1986; 4:710–715.
6. The Lung Cancer Study Group. Effects of postoperative mediastinal radiation on completely resected stage II and stage III epidermoid cancer of the lung. N Engl J Med 1986; 315:1377–1381.
7. The Lung Cancer Study Group. The benefit of adjuvant treatment for resected locally advanced non-small-cell lung cancer. J Clin Oncol 1988; 6:9–17.
8. Dautzenberg B, Chastang C, Arriagado R, Le Chevalier T, Belpomme D, Hurdebrourcq M, Lebeau B, Fabre C, Charvolin P, Guerin RA, for the GETCB (Groupe d'Etude et de Traitement des Cancers Bronchiques). Adjuvant radiotherapy versus combined sequential chemotherapy followed by radiotherapy in the treatment of resected non–small cell lung carcinoma. Cancer 1995; 76:779–786.
9. Ohta M, Tsuchiya R, Shimoyama M, Sawamura K, Mori T, Miyazawa N, Suemasu K, Watanabe Y, Tomita M, Terashima M, and the Japan Clinical Oncology Group. Adjuvant chemotherapy for completely resected stage III non–small-cell lung cancer. J Thorac Cardiovasc Surg 1993; 106:703–708.
10. Wada H, Hitomi S, Teramatsu T, the West Japan Study Group for Lung Cancer Surgery. Adjuvant chemotherapy after complete resection on non–small-cell lung cancer. J Clin Oncol 1996; 14:1048–1054.
11. The Study Group of Adjuvant Chemotherapy for Lung Cancer (Chuba, Japan). A randomized trial of postoperative adjuvant chemotherapy in non-small cell lung cancer (the second cooperative study). Eur J Surg Oncol 1995; 21:69–77.

12. Mayer R, Smoole-Juettner FM, Szolar D, Stuecklschweiger GF, Quehengerger F, Friehs G, Hackl A. Postoperative radiotherapy in radically resected non–small cell lung cancer. Chest 1997; 112:954–959.

13. Keller SM, Adak S, Wagner H, Kerskovic A, Brooks BJ, Perry MC, Livingston RB, Johnson DH. Prospective randomized trial of postoperative adjuvant therapy in patients with completely resected stages II and IIIA non-small cell lung cancer: an intergroup trial (E3590). Proc ASCO 1999; 18:465a.

14. LeLorier J, Gregoire G, Benhaddad A, Lapierre J, Derderian F. Discrepancies between meta-analyses and subsequent large randomized, controlled trials. N Engl J Med 1997; 337:536–542.

15. Bailar JC. The promise and problems of meta-analysis. N Engl J Med 1997; 337: 559–560.

16. Non-small Cell Lung Cancer Collaborative Group. Chemotherapy in non–small cell lung cancer: a meta-analysis using updated data on individual patients from 52 randomised clinical trials. Br Med J 1995; 311:899–909.

17. PORT Meta-analysis Trialists Group. Postoperative radiotherapy in non-small cell lung cancer: systematic review and meta-analysis of individual patient data from nine randomized controlled trials. Lancet 1998; 352:257–263.

18. Gunduz N, Fisher B, Saffer EA. Effect of surgical removal of the growth and kinetics of residual tumor. Cancer Res 1979; 39:3861–3865.

19. Fisher B, Gunduz N, Saffer EA. Influence of the interval between primary tumor removal and chemotherapy on kinetics and growth of metastases. Cancer Res 1983; 43:1488–1492.

20. Surbone A, Gilewski TA, Norton L. Cytokinetics. In: Holland JF, Frei E, Bast RC Jr, Kufe DW, Morton DL, Weichselbaum RR eds. Cancer Medicine. Baltimore: Williams Wilkins, 1997:769–798.

21. Goldie JH, Coldman AJ, Gudauskes GA. Rationale for the use of alternating non-cross-resistant chemotherapy. Cancer Treat Rep 1982; 66:439–449.

12

Surgery for Potentially/Marginally Resectable Pathological N₂ NSCLC: Pro

William H. Warren
Rush-Presbyterian-St. Luke's Medical Center, Chicago, Illinois

INTRODUCTION

Complete surgical resection has provided the best local control and the best 5-year survivals for stage I and stage II carcinoma of the lung. Many studies have failed to prove a survival advantage with the addition of immunotherapy, chemotherapy, or radiotherapy, either alone, or in any combination. Surgical resection alone is adequate for these stages of malignancy and reflects the relative ineffectiveness of other modes of therapy.

Stage III lung cancer, however, presents a different clinical challenge. While, by definition, the tumor is still localized to the thorax, complete surgical extirpation is much more difficult to accomplish. Even in patients assessed to have undergone a complete resection (as determined by a pathological assessment of the specimen), the development of local/regional recurrence and/or distant metastases is a frequent occurrence. Early data documented that the 5-year survival of all stage III patients undergoing resection alone is only 5%. This sobering statistic has instigated a nihilistic approach to this stage of disease with the advocation of palliative radiotherapy alone as an alternative to surgical resection. This attitude may still persist. Nevertheless, surgeons have continued to advise that, within the entire population of stage III patients, there is a subset for which surgical resection plays an important role.

Recognizing that stage III was simply too heterogeneous to address this controversy, the early TNM staging system was modified in 1986 (1). Stage III was subdivided into stage IIIA and stage IIIB on the basis of ''resectability'' versus ''unresectability'' using the conventional criteria of the day. Many T_4 tumors (stage IIIB), by virtue of involvement of the carina, superior vena cava, and left atrium, can now be resected safely with a long-term survival advantage over nonoperative care. Nevertheless, most patients with stage IIIB lung disease are not surgical candidates, particularly those with N_3 nodal involvement (2–5).

Over the past 25 years, several studies have been published to attempt to define the best management of patients with stage IIIA lung carcinoma. The result of surgical therapy alone, while better than that of stage IIIB, has still been disappointing regardless of the scope of the resection. While generally the unaltered natural history of stage IIIA disease may be the same, evidence suggests that not all subtypes of this stage respond equally to therapeutic intervention. Encouraging results have been reported in surgically resected stage IIIA disease particularly in the absence of N_2 involvement (3,6,7).

Many authors have demonstrated that T_3N_1 tumors (be they peripheral or central T_3 carcinomas) respond better to surgical resection, with or without adjuvant therapy, than $T_{1-2}N_2$, and especially T_3N_2 tumors, even though all are staged as IIIA tumors (8). Ichinose et al. observed that the 5-year survival after resection of stage IIIA (N_0, N_1) tumors was 62.1% versus a 5-year survival of only 22.7% after resection of stage IIIA (N_2) tumors (9). The focus on stage IIIA (N_2) as a specific subset within stage IIIA is a more recent development and this distinction is increasingly being adopted in current clinical reports (10).

This functional refinement in staging has realized that the majority of cases of surgically resected stage IIIA (N_2) recur with distant metastatic spread. Moreover, completely resected patients had an unacceptably high local/regional recurrence rate. These features have led to the incorporation of various local and systemic adjuvant therapies attempting to modify patterns of failure and/or to improve the long-term survival. The interpretation of the results of the many clinical trials has been problematic. The subject matter derives from many disciplines including radiation biology, pharmacokinetics, and immunology, and the trials are often retrospective, nonrandomized, and subject to considerable selection bias. Earlier reports failed to address specifically the subpopulation of stage IIIA disease with N_2 involvement. Nevertheless, many observations were made that help to define the role of surgical resection in this particular subset.

PREDICTORS FOR FAVORABLE PROGNOSIS FOR SURGICAL RESECTION OF STAGE IIIA (N$_2$) DISEASE

Over the past 25 years, several reports have attempted to define features that predict favorable outcome after surgical resection (11–17). These include patient characteristics, the scope of the surgical resection, and various tumor parameters, including mediastinal lymph node involvement.

The performance status and overall health of a patient may determine whether a patient may participate in a given therapeutic intervention. This is important when comparing results of a trial of preselected patients and historical results of a patient population. In a radiotherapy series of ''inoperable'' patients considered to be ''favorable'' (i.e., Karnofsky Performance Status of 70 or greater and little or no weight loss), favorable patients had a better response to therapy than ''unfavorable'' patients (18). In a series comparing combined chemotherapy and radiotherapy with resection in patients identified as ''eligible'' or ''ineligible'' for resection, ''eligible'' and resected patients had a 3-year survival of 39% versus ''ineligible'' patients denied a resection with a 3-year survival of 18% (19). Another report compared the outcomes of patients receiving combined therapy with or without surgery, assessing patients eligible for surgery versus patients considered initially ineligible for surgery. In patients eligible for surgery who elected to undergo surgery, the 3-year survival was 52%; in contrast, those eligible, but who declined surgery, had a 3-year survival, no different than those ineligible for surgery (25% vs. 19%) (20). In these series, however, stage III (N$_2$) was not separately analyzed. Intuitively, patients with a better performance status present a lower operative risk and have a better long-term prognosis, even among patients with the same TNM stage. The selection bias to enlist only the favorable patients for aggressive therapy confounds interpretation of the results of most nonrandomized and randomized clinical trials.

Complete surgical resection is also an important prognostic factor. Complete resection mandates that all microscopic margins are free of tumor after a complete mediastinal lymph node dissection. Sabanathan et al. demonstrated a 5-year survival of 42% in stage III patients undergoing a complete surgical resection, and a 0% 5-year survival in those undergoing ''incomplete'' resections (21). In two similar series of patients with stage IIIA (N$_2$) disease, the 5-year survival in patients undergoing a complete resection was significantly better than in those undergoing an incomplete resection (16,17). Suzuki et al. observed that complete resection (vs. incomplete resection) was one of four statistically significant and independent prognostic factors (15). The Lung Cancer Study Group (LCSG) extended the definition of complete resection to include the absence of metastatic tumor in the highest mediastinal lymph node. In a LCSG trial of preoperative chemoradiotherapy, Weiden and Piantadosi observed that the best local control was achieved after complete resection (vs. incomplete resection), especially if the tumor had undergone a complete histological response (22).

The size and location of the primary tumor is another independent prognostic factor. Several series have reported that the T status impacts on prognosis, with T_3N_2 tumors having a 5-year survival of 0–20% (11–14,21,23,24). Size and location of the primary tumor may reflect the extent of the operation required for its removal. One study observed that patients with stage III (N_2) tumors requiring a pneumonectomy to accomplish complete resection had a worse prognosis that those undergoing a lobectomy (16). Some authors have been unable to confirm that the size of the primary tumor influences the long-term survival (25,26). According to Asamura et al., peripheral T_1 tumors with N_2 metastases have a 44.5% 5-year survival after a complete resection (27). Additionally, Daly et al. found that patients with microscopically positive N_2 disease and whose primary tumor was peripheral had a survival advantage over similar patients in whom the tumor was central (28).

Most investigators have recognized that the size and number of involved mediastinal lymph nodes impact on the results of surgical resection and long-term outcome. Several authors have distinguished between ''clinically'' positive, bulky or grossly involved nodes and ''microscopically'' positive or occult metastases discovered at the time of routine mediastinoscopy or surgical resection (10,29,31). Pearson et al. reported that in patients who had positive mediastinal nodes at the time of resection and negative nodes by mediastinoscopy, the 5-year survival after a complete resection was 41%; those who had positive nodes by mediastinoscopy and a ''curative'' resection had a 5-year survival of 15% (32). Nakanishi et al. reported a 21% 5-year survival in a group of patients with radiologically unsuspicious, but surgically discovered stage III (N_2) disease (17). Martini et al. and Watanabe et al. both reported a 33% 5-year survival in patients whose N_2 disease first became apparent at the time of thoracotomy and underwent a curative resection (11,33). Cybulsky et al. reviewed the preoperative CT scans of patients with completely resected stage IIIA (N_2) disease. In those patients found to have mediastinal nodes greater than or equal to 1 cm, the 5-year survival was 6.6% compared to 13.5% in those patients with mediastinal nodes 1 cm or less (34). Several authors have found that patients with disease limited to the lower mediastinal nodes had a better prognosis than those with disease in the upper mediastinal nodes. Patients with multiple levels of involvement had the worse survival (35–38). Upon reviewing their experience with surgical resection of stage IIIA (N_2) lung carcinoma, other investigators discovered that patients who had involvement at only one level had a significantly better 3-year survival than those with involvement at multiple levels (11,37,39,40). However, in all of these studies, there was no significant difference in survival 4 years after surgery.

Patients with N$_2$ metastatic disease confined to the subaortic nodes (level 5,6) have a better prognosis than those with any other single level of mediastinal nodal involvement. Patterson et al. reported 23 patients undergoing a complete resection with N$_2$ disease confined to the subaortic nodes and the 5-year survival was 42% (41). Cybulsky et al. and Nakanishi et al. also reported that patients with carcinomas in the left upper lobe and N$_2$ nodal involvement limited to the subaortic nodes had a significantly better 5-year survival than other patients with more extensive N$_2$ disease (17,34). Others have been unable to validate this observation (25). On the other hand, patients with subcarinal nodal involvement (level 7) have a worse prognosis than other patients with N$_2$ disease in other locations (36). Naruke et al. observed that in patients with resected N$_2$ disease the 5-year survival was 29% with uninvolved subcarinal nodes and 9% if the subcarinal nodes were involved (42).

Several histological characteristics have been identified as having prognostic significance. In an early report, Pearson et al. recognized that if the tumor had squamous differentiation, was intracapsular, and was microscopic, the 5-year survival of patients undergoing radiotherapy followed by complete resection was 31% (31). The distinction between intracapsular and extracapsular disease is easier to make on a mediastinal node dissected at the time of thoracotomy as opposed to nodal biopsy by mediastinoscopy (43).

While the above data support the position that there are patients with stage IIIA (N$_2$) who would predictably do better in the short term with a complete surgical resection than with palliative radiotherapy, the overall long-term survival statistics after surgery alone are poor. The patterns of failure, site of first recurrence, and 5-year survival have all been documented and considered in devising adjuvant therapies. Over the last 25 years, numerous clinical trials have been conducted to attempt to improve these results. The outcomes of these trials will be outlined.

ADJUVANT RADIOTHERAPY

Preoperative external-beam radiotherapy was the first adjuvant therapy to be used in conjunction with surgical resection. In 1975, a large cooperative study was published that compared the results of 40-Gy external-beam radiotherapy to the mediastinum and primary tumor followed by surgical resection to surgical resection alone. Although no staging system was in use, survival in the two groups was almost identical (44). Another part of this study assessed the value of preoperative therapy in patients initially thought to be unresectable. Those patients who responded to radiotherapy and upon reassessment were considered to be potentially resectable were randomized to surgery versus no surgery. Survival in these two groups was also not significantly different (44). In 1990, a similar, but nonrandomized trial was performed. Patients with stage III tumors underwent preoperative 40 Gy to the primary tumor and mediastinum over a 4-week period. Patients with (N_2) disease had a 5-year survival of 20%. Of the cases considered to be inoperable after radiotherapy, there were no 5-year survivors (45).

Postoperative radiotherapy after complete resection for stage IIIA disease has also been studied. In 1990, Astudillo and Conill studied 146 patients with stage IIIA carcinoma treated by complete resection. Some patients were treated with postoperative radiotherapy in a nonrandomized fashion. The incidence of local/regional recurrence was marginally lower with the addition of postoperative radiotherapy, but there was no impact on survival (23). In 1980, Van Houtte reported on the effect of the administration of 60 cGy to the mediastinum after a complete resection. Not only was survival unaffected, but there was an additional detrimental effect in patients with squamous carcinoma undergoing a pneumonectomy (46). Nevertheless, others continued to find some improvement in local/regional control and improvement in 3-year survival (47). In 1986, another trial for completely resected stage IIIA (N_2) disease randomized patients to receive 50 cGy radiation postoperatively to the mediastinum versus no additional therapy. There was some benefit with local/regional recurrence but there was no survival advantage with radiotherapy (48). All of these trials conclude that survival in completely resected stage III (N_2) patients was primarily determined by recurrence at distant sites, and that future trials should encompass effective systemic adjuvant therapy.

ADJUVANT CHEMOTHERAPY

The poor survival statistics for patients with stage IIIA (N_2) disease with local therapies of surgical resection and radiation, either in concert or alone, was a reflection of the high incidence of tumor recurrence at distant sites, often after good local control had been achieved. This is assumed to be on the basis of subclinical micrometastases at the time of diagnosis and unaffected by local therapies. This naturally led to the search for effective systemic therapy.

Although immunotherapy has had many proponents and many theoretical advantages over conventional chemotherapy, the vast majority of the studies to date, especially those pertaining to patients with stage III carcinomas, have failed to demonstrate any survival benefit. In fact, several studies found a deleterious effect upon combining immunotherapy with conventional chemotherapy (49,50).

Numerous studies have assessed the value of postoperative chemotherapy after complete resection of lung cancer (51–54). Unfortunately, many early trials failed to stratify for the TNM stage. Moreover, the agents available were only marginally effective against primary lung cancer. The mid-1980s marked a new era with the more consistent application of clinical staging and reporting. Furthermore, clinical trials focused on more uniform patient subpopulations. In addition, this period marks the advent of newer and more effective systemic agents. The combination of cyclophosphamide, doxorubicin, and cisplatin (CAP), or cisplatin, etoposide, and 5-FU evolved as standards against which other regimens have come to be measured.

In the early 1980s, the LCSG assessed the potential benefit of adding cisplatin-based multiagent chemotherapy to radiotherapy after ''incomplete'' resections versus postoperative radiotherapy alone (55). A total of 119/151 patients had been identified as having stage IIIA (N_2) tumors, but this population was not analyzed separately. Although there was a survival advantage and a decrease in distant metastases at 1 year in the arm combining postoperative chemotherapy and radiotherapy, the advantage abated after 3 years. Other trials utilizing postoperative chemotherapy, either alone or in combination with radiotherapy, have also reported no long-term survival advantage over complete surgical resection alone (51,52).

PREOPERATIVE ADJUVANT CHEMOTHERAPY WITH/WITHOUT RADIOTHERAPY

Early experience with neoadjuvant chemotherapy (with or without radiotherapy) was disappointing, owing to the ineffective chemotherapeutic agents available prior to the advent of cisplatin. In contrast to the experience of postoperative adjuvant therapy, the administration of induction cisplatin-based chemo/radiotherapy preoperatively has yielded encouraging results (6,14,30,56–70). There are several theoretical advantages in administering chemoradiotherapy in the preoperative setting. Chemotherapy treats not only the primary tumor, but also subclinical micrometastatic disease. In addition, several agents, including cisplatin and 5-FU, have been shown to have radiosensitizing properties, enhancing the effect of a given dose of radiotherapy. The addition of radiotherapy is designed to reduce the size of the primary tumor to provide a wider resection margin, and in some cases, to provide the opportunity to perform more conservative resections. Studies have shown that an excellent radiological response does not necessarily correlate with a complete pathological response. On the other hand, patients with only a partial or minimal radiological response may have undergone a complete histological response with only scar tissue remaining in the lung and mediastinal nodes (6,30). In other instances, metastatic disease evolves during the course of adjuvant therapy, often only discovered by restaging the patient prior to surgery. Hence, it is important to routinely reassess these patients with CT scan of the brain, chest, and upper abdomen, and with a nuclear bone scan after adjuvant therapy and prior to resection. The exclusion of patients developing metastatic disease introduces a selection process that undoubtedly has helped to improve the results in the surgical arm.

A multitude of phase I and II trials have documented that patients can tolerate these regimens with acceptable toxicity and operative mortality (56,58). In every study where patients with stage IIIA (N_2) carcinomas could be evaluated, the results favored the use of preoperative cisplatin-based adjuvant chemotherapy. Encouraging reports documented a higher rate of complete resection at the time of thoracotomy than historical controls of surgery with or without preoperative radiotherapy. The incidence of complete resection was also higher than seen historically with surgery alone. Complete surgical resection was found to be an important prognostic factor (5,6,8,10,15–17,19,21,22,30,56,70). The incidence of local/regional recurrence after a complete resection was also lower even though most patients died with distant recurrent disease (71–73). The brain was not only a common site for distant metastatic disease, but it was the most frequent site when distant metastatic disease was limited to a solitary site (56,60,74). Although this incidence could be reduced with prophylactic cranial radiotherapy, it did not seem to influence the long-term survival.

Several phase III prospective randomized trials comparing induction chemotherapy and surgery to surgery alone have yielded encouraging results in stage IIIA N_2 disease (22,75–77). Rosell et al. did not separately analyze patients with N_2 disease, but the majority of patients in both treatment arms had documented stage III (N_2) carcinomas (78). There were no 3-year survivors in the surgery-alone arm compared with 7/30 patients surviving beyond 3 years undergoing preoperative chemotherapy. In a small study of remarkably uniform patients, Pass et al. also demonstrated a trend toward increased disease-free interval and survival time in patients treated with preoperative cisplatin-based chemotherapy and postoperative radiotherapy versus surgical resection and postoperative radiotherapy alone (75). Roth et al. compared cisplatin-based chemotherapy followed by surgical resection with surgical resection alone (79). Unfortunately, the course of stage IIIA (N_2) patients was not analyzed separately, but they represented the majority of cases in both arms of the trial. This trial, also, showed a clear advantage in favor of preoperative chemotherapy.

Insight into the role of surgical resection in N_2 disease has been provided in a phase II study that identified 12 patients who had undergone preoperative chemoradiotherapy and were assessed to be resectable, but who refused surgery. Seven of the 12 patients refusing a thoracotomy underwent additional nonoperative therapy. Their clinical course was compared with that of 62 similar patients who completed the neoadjuvant therapy and underwent a thoracotomy (20). Approximately one-half of the patients in the study were assessed to have mediastinal nodal involvement. Although conclusions are soft from this small number of patients, the 3-year survival in those patients electing to have surgery was 52%

compared with 25% in those patients who refused. Unfortunately, such follow-up and analysis of patients refusing surgery has been uncommon.

PROGNOSTIC FACTORS IN STAGE IIIA (N₂) DISEASE AFTER PREOPERATIVE CHEMOTHERAPY (WITH OR WITHOUT RADIOTHERAPY)

Those factors cited favoring a good prognosis after surgical resection alone presumably also apply after induction chemotherapy. Good performance status, underlying good health, smaller primary tumors, and minimal mediastinal node involvement can all be expected to favor a better long-term survival. A complete surgical resection has also been found to have prognostic significance after adjuvant preoperative chemotherapy. In addition, several reports have identified that patients with a complete pathological response (no viable tumor in specimen) have a better prognosis than similar patients found to have viable tumor in the resected specimen (45,56,80). The incidence of complete histological response among those subjected to thoracotomy after neoadjuvant therapy has ranged from 0 to 39% (5,6,22,30,62,68,69,81,82). Although complete response had occasionally been seen in patients undergoing preoperative radiotherapy alone, no survival advantage could be demonstrated in that setting, presumably because the patients had not undergone systemic therapy. Some authors have suggested that sterilization of previously involved mediastinal nodes (even with residual tumor in the lung and/or in N₁ nodes) may still have some prognostic significance (82).

PROBLEMS ASSOCIATED WITH NEOADJUVANT CHEMORADIOTHERAPY

Although the prognosis for patients with completely resected stage IIIA (N₂) carcinoma can be improved with the use of preoperative chemoradiotherapy, the operative morbidity and mortality may be increased. At thoracotomy the dissection may be tedious with tissue planes obliterated by an intense inflammatory reaction. Commonly the primary tumor has been "downstaged" by preoperative therapy, and a more conservative resection, including bronchial sleeve resection, can be performed provided it accomplishes a complete resection. Rendina et al. documented that the use of preoperative neoadjuvant therapy does not increase the incidence of complications with bronchial or vascular reconstruction (83). Nevertheless, there is an increase in postoperative morbidity, including pneumonia, atelectasis, deep venous thrombosis, atrial arrhythmias, and prolonged bronchopleural fistula.

In the various phase II and III trials, the overall "treatment-related" mortality has been approximately 5% (1–15%). The incidence of "induction-related" mortality ranged from 0 to 7%; the 30-day perioperative mortality ranged from

0 to 10% (56). Of those patients who died in the postoperative period, most had undergone a pneumonectomy, and many developed ARDS and/or a bronchopleural fistula (6,84,85). In several series, the relatively high perioperative mortality has been linked to the incidence of pneumonectomy (66,84). An attempt to perform a curative resection with less than a pneumonectomy is preferable, especially after neoadjuvant therapy.

Although the overall survival of patients with stage IIIA (N_2) carcinoma remains disappointingly low, complete surgical resection may still provide the best form of local/regional control. The incidence of local/regional recurrence is much lower than in those patients who have not undergone a resection. Other advantages of resection include obtaining tissue for tumor marker assay and chemosensitivity analysis. To date, neither of these has been found to be clinically valuable but may in the near future help determine prognosis and further management strategies.

CONCLUSION

Although the overall long-term prognosis for patients with stage IIIA (N_2) carcinoma of the lung remains poor, surgical resection (with or without adjuvant therapy) has certainly provided the best results for the minority of patients with minimal mediastinal lymphadenopathy. More effective systemic control is necessary, and at present, surgical resection offers the best local/regional control. Even with a large mediastinal tumor burden, ''complete'' surgical resection has provided the best means of local/regional control. It can be performed with acceptable morbidity and mortality. The long-term survival has been shown to be improved by the addition of chemoradiotherapy. The advantage of surgical resection in stage IIIA (N_2) patients after induction chemoradiotherapy over chemoradiotherapy alone remains to be proven. Currently, there are several prospective randomized clinical trials (RTOG 9309, CALGB 9531, CALGB 9592) comparing neoadjuvant chemoradiotherapy followed by surgical resection versus chemoradiotherapy alone. The results of these trials are anxiously awaited.

REFERENCES

1. Mountain CF. A new international staging system for lung cancer. Chest 1986; 89: 225–233s.
2. Warren WH, Faber LP. Extended resections for locally advanced pulmonary carcinomas. In: Pass HI, Mitchell JB, Johnson DH, Turrisi AT, eds. Lung Cancer: Principles and Practice. Philadelphia: Lippincott-Raven, 1996:567–584.
3. Martini N, Yellin A, Ginsberg RJ, Bains MS, Burt ME, McCormack PM, Rusch VW. Management of non–small cell lung cancer with direct mediastinal involvement. Ann Thorac Surg 1994; 58:1447–1451.

4. Macchiarini P, Chapelier AR, Monnet I, Vannetzel JM, Rebischung JL, Cerrina J, Parquin F, Ladurie FLR, Lenot B, Dartevelle PG. Extended operations after induction therapy for stage IIIB (T₄) non–small cell lung cancer. Ann Thorac Surg 1994; 57:966–973.

5. Rusch VW, Albain KS, Crowley JJ, Rice TW, Lonchyna V, McKenna R, Livingston RB, Griffin BR, Benfield JR. Surgical resection of stage IIIA and stage IIIB non–small cell lung cancer after concurrent induction chemoradiotherapy. A Southwest Oncology Group trial. J Thorac Cardiovasc Surg 1993; 105:97–106.

6. Faber LP, Kittle CF, Warren WH, Bonomi PD, Taylor IV SG, Reddy S, Lee MS. Preoperative chemotherapy and irradiation for stage III non–small cell lung cancer. Ann Thorac Surg 1989; 47:669–677.

7. Burt ME, Pomerantz AH, Bains MS, McCormack PM, Kaiser L, Hilaris BS, Martini N. Results of surgical treatment of stage III lung cancer invading the mediastinum. Surg Clin North Am 1987; 67:987–1000.

8. Bonomi P, Faber LP. Neoadjuvant chemoradiation therapy in non-small lung cancer: the Rush University experience. Lung Cancer 1993; 9:383–390.

9. Ichinose Y, Yano T, Asoh H, Yokoyama H, Yoshino I, Katsuda Y. Prognostic factors obtained by a pathologic examination in completely resected non–small cell lung cancer. An analysis in each pathologic stage. J Thorac Cardiovasc Surg 1995; 110:601–605.

10. Vansteenkiste JF, De Leyn PR, Deneffe GJ, Stalpaert G, Nackaerts KL, Lerut TE, Demedts MG. Survival and prognostic factors in resected N₂ non–small cell lung cancer: a study of 140 cases. Ann Thorac Surg 1997; 63:1441–1450.

11. Martini N, Flehinger BJ, Zaman MB, Beattie EJ. Results of resection in non-oat cell carcinoma of the lung with mediastinal lymph node metastases. Ann Surg 1983; 198:386–397.

12. Martini N. Flehinger BJ, Zaman MB, Beattie EJ. Results of surgical treatment in N₂ lung cancer. World J Surg 1981; 5:663–666.

13. Naruke T, Goya T, Tsuchiya R, Suemasu K. The importance of surgery to non–small cell carcinoma of lung with mediastinal lymph node metastasis. Ann Thorac Surg 1988; 46:603–610.

14. Cangemi V, Volpino P, D'Andrea N, Chiarotti F, Tomassini R, Piat G. Results of surgical treatment of stage IIIA non–small cell lung cancer. Eur J Cardio-thorac Surg 1995; 9:352–359.

15. Suzuki K, Nagai K, Yoshida J, Nishimura M, Takahashi K, Nishiwaki Y. The prognosis of surgically resected N₂ non–small cell lung cancer: the importance of clinical N status. J Thorac Cardiovasc Surg 1999; 118:145–153.

16. Miller DL, McManus KG, Allen MS, Ilstrup DM, Deschamps C, Trastek VF, Daly RC, Pairolero PC. Results of surgical resection in patients with N₂ non–small cell lung cancer. Ann Thorac Surg 1994; 57:1095–1101.

17. Nakanishi R, Osaki T, Nakanishi K, Yoshino I, Yoshimatsu T, Watanabe H, Nakata H, Yasumoto K. Treatment strategy for patients with surgically discovered N₂ stage IIIA non–small cell lung cancer. Ann Thorac Surg 1997; 64:342–348.

18. Cox JD, Azarnia N, Byhardt RW, Shin KH, Emami B, Perex CA. N₂ (clinical) non–small cell carcinoma of the lung: prospective trials of radiation therapy with total

doses 60 Gy by the Radiation Therapy Oncology Group. Int J Radiat Oncol Biol Phys 1991; 20:7–12.

19. Taylor MA, Reddy S, Lee MS, Bonomi P, Taylor IV SG, Kaplan E, Faber LP, Warren W, Hendrickson FR. Combined modality treatment using BID radiation for locally advanced non-small cell lung carcinoma. Cancer 1994; 73:2599–2606.

20. Reddy S, Lee MS, Bonomi P, Taylor IV SG, Kaplan E, Gale M, Faber LP, Warren WH, Kittle CF, Hendrickson FR. Combined modality therapy for stage III non–small cell lung carcinoma: results of treatment and patterns of failure. Int J Radiat Oncol Biol Phys 1992; 24:17–23.

21. Sabanathan S, Richardson J, Mearns AJ, Goulden C. Results of surgical treatment of stage III lung cancer. Eur J Cardio-thorac Surg 1994; 8:183–187.

22. Weiden PL, Piantadosi S. Preoperative chemotherapy (cisplatin and fluorouracil) and radiation therapy in stage III non–small cell lung cancer: a phase II study of the Lung Cancer Study Group. J Natl Cancer Inst 1991; 83:266–272.

23. Astudillo J, Conill C. Role of postoperative radiation therapy in stage IIIA non–small cell lung cancer. Ann Thorac Surg 1990; 50:618–623.

24. Inoue K, Sato M, Fujimura S, Sakurada A, Takahashi S, Usuda K, Kondo T, Tanita T, Handa M, Saito Y, Sagawa M. Prognostic assessment of 1210 patients with non–small cell lung cancer who underwent complete resection from 1980–1993. J Thorac Cardiovasc Surg 1998; 116:407–411.

25. Riquet M, Manac'h D, Saab M, Le Pimpec-Barthes F, Dujon J, DeBesse B. Factors determining survival in resected N_2 lung cancer. Eur J Cardio-thorac Surg 1995; 9:300–304.

26. Skarin A, Jochelson M, Sheldon T, Malcolm A, Oliynyk P. Overholt R, Hunt M, Frei E. Neoadjuvant chemotherapy in marginally resectable stage III M_0 non–small cell lung cancer: long-term follow-up in 41 patients. J Surg Oncol 1989; 40:266–274.

27. Asamura H. Nakayama H, Kondo H, Tsuchiya R, Shimosato Y, Naruke T. Lymph node involvement, recurrence and prognosis in resected, small, peripheral, non–small cell lung carcinomas: are these carcinomas candidates for video-assisted lobectomy? J Thorac Cardiovasc Surg 1996; 111:1125–1134.

28. Daly DBT, Mueller JD, Faling LJ, Diehl JT, Bankoff MS, Karp DD, Rand WM. N_2 lung cancer: outcome in patients with false-negative computed tomographic scans of the chest. J Thorac Cardiovasc Surg 1993; 105:904–911.

29. Shields TW. The significance of ipsilateral mediastinal lymph node metastasis (N_2 disease) in non–small cell carcinoma of the lung. A commentary. J Thorac Cardiovasc Surg 1990; 99:48–53.

30. Martini N, Kris MG, Gralla RJ, Bains MS, McCormack PM, Kaiser LR, Burt ME, Zaman MB. The effects of preoperative chemotherapy on the resectability of non–small cell lung carcinoma with mediastinal lymph node metastases (N_2M_0). Ann Thorac Surg 1988; 45:370–379.

31. Pearson FG, Nelems JM, Henderson RD, Delarue NC. The role of mediastinoscopy in the selection of treatment for bronchial carcinoma with involvement of the superior mediastinal nodes. J Thorac Cardiovasc Surg 1972; 64:382–390.

32. Pearson FG, Delarue NC, Ilves R, Todd TRJ, Cooper JD. Significance of positive

superior mediastinal nodes identified at mediastinoscopy in patients with resectable cancer of the lung. J Thorac Cardiovasc Surg 1982; 83:1–11.

33. Watanabe Y, Shimizu J, Oda M, Hayashi Y, Watanabe S. Tatsuzawa Y, Iwa T, Suzuki M, Takashima T. Aggressive surgical intervention in N₂ non–small cell cancer of the lung. Ann Thorac Surg 1991; 51:253–261.

34. Cybulsky IJ, Lanza LA, Ryan B, Putnam JB, McMurtrey MM, Roth JA. Prognostic significance of computed tomography in resected N₂ lung cancer. Ann Thorac Surg 1992; 54:553–557.

35. Mountain CF. Surgery for stage IIIA-N₂ non–small cell lung cancer. Cancer 1994; 73:2589–2598.

36. Thomas PA, Piantadosi S, Mountain CF. Should subcarinal nodes be routinely examined in patients with non–small cell lung cancer? J Thorac Cardiovasc Surg 1988; 95:883–887.

37. Maggi G, Casadio C, Mancuso M, Oliaro A, Cianci R, Ruffini E. Resection and radical lymphadenectomy for lung cancer: prognostic significance of lymphatic metastases. Int Surg 1990; 75:17–21.

38. Okada M, Tsubota N, Yoshimura M, Miyamoto Y, Matsuoka H. Prognosis of completely resection pN₂ non–small cell lung carcinomas: what is the significant node that affects survival? J Thorac Cardiovasc Surg 1999; 118:270–275.

39. Goldstraw P, Mannam GC, Kaplan DK, Michail P. Surgical management of non–small cell lung cancer with ipsilateral mediastinal node metastasis (N₂ disease). J Thorac Cardiovasc Surg 1994; 107:19–28.

40. Conill C, Astudillo J, Verger E. Prognostic significance of metastases to mediastinal lymph node levels in resected non–small cell lung carcinoma. Cancer 1993; 72: 1199–1202.

41. Patterson GA, Piazza D. Pearson FG, Todd TRJ, Ginsberg RJ, Goldberg M, Waters P, Jones D, Ilves R, Cooper JD. Significance of metastatic disease in subaortic lymph nodes. Ann Thorac Surg 1987; 43:155–159.

42. Naruke T, Suemasu K, Ishikawa S. Lymph node mapping and curability at various levels of metastasis in resected lung cancer. J Thorac Cardiovasc Surg 1978; 76: 832–839.

43. Theunissen PHMH, Bollen ECM, Koustaal J, Thunnissen FBJM. Intranodal and extranodal tumor growth in early metastasised non–small lung cancer: problems in histological diagnosis. J Clin Pathol 1994; 47:920–923.

44. Warram J. Preoperative irradiation of cancer of the lung: final report of a therapeutic trial: a collaborative study. Cancer 1975; 36:914–925.

45. Reddy S, Faber LP, Baumann LA, Lee MS, Jensik RJ, Kittle CF, Bonomi PD, Taylor SG IV, Hendrickson FR. Preoperative radiation therapy in regionally localized stage III non–small cell lung carcinoma: long-term results and patterns of failure. Int J Radiat Oncol Biol Phys 1990; 19:287–292.

46. Van Houtte P, Rocmans P, Smets P, Goffin JC, Lustman-Marechal J, Vanderhoeft P, Henry J. Postoperative radiation therapy in lung cancer: a controlled trial after resection of curative design. Int J Radiat Oncol Biol Phys 1980; 6:983–986.

47. Chung CK, Stryker JA, O'Neill M, DeMuth WE. Evaluation of adjuvant postoperative radiotherapy for lung cancer. Int J Radiat Oncol Biol Phys 1982; 8:1877–1880.

48. Weisenburger TH, Gail M. Effects of postoperative mediastinal radiation on com-

pletely resected stage II and stage III epidermoid cancer of the lung. N Engl J Med 1986; 315:1377–1381.

49. Anthony HM, Mearns AJ, Mason MK, Scott DG, Moghissi K, DeVerall PB, Rozycki ZJ, Watson DA. Levamisole in surgery of bronchial carcinoma patients: increase in deaths from cardiorespiratory failure. Thorax 1979; 34:4–12.

50. Ruchdeschel JC, McNeally MF, Baxter DH, De Vore C, Kellar S, Killam D, Caradonna R, Sedransk N, McIlduff JB, Horton J. Regional immunotherapy has a detrimental effect on the response to combined irradiation and chemotherapy in locally advanced non–small cell lung cancer. Cancer Immunol Immunother 1981; 11:227–282.

51. Holms EC, Gail M. Surgical adjuvant therapy for stage II and stage III adenocarcinoma and large-cell undifferentiated carcinoma. J Clin Oncol 1986; 4:710–715.

52. Ohta M, Tsuchiya R, Shimoyama M, Sawamura K, Mori T, Miyazawa N, Suemasu K, Watanabe Y, Tomita M, Terashima M. Adjuvant chemotherapy for completely resected stage III non–small cell lung cancer. Results of a randomized prospective study. J Thorac Cardiovas Surg 1993; 106:703–708.

53. Katsuki H, Shimada K, Koyama A, Okita M, Yamaguchi Y, Okamoto T. Long-term intermittent adjuvant chemotherapy for primary resected lung cancer. J Thorac Cardiovasc Surg 1975; 70:590–605.

54. Wada H, Hitomi S, Teramatsu T. Adjuvant chemotherapy after complete resection in non–small cell lung cancer. J Clin Oncol 1996; 14:1048–1054.

55. Lad T, Rubenstein L, Sadeghi A. The benefit of adjuvant treatment for resected locally advanced non-small-cell lung cancer. J Clin Oncol 1988; 6:9–17.

56. Eberhardt W, Wilke H, Stamatis G, Stuschke M, Harstrick A, Menker H, Krause B, Mueller MR, Stahl M, Flasshove M, Budach V, Greschuchna D, Konietzko N, Sack H, Seeber S. Preoperative chemotherapy followed by concurrent chemoradiation therapy based on hyperfractionated accelerated radiotherapy and definitive surgery in locally advanced non–small cell lung cancer. Mature results of a phase II trial. J Clin Oncol 1998; 16:622–634.

57. Vokes EE, Bitran JD, Hoffman PC, Ferguson MK, Weichselbaum RR, Golomb HM. Neoadjuvant vindesine, etoposide, and cisplatin for locally advanced non-small cell lung cancer. Final report of a Phase II study. Chest 1989; 96:110–113.

58. Bitran JD, Golomb HM, Hoffman PC, Albain K, Evans R, Little AG, Purl S, Skosey C. Protochemotherapy in non–small cell lung carcinoma. An attempt to increase surgical resectability and survival. A preliminary report. Cancer 1986; 57:44–53.

59. Strauss GM, Herndon JE, Sherman DD, Mathisen DJ, Carey RW, Choi NC, Rege VB, Modeas C, Green MR. Neoadjuvant chemotherapy and radiotherapy followed by surgery in stage IIIA non–small cell carcinoma of the lung: report of a Cancer and Leukemia Group B phase II study. J Clin Oncol 1992; 10:1237–1244.

60. Kim DH, Lynch TJ, Mentzer SJ, Lee TH, Strauss GM, Elias AD, Skarin A, Sugarbaker DJ. Multimodality therapy of patients with stage IIIA, N_2 non–small cell lung cancer. Impact of preoperative chemotherapy on resectability and downstaging. J Thorac Cardiovasc Surg 1993; 106:696–702.

61. Burkes RL, Ginsberg RJ, Shephard FA, Blackstein ME, Goldberg M, Waters PF, Patterson GA, Todd T, Pearson FG, Cooper JD, Jones D, Lockwood G. Induction chemotherapy with mitomycin, vindesine, and cisplatin for stage III unresectable

non–small cell lung cancer: results of the Toronto phase II trial. J Clin Oncol 1992; 10:580–586.

62. Sugarbaker DJ, Herndon J, Kohman LJ, Krasna MH, Green MR. Results of Cancer and Leukemia Group B protocol 8935. A multiinstitutional phase II trimodality trial for stage III (N₂) non–small cell lung cancer. J Thorac Cardiovasc Surg 1995; 109: 473–485.

63. Taylor IV SG, Murthy AK, Bonomi P, Reddy S, Lee MS, Faber LP, Mathisen DJ. Concomitant therapy with infusion of cisplatin and 5-fluorouracil plus radiation in stage III non–small cell lung cancer. NCI Monogr 1988; 6:327–329.

64. Takita H, Regal AM, Antkowiak JG, Rao UNM, Botsoglou NK, Lane WW. Chemotherapy followed by lung resection in inoperable non-small cell lung carcinomas due to locally far-advanced disease. Cancer 1986; 57:630–635.

65. Bonomi P, Rowland K, Taylor IV SG, Reddy S, Lee MS, Faber LP, Warren W. Phase II trial of etoposide, cisplatin, continuous infusion 5-fluorouracil, and simultaneous split-course radiation therapy in stage III non–small cell bronchogenic carcinoma. Semin Oncol 1986; 13(suppl 3):115–120.

66. Rusch VW, Benfield JR. Neoadjuvant therapy for lung cancer: a note of caution. Ann Thorac Surg 1993; 55:820–821.

67. Sridhar KS, Thurer R, Kim Y, Fountzilas G, Davila E, Donnelly E, Charyulu KKN, Saldana MJ, Thompson T, Benedetto P, Raskin N, Beattie EJ. Multimodality treatment of non–small cell lung cancer: response to cisplatin, VP-16, and 5-FU chemotherapy and to surgery and radiation therapy. J Surg Oncol 1988; 38:193–215.

68. Recine D, Rowland K, Reddy S, Lee MS, Bonomi P, Taylor IV SG, Faber LP, Warren W, Kittle CF, Hendrickson FR. Combined modality therapy for locally advanced non–small cell lung cancer. Cancer 1990; 66:2270–2278.

69. Rice TW, Adelstein DJ, Ciezki JP, Becker ME, Rybicki LA, Farver CF, Larto MA, Blackstone EH. Short-course induction chemoradiotherapy with paclitaxel for stage III non–small cell lung cancer. Ann Thorac Surg 1998; 66:1909–1914.

70. Martini N, Kris MG, Flehinger BJ, Gralla RJ, Bains MS, Burt ME, Heelan R, McCormack PM, Pisters KMW, Rigas JR, Rusch VW, Ginsberg RJ. Preoperative chemotherapy for stage IIIA (N₂) lung cancer: the Sloan-Kettering experience with 136 patients. Ann Thorac Surg 1993; 55:1365–1374.

71. Eagan RT, Ruud C, Lee RE, Pairolero PC, Gail MH. Pilot study of induction therapy with cyclophosphamide, doxorubicin, and cisplatin (CAP) and chest irradiation prior to thoracotomy in initially inoperable stage III M₀ non–small cell lung cancer. Cancer Treat Rep 1987; 71:895–900.

72. Holmes EC. Surgical adjuvant therapy of non–small cell lung cancer. J Surg Oncol 1989; I(suppl):26–33.

73. Ciriaco P, Rendina EA, Venuta F, DeGiacomo T, Della Rocca G, Flaishman I, Baroni C, Cortesi E, Bonsignore G, Ricci C. Preoperative chemotherapy and immunotherapy for locally advanced stage IIIA and IIIB non–small cell lung cancer. Preliminary results. Eur J Cardio-thorac Surg 1995; 9:305–309.

74. Albain KS, Rusch VW, Crowley JJ, Rice TW, Turrisi III AT, Weick JK, Lonchyna VA, Presant CA, McKenna RJ, Gandara DR, Fosmire H, Taylor SA, Stelzer KJ, Beasley KR, Livingston RB. Concurrent cisplatin/etoposide plus chest radiotherapy followed by surgery for stages IIIA (N₂) and IIIB non–small cell lung cancer: mature

results of South Oncology Group phase II study 8805. J Clin Oncol 1995; 13:1880–1892.

75. Pass HI, Pogrebniak HW, Steinberg SM, Mulshine J, Minna J. Randomized trial of neoadjuvant therapy for lung cancer: interim analysis. Ann Thorac Surg 1992; 53: 992–998.

76. Dillman RO, Seagren SL, Propert KJ, Guerra J, Eaton WL, Perry MC, Carey RW, Frei EF, Green MR. A randomized trial of induction chemotherapy plus high-dose radiation versus radiation alone in stage III non–small cell lung cancer. N Engl J Med 1990; 323:940–945.

77. Dillman RO, Herndon J, Seagren SL, Eaton WL, Green MR. Improved survival in stage III non–small cell lung cancer: Cancer and Leukemia Group B (CALGB) 8433 trial. J Natl Cancer Inst 1996; 88:1210–1215.

78. Rosell R, Gomez-Codina J, Camps C, Maestre J, Padille J, Canto A, Mate JL, Li S, Roig J, Olazabal A, Canela M, Ariza A, Skacel Z, Morera-Prat J, Abad A. A randomized trial comparing preoperative chemotherapy plus surgery with surgery alone in patients with non–small cell lung cancer. N Engl J Med 1994; 330:153–158.

79. Roth JA, Fossella F, Komaki R, Ryan MB, Putnam JB, Lee JS, Dhingra H, DeCaro L, Chasen M, McGavran M, Atkinson EN, Hong WK. A randomized trial comparing perioperative chemotherapy and surgery with surgery alone in resectable stage IIIA non–small cell lung cancer. J Natl Cancer Inst 1994; 86:673–680.

80. Pisters KMW, Kris MG, Gralla RJ, Zaman MB, Heelan RT, Martini N. Pathologic complete response in advanced non–small cell lung cancer following preoperative chemotherapy: implications for the design of future non–small cell lung cancer combined modality trials. J Clin Oncol 1993; 11:1757–1762.

81. Choi NC, Carey RW, Daly W, Mathisen D, Wain J, Wright C, Lynch T, Grossbard M, Grillo H. Potential impact on survival of improved tumor downstaging and resection rate by preoperative twice-daily radiation and concurrent chemotherapy in stage IIIA non–small cell lung cancer. J Clin Oncol 1997; 15:712–722.

82. Mathisen DJ, Wain JC, Wright C, Choi N, Carey R, Hilgenberg A, Grossbard M, Lynch T, Grillo H. Assessment of preoperative accelerated radiotherapy and chemotherapy in stage IIIA (N_2) non–small cell lung cancer. J Thorac Cardiovasc Surg 1996; 111:123–133.

83. Rendina EA, Venuta F, DeGiacomo T, Flaishman I, Fazi P, Ricci C. Safety and efficacy of bronchovascular reconstruction after induction chemotherapy for lung cancer. J Thorac Cardiovasc Surg 1997; 114:830–837.

84. Rice TW, Adelstein DJ, Koka A, Tefft M, Kirby TJ, VanKirk MA, Taylor ME, Olencki TE, Peereboom D, Budd GT. Accelerated induction therapy and resection for poor prognosis stage III non–small cell lung cancer. Ann Thorac Surg 1995; 60: 586–592.

85. Fowler WC, Langer CJ, Curran WJ, Keller SM. Postoperative complications after combined neoadjuvant treatment of lung cancer. Ann Thorac Surg 1993; 55:986–989.

13

Surgery for Potentially/Marginally Resectable Pathological N_2 NSCLC: Con

Elizabeth M. Gore and Roger W. Byhardt
Medical College of Wisconsin, Milwaukee, Wisconsin

INTRODUCTION

Patients with ipsilateral mediastinal lymphadenopathy (N_2) non–small cell lung cancer (NSCLC) are a heterogeneous group with varying prognoses. When N_2 disease is diagnosed preoperatively by CT scan or chest x-ray (clinical N_2), the prognosis is worse than when N_2 involvement is microscopic, diagnosed with mediastinoscopy or at the time of thoracotomy (minimal N_2). Additional prognostic factors include extent of tumor within the nodes, extracapsular extension, multiple nodal levels, multiple nodes at a single level, nodal station, and histology (1,2). Controversy exists over the most appropriate management of N_2 disease owing to inconsistent pathological documentation and grouping of patients with other T and N stages. The majority of patients with N_2, M_0 disease are grouped into stage IIIA, which is potentially resectable, locally advanced disease. T_4, N_2 (in addition to T_4, N_{0-1}, and N_3) is IIIB disease. Subclassification of IIIA disease, based on T stage and degree of N_2 involvement, has been proposed (3). Outcome with multimodality therapy differs between subsets making the distinctions relevant when choosing and comparing different therapies.

Comparing surgical and nonsurgical trials for NSCLC is particularly difficult. Generally patients treated with radiation are referred by surgeons not recommending resection because of disease bulk or medical contraindication. This group is clearly not comparable to those receiving an operation.

Distant micrometastases are present in $\geq 60\%$ of patients with N_2 disease (3), emphasizing the need for effective systemic treatment. Adjuvant chemotherapy has been shown to decrease distant metastases. In addition, chemotherapy as part of multimodality therapy is effective in improving local control in both surgical and nonsurgical management of stage III disease. Studies with the most encouraging results use multimodality therapy.

The current recommendation for minimal N_2 disease is resection (1,4,5), but controversy exists over whether pre- or postoperative chemotherapy and/or radiation improves survival. This recommendation is based on superior surgical results compared to standard radiotherapy for unresectable or medically inoperable disease. For bulky or clinical N_2 disease chemoradiotherapy is standard of care. One question must be addressed: does surgical resection after induction chemoradiotherapy in a select group of clinical N_2 patients improve outcome over chemoradiotherapy alone?

Intergroup trial 0139 is a phase III trial designed to assess whether concurrent chemotherapy and radiotherapy followed by surgical resection results in a significant improvement in progression-free, median, and long-term survival compared to the same chemotherapy plus standard radiotherapy in patients with biopsy-proven T_{1-3}, N_2 NSCLC. This study is currently accruing patients. The results should help resolve these controversies.

MINIMAL N_2 DISEASE

Surgery

Surgical resection of minimal N_2 NSCLC results in 5-year survival rates of 10–34%. Martini and Flehinger reported 3- and 5-year survivals of 47 and 34% after complete resection of clinical N_{0-1}/pathological N_2 disease (1). This was a retrospective review of 151 patients who had complete resections for N_2 NSCLC. Of the original 404 patients surgically explored, 224 had clinical N_{0-1} disease. In 53% (119/224) complete resection was possible. Survival rates are based on this very select group of patients with completely resected tumors. Ninety percent of the patients were treated with postoperative radiation. Locoregional failure was only 20%. In the series reported by Naruke et al., the 5-year survival for resected N_2 disease was 19.2% (4). Pearson et al. reported 9% and 24% 5-year survival after resection of N_2 disease with positive and negative mediastinoscopy, respectively (6).

Randomized combined modality trials for minimal N$_2$ disease include a National Cancer Institute (NCI) trial reported in 1992 comparing pre- and postoperative chemotherapy and postoperative radiation alone (7) and a Japanese trial of preoperative chemoradiotherapy versus resection alone (8). Neither study showed a survival advantage with induction therapy. Two- to 3-year survival in the Japanese trial was 37–40% and 21–46% in the NCI trial.

Radiation Therapy

Patients without clinical N$_2$ disease, medically unfit for surgery and referred for radiation, are, unfortunately, not routinely mediastinoscoped and therefore not accurately staged. The incidence of occult mediastinal lymphadenopathy in clinical T$_{1-3}$, N$_1$ disease is approximately 25%. Radiation results in patients with clinically occult N$_2$ disease are difficult to obtain. In "higher"-performance-status patients and clinical N$_1$ disease, treated with "standard" radiation (60 Gy given in 30 daily fractions 5 days per week), 5-year survival of 28% has been reported (9).

Local control rates with "standard" radiation are poor. Evidence suggests that increasing the biological total dose of radiation improves local control. This can theoretically be accomplished with hyperfractionated radiation (10), three-dimensional conformal radiation, and noncytotoxic radiosensitizers or low-dose cytotoxic chemotherapy given with radiation. It is expected that with conformal radiation, total doses can safely be escalated, improving local control while avoiding unacceptable doses to normal tissue volumes. This is now being evaluated by the RTOG. Hyperfractionated radiation can be used to increase the total dose of radiation given to the tumor without increasing normal tissue toxicity. With optimal radiation therapy in good-performance-status patients, local control and survival may be similar to that achieved with surgery and postoperative irradiation. As with surgical series, effective systemic therapy is necessary to improve the rate of response of distant metastases.

CLINICAL N$_2$ DISEASE

As with minimal N$_2$ disease, there is no completed prospective randomized trial that identifies whether surgery is beneficial after induction chemotherapy or chemoradiotherapy. Available studies have used heterogeneous patient populations. The surgical series include patients who are medically fit for surgery and have less bulky, technically resectable disease. Other patients with clinical N$_2$ disease are generally referred for radiation. Historically, owing to poor results, radiation is frequently considered palliative. With the introduction of effective systemic chemotherapy, radiosensitizing chemotherapy, and new radiotherapy techniques, more patients are receiving preoperative chemotherapy or chemoradiotherapy for downstaging followed by resection or various combinations of chemotherapy and radiation as definitive treatment.

Surgery alone and radiation alone will be discussed to emphasize the similar poor results with single-modality therapy. Multimodality therapy with and without surgery will then be discussed.

Surgery

Martini and Flehinger have reported survival rates for clinical N_2 disease, detected radiographically or by mediastinoscopy, treated with surgery and postoperative irradiation (1). In this retrospective review, 179 patients with clinical N_2 disease were considered to have operable tumors. Only 32 (18%) had complete resections producing 3- and 5-year survival rates of 9%.

Two small prospective randomized trials comparing surgery to preoperative chemotherapy and surgery for IIIA disease have been published (11,12). Ipsilateral mediastinal lymphadenopathy was clinically obvious on CT scans. Pathological confirmation of N_2 disease was not required. It is important to note that as many as 35% of patients with positive mediastinal lymph nodes on CT scan will have negative nodes by mediastinoscopy (13). Median survivals for surgery alone were 8 and 11 months in both studies and 3-year survivals were 15% and 15% (Table 1). Both studies showed a survival advantage with preoperative chemotherapy.

TABLE 1   Single Modality Therapy

Survival	Median	1 year	2 year	3 year	5 year
Standard RT					
Perez (14)			20%		
Dillman (16)	9.6	40%	13%	10%	6%
Sause (15)	11.4	46%	19%	6%	
Cox (17)		30%		7%	
Hyperfractionated RT					
Sause (15)	12.3	51%			
Cox (10)	13		29%		
Cox (17)		58%		20%	
Surgery					
Martini (1)				9%	9%
Rosell (11)	8			15%	
Roth (12)	11		25%	15%	

In the study reported by Rosell et al. 60 patients with stage II and III NSCLC were randomly assigned to either three cycles of preoperative chemotherapy (mitomycin and cisplatin) or surgery alone (11). Eighty-three percent of patients in the chemotherapy arm had clinical N_2 disease and 63% in the surgery-alone group. There was one pathological complete response to chemotherapy. Complete resection rate was 76% in the chemotherapy group and 90% in the surgery-only group. Median survival with preoperative chemotherapy was 26 months and 8 months with surgery alone. Three-year survival was 30% for preoperative chemotherapy and 0% for surgery alone. Prevalence of mutated K-ras oncogene was 15% in patients receiving preoperative chemotherapy and 42% in those treated with surgery alone. This may partly explain the different outcomes between the two groups.

At MDACC 60 patients with stage IIIA NSCLC were randomized to surgery alone or six cycles of perioperative chemotherapy (cyclophosphamide, etoposide, and cisplatin) (12). Three cycles were given preoperatively and three cycles postoperatively in responders. Sixty-nine percent of the surgery-only group and 71% of the chemotherapy group had clinical stage IIIA disease. Only 20/28 patients in the chemotherapy arm went on to thoracotomy. There was one complete responder and eight partial responders to preoperative chemotherapy. Complete resection rates were 61 and 66% and were not statistically different. Estimated median survival in the chemotherapy group was 64 months compared to 11 months in the surgery-alone arm ($p < 0.008$). Estimated 2- and 3-year survivals were 60% and 56% respectively, for the perioperative chemotherapy patients and 25% and 15% for those who had surgery alone. Most recurrences following resection were distant metastases. There was one local recurrence after complete resection in the chemotherapy arm and three in the surgery-alone arm. Including patients with unresectable disease, local control was not achieved in 43% (12/28) of patients in the chemotherapy arm and 44% (14/32) of patients in the surgery arm.

Radiation Therapy

The results of RTOG 73-01 established a "standard" for definitive radiation for medically inoperable or technically unresectable NSCLC (14). This study showed survival rates with continuous-course radiation to 60 Gy in 30 fractions to be superior to lower total doses. Survival at 2 years was 20% with a local control of 50%. The "standard" radiation-only arms of RTOG 88-08 and CALGB 8433 both reported similar results (15,16). Patients in these studies had IIIA or IIIB disease, KPS ≥ 70, and <5% weight loss in the 3 months prior to entry. In the RTOG study, median survival was 11.4 months and 1-year survival 46%. Fifty-six percent of patients had N_2 disease, 20% had N_3 disease, and only 24% had

N_{0-1} disease (15). In the CALGB study median survival was 9.6 months and 1-, 3-, and 5-year survivals were 40%, 10%, and 6%, respectively (16). Despite the more advanced stage in the radiation series the results are similar to those in the surgical series. Survival in these studies was superior in the induction chemotherapy arms due mostly to decreased distant metastases. Locoregional progression was high, emphasizing the need for more aggressive local treatment.

A phase I/II dose escalation trial of hyperfractionated radiation with total doses of 60–79.2 Gy for unresectable NSCLC demonstrated a dose response for survival (10). Survival with 69.6 Gy given at 1.2 Gy per fraction twice daily was significantly better than with lower doses. Two-year survival was 29% and median survival was 13 months. These results were confirmed in the hyperfractionation arm of RTOG 88-08, showing a 1-year survival of 51% and median survival of 12.3 months (15).

Cox et al. evaluated only patients with clinical N_2 disease with <5% weight loss and KPS $\geq$ 70 treated with hyperfractionated radiation on RTOG 83-11 and compared them to similar patients treated with "standard" radiation on RTOG protocols 73-01, 78-11, and 79-11 (17). Patients treated with 1.2 Gy twice daily to 69.6 Gy had significantly longer 1- and 3-year survivals (58% and 20%, respectively) compared to 2 Gy per fraction to 60 Gy (30% and 7%). More than half of the patients had T_3 or T_4 primary tumors. Patients with technically unresectable disease were not excluded. Despite differences in patient population compared to surgical series, these results compare favorably to those with surgery alone or surgery plus postoperative radiation. They are also similar to those in surgical series using perioperative chemotherapy or chemoradiotherapy.

Multimodality Therapy-Surgery

Preoperative Chemotherapy

Preoperative chemotherapy or chemoradiotherapy in responsive tumors can increase resectability rates and control micrometastases. It is important that studies evaluating induction therapy followed by surgery for N_2 disease use pathological staging prior to induction therapy. Studies from Memorial Sloan-Kettering (18), the CALGB (19), and Toronto (20) used preoperative chemotherapy and postoperative irradiation in pathologically documented clinical N_2 disease. Complete resection rates were 51–65%, locoregional relapse 25%, and median survivals 15–21 months (Table 2).

The 136 patients in the Sloan-Kettering study had clinical N_2 disease defined as bulky mediastinal lymph node metastases or multiple levels of lymph node involvement in the ipsilateral mediastinum or subcarinal space on chest x-rays, computed tomographic scans, or mediastinoscopy (18). Patients received two to three cycles of MVP (mitomycin + vindesine or vinblastine + high-dose cisplatin) preoperatively. The complete resection rate was 65% and the complete

TABLE 2   Multimodality Therapy

Survival	Median	1 year	2 year	3 year	5 year
Preop CT					
Martini (1)	19			28%	17%
Sugarbaker (19)	15			23%	
Burkes (20)	21			34%	
Preop CT/RT					
Strauss (22)	15.5	58%			
Albain (21)	15			26%	
Weiden (24)	13				
CT/RT					
Dillman (16)	13.7	54%	26%	24%	17%
Sause (15)	13.8	60%			
Byhard (27)	12.2	54%	28%		

pathological response rate was 14%. After complete resection, local regional recurrences occurred only in patients who did not have complete pathological responses. Median survival was 19 months and overall 3- and 5-year survival rates were 28% and 17%, respectively. The CALGB used vinblastine and cisplatin preoperatively followed by postoperative irradiation (19) with a complete resection rate of 62%. Median survival was 15 months. Burkes et al. published a similar series from Toronto, using preoperative chemotherapy. The resection rate was 51% and the median survival 21 months (20). There was a plateau in overall survival between 3 and 5 years of 34% (21). In these studies, the majority of recurrences in patients with complete resections were distant metastases. Most patients with unresectable disease died of locoregional progression.

Preoperative Chemoradiotherapy

Preoperative chemoradiotherapy has been assessed in phase II studies by CALGB (22), SWOG (23), and LCSG (24). These studies were intended for marginally resectable or potentially unresectable disease. This may be the most appropriate group to compare to patients treated with definitive chemoradiation (Table 2).

The CALGB trial treated 41 patients with histologically confirmed T_3 and/ or N_2 disease (22). Eighty percent of patients had N_2 disease. Both preoperatively and postoperatively, patients were treated with two cycles of cisplatin, vinblastine, and 5-FU, and radiation starting concurrently with the first cycle of chemotherapy. Each cycle of radiation was 30 Gy given in 15 fractions. Resection rate was 57% with a complete response rate of 22.5%. Median survival was 15.5 months and 1-year survival 58%. There were six (14%) treatment-related deaths. In the SWOG study, eligible patients had histologically proven N_2 or N_3 nodal disease or T_4 primary lesions (23). Patients were treated with 45 Gy given at 1.8 Gy per fraction concurrently with two cycles of cisplatin and etoposide. Resectability was 83%. Locoregional relapse was 11%. Three-year survival was 26% and median survival 15 months. Treatment-related mortality was 10%. Median survival time and 3-year survival rate were significantly better if mediastinal nodes were negative in the surgical specimen (30 months vs. 10 months and 44% vs. 18%). The LCSG treated 85 patients with technically unresectable disease (24). They received two cycles of cisplatin and 5-FU with 30 Gy at 2 Gy per fraction starting concurrently with the first cycle of chemotherapy. Complete pathological response was 9%. Complete resection rate was 34%. Median survival was 13 months. Postoperative mortality was 7%. Treatment-related deaths with induction chemotherapy and chemoradiotherapy were between 4 and 10%.

Multimodality Therapy—Radiation

The CALGB 8433 and RTOG 8808 have established standard of care for patients with unresectable stage IIIA and IIIB NSCLC with KPS $\geq$ 70 and <5% weight loss. These trials demonstrated median and overall survival advantage of induction chemotherapy with two cycles of vinblastine and cisplatin followed by "standard" radiation over "standard" radiation alone or hyperfractionated radiation alone (Table 2).

RTOG 8808 included medically or surgically inoperable clinical stage II, IIIA, and IIIB disease (15). This was a three-arm study comparing induction chemotherapy followed by 60 Gy radiation given at 2 Gy per fraction, 60 Gy radiation alone, and 69.9 Gy given at 1.2 Gy twice daily. Only 5–7% of patients in each arm were stage II, and 18–24% of patients had N_{0-1} disease. The remaining patients had N_2–N_3 disease. One-year survival was 60% in the induction chemotherapy arm, 46% for standard radiation, and 51% for hyperfractionated radiation. Median survivals were 13.8, 11.4, and 12.3, respectively. These differences were significant. CALGB 8433 compared the same induction chemotherapy arm to standard radiation (16). Patients had to have clinical T_3 or N_2 disease with <5% weight loss and Zubrod performance status of 0 or 1. Median survival for CT-RT was 13.7 months compared to 9.6 months for radiation alone. Three- and 5-year survival rates were 24 and 17%, respectively, in the chemotherapy arm and 10 and 6% in the radiation-only arm. Local failure rates in both trials were high, emphasizing the need for more aggressive local treatment.

Concurrent chemotherapy and radiation has demonstrated promising local response rates. Radiosensitizing chemotherapy improves local control (25). The EORTC conducted a phase III trial with nonstandard radiation of 30 Gy in 10 fractions with a 3-week break followed by 25 Gy in 10 fractions with either weekly or daily cisplatin. Survival due to improved local control was superior in the radiotherapy-plus-weekly-cisplatin group. One-, 2-, and 3-year survival rates were 54%, 26%, and 16%, respectively. Two-year survival without local failure was 31% with weekly cisplatin compared to 19% without. Jeremic et al. randomized patients to 64.8 Gy at 1.2 Gy twice daily alone or with weekly or every-other-week carboplatin and VP16 (26). Five-year overall survival, median survival, and local control were improved with weekly chemotherapy. Five-year survival was 21% versus 4.9%, median survival 18 versus 8 months, and 5-year local recurrence-free survival 34% versus 12%. There was a plateau from 3 to 5 years in overall survival and local recurrence-free survival. RTOG conducted a phase II trial of hyperfractionated radiation given concurrently with cisplatin and vinblastine (27). Inoperable stage II, IIIA, and IIIB patients were eligible, the majority of whom had >5% weight loss over 3 months prior to therapy. Concurrent chemotherapy and hyperfractionated radiation had more intense acute toxicity than hyperfractionation alone, but late toxicity was acceptable. One- and 2-year survival rates were 54% and 28%, respectively, and median survival was 12.2 months (27).

RTOG 94-10 is a three-arm phase III study comparing induction chemotherapy followed by standard radiation to concurrent chemotherapy and daily radiation or concurrent chemotherapy and hyperfractionated radiation in "good risk" patients with medically inoperable stage II and IIIA or unresectable stage IIIA and IIIB NSCLC. This phase III trial with over 600 patients compared 3 arms: (1) induction CT (cisplatin/vinblastine) plus RT (60 Gy/qd); (2) the same regimen administered concurrently; and (3) concurrent cisplatin and oral VP-16 with hyperfractionated RT (BID to 69.6 Gy). The median survival times were 14.6 months, 17.0 months, and 15.6 months, respectively. These preliminary results demonstrated a trend (p = 0.08) supporting the benefit of concurrent chemo/RT (using daily RT) (28).

CONCLUSION

The best chemoradiotherapy regimens in good-risk patients yield similar results to preoperative chemoradiotherapy trials, despite the fact that there is a selection bias with more extensive IIIA and IIIB being excluded form the surgical trials. Chemoradiotherapy alone results in significant myelosuppression, esophagitis, and pneumonitis. Morbidity from induction chemoradiotherapy followed by surgery is significant. The dissection may be more difficult after radiation and/or chemotherapy due to fibrosis in the tumor area, especially if there has been a dramatic response. Surgery following induction therapy increases the frequency of pulmonary complications over that expected for surgery alone, radiotherapy alone, or chemoradiotherapy. Quality of life is a necessary part of evaluating treatment outcomes in this population.

Local control rates in patients undergoing complete resection after induction therapy are high. These are a select group of patients who have responded to induction therapy. With the best available chemotherapy and radiotherapy combinations surgical resection may not further improve results in clinical N_2 disease but may only serve to increase complications and have a negative impact on quality of life.

In patients with minimal N_2 disease, the best available chemotherapy and radiotherapy combinations in comparable patient groups may yield similar results as surgery. This may be an acceptable alternative to surgery in patients who refuse surgery or are medically unfit for surgery.

REFERENCES

1. Martini N, Flehinger BJ. The role of surgery in N_2 lung cancer. Surg Clin North Am 1987; 67(5):1037–1049.
2. Shields TW. The significance of ipsilateral mediastinal lymph node metastasis (N_2 disease) in non–small cell carcinoma of the lung. A commentary. J Thorac Cardiovasc Surg 1990; 99:48–53.
3. Greco FA, Hainsworth JD. Multidisciplinary approach to potentially curable non–small cell carcinoma of the lung. Oncology 1997; 11(1):27–36.
4. Naruke T, Goya T, Tsuchiya R, Suemasu K. The importance of surgery to non–small cell carcinoma of lung with mediastinal lymph node metastasis. Ann Thorac Surg 1988; 46:603–610.
5. Ginsberg RJ, Vokes EE, Raben A. Non-small cell lung cancer. In: DeVita VT, Hellman S, Rosenberg SA, eds. Cancer: Principles and Practice of Oncology. Philadelphia: Lippincott-Raven, 1997:856–911.
6. Pearson FG, DeLarue NC, Ilves R, Todd TR, Cooper JD. Significance of positive superior mediastinal nodes identified at mediastinoscopy. J Thorac Cardiovasc Surg 1982; 83:1–11.
7. Pass HI, Pogrebniak HW, Steinberg SM, Mulshine J, Minna J. Randomized trial of neoadjuvant therapy for lung cancer: interim analysis. Ann Thorac Surg 1992; 53: 992–998.
8. Yoneda S, Hibino S, Gotoh I, Sakai H, Noguchi Y, Yamamoto M, Nishimura H, Izumo T, Sakura M. A comparative trial on induction chemoradiotherapy followed by surgery (CRS) or immediate surgery (IS) for stage III non–small cell lung cancer (NSCLC). Proc Asco 1995; 14:367.
9. Rosenthal SA, Curran WJ, Herbert SH, Hughes EN, Sandler HM, Stafford PM, McKenna WG. Clinical stage II non–small cell lung cancer treated with radiation therapy alone. Cancer 1992; 70(10):2410–2417.
10. Cox JD, Azarnia N, Byhardt RW, Shin KH, Emami B, Pajak TF. A randomized phase I/II trial of hyperfractionated radiation therapy with total doses of 60.0 Gy to 79.2 Gy: possible survival benefit with ≥69.6 Gy in favorable patients with radiation therapy oncology group stage III non–small cell lung carcinoma: report of radiation therapy oncology group 83-11. J Clin Oncol 1990; 8(9):1543–1555.
11. Rosell R, Gomez-Codina J, Camps C, Maestre J, Padille J, Canto A, Mate JL, Li S, Roig J, Olazabal A, Canela M, Ariza A, Skagel Z, Morera-Prat J, Abad A. A randomized trial comparing preoperative chemotherapy plus surgery with surgery

alone in patients with non–small cell lung cancer. N Engl J Med 1994; 330(3):153–158.

12. Roth JA, Fossella F, Komaki R, Ryan MB, Putnam Jr. JB, Lee JS, Dhingra H, De Caro L, Chasen M, McGavran M, Atkinson EN, Kong WK. A randomized trial comparing perioperative chemotherapy and surgery with surgery alone in resectable stage III non–small cell lung cancer. J Natl Cancer Inst 1994; 86:673–680.

13. Jolly PC, Hutchinson BS, Detterbeck F, Guyton SW, Hofer B, Anderson RP. Routine computed tomographic scans, selective mediastinoscopy, and other factors in evaluation of lung cancer. J Thorac Cardiovasc Surg 1991; 102:266–271.

14. Perez C, Stanley K, Rubin P, Kramer S, Brady L, Pere-Tamayo R, Brown GS, Concannon J, Rotman M, Seydel HG. A prospective randomized study of various irradiation doses and fractionation schedules in the treatment of inoperable non–oat cell carcinoma of the lung. Preliminary report by the Radiation Oncology Therapy Group. Cancer 1980; 45(11):2744–2753.

15. Sause WT, Scott C, Taylor S, Johnson D, Livingston R, Komaki R, Emami B, Curran WJ, Byhardt RW, Turrisi AT, Dar AR, Cox JD. Radiation Therapy Oncology Group (RTOG) 88-08 and Eastern Cooperative Oncology Group (ECOG) 4588: preliminary results of a phase III trial in regionally advance, unresectable non–small cell lung cancer. J Natl Cancer Inst 1995; 87(3):198–205.

16. Dillman RO, Herdon J, Seagren SL, Eaton WL Jr, Green MR. Improved survival in stage III non–small cell lung cancer: seven-year follow-up of Cancer and Leukemia Group B (CALGB) 8433 trial. J Natl Cancer Inst 1996; 88(17):1210–1215.

17. Cox JD, Azarnia N, Byhardt RW, Shin KH, Emami B, Perez CA. N₂ (clinical) non–small cell carcinoma of the lung: prospective trials of radiation therapy with total doses 60 Gy by the radiation therapy oncology group. Int J Radiat Oncol Biol Phys 1991; 20:7–12.

18. Martini N, Kris MG, Flehinger BJ, Gralla RJ, Bains MS, Burt ME, Heelan R, McCormack PM, Pisters KMW, Rigas JR, Rusch VW, Ginsberg RJ. Preoperative chemotherapy for stage IIIA (N₂) lung cancer: the Sloan-Kettering experience with 136 patients. Ann Thorac Surg 1993; 55:1365–1374.

19. Sugarbaker DJ, Herndon J, Kohman LJ, Krasna MJ, Green MR, Cancer and Leukemia Group B Thoracic Surgery Group. Results of Cancer and Leukemia Group B protocol 8935. A multi-institutional phase II trimodality trial for stage IIIA non–small cell lung cancer. J Thorac Cardiovasc Surg 1995; 109:473–485.

20. Burkes RL, Shepherd FA, Ginsberg RJ, Blackstein ME, Goldberg M, Todd T, Pearson FG, Jones C, Greenwood C. Induction chemotherapy with MVP for stage III (N₂) unresectable non–small-cell lung cancer: results of Toronto phase II trial. J Clin Oncol 1992; 10:580–586.

21. Albain KS. Induction chemotherapy with/without radiation followed by surgery in stage III non–small-cell lung cancer. Oncology 1997; 11(suppl 9):51–57.

22. Strauss GM, Herndon JE, Sherman DD, Mathisen DJ, Carey RW, Choi NC, Rege VB, Modeas C, Green MR. Neoadjuvant chemotherapy and radiotherapy followed by surgery in stage IIIA non–small-cell carcinoma of the lung: report of a Cancer and Leukemia Group B phase II study. J Clin Oncol 1992; 10(8):1237–1244.

23. Albain KS, Rusch VW, Crowley JJ, Rice TW, Turrisi AT, Weick JK, Lonchyna VA, Presant CA, McKenna RJ, Gandara DR, Fosmire H, Taylor SA, Stelzer KJ,

Beasley KR, Livingston RB. Concurrent cisplatin/etoposide plus chest radiotherapy followed by surgery for stages IIIA (N$_2$) and IIIB non–small-cell lung cancer: mature results of Southwest Oncology Group phase II study 8805. J Clin Oncol 1995; 13(8): 1880–1892.

24. Weiden PL, Piantadosi S. Preoperative chemotherapy (cisplatin and fluorouracil) and radiation therapy in stage III non–small-cell lung cancer: a phase II study of the Lung Cancer Study Group. J Natl Cancer Inst 1991; 83(4):266–272.

25. Schaake-Koning C, van den Bogaert W, Dalesio O, Festen J, Hoogenhout J, van Houtte P, Kirkpatrick A, Koolen M, Maat B, Nijs A, Renaud A, Rodrigus P, Schuster-Uitterhoeve L, Sculier J, van Zandwijk N, Bartelink H. Effects of concomitant cisplatin and radiotherapy on inoperable non–small-cell lung cancer. N Engl J Med 1992; 326(8):524–530.

26. Jeremic B, Shibamoto Y, Acimovic L, Djuric L. Randomized trial of hyperfractionated radiation therapy with or without concurrent chemotherapy for stage III non–small-cell lung cancer. J Clin Oncol 1995; 13(2):452–458.

27. Byhardt RW, Scott CB, Ettinger DS, Curran WJ, Doggett RLS, Coughlin C, Scarantino C, Rotman M, Emami B. Concurrent hyperfractionated irradiation and chemotherapy for unresectable non–small cell lung cancer. Cancer 1995; 75(9):2337–2344.

28. Curran WJ, Jr, Scott C, Langer C, Komaki R, Lee J, Hauser S, Movsas B, Wasserman TH, Rosenthal S, Byhardt R, Sause W, Cox J. Phase III comparison of sequential vs. concurrent chemoradiation for PTS with unresected stage III non–small cell lung cancer (NSCLS): Initial report of Radiation Therapy Oncology Group (RTOG) 9410. Proc ASCO 2000; 19, 484a.

14

Management of Superior Sulcus Tumors

**Garrett L. Walsh, Sunil Gandhi, and
Ritsuko Komaki**
University of Texas M. D. Anderson Cancer Center, Houston, Texas

INTRODUCTION

Controversy and confusion are terms that appropriately describe the diagnosis, workup, and management of superior sulcus tumors, first described over a century and a half ago. As a relatively rare bronchogenic malignancy, accounting for less than 3% of all lung cancers, there have been no randomized, controlled trials evaluating treatment modalities. Most of the progress has been made through single-institution phase II trials using historical controls as a measure of success. Advances in surgical and radiation therapy techniques have improved local control and long-term survival to the point where the expected cure rates are comparable to those of non–superior sulcus lung cancers. Despite treatment advances, locoregional recurrence following treatment can cause debilitating problems from invasion into surrounding musculoskeletal and neurovascular structures that can lead to severe pain, often difficult to control with narcotics. Tumor growth can lead to the progressive loss of function of the upper extremity on the affected side. A thoracic surgeon need only encounter one such patient in his career, who has lost limb function, to serve as an impetus to develop aggressive surgical and multimodality treatments to deal both with the devastating local problems and the systemic metastatic disease that these tumors inflict. In this chapter we will examine the clinical changes in evaluation, management, and multimodality approaches that have evolved over the past 50 years in caring for these patients.

HISTORICAL CONTROVERSIES RELATED TO PRESENTATION AND ORIGIN

A patient with a tumor involving the apex of the lung associated with localized pain and an ulnar neuropathy was first described by Edwin Hare in the *London Medical Gazette* in 1838 (1). The etiology of this mass was felt to be infectious. In 1924 and 1932, Henry Pancoast described a clinical syndrome that he had seen in seven patients with small opacities in their chest apices with local rib destruction and often vertebral infiltration (2,3). The clinical constellation of symptoms (Pancoast syndrome) included pain around the shoulder with or without radiation to the axilla, scapula, and down the arm, Horner's syndrome, and atrophy of the muscles of the hand. Death occurred as a result of what seemed to be a comparatively trivial growth in the thoracic inlet without detectable metastases. He had attributed the etiology of the destructive radiographic process to an embryonic rest. It was not until 1932 that Tobias in Argentina correctly identified this process as a bronchogenic cancer (4).

RADIOGRAPHIC CONTROVERSY: WHAT LESIONS ACTUALLY MEET THE CRITERIA OF A SUPERIOR SULCUS TUMOR?

Pancoast in his original paper was very specific in his description of the superior pulmonary sulcus tumors as always occurring at a definite location in the thoracic inlet producing constant and the characteristic clinical presentation of pain in the eighth cervical and first and second thoracic root distribution. Pancoast, who was a radiologist and at that time the chairman of the section of radiology of the American Medical Association, described the lesion radiographically as "a small, homogeneous density at the extreme apex with more or less local rib destruction and often vertebral infiltration." There was no description of involvement of the superior vena cava or the phrenic or recurrent laryngeal nerves (5). Large tumors with their epicenter in the center of the upper lobe with extension into the apex can also produce a clinical Pancoast syndrome but do not meet his strict radiographic definition. True superior sulcus tumors can often be overlooked as thickening of the apical pleura and are often small tumors, leading to a delay in diagnosis in many patients.

Many series do not follow these strict definitions and therefore would include bulky upper-lobe tumors in their patient population. This often makes it difficult to compare one series results to the next. The larger tumors may be associated with symptoms of cough, hemoptysis, and superior vena caval obstruction that are not typically associated with these smaller apical tumors, which produce pain and a subtle thickening of the apical pleura. Today, better clinical appreciation of these tumors often will lead to a diagnosis of a superior sulcus tumor prior to the development of advanced wasting of the hypothenar hand muscles or ulnar neuropathy as was seen 60 years ago. By definition, these tumors are T_3 or T_4 and therefore are associated with pain around the shoulder, axilla, or arm and varying degrees of neurological involvement or loss of function depending on the extent of nerve root, sympathetic nerve, rib, or vertebral body involvement. Similarly, an apical tumor without the clinical presentation of pain would not qualify as a superior sulcus tumor.

INITIAL CONTROVERSIAL TREATMENT APPROACHES

The opinion of the medical community in the 1930s and 1940s was that these lesions were uniformly fatal with no known 5-year survivors, with death usually occurring within 10–14 months from the time of diagnosis (6). Pancoast stated that these tumors were clearly not amenable to surgical resection and were also considered radioresistant. Fifty years later we know that both of these statements were incorrect. Surgeons had been reluctant to attempt resection because of the typical dense infiltration of the tumor into the surrounding tissue. While it was felt that radiation therapy could not cure a patient, in the early 1950s Haas et al. described a patient who had not only survived nearly 3 years after radiation therapy but also, more importantly, had significant improvement in symptoms (7). It was not until 1956 that Chardack and MacCallum published the first successful report of a combined-modality (surgery followed by 65-Gy radiation therapy) cure of a patient (8). In the 1960s, with higher dosage and wider portals including the mediastinum, vertebral bodies, and supraclavicular fossae, reports were published with 5-year survivors after radiation therapy alone.

Shaw and colleagues in 1961 described a fortuitous case where a patient with an ''unresectable'' Pancoast tumor responded dramatically with a 50% decrease in the tumor volume after an initial 30 Gy of radiation therapy (9). This was sufficient to permit a complete resection of the lesion. This patient lived for 27 years without recurrence of the tumor. Their approach was popularized by Paulson and has remained the ''standard'' approach for this lesion for over 30 years in many centers (10). Surgical techniques have also evolved over the past 50 years, and tumors that involve the subclavian vessels or the vertebral body, previously considered an absolute contraindication to resection, can now be safely resected and reconstructed with minimal morbidity and mortality (11). We will now examine some of the specific details of these changing treatment modalities that have occurred and the present-day evaluation of these lesions.

EVALUATION OF A PATIENT

The early diagnosis of a superior sulcus tumor often requires an astute clinician. The periscapular and shoulder pain is frequently misdiagnosed as bursitis or arthritis or cervical degenerative disc disease with secondary radicular pain into the arm. The mean delay in diagnosis is usually 5–7 months but can vary from 1 to 48 months (12). Pain or symptoms along an ulnar nerve distribution should prompt a chest radiograph regardless of the age of the patient and especially if there is a smoking history. We have seen advanced Pancoast tumors in individuals even in their twenties. Many have been erroneously diagnosed as ulnar entrapment syndrome or carpal tunnel syndrome and have undergone transposition and decompressive procedures on these nerves with persistent postoperative pain that usually prompts a more detailed evaluation. A good-quality plain chest radiograph with a special emphasis on the symmetry of the apices will often be the first step to appropriate diagnosis of the problem. Horner's syndrome [ptosis, enophthalmos, and a meiotic (small) pupil because of unopposed parasympathetic innervation] and dryness and inability to sweat on the side of the face usually are seen in more locally advanced tumors that have invaded the stellate ganglion on the vertebral body. This usually occurs in 20–40% of the patients (11,13). Although recognized as a poor prognostic clinical sign, this does not necessarily rule out surgery (12).

These patients, on presentation, are often debilitated because of chronic pain and have lost a fair amount of weight because of the secondary anorexia that results. While their presenting performance (Karnofsky) status can be so poor to the point that they are felt not to be a surgical candidate, an intense program of appropriately dosed narcotics, either orally or by patch administration, can dramatically improve their quality of life and appetite. We have used Megace over a short time frame as an appetite stimulant to help patients regain weight and muscle mass that they have lost over several months secondary to anorexia and pain. Some patients can be nutritionally optimized within 2–3 weeks to a point where a major resection can be performed safely.

The medical history must also focus on other bone symptoms away from the tumor and a detailed review of systems trying to discern new neurological findings. The physical examination will focus on the general physical appearance of the patient, the supraclavicular fossa that often reveals the asymmetry and firmness on the side of the tumor, a search for palpable lymph nodes on both sides of the neck and axilla, and the degree of neurological changes in the arm. Sensory changes usually occur at the T1 level and can extend equally cephalad and caudally into the C8 and T2 levels and less commonly into the T3 and C7 levels. Progressive neurological changes occur as these lesions initially abut, displace, and finally invade these intercostal nerves and the roots of the brachial plexus. Patients with more prolonged symptoms will also begin to show atrophy of the hypothenar muscles. Progressive motor loss in the hand, wrist, and arm usually indicates a more advanced tumor with progressive cephalad infiltration rather than displacement of the brachial plexus (14). We would view upper-trunk involvement with motor loss as a contraindication to a surgical approach.

IS THE RADIOGRAPHIC WORKUP ANY DIFFERENT FROM THAT DONE FOR ROUTINE LUNG CANCERS?

Most bronchogenic malignancies can be fully evaluated with a plain chest radiograph and a CT scan of the chest (which includes a few cuts of the upper abdomen) with bone scans and brain scans requested only if clinical symptoms exist. The chest radiograph is also very important in the initial diagnosis of a superior sulcus tumor. Special attention must be focused on the lung apices, above the medial portion of the clavicle within the arc of the first rib on the posteroanterior film. Asymmetrical pleural thickening is usually the first subtle radiographic finding. An elevation of the hemidiaphragm on the affected side may indicate a more advanced lesion that has involved the phrenic nerve.

CT scans of the chest are important to assess for enlarged hilar or mediastinal nodes and for other parenchymal metastases. Patients with superior sulcus tumors in addition require MRI evaluations as the coronal and sagittal imaging techniques yield important details for surgical planning, including the involvement of the subclavian vessels, the extent of infiltration of the brachial plexus, and the number of bony structures invaded including the ribs, clavicle, sternum, and vertebral body. These details cannot be as readily appreciated by computed tomography. The extent of vertebral body involvement is critical for surgical planning including the extension into the neural canal, with or without epidural extension and dural sac compression. This anatomical location of a lung cancer is the only site where we routinely obtain an MRI for evaluation, which yields more information than a CT scan for preoperative evaluation. Positron emission tomography (PET) will likely be more frequently utilized in the workup and follow-up of patients following surgery and radiation therapy in the next 5 years but there is little information in this subset of lung cancer patients now.

While the biological behavior of superior sulcus tumors is considered by some to remain more locally aggressive for a longer period of time prior to metastasis, many patients will eventually die from metastatic disease. As the brain is the most common site of systemic failure, we routinely perform MRI imaging of the brain prior to considering treatment options and embarking on major surgical resections. Bone scans are also done to complete the metastatic workup and help evaluate the extent of bony involvement of the ribs, clavicle, sternum, and vertebral bodies.

PHYSIOLOGICAL TESTING

All patients undergo physiological pulmonary testing with a baseline spirometry, pre- and postbronchodilators, and diffusion capacity measurements. Exercise oxygen consumption testing can be performed in patients with marginal respiratory parameters (15). Xenon ventilation and perfusion scans help to predict if a formal lobectomy can be tolerated or if a more limited segmental or nonanatomical wedge resection is required. It is hard to predict the physiological compromise to a patient's respiratory function following the en bloc resections that usually require one to three ribs and an extended posterolateral thoracotomy. Although the chest wall defect does not usually require formal reconstruction (as it is very well covered by the scapula and chest wall musculature), these patients seem to experience a fair amount of lung volume loss on the operative hemithorax. Resection of the scalene muscles and on occasion the clavicle further leads to rotation of the shoulder and loss of some of these accessory muscles of respiration. These are important considerations when trying to decide to proceed to an anatomical lobectomy in these patients. Many require assisted ventilation and are prone to collapse of the remaining lobe or lobes on the operative side for a few days, postoperatively, until better pulmonary mucous clearance and chest wall movement are possible on the operative side.

PRETREATMENT HISTOLOGICAL DIAGNOSIS: IS IT NECESSARY AND HOW SHOULD IT BE OBTAINED?

There are several conditions, including fungal and bacterial infections (*Staphylococcus*, *Cryptococcus*, *Echinococcus*, and *Actinomyces*), lymphomas, and plasmacytomas, that can mimic a superior sulcus tumor; therefore, we feel it is essential to obtain tissue for diagnosis prior to treatment or enrollment on a protocol (16). Occasionally these tumors can be of small cell histology, which is better treated nonsurgically. Transthoracic fine-needle aspiration (FNA) has yielded the best results with a positive diagnostic yield in >90% of patients (14). Pneumothorax is rare as these tumors are often invading the surrounding structures and the lung cannot fall away from the chest wall. If a pneumothorax does result and the tumor does in fact "fall away" from the thoracic apex, it is not a Pancoast tumor and will be at worst a T2 (visceral pleural involvement) lesion. Palpable scalene or supraclavicular nodes can be biopsied directly in the outpatient clinic. Because of the peripheral location, sputum cytology and bronchoscopy are usually less rewarding with positive results in only 20–40% of patients. Thoracoscopy, while useful for the evaluation of the pleural cavity, is not generally utilized to avoid tumor spill that may result from manipulation of the adhesions at the apex of the chest. Mediastinoscopy should be used in patients with clinically enlarged nodes by CT scan (>1 cm) because of the poor outcome in many series in patients with N_2 disease with superior sulcus tumors.

The histology of superior sulcus tumors in most series demonstrates 25–40% squamous, 25–60% adenocarcinoma (with adenocarcinomas representing nearly twice the incidence of squamous histology in more recent studies over the past 10 years) with the remaining 5–15% large cell, mixed, and approximately 2–5% small cell histologies.

NODAL INVOLVEMENT: SHOULD STANDARD N_2 AND N_3 NODAL DEFINITIONS APPLY TO SUPERIOR SULCUS TUMORS?

All of the Pancoast tumors are at minimum T3 (parietal pleura, rib involvement) or T4 (vertebral body or mediastinal structure). Patients with N_2 disease are known to have a poor overall survival. Therefore, in the face of radiographically enlarged (>1 cm) mediastinal nodes, we would first proceed to mediastinoscopy prior to resection to confirm or rule out N_2 disease. Even in the setting of a normal mediastinum by CT scan, many would argue that mediastinoscopy should be routine as the long-term survival of these patients with N_2 disease is so poor that it would not be warranted to proceed with a major en bloc resection with no survival advantage (17). If positive paratracheal or subcarinal nodes were demonstrated preoperatively, then surgery would be abandoned as a treatment option in favor of radiation therapy.

By definition, a supraclavicular node or scalene node on the same side of the tumor is an N_3 node. We would, however, consider a node in this setting to be more of a locoregional node and would not exclude a patient from surgery on this basis if the surgeon felt all disease could be resected at the time of surgery. Some studies show an obvious survival difference in N_1 disease versus N_2 or N_3 but no difference between N_2 and N_3 patients (18). Muscolino et al., however, have demonstrated that the presence of an ipsilateral supraclavicular metastasis was not a contraindication to operation (19). Hilaris et al. demonstrated improved survival in patients with N_0, N_1, or N_3 disease compared to N_2 (20).

Other European authors, Grunenwald and Spaggiari, who have experience with radical resections for superior sulcus tumors, also adopt this philosophy toward cervical nodes (21).

DIFFERENT SURGICAL APPROACHES AND WHEN THEY ARE USED

A patient is considered to be a surgical candidate unless: (1) he has documented metastatic disease to the mediastinum or other organs, (2) he has pronounced

motor loss of the arm with MRI evidence of extensive brachial plexus, or (3) he
has direct invasion of the trachea or esophagus. The CT scans and the MRI are
extremely important in planning the surgical approach. A surgeon should consider an operation only in patients in whom he feels a complete surgical resection
of all gross disease is possible. Debulking of Pancoast tumors is of no benefit
and does not improve local control.

We have utilized Dartevelle's classification of tumor location along the
first rib as anterior, middle, or posterior to guide our surgical approach (22,23).
We utilize one of three surgical approaches to resect these lesions: (1) an anterior
neck approach only, (2) a posterior approach only, or (3) a combined anterior and
posterior approach. Anteriorly placed tumors often abut or invade the subclavian
vessels. If the subclavian vein is involved by MRI, a hockey-stick incision is
made along the anterior border of the sternocleidomastoid muscle and extended
along the clavicle. The clavicle is resected with a Gigli saw to improve the exposure to the subclavian vessels (Figure 1). No attempt is made to salvage, plate,
or reconstruct the clavicle. Removal of the clavicle affords excellent exposure
of the thoracic inlet. Tumors that involve the vein have usually resulted in collat-
eralization around the scapula and chest wall over many months; therefore, it is
not necessary to reconstruct the subclavian vein and simple ligation of the subcla-

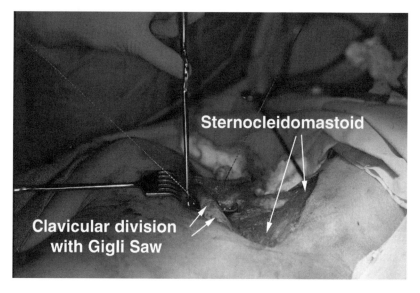

FIGURE 1   Initial dissection of an anteriorly positioned superior sulcus tumor with
an L-shaped incision along the anterior border of the sternocleidomastoid and
along the inferior margin of the right clavicle.

vian and usually the jugular vein is well tolerated. Occasionally, mild arm swelling can result if the vein was not previously fully obstructed, but this edema quickly improves once collaterals develop. On the left, the thoracic duct is carefully identified and ligated at its junction with the internal jugular and subclavian veins. This will prevent the development of a postoperative chyle leak, which will either drain into the neck wound or track into the chest requiring reoperation in most instances. When the tumor appears to displace rather than involve the subclavian vessels, the clavicle can often be left in place. We have modified Dartevelle's anterior approach and have tried to maintain the clavicle as much as possible. The cosmetic and functional deformity that results when the clavicular support is removed, with the secondary internal rotation and drooping of the arm, can be avoided. If the oncological dissection is compromised, however, the clavicle is removed. The anterior scalene muscle requires division next and the course of the phrenic nerve along the anterior border of scalenus anterior is identified and preserved if uninvolved or transected if infiltrated with tumor.

Dissection of the subclavian artery in the subadventitial plane often permits elevation of the subclavian artery away from the tumor mass. Care must be taken to divide the internal mammary artery to permit elevation of the subclavian artery off of the first rib. If the patient has been radiated prior to resection, care must be taken to ligate this vessel and avoid a suture cutting through the vessel, which is extremely soft and fragile (even in a nonradiated field). Dissection proximally of the right subclavian at its junction with the takeoff of the carotid from the innominate artery must avoid injury to the recurrent nerve, which branches from the vagus at this point and loops inferiorly around the subclavian artery. Significant morbidity can result if the recurrent is injured resulting in poor vocal cord apposition and a poor cough postoperatively increasing the risk of atelectasis and pneumonia. The thyrocervical trunk often requires ligation and the dissection proceeds laterally attempting to elevate the subclavian artery from the first rib. The vertebral artery may also require ligation. With the subclavian artery mobilized, it is possible to divide the anterior portion of the first and second ribs from the front (Figure 2). If the subclavian artery is invaded rather than displaced by the tumor, it is resected and primarily reanastomosed if the segment is short, or an interposition graft of PTFE utilized for the reconstruction if a greater length is resected. Invasion of the subclavian artery should not be considered a contraindication to resection as this vessel can easily be resected through this anterior approach (Figure 3).

The brachial plexus can now be easily identified as it courses at an angle just lateral to the scalene anterior. Direct neurolysis is usually possible to free the plexus from the tumor. If required, the lower trunk of the plexus can be sharply divided if tumor infiltrates rather than displaces the nerve.

In some patients with small tumors, it is possible to divide the ribs posteriorly from the front and deliver the specimen into the neck wound, amputating a

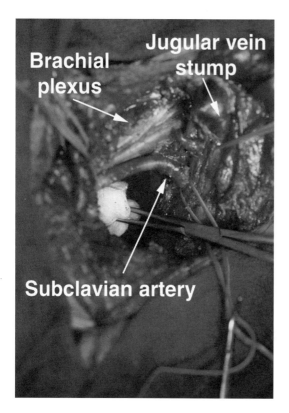

FIGURE 2   This dissection demonstrates the division of the first and second ribs from the anterior approach with resection of the subclavian vein and jugular vein. In this case the subclavian artery has been dissected along the plane of Leriche and spared. The brachial plexus is also demonstrated.

generous wedge of the upper lobe with a GIA or TA stapling device and allowing the lung to retract into the hemithorax. As such, a posterolateral thoracotomy is avoided. Anterior thoracotomies can also be performed with the patient supine and a formal lobectomy performed from the front.

For tumors that are extensive involving both the vessels anteriorly and the spine posteriorly, following mobilization of the vessels and plexus, and anterior division of one or two ribs, the neck incision can be closed and the patient repositioned for the posterior resection and lobectomy.

In patients with tumors that are posteriorly situated only, with a clear plane by MRI away from the subclavian vessels, the surgical approach can be in a standard manner, entirely from the back with an extended posterolateral thoracotomy. If the tumor involves the vertebral body and will require resection, the head

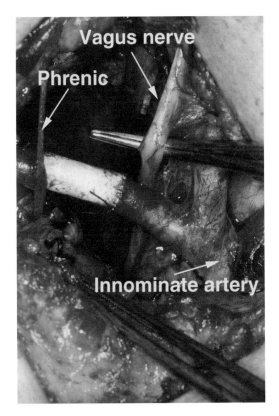

FIGURE 3   In this patient the tumor involved subclavian artery and required a 6-mm PTFE interposition graft to reconstruct the resected subclavian artery resected en bloc with the tumor. The vagus nerve has been transposed with the recurrent nerve behind the stump of the subclavian artery. The phrenic nerve has been preserved.

is positioned in cervical tongs at the time of lateral positioning (Figure 4). A generous posterolateral thoracotomy, with extension to the base of the neck by dividing the latissimus dorsi, trapezius, and rhomboids, is performed. A chest spreader is placed beneath the scapula and stabilized into one of the interspaces inferiorly. This permits the scapula to be elevated away from the chest wall and provides superb exposure to the superior sulcus of the chest. An interspace is chosen one below those involved with tumor to obtain a clear inferior margin. If this is not clear from the external examination of the hemithorax, an anterior interspace is initially opened to permit digital palpation of the chest from within. The anterior ribs are first divided. If a previous anterior approach has been performed, it is now safer and quicker to divide the first rib, if it was not previously

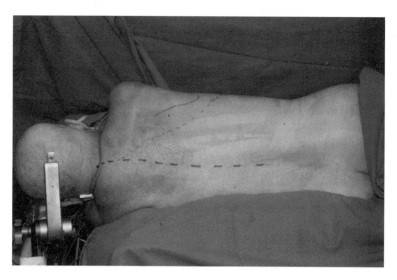

Figure 4 Patient positioned for an extended posterolateral thoracotomy with a chest wall resection and vertebral body resection for a superior sulcus tumor. The head is held in place with cervical tongs during the procedure to avoid movement in the spinal axis.

divided, knowing that the neurovascular structures have been safely elevated and mobilized away from the first rib. Otherwise, care must be taken to stay precisely in the subperiosteal plane, to avoid injury to these vital structures. If the paraspinal muscles are not involved, they are elevated from the transverse processes. The ribs are disarticulated from each of the transverse processes and the vertebral body taking care not to place excessive traction on the nerve roots, which can result in a dural tear where the nerve root exits the dural sac. If this tear at the "axilla" of the nerve root goes unrecognized, this will result in a serious postoperative cerebrospinal fluid leak that generally does not seal with conservative maneuvers such as the placement of a lumbar drain. Often, a re-do thoracotomy, drilling out the neural foramen and direct suture repair of the dural sac and coverage with autogeneous tissue, is required. Each of the neurovascular bundles is individually ligated as one proceeds cephalad. Dissection of the T1 nerve root must proceed slowly. This is a large root that courses just above the angle of the second rib, and runs beneath the first rib to join the C8 root. The neck of the first rib essentially bisects these two nerve roots. To safely remove the first rib without injury to these nerves, it is sometimes easier to divide the first rib at its angle. This now permits sharp dissection along the T1 root and the C8 root until a decision is made regarding the need to sacrifice or spare these roots. At this point the stellate ganglion is visualized and often has to be resected with the specimen. Patients who do not have a Horner's syndrome preoperatively often develop one postoperatively because of the extent of the required resection. When the preoperative consent is obtained, they must be informed that this will likely occur.

INVOLVEMENT OF THE VERTEBRAL BODY: SHOULD THIS BE CONSIDERED RESECTABLE OR UNRESECTABLE?

By many, clear-cut involvement of the vertebral body is considered a contraindication to surgery, as the results have been dismal with no patients surviving more than 1 year with most series demonstrating a median survival of only 7 months (5). We now have experience in over 200 resections of the vertebral bodies with immediate reconstruction for metastatic disease to the spine (24). We have applied these techniques to primary bronchogenic malignancies such as the Pancoast tumors when they directly invade the vertebral body (Figure 5). We recently

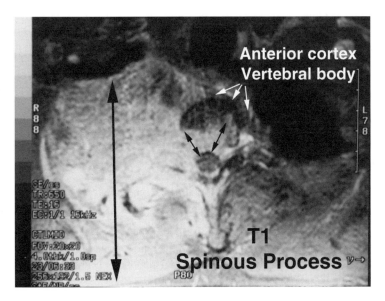

FIGURE 5 An extensive superior sulcus tumor presenting in a 32-year-old man with a 25-pack-year cigarette smoking history. Long arrow demonstrates extension of tumor into paraspinous musculature. Short arrows demonstrate vertebral body involvement with compression of spinal cord circumferentially. This patient required a three-level vertebrectomy and reconstruction with anterior and posterior instrumentation for resection of this tumor.

reported our experience with 17 patients from 1990 to 1998 with Pancoast tumors with T4 involvement of the vertebral body. Seven patients had total vertebrectomies with immediate reconstruction, seven with partial vertebrectomies, and three with neural foramina or transverse process resection (Figure 6). The median hospital stay was 11 days, with no perioperative deaths and all patients remaining ambulatory. Morbidity occurred in seven patients (42%) including pneumonia in six patients, arrhythmias in two, CSF leaks in two, and one wound breakdown. The actuarial 2-year survival was 54% with 11 patients alive 2–50 months following resection. The locoregional tumor recurrence was noted in six patients, all of whom had positive surgical margins as opposed to 1/11 patients who had negative margins ($p < 0.006$). The 2-year actuarial survival was 80% in the 11 patients in whom we obtained negative margins compared to 0% for the six with positive margins ($p < 0.006$). Our present technique is to separately resect the involved vertebrae once the tumor with disarticulated ribs and chest wall has been removed. All areas are resected with reconstruction performed when the support function of the vertebrae has been compromised. We use a combination of an anterior methylmethacrylate column created around a chest tube supplemented with lateral titanium plating. If more levels or structure is sacrificed by wider resection, or anterior plating is not possible, then an extensive posterior instrumentation is performed (Figures 7–9). This requires a careful transition from the skin incision of the thoracotomy to the midline incision for posterior instrumentation to avoid ischemic skin flaps that can result in serious wound dehiscence and contamination of the spinal hardware if breakdown occurs. Dartevelle and Grunenwald have also published hemivertebrectomy and total vertebrectomy techniques that are somewhat different from our technique although long-term outcome and survival have yet to be reported (25).

FIGURE 6   (Inset) Drawing demonstrating the surgical incisions: a standard posterolateral thoracotomy is performed to gain access to the chest cavity, whereas posterior midline exposure is needed for the laminectomy and dorsal instrumentation and fusion. The primary illustration depicts the surgical field after the tumor (along with the invaded chest wall) has been completely mobilized from the surrounding structures and reflected inferiorly. Complete laminectomy and partial vertebrectomy at the T1–3 levels are visualized through the defect. The first through fifth ribs have been transected laterally and disarticulated medially from the spinal column. The C8 and T1 nerve roots are preserved, whereas the T2 and T3 nerve roots are sectioned proximal to the dorsal root ganglia. At the apex of the surgical cavity, brachial plexus, subclavian, and vertebral arteries are visualized. The azygos vein is observed crossing the surgical field at the inferior half of the surgical defect, and the esophagus and trachea are seen anterior to the thoracic spinal column.

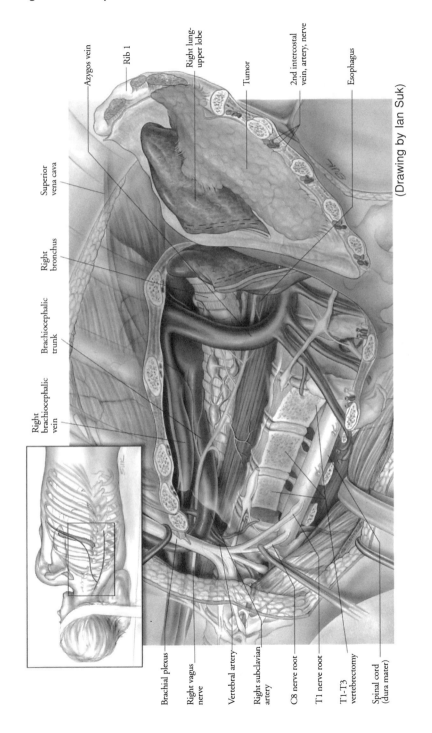

(Drawing by Ian Suk)

Azygos vein

Rib 1

Right lung-upper lobe

Tumor

2nd intercostal vein, artery, nerve

Esophagus

Superior vena cava

Right bronchus

Brachiocephalic trunk

Right brachiocephalic vein

Brachial plexus

Right vagus nerve

Vertebral artery

Right subclavian artery

C8 nerve root

T1 nerve root

T1-T3 vertebrectomy

Spinal cord (dura mater)

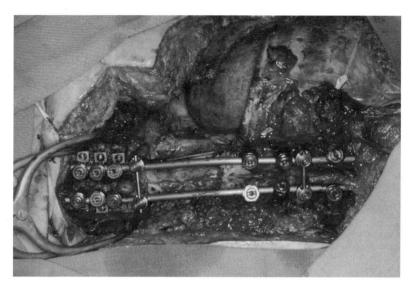

FIGURE 7 Extensive posterior instrumentation in a patient with a two-level verte-brectomy.

HOW MUCH LUNG PARENCHYMA SHOULD BE RESECTED: A LOBECTOMY OR WEDGE RESECTION?

The extent of pulmonary resection, lobectomy versus segmentectomy/wedge, has been the subject of debate. Studies by Paulson, Shahian, and Dartevelle did not demonstrate any significant survival advantage whether the patient had a complete lobectomy or more limited pulmonary resection (5,13). Sartori et al. feel that extended lobectomies are not necessary as these tumors occur in the periphery and in 35 segmentectomies they had performed for resection of Pancoast tumors neither positive parenchymal margins nor ipsilateral lung relapse was observed (5). Hilaris and Ginsberg, however, feel that there is a survival advantage in patients who received lobectomies when compared to wedge (20,26). In Ginsberg's study, the 5-year survival of patients with lobectomy was 60% compared to 33% in patients who underwent a wedge resection only. In this study, locoregional recurrence accounted for the majority of the tumor relapses and only patients who underwent lobectomy, mediastinal node dissection, and en bloc chest wall resection had a decrease in locoregional recurrence. This is consistent with other studies comparing lobe to lesser resections.

Our approach is tailored more to a patient's estimated postoperative pulmonary reserve. For patients with more limited pulmonary function and smaller

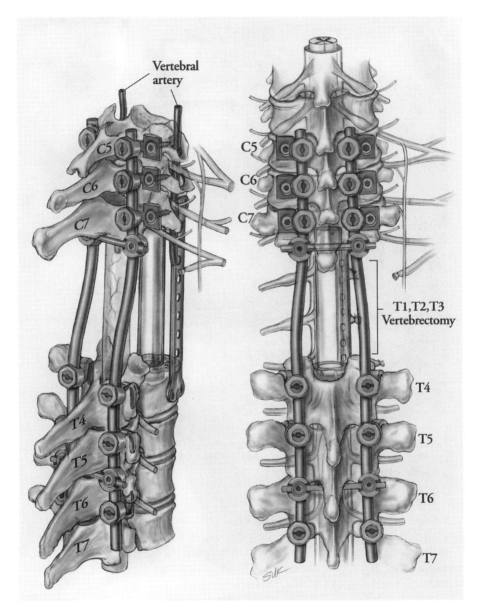

FIGURE 8   Dorsal and dorsolateral view of the spinal column showing T1–3 laminectomy and corpectomy as well as an anterior column reconstruction with methylmethacrylate after extensive resection of a Pancoast tumor. (Drawing by Ian Suk)

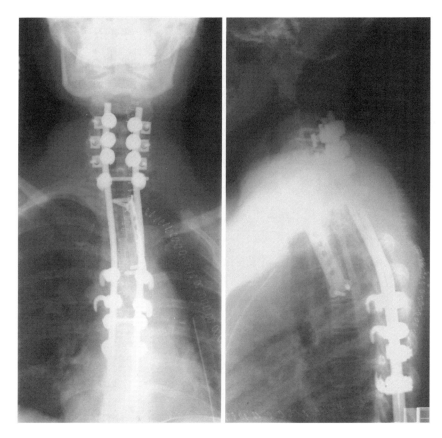

FIGURE 9 Posteroanterior and lateral radiograph demonstrating both anterior and posterior instrumentation required for a two-level vertebrectomy in a patient with an advanced superior sulcus tumor.

tumors, a generous wedge and mediastinal node dissection would be sufficient. For patients with otherwise good lung function or larger tumors, we would normally proceed to a formal lobectomy with full and complete mediastinal lymphadenectomy. If a formal thoracotomy is performed, then the inferior pulmonary ligament is divided to permit the remaining lung to rotate into the upper hemithorax.

HOW TO MANAGE THE ASSOCIATED CHEST WALL DEFECT

The chest wall defect of only the first three ribs is usually not reconstructed, as the scapula will cover this nicely without obvious paradoxical motion. If more of the chest wall is resected, then reconstruction with Marlex mesh is usually performed. If an extensive paraspinal muscle resection was performed with posterior instrumentation, then the Marlex can be attached directly to the posterior hardware or the supraspinous ligament. Care must be taken to ensure that the scapular tip will not become entrapped in the chest wall resection defect. If it does, then removing the tip of the scapula will prevent this complication.

THE USE OF CHEMOTHERAPY ALONE OR PRIOR TO SURGERY

There has been interest over the past 15 years in the use of chemotherapy in patients with locally advanced lung cancer, prior to resection, in an attempt to control both gross and microscopic disease, reduce the size of the tumor to facilitate the resection, and improve the margins (27). There have been two randomized trials, including one from our institution in patients with IIIA disease that demonstrated prolonged survival in patients who received chemotherapy first followed by resection rather than resection alone (28,29). Based on our success with this approach, we then used a similar combination of drugs in patients with superior sulcus tumors. We did not see a similar response and had to stop the study after only 16 patients because of disease progression in most patients (30). This was also recognized by Ginsberg et al. in 10 patients in whom they utilized a preoperative platinum regimen (26). None of four patients treated with chemotherapy alone survived more than 2 years in a series by Komaki et al. (31) Perhaps as newer agents and more active chemotherapeutics are developed, this trial may be repeated. For the present, chemotherapy for the treatment of patients with superior sulcus tumors has been used more in its role as a radiosensitizer.

RATIONALE FOR PREOPERATIVE RADIATION THERAPY

Theoretically, preoperative radiation therapy might improve results over resection alone: (1) by destroying tumor that has extended into the critical adjacent structures, such as major blood vessels, the brachial plexus, chest wall, or mediastinum to improve a surgeon's ability to obtain clear margins at a subsequent operation; and (2) by killing tumor cells that otherwise might be seeded in the operative field or disseminated via the blood or lymphatics (32,33). During the 1950s, interest was directed toward the various combinations of therapy, particularly radiotherapy and surgery, for lung cancer. Originally, Bloedorn and Cowley reported encouraging results with preoperative radiation therapy for bronchogenic carcinoma (34). However, this was a retrospective study of 192 patients who met the criteria for selection; the 1-year survival rate was 13.5% overall, and 23% for those who had complete resections after radiation therapy with cobalt 60 (35).

Shaw and co-workers first reported preoperative radiation therapy and surgical resection in 1961 (9). This original series has been continued by Paulson and updated on several occasions (10,36,37). The treatment regimen consists of delivering 3000 cGy using megavoltage equipment in 10 fractions over 12 elapsed days to the area of the tumor in the superior pulmonary sulcus, the chest wall, and the superior mediastinum beyond the midline. Three weeks after completion of the radiotherapy, the patients undergo an en bloc surgical resection of all involved structures. As of 1983, Paulson's series totaled 131 patients (37). Of the 79 patients operated on after the preoperative radiation, only one had an unresectable tumor. Therefore, 78 of these patients (60%) completed the combined treatment. The operative mortality rate was 2.6% and the survival rate for those completing combined treatment was 31% at 5 years, 26% at 10 years, and 22% at 15 years (Figure 10) (Table 1). Only three of 17 patients who had either hilar or mediastinal nodal involvement survived 1 year, and none survived 2 years. Forty-four percent of those who did not have nodal involvement at operation survived 5 years or more, 33% for 10 years and 30% for 15 years.

A range of preoperative radiation therapy dosages have been used in several trials. Other surgical series have reported on combined preoperative radiation and surgical resection using the Paulson technique. Miller and colleagues utilized

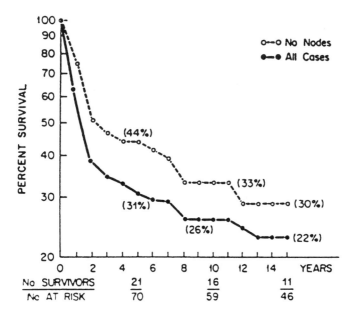

FIGURE 10   Five-, 10-, and 15-year actuarial survival curves of 78 patients after combined preoperative radiation, followed by en bloc surgical resection (1956–83) in patients with no lymph nodes involved and including those with nodal involvement. (From Ref. 37.)

TABLE 1 Results of Treatment of Superior Sulcus Tumors[a]

Treatment	Local control (%)	Survival (%)				
		2-year	3-year	5-year	10-year	15-year
Preop radiation and resection	31–70	29–40	23	13–50	26	22
Resection only	53	—	—	15–60	—	—
Resection, postop radiation	0–56	—	7	15	—	—
Radiation only	33–55	17	7–28	3.5–23	—	—

[a] Large range of results reflects varying stages of carcinoma among institutions.
From Ref. 37.

2000–4000 cGy over a time span of 4 days to 4 weeks, but the most common regimen was that of Paulson (37,38). Attar and colleagues initially gave 5500–6000 cGy preoperatively over a 4-week period, but after noting a high rate of morbidity and mortality, decreased the dose of radiation to that used by Paulson and colleagues (11). Ginsberg also used a dose of 3000 cGy preoperatively (39). Beyer and Weisenburger noted that patients who received at least 5500 cGy showed a better response and appeared to have increased survival (40). The preoperative radiation dosage employed by Devine and associates was 3000–3500 cGy over 2 weeks in 25 of their patients and 4500–5000 cGy over 5–5.5 weeks in 15 of their patients (41). They noted no difference in resectability or survival between the two groups receiving the different dose levels.

The survival in these preoperative regimens varied. Attar and associates reported 19 patients who underwent preoperative radiation followed by en bloc resection and noted a 23% 3-year survival rate (11). Miller and colleagues reported on 26 patients who underwent combined radiation treatment and en bloc resection (38). There was one early postoperative death, and 32% survived for 5 years. Stanford and colleagues noted a 5-year survival rate of 49.7% in patients with a similar treatment regimen (42). Beyer and Weisenburger treated 28 patients who had localized disease with megavoltage radiation with or without surgical resection and had an actuarial survival rate of 22% at 5 years (40). They noted, however, that the 15 patients who received combined radiation and surgery had a 45% 5-year survival rate. Ginsberg reported that 72 patients with Pancoast tumors were seen between 1966 and 1976 at the University of Toronto (39). Fifty were deemed inoperable after staging. Ten underwent preoperative radiation and resection with a 40% 2-year survival rate. Twelve patients also had limited disease with no evidence of metastasis and, although potentially surgical candidates, were never referred for surgery and received only radiation therapy. Only two of those patients (17%) survived 24 months.

Martini treated 145 patients at Memorial Sloan-Kettering Cancer Center over a 36-year period, 29 of whom were treated by external radiation alone, 68 by operation without preoperative radiation, and 48 by preoperative radiation followed by resection (43). Only 9% treated by operation alone had resectable tumors compared with 23% who received preoperative radiation. He noted that a large group of patients did not have resectable tumors at exploration, with or without preoperative radiation therapy. This is perhaps because many patients were explored without preoperative mediastinoscopy and more sophisticated imaging evaluation, such as CT or MRI. The mean survivals were 6 months with external radiation alone, 30 months with preoperative radiation followed by resection, and 10 months with operation alone. If the tumor was not resectable, the combination of implantation of radon seeds and external radiation (4000 cGy in 4 weeks) provided a better survival rate than external radiation therapy alone (12 months vs. 6 months), although patients treated with postoperative radiation alone had more extensive tumors. Devine and colleagues reported a 2-year survival of 29% and a 5-year survival of 14% in patients who completed preoperative radiation and surgery (41). They noted, however, that 30% of patients in whom preoperative radiation therapy followed by surgical therapy was planned, did not undergo surgical resection.

Over the past several years, there have been several other reports of sizable series treated with a combination of preoperative radiation and surgical resection (44). Anderson et al. reported the UCLA experience in which 21 patients received preoperative radiation followed by resection, resulting in a 5-year survival rate of 34% (12). They also advocated radiation by iridium implants postoperatively to 3000 cGy if the tumor was close to the vertebral bodies and nerve roots at the time of operation. Mathisen's group reported on 21 patients who underwent combined therapy at the Massachusetts General Hospital and noted three operative deaths with a median survival time of 24 months and an actuarial survival rate of 55% in 3 years and 27% at 5 years (45). Long-term palliation of pain was achieved in 72% of the patients. Shahian et al. reported on 18 patients treated with preoperative radiation and resection, 14 of whom underwent supplemental postoperative radiotherapy because of positive lymph nodes, tumor at the resection margins, or both (13). There were no hospital deaths and the overall 5-year observed survival rate for the entire series was an impressive 56%. These authors believed that the addition of postoperative radiotherapy for those with unfavorable operative findings (positive margins, positive lymph nodes) resulted in long-term survivals that were comparable to those with negative nodes and margins. Ricci and his colleagues reported on 56 patients with superior sulcus tumors, 32 of whom received preoperative radiation and four of whom also received postoperative radiotherapy (46). This group used Paulson's approach in 30 cases and Dartevelle's in 11, and the 5-year survival rate was 34%. Sartori and his colleagues reported on 42 patients with superior sulcus tumors who received preoperative radiation followed by en bloc resection of the tumor, chest wall, and adjacent structures with one perioperative death, a median survival time of 14 months, and a 5-year actuarial survival rate of 25% (5). They also observed poor results in patients with vertebral invasion, subclavian artery invasion, or N_2 disease.

COMBINING CHEMOTHERAPY WITH PREOPERATIVE RADIATION THERAPY

Chemotherapy given alone or concurrently with radiation therapy prior to surgery has the potential advantage of immediate treatment of subclinical metastatic disease as well as potential radiation sensitization to downstage the lesion and perhaps improve the ability of a surgeon to obtain clear surgical margins intraoperatively. This is the subject of a Southwest Oncology Group (SWOG) phase II trial utilizing cisplatin (50 mg/m^2), etoposide (50 mg/m^2), and concurrent radiation therapy to a dose of 45 Gy preoperatively. The combined induction therapy was well tolerated and yielded an impressive 50% complete pathologic response rate and approximately 50% 3-year survival rate in patients with T3/T4 N0M0 Pancoast tumors (16).

POTENTIAL DISADVANTAGES TO PREOPERATIVE RADIATION THERAPY

There are disadvantages to preoperative radiation therapy. (1) There may be increased operative morbidity including bronchopleural fistulas. (2) The tumor extensions into surrounding structures could be obscured by edematous, inflammatory, or fibrotic changes after induction radiation therapy. Most surgeons believe that preoperative radiation therapy results in a better-delineated tumor mass facilitating dissection. (3) The initial stage of the tumor is not known and staging is dependent on radiographic studies for the T and N status if mediastinoscopy is not done. (4) If there is viable residual tumor beyond the resected specimen, few meaningful treatment options remain. Further radiation is usually delayed owing to the interval from irradiation to operation plus the period required for adequate healing of the surgical wounds. This total interruption of radiation therapy is often 2–3 months. These patients have already received 30–50 Gy preoperatively. Meaningful local control with radiation therapy usually requires at least 60 Gy. These patients, therefore, require an additional 10–30 Gy of treatment but this is a split course sandwiched on either side of the operation. Split-course regimens have been demonstrated to be less effective than a continuous course by Perez and associates, who reported a Radiation Therapy Oncology Group (RTOG) study comparing rapid-fractionation, split-course radiation therapy with continuous-course therapy in non–small cell lung cancer (47,48). The 40-Gy split course was definitely inferior to the 50-Gy and 60-Gy continuous courses. However, Shahian and colleagues advocate preoperative and postoperative radiotherapy to improve the survival of patients with Pancoast tumors (13). The majority of thoracic surgeons still advocate preoperative irradiation, emphasizing its value in accomplishing complete resections.

SURGERY WITH INTRAOPERATIVE BRACHYTHERAPY

Although advocated by Hilaris et al., there is little evidence that intraoperative brachytherapy improves outcome with unresectable tumors. Ginsberg in 1994 reviewed a 17-year experience (1974–91) with 124 patients who underwent a thoracotomy for attempted resection of Pancoast tumors at Memorial Sloan-Kettering Cancer Center. One hundred patients who underwent complete en bloc resections with anatomical lobectomies had the best outcome with a 41% 5-year survival. Intraoperative brachytherapy did not improve survival in these who had complete resections. In patients who had incomplete resections, survival was poor (9%, 5-year) with either form of radiotherapy regardless of whether preoperative radiation therapy or intraoperative brachytherapy treatment was used. If a patient is unresectable at operation, the value of brachytherapy for palliation is unknown (26).

EXPERIENCE WITH POSTOPERATIVE
RADIATION THERAPY

The value of postoperative radiation therapy in patients with carcinoma of the lung who have had complete surgical resection and have no metastasis to the regional lymph nodes has not been established. This applies to any site of cancer of the lung including superior sulcus tumors.

Martini and McCormack reported on 170 patients with superior sulcus tumors treated from 1938 to 1978 (49). The 5-year survival of 127 patients who underwent surgery was 17% compared with 3.4% for the inoperable patients. Twenty patients with curative surgery had a 5-year survival rate of 28.9%. Hilaris and associates reported on 116 patients with superior sulcus tumors treated by irradiation alone or combined surgical resection and irradiation (implant, external irradiation alone, or implant and external irradiation) (50). Twelve patients survived longer than 5 years after the treatment, 10 (83%) of whom had resection of the tumor, implantation, and postoperative external irradiation (4000 cGy in 4 weeks).

A more recent report on 85 patients with superior sulcus tumors by Komaki and colleagues revealed that surgery and radiotherapy was more effective in controlling the superior sulcus tumor and improving survival compared with the results with the use of either modality alone (31). There were 43 patients with superior sulcus tumors categorized as stage IIIA and 42 patients as stage IIIB. Surgery was a component of treatment more frequently in patients with stage IIIA than in Stage IIIB disease ($p < .05$), and chemotherapy was used significantly more often in patients with stage IIIB disease ($p < .01$). Stage IIIA patients had a 46.5% 1-year survival rate compared with 21% for stage IIIB ($p = .0042$). When surgery was a component of treatment, 52% (13/25) lived longer than 2 years compared with 22% (13/60) when radiation therapy was used for unresectable tumors. Fifty-two patients (61%) had local control, and their survival was significantly better than those who did not achieve local control ($p < .01$). High performance status, less than 5% weight loss, and lack of direct extension into vertebral bodies were highly significant factors for better survival. These data support the recommendation that surgical resection should be used whenever possible for superior sulcus tumors. Patients with unresectable lesions should receive high-dose radiation therapy with no interruptions.

Dartevelle and his colleagues in 1993 reported 2- and 5-year actuarial survival rates of 50% and 31%, respectively, with a median follow-up time of 2.5 years (22). None of their patients received preoperative radiation, 14% had surgery alone, and 86% had surgery followed by postoperative irradiation. This represents a group of patients who had extensive invasion of the superior sulcus and were resected without preoperative radiation. The resectability rate is high owing to the exposure that the anterior transcervical thoracic approach provides, and the more adequate preoperative evaluation by modern imaging studies.

No randomized trials of carefully staged patients with superior sulcus tumors comparing preoperative radiation followed by surgical resection; surgical resection alone; surgical resection with postoperative radiation; or radiation therapy alone have been performed. Indeed, the low incidence of superior sulcus tumors makes such a trial virtually impossible. The Lung Cancer Study Group projected that even in a multicenter trial, such a study would require more than 10 years of patient accrual, and this would be impractical (51).

MANAGEMENT OF PATIENTS WITH INOPERABLE DISEASE

Morris and Abadir recommended radiotherapy alone for superior sulcus tumors (52). They reported 26 cases and showed that high-dose radiation therapy [nominal single dose (NSD) 1900 rets (equivalent to 7000 cGy in 7 weeks) or higher] controlled direct bony invasion better than lower doses (less than 1900 rets). Ahmad and colleagues treated 48 patients by irradiation alone using either cobalt 60 or cesium 137 teletherapy to dose between 5000 cGy and 6000 cGy in 5–6 weeks (53). Their actuarial survival rate was 28% at 3 years and 21% at 5 years. They encountered no severe complications among the patients who received radiation therapy alone, except for asymptomatic scarring on chest films. Van Houtte and colleagues reported 31 patients with superior sulcus tumors treated with external radiation therapy in doses ranging from 2000 cGy to 7000 cGy, with an overall 5-year survival rate of 18% (54). They found that doses below 5000 cGy and bone invasion were each associated with a higher rate of local recurrence.

At the Medical College of Wisconsin, 36 patients with superior sulcus tumors were treated by external irradiation alone between 1963 and 1977 (55). Local control correlated positively with median survival. The patients who failed locally did not survive beyond 2 years. Larger field size was also a favorable treatment factor. Between 1978 and 1983, an additional 32 patients with inoperable superior sulcus tumors were studied with similar results.

Relief of pain was achieved in 91% of all patients presenting with pain. Three-fourths of the patients with Horner's syndrome responded to the irradiation. The disease-free survival rates were 65%, 38%, 25%, and 15% at 12 months, 24 months, 36 months, and 48 months, respectively (Figure 11). No patients survived beyond 24 months if the primary tumor was not controlled in the chest. The pattern of failure showed the brain to be the most common site of distant metastases (23 of 68 patients, 34%). No fatal complications occurred as a result of external radiation therapy alone.

In the series studied by Anderson et al., 27 patients received radiation only and this group had no 5-year survivors (12). The majority of these patients received 4000–6000 cGy because they were either unresectable, refused surgery, were medically too ill to undergo resection, or had distant metastasis. Ricci and

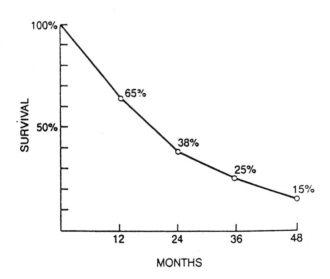

FIGURE 11   Disease-free survival in patients with superior sulcus tumor treated by external irradiation alone. (From Ref. 55.)

his colleagues reported on 15 inoperable patients who were treated by 6000 cGy with a 2-year survival rate of 6% (46).

High-energy external radiotherapy is therefore recommended for patients proved to have superior sulcus tumors by means of CT-guided aspiration cytological techniques or biopsy who are unable to have surgical resection because of the extent of the disease or are inoperable for medical reasons. The field must be generous enough to encompass the upper mediastinum and the vertebral bodies as well as the supraclavicular region. The total minimum tumor dose should be 6000 cGy administered in 6–6.5 weeks. CT-planning dosimetry techniques (Figure 12) are helpful in determining the adequate tumor dosing. The three-dimensional displays of the tumor permit conformal radiation therapy to higher total doses to the tumor but avoid critical normal tissues such as the spinal cord, esophagus, and excessive volume of the lung (Figure 13, A and B) (56). As with other sites of inoperable non–small cell lung cancer, additional chemotherapy has shown improvement of survival to radiation, but clinical trials focused on superior sulcus tumors are lacking (57). If chemotherapy and radiotherapy are given for inoperable superior sulcus tumors, concurrent chemotherapy and radiotherapy is preferable (58).

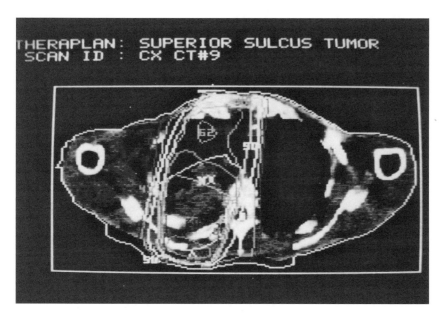

FIGURE 12 Computed tomography was performed for treatment planning. The dose to the tumor is 65 Gy and that to the spinal cord is 45 Gy by 2:1 loading more posteriorly. (From Ref. 56.)

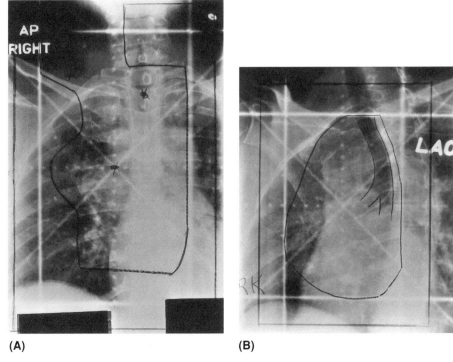

(A)   **(B)**

FIGURE 13   Radiation portals. (A) A typical radiation therapy port using anteroposterior parallel opposed fields, 2 Gy/fraction, up to 40 Gy at the central axis. (B) Boost for definitive radiotherapy using parallel oblique fields to give an additional 20–24 Gy at 2 Gy/fraction at the central axis. The total dose to the apical lesion will be 66–72 Gy for definitive purposes. (From Ref. 56.)

THE ROLE OF CRANIAL IRRADIATION

The longer the survival after the initial treatment of lung cancer, the greater the incidence of brain metastases. Komaki et al. demonstrated that 44% of patients surviving more than 2 years develop brain metastases (55). Brain metastases were more common in patients with tumors that were poorly differentiated or undifferentiated (56%). Their recommendation was prophylactic whole-brain irradiation in these patient subgroups. Over the past decade, because of the discovery of the neuropsychological changes that result from cranial radiation, the pendulum swung to the other side, reserving treatment for documented, symptomatic metastases. However, the continued demonstration in numerous series of a high rate of brain metastases suggests further consideration of prophylactic cranial irradiation. Also, more recent meta-analysis has shown survival improvement by application of prophylactic cranial irradiation (PCI) for patients who achieved complete response to the treatment of small cell lung cancer without adverse neurological effect from PCI (59).

SUMMARY

Superior sulcus tumors without distant metastases, and without lymph node involvement, can be treated with similar results as with other non–small cell bronchogenic carcinomas. The extent of the disease should be defined clinically by a detailed history and physical examination and by CT, MR imaging, and mediastinoscopy when indicated. If the lesion is grossly resectable and the patient's cardiopulmonary reserve is adequate, the lesion can be resected directly without preoperative radiation therapy. If the lesion is marginally resectable, preoperative radiation (50 Gy in 25 fractions) or concurrent chemotherapy (cisplatin, etoposide) and radiation therapy (40–44 Gy) may be followed by reevaluation and consideration for total resection. A complete surgical resection is the most important predictor of long-term survival and quality of life, and therefore, we have developed an aggressive surgical approach to these lesions. Involvement of the subclavian vessels, vertebral bodies, and lower cord of the brachial plexus with limited extension into the neural foramina does not preclude resection. Ipsilateral scalene or supraclavicular nodes are considered locoregional disease and would be removed initially by anterior neck dissection. Frequently these tumors are approached through an anterior neck incision to safely dissect and resect when necessary the subclavian vessels and lower cords of the brachial plexus. Posterolateral thoracotomies are required when the lesion involves the vertebral bodies. Our experience with resections and reconstructions of vertebral bodies has been applied to tumors in the superior sulcus with resultant good palliation of symptoms and prolonged survival. We prefer, when possible, to initially treat these patients surgically and give concurrent radiation therapy and chemotherapy in the postoperative setting, in an uninterrupted course of radiotherapy.

While we feel that local control has been improved with aggressive en bloc resections with high-dose concurrent chemoradiation therapy postoperatively, patients often die with distant, systemic metastases similar to other patients with lung cancer. This highlights the importance of our continued search for agents that will control these occult metastases that result in the ultimate death of most patients with this disease. Without these systemic therapies, the role of surgery and radiation therapy continues to palliate the devastating local effects, with the occasional cure of those with truly localized disease.

REFERENCES

1. Hare ES. Tumor involving certain nerves. London Med Gazette 1838; 23:16.
2. Pancoast HK. Importance of careful roentgenray investigations of apical chest tumors. JAMA 1924; 86:1407–1411.

3. Pancoast HK. Superior pulmonary sulcus tumors. JAMA 1932; 99:1391–1396.

4. Tobias JW. Sindrome apico-costovertebral dolorosa por tumors apexicano. Su valor diagnostico el el cancer primitivo pulmonar. Rev Med Lat Am 1932; 19:1552–1556.

5. Sartori F, Rea F, Calabro F, Mazzucco C, Bortolotti L, Tomio L. Carcinoma of the superior pulmonary sulcus: results of irradiation and radical resection. J Thorac Cardiovasc Surg 1992; 104:679–683.

6. Herbut PA, Watson TS. Tumor of the thoracic inlet producing the Pancoast syndrome. Arch Pathol 1946; 42:88–103.

7. Haas LL, Harvey RA, Langer SS. Radiation management of otherwise hopeless thoracic neoplasms. JAMA 1954; 154:323–326.

8. Chardack WM, MacCallum JD. Pancoast tumor: five-year survival without recurrence or metastases following radical resection and postoperative irradiation. J Thorac Surg 1956; 31:535–542.

9. Shaw RR, Paulson DL, Kee JL. Treatment of the superior sulcus tumor by irradiation followed by resection. Ann Surg 1961; 154:29–40.

10. Paulson DL. Carcinomas in the superior pulmonary sulcus. J Thorac Cardiovasc Surg 1975; 70:1095–1104.

11. Attar S, Miller JE, Satterfield J, Ho CK, Slawson RG, Hankins J, et al. Pancoast's tumor: irradiation or surgery? Ann Thorac Surg 1979; 28:578–586.

12. Anderson TM, Moy PM, Holmes EC. Factors affecting survival in superior sulcus tumors. J Clin Oncol 1986; 4:1598–1603.

13. Shahian DM, Neptune WB, Ellis FH Jr. Pancoast tumors: improved survival with preoperative and postoperative radiotherapy. Ann Thorac Surg 1987; 43:32–38.

14. Maggi G, Casadio C, Pischedda F, Giobbe R, Cianci R, Ruffini E, et al. Combined radiosurgical treatment of pancoast tumor. Ann Thorac Surg 1994; 57:198–202.

15. Walsh GL, Morice RC, Putnam JB Jr, Nesbitt JC, McMurtrey MJ, Ryan MB, et al. Resection of lung cancer is justified in high-risk patients selected by exercise oxygen consumption. Ann Thorac Surg 1994; 58:704–711.

16. Kraut MJ; Rusch VW, Crowley, JJ, Gandara DR. Induction chemoradiation plus surgical resection is a feasible and highly effective treatment for pancoast tumors: initial results of SWOG 9416 (Intergroup 0160) Trial. Proc ASCO 2000; 19:487a.

17. Wright CD, Moncure AC, Shepard JO, Wilkins EW Jr, Mathisen DJ, Grillo HC. Superior sulcus lung tumors: results of combined treatment (irradiation and radical resection). J Thorac Cardiovasc Surg 1987; 94:69–74.

18. Attar S, Krasna MJ, Sonett JR, Hankins JR, Slawson RG, Suter CM, et al. Superior sulcus (Pancoast) tumor: experience with 105 patients. Ann Thorac Surg 1998; 66:193–198.

19. Muscolino G, Valente M, Andreani S. Pancoast tumors, clinical assessment and long term results of combined radiosurgical treatment. Thorax 1997; 52:284–286.

20. Hilaris BS, Martini N, Wong GY. Treatment of superior sulcus tumor (Pancoast tumor). Surg Clin North Am 1987; 67:965–977.

21. Spaggiari L, Rusca M, Carbognani P, Solli P. Hemivertebrectomy for apical chest tumors: is the risk justified by the outcome? (Letter to the editor). Ann Thorac Surg 1998; 65:1515–1516.

22. Dartevelle PG, Chapelier AR, Macchiarini P, Lenot B, Gerrina J, Ladurie FLR, et al. Anterior transcervical-thoracic approach for radical resection of lung tumors invading the thoracic inlet. J Thorac Cardiovasc Surg 1993; 105:1025–1034.

23. Dartevelle PG. Extended operations for the treatment of lung cancer. Ann Thorac Surg 1997; 63:12–19.

24. Walsh GL, Gokaslan ZL, McCutcheon IE, Mineo MT, Yasko AW, Swisher SG, et al. Anterior approaches to the thoracic spine in patients with cancer—indications and results. Ann Thorac Surg 1997; 64:1611–1618.

25. Grunenwald D, Mazel C, Girard Ph, Berthiot G, Dromer C, Baldeyrou P. Total vertebrectomy for en bloc resection of lung cancer invading the spine. Ann Thorac Surg 1996; 61:723–726.

26. Ginsberg RJ, Martini N, Zaman M, Armstrong JG, Bains MS, Burt ME, et al. Influence of surgical resection and brachytherapy in the management of superior sulcus tumor. Ann Thorac Surg 1994; 57:1440–1445.

27. Macchiarini P, Chapelier AR, Monnet I, Vannetzel JM, Rebischung JL, Cerrina J, et al. Extended operations after induction therapy for stage IIIB (T_4) non–small cell lung cancer. Ann Thorac Surg 1994; 57:966–973.

28. Roth JA, Fossella J, Komaki R, et al. A randomized trial comparing perioperative chemotherapy and surgery with surgery alone in resectable Stage IIIA non–small cell lung cancer. J Natl Cancer Inst 1994; 86:673–680.

29. Rosell R, Gomez-Condina J, Camps C, Maestre J, Padilla J, Canto A, et al. A randomized trial comparing preoperative chemotherapy plus surgery with surgery alone in patients with non–small-cell lung cancer. N Engl J Med 1994; 330:153–158.

30. Ryan B, Glisson B, Putnam JB Jr, Roth JA. A prospective trial of neoadjuvant chemotherapy in superior sulcus carcinomas of the lung. Ann Surg Oncol 1994; 68:182 (abstr).

31. Komaki R, Mountain CF, Holbert JM, Garden AS, Shallenberger R, Cox JD, et al. Superior sulcus tumors: treatment selection and results for 85 patients without metastasis (MO) at presentation. Int J Radiat Oncol Biol Phys 1990; 19:31–36.

32. Komaki R. Preoperative and postoperative irradiation for cancer of the lung. J Belge Radiol 1985; 68:195–198.

33. Widow W. Preoperative irradiation of bronchial carcinoma. Cancer 1971; 28:798–801.

34. Bloedorn FG, Cowley RA. Irradiation and surgery in treatment of bronchogenic carcinoma. Surg Gynecol Obstet 1960; 111:141–146.

35. Bloedorn FG, Cowley RA, Cuccia C, et al. Preoperative irradiation in bronchogenic carcinoma. Am J Roentgenol Radiat Ther Nucl Med 1964; 92:77–87.

36. Paulson DL. Stage III superior sulcus carcinomas. In: Sabiston D, Spencer F, eds. Gibbons Surgery of the Chest. Vol 1. Philadelphia: WB Saunders, 1983:506–515.

37. Paulson DL. Technical considerations in stage III disease: the "superior sulcus" lesion. In: Delarue NC, Eschapasse H, eds. International Trends in General Surgery. Philadelphia: WB Saunders, 1985:121–131.

38. Miller JL, Mansour KA, Hatcher CR. Carcinoma of the superior pulmonary sulcus. Ann Thorac Surg 1979; 28:44–47.

39. Ginsberg RJ. Pancoast's tumor: irradiation or surgery? Ann Thorac Surg 1979; 28: 578–586.

40. Beyer DC, Weisenburger T. Superior sulcus tumors. Am J Clin Oncol 1985; 8:24–25.

41. Devine JW, Mendenhall WM, Million RR, Carmichael MJ. Carcinoma of the superior pulmonary sulcus treated with surgery and/or radiation therapy. Cancer 1986; 57:941–943.

42. Stanford W, Barnes RP, Tucker AR. Influence of staging in superior sulcus (Pancoast) tumors of the lung. Ann Thorac Surg 1980; 29:406–410.

43. Martini N. Pancoast's tumor: irradiation or surgery? Ann Thorac Surg 1979; 28: 578–586.

44. Fuller DB, Chambers JS. Superior sulcus tumors: combined modality. Ann Thorac Surg 1994; 57:1133–1139.

45. Mathisen DJ, Grillo HC, Wright CD, et al. Superior sulcus tumors: results of combined treatment (irradiation and radical resection). J Thorac Cardiovasc Surg 1987; 94:69–74.

46. Ricci C, Rendina EA, Venuta F, et al. Superior pulmonary sulcus tumors: radical resection and palliative treatment. Int Surg 1989; 74:175–179.

47. Perez CA, Stanley K, Rubin P, Kramer S, Brady LW, Marks JE, et al. Patterns of tumor recurrence after definitive irradiation for inoperable non–oat cell carcinoma of the lung. Int J Radiat Oncol Biol Phys 1980; 6:987–994.

48. Perez CA, Stanley K, Grundy G, Hanson W, Kramer S, Brady LW, et al. Impact of irradiation technique and tumor extent in tumor control and survival of patients with unresectable non-oat cell carcinoma of the lung: report by the Radiation Therapy Oncology Group. Cancer 1982; 50:1091–1099.

49. Martini N, McCormack P. Therapy of stage III (nonmetastatic disease). Semin Oncol 1983; 10:95–110.

50. Hilaris BS, Martini N, Luomanen RKJ, et al. The value of preoperative radiation therapy in apical cancer of the lung. Surg Clin North Am 1974; 54:821–831.

51. Lung Cancer Study Group. Effects of postoperative mediastinal radiation on completely resected stage II and stage III epidermoid cancer of the lung. N Engl J Med 1986; 315(22):1377–1381.

52. Morris RW, Abadir R. Pancoast tumors: the value of high-dose radiotherapy. Radiology 1979; 132:717–719.

53. Ahmad K, Fayos JV, Kirsch MM. Apical lung carcinoma. Cancer 1984; 54:913–917.

54. van Houtte P, MacLennan I, Poulter C, et al. External radiation in the management of superior sulcus tumor. Cancer 1984; 54:223–228.

55. Komaki R, Roh J, Cox JD, Lopesda Conceicao A. Superior sulcus tumors: results of irradiation of 36 patients. Cancer 1981; 48:1563–1569.

56. Grover FL, Komaki R. Special considerations: superior sulcus tumors. In: Roth JA, Ruckdeschel JC, Weisenburger TH, eds. Thoracic Oncology. Philadelphia: WB Saunders, 1989:263–279.

57. Dillman RO, Herndon J, Seagren SI, et al. Improved survival in stage III non–small cell lung cancer: seven year follow-up of Cancer and Leukemia Group B trial 8433. J Natl Cancer Inst 1996; 88:1210–1215.

58. Furuse K, Fukuoka M, Kawahara M, et al. Phase III study of cocurrent versus sequential thoracic radiotherapy in combination with mitomycin, vindesine, and cisplatin in unresectable stage III non–small cell lung cancer. J Clin Oncol 1999; 17: 2692–2699.

59. Auperin A, Arriagada R, Pignon JP, et al. Prophylactic cranial irradiation for patients with small cell lung cancer in complete remission. N Engl J Med 1999; 341:476–484.

15

Extended Resections in Stage T_4 NSCLC: Pro

Chong Hee Lim, Thomas W. Rice, and Eugene H. Blackstone
Cleveland Clinic Foundation, Cleveland, Ohio

INTRODUCTION

Stage IIIB lung cancer comprises a large, heterogeneous group of locally advanced tumors. Stage IIIB is defined by presence of a T_4 tumor or any tumor with N_3 nodal metastases (Table 1). Because these tumors are generally unresectable and incurable, palliation with supportive therapy or radiation is the principal means of treatment. For patients with good performance status and adequate pulmonary function, the addition of cisplatin-based chemotherapy to definitive radiation prolongs survival when compared to radiation alone (1). In two large retrospective series of patients with resected stage IIIB lung cancer, 5-year survival ranged from 7% to 8.4% for T_4 carcinomas and 0% to 3% for N_3 (2,3). However, in patients with specific anatomical conditions, resection has prolonged survival and, on occasion, resulted in cure. Induction chemotherapy and chemoradiotherapy can downstage some patients with stage IIIB tumors and permit aggressive resection with limited mortality and good outcome.

Resection of locally advanced lung cancer usually requires en bloc removal of adjacent structures. An extended resection implies removal of tissues beyond

TABLE 1 Stage IIIB Descriptors and Groupings

Descriptors
  T_4 primary tumor
    A tumor of any size with one of the following:
      1. Invasion of
          trachea
          carina
          heart
          great vessels
          vertebral body
          esophagus
          mediastinum
      2. Satellite tumor nodule same lobe
      3. Malignant pleural effusion
  N_3 regional lymph nodes
    Metastasis to:
      contralateral mediastinal lymph nodes
      contralateral hilar lymph nodes
      ipsilateral or contralateral scalene lymph nodes
      ipsilateral or contralateral supraclavicular lymph nodes
Groupings
  $T_4N_0M_0$
  $T_4N_1M_0$
  $T_4N_2M_0$
  $T_1N_3M_0$
  $T_2N_3M_0$
  $T_3N_3M_0$
  $T_4N_3M_0$

---

the physical boundaries of a standard lobectomy or pneumonectomy. Induction chemotherapy and chemoradiotherapy extends the use of surgery to previously inoperable patients. It may be contended that any operation for a stage IIIB lung cancer is, in fact, extended because it has the potential to increase surgery to the extreme.

EXTENDED RESECTIONS OF T_4 AND N_3 LUNG CANCERS

Invasion of Adjacent Structures

Trachea or Carina

The greatest experience with extended resections for stage IIIB carcinomas has been documented in patients with involvement of the distal trachea. An in-depth review of these reports provides an understanding of this uncommon clinical problem. More importantly, the lessons learned from these experiences are helpful in developing treatment strategies and setting guidelines for the extended resections of other less common stage IIIB carcinomas.

Primary carcinomas of the carina and bronchogenic carcinomas with tracheal involvement are generally unresectable. They are usually bulky, locally extensive, and associated with metastatic subcarinal and paratracheal lymphadenopathy. Early series of resection of these airway tumors reported significant operative mortalities and few long-term survivors (4–7). Operative deaths were the result of pneumonia, adult respiratory distress syndrome (ARDS), cardiac complications, and anastomotic catastrophes. However, careful patient selection and preparation, reassessment of surgical techniques, development of strategies for intraoperative ventilation, and conscientious perioperative care have permitted successful resection of $T_4N_0M_0$ carcinomas of the main airways in some institutions (8–12).

Patient selection is crucial. Cardiopulmonary assessment of these high-risk patients should include arterial blood gases, spirometry, diffusion capacity, quantitative ventilation-perfusion scans, maximal oxygen uptake during exercise, echocardiography, thallium stress testing, and, when indicated, coronary arteriography (12). Exclusion of distant metastatic disease is imperative regardless of the presence or absence of extrathoracic symptoms. Silent stage IV disease may be best detected by whole body ^{18}F-fluorodeoxyglucose positron emission tomography (FDG PET), which should be considered for any patient being evaluated for extended resection.

Bronchial and mediastinal assessments include bronchoscopy with biopsy and mediastinoscopy. Recurrence of bronchogenic carcinoma at a pneumonectomy stump is associated with increased operative mortality and negates reoperation by tracheal sleeve resection (4). These patients should receive radiation. The preferred candidate has a right upper lobe or right main bronchial tumor with invasion of the right lateral tracheal wall or carina. Isolated carinal or left main bronchial carcinomas are uncommon and usually secondary to airway invasion from subcarinal or peribronchial nodal metastases. Bronchoscopy, with biopsy of normal mucosa at least 2 cm proximal to and distal from the primary tumor, will exclude microscopic submucosal spread. The distance considered a safe limit between proximal tracheal and distal main bronchial margins is 4 cm. This should not be exceeded if anastomotic tension is to be minimized (12). Mediastinoscopy is mandatory. The presence of N_2 or N_3 disease precludes resection because no early survivors (less than 2 years) have been reported following extended tracheal resection of $T_4N_2M_0$ or $T_4N_3M_0$ carcinomas (13). Mediastinoscopy should be done immediately before or at the time of tracheal sleeve pneumonectomy to avoid excessive scarring at the operative site.

One of the main causes of postoperative mortality is pulmonary complications. To help prevent these complications, patient preparation is critical. Smoking cessation, bronchodilation, and treatment of bronchitis and/or pneumonia optimize pulmonary function. Endobronchial laser ablation may be required to relieve airway obstruction and treat distal pneumonia. During patient evaluation and preparation, 6 weeks of cardiopulmonary rehabilitation is helpful.

The best approach for right tracheal sleeve pneumonectomy is through a right posterior lateral thoracotomy. Median sternotomy is used for the uncommon left tracheal sleeve resection or pneumonectomy. Left-sided resections have been staged with pneumonectomy via thoracotomy being followed 2–3 weeks later by a sleeve tracheal resection through a median sternotomy (7). Preservation of the tracheal blood supply, which enters from the lateral aspect, is required to minimize anastomotic complications. Mobilization should be limited to the anterior and posterior surfaces of the trachea. Tension at the anastomosis may be reduced by hilar releases and by division of the ligamentum arteriosum, dissection of the aortopulmonary window, and mobilization of the first centimeter of the descending aorta during left tracheal sleeve pneumonectomy (12). Upper airway and laryngeal releases are not generally helpful with these distal tracheal operations.

Ventilation is performed by one of two methods: continuous jet ventilation through a small catheter passed through the field into the contralateral main bronchus or intermittent ventilation with cross-field periodic intubation of the main bronchus alternating periods of apnea with ventilation. Either of these two options exposes the airway to contamination with blood and debris from the operative field. Every attempt to avoid airway soiling must be made. Aggressive suctioning of the trachea and distal airway with removal of secretions, blood, and debris is vital to prevent pulmonary complications. Cardiopulmonary bypass is rarely required for these operations, but should be available.

Techniques of airway anastomosis are identical to those applied in bronchoplastic procedures and lung transplantation. The anastomosis must be continuously tailored to compensate for size discrepancies. Telescoping of the distal airway into the trachea is recommended (12). The anastomosis should be wrapped or partitioned from nearby vascular structures with autologous vascularized tissue. On completion of the procedure and prior to extubation, bronchoscopic inspection of the anastomosis and, more importantly, removal of blood and secretions are performed. Extubation in the operating room or immediately in the intensive care unit is optimum. The requirement of a chin stitch in distal tracheal operations is debatable. Excessive neck flexion may impair cough and promote aspiration (12).

Meticulous postoperative respiratory care and careful attention to fluid balance is critical, but may not be sufficient to prevent noncardiogenic pulmonary edema (ARDS). This complication may be fostered by extended resections where extensive airway mobilization damages pulmonary lymphatics. Injury to the alveolar-capillary interface is probably multifactorial and promoted by the inability of the pulmonary lymphatics to clear interstitial fluid. Aggressive pulmonary care, fluid restriction, and early institution of nitric oxide therapy may prevent this complication. Once established, ARDS in the postpneumonectomy patient is generally lethal.

For carefully selected patients who have undergone carinal resections and tracheal sleeve pneumonectomy, 5-year survival ranges from 0% to 43%; operative mortality ranges from 5% to 29% (Table 2). Meta-analysis of 312 patients included in eight series demonstrated median and 5-year survivals of 23 months and 31% (Figure 1). The hazard function depicts an exponential decay in the instantaneous risk of death for patients undergoing extended resections of lung cancers with distal tracheal or carinal invasion (Figure 2). This biphasic risk is composed of an early, rapidly declining component that is the result of significant postoperative mortality. After 3 months the hazard curve slowly declines to reach a plateau. The risk of death is then constant over time, mainly the consequence of death from recurrent lung cancer.

Heart or Great Vessels

The left atrium may be involved by direct invasion or by tumor emboli via the pulmonary vein. In 44 patients with atrial involvement, extended resection without cardiopulmonary bypass resulted in a 22% 5-year survival (14). In 31 patients with left atrial involvement, 17 by direct invasion and 14 by tumor embolization, resection was associated with a 22% 5-year survival (15). However, all patients with embolic left atrial involvement died of distant hematogenous metastasis after a median disease-free interval of 6 months. In four patients undergoing atrial resection with cardiopulmonary bypass there was one long-term survivor at 54

TABLE 2 Sleeve Pneumonectomy and Carinal Resection for Lung Cancer: Operative Mortality and Survival

Author	Patients (N)	Operative mortality (%)	5-year survival (%)
Jensik (4)	34	29	15
Fujimura (5)	7	14	—
Deslauriers (7)	38	29	13
Tsuchiya (8)	20	30	59 (2yr)
Vogt-Moykopf (9)	78	17	0
Mathisen (10)	37	19	19
Roviaro (11)	28	5	25
Dartevelle (12)	70	10	43
Total	312		

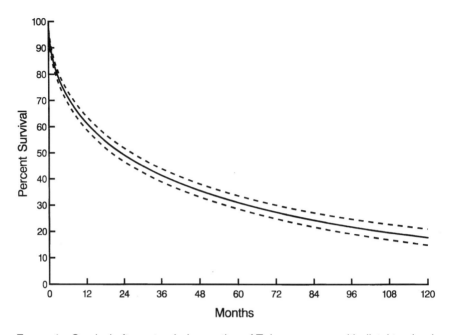

FIGURE 1 Survival after extended resection of T_4 lung cancers with distal tracheal or carinal invasion. Meta-analysis of 312 patients included in eight series. The dashed lines represent asymmetrical confidence limits equivalent to 1 standard deviation. Median survival is 23 months (95% CI, 17–30).

months (16). Two early deaths occurred at 54 days (operative death) and 11 months (cerebral metastases). Shirakusa and colleagues (17) in a recent report of a 4-year experience of extended resections of T_4 cancers, documented six patients who underwent extended resections including the left atrium; four died at 3, 4, 4, and 15 months postoperatively and two are alive at 4 and 13 months. In their entire experience, there are two long-term survivors at 8 and 11 years following left atrial resection requiring cardiopulmonary bypass (16,17).

Resection and reconstruction of the pulmonary artery in patients with central bronchogenic carcinoma is technically feasible using cardiopulmonary bypass. However, all reported postoperative survivors died soon after resection owing to recurrent cancer. Resection of the pulmonary artery bifurcation in seven patients resulted in one operative death (14%) (14). The deaths of the remaining six patients occurred within 30 months. In a smaller series, all three patients successfully resected with main pulmonary artery invasion died within 25 months of operation: one postoperative death and two deaths at 3 months and 25 months from distant metastases (18).

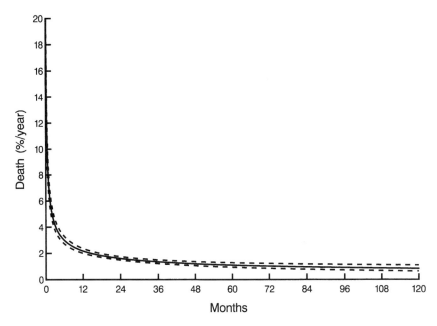

FIGURE 2 Instantaneous risk of death (hazard function) after extended resection of T₄ lung cancers with distal tracheal or carinal invasion.

Extended resections of the aorta have included intra-adventitial dissection and excision of superficially invading tumors and resection and replacements of portions of the aorta. In a report with limited follow-up, enbloc resection of bronchogenic carcinomas with involvement of the aortic arch and left subclavian artery resulted in two deaths from systemic metastases within 12 months of operation; one patient was alive at 17 months (19). Of 20 patients with aortic invasion, only one was alive 5 years following resection (20). This patient was incompletely resected and received brachytherapy. In 28 patients with aortic invasion, 21 involving the adventitia and seven the complete aortic wall, en bloc resection was attempted (14). Intra-adventitial dissection and peeling of the bronchogenic carcinoma resulted in incomplete resection in 11 patients (52%). These results led Tsuchiya and colleagues (14) to conclude this procedure an inadequate operation for lung cancer with aortic invasion. However, 3-year survival was identical in 28 patients: 14% (3/21) for patients undergoing adventitial peel and 14% (1/7) for those undergoing resection and aortic replacement. Five patients underwent resection of the thoracic aorta, four with cardiopulmonary bypass and one with a temporary shunt (21). Three patients died of systemic metastases at 17, 26, and 27 months after surgery. Two patients were alive at 14 and 50 months following resection, with 1-, 2-, and 4-year survival of 100%, 75%, and 25%, respectively. The only intraoperative complication occurred in the patient who as resected using a temporary shunt and prompted Klepetko and associates (21) to suggest cardiopulmonary bypass in all patients undergoing extended pulmonary resections with aortic invasion. They recommend normothermic partial bypass for tumors involving the descending thoracic aorta and cardiopulmonary bypass with selective cerebral perfusion or deep hypothermia and circulatory arrest for tumors involving the aortic arch. In a small series with short-term follow-up, four of five patients are alive at 8, 14, 32, and 41 months following extended resection including the aorta. One patient died 21 months postoperatively (17).

The superior vena cava may be involved by direct extension from right upper lobe tumors or by metastases to pericaval mediastinal nodes (lymph node stations R2, R4, and 3). The majority of these tumors are unresectable. When feasible, resection usually includes pneumonectomy or carinal pneumonectomy. Options of reconstruction include direct suture closure if 30% or less of the circumference is involved, patch reconstruction using autologous or bovine pericardium, or replacement using polytetrafluoroethylene (PTFE) conduits. Invasion of the origin of the superior vena cava typically precludes resection; however, reconstruction at the level of one or both brachiocephalic veins has been reported (15). Partial caval clamping or clamping of a chronically obstructed vena cava is well tolerated. However, occultation of the patent superior vena cava may produce intracranial bleeding, brain damage, and potentially lethal reductions of cardiac output. These complications can be avoided by intraliminal shunting (22) or judicious fluid loading and peripheral vasoconstriction (15). Graft patency using PTFE is excellent and has been reported to be 92% at 1 year (23). Operative mortality of 7.1% has been reported (15). The largest experience reported is 21 patients undergoing partial resection with side clamping of the superior vena cava and direct suture repair, seven having PTFE replacement and four with pericardial patch closure. While operative mortality and survival for these patients is not reported separately, it is reported for a group of patients with heart and great vessel involvement (14). Of 14 patients undergoing extended resections for superior vena caval invasion the 5-year survival has been 31%, with five patients alive and disease free at 13–73 months postoperatively (15). Three reports include a total of seven patients with a median survival of 18 months and one long-term survivor at 64 months (19,22,24).

The inferior vena cava is protected from frequent invasion by lower lobe lung cancer and its involvement is generally an end-stage event. Extended resection of the inferior vena cava was reported once (25). The reconstruction was done with simple clamping and resulted in hemodynamic and renal instability, requiring 3 L of fluid replacement and inotropic support. The patient, who had had a previous laryngectomy and partial glossectomy, was reported alive 6 months after the resection of this right lower lobe tumor, which could have been a metachronous lung primary or a metastasis from the previous head and neck primaries.

For extended resection of lung cancers involving the heart and great vessels, postoperative pneumonia, bleeding, incomplete resection, and mediastinal lymph node metastases (N$_2$ and N$_3$) have been identified by multivariable analysis as predictors of reduced survival (14).

Vertebral Body

Invasion of the thoracic vertebrae by bronchogenic carcinoma is uncommon below T5. It is most frequently seen in the apex of the chest. Massive invasion is well documented by preoperative CT and MRI scanning. However, minimal vertebral invasion is difficult to diagnose pre- or intraoperatively. DeMeester and colleagues (26) studied patients with minimal vertebral involvement, defined by persistent chest wall pain, fixation to the vertebral body with minimal or no vertebral erosion by preoperative roentgenographic studies, and absence of invasion of the costotransverse foramen (the triangle formed by the rib, transverse process, and pedicle of the vertebral body). They reported a 42% 5-year survival in 12 patients treated with preoperative radiation therapy (30 Gy) and en bloc resection including a tangential excision of the involved vertebral body. Following radiation and resection, depth of invasion was visceral pleura in one patient, parietal pleura in three, periosteum in six, and cortex in two. Six patients died: one without recurrent disease, one with local disease only, two with distant disease only, and two with both local and distant disease. Distant disease was reported in the two patients with vertebral cortex invasion, one with N$_2$ disease.

Dartevelle and colleagues (27) have employed extended resection that included vertebrectomy in four patients (partial in two patients, total in two). At 5 months one patient died of complications (esophageal fistula). Three are alive, two free of disease at 5 and 25 months and one with brain metastases at 13 months.

Recent advances in surgical technique and improved spinal instrumentation have allowed gross-total resection with vertebrectomy. Although the curative value of this extended resection is theoretical, prevention of paralysis and pain relief was reported in one patient at 32 months (28). In nine patients, paralysis was prevented and in four pain was reduced by extended resection including the chest wall resection and vertebrectomy with spinal stabilization (29). Three patients died at 4 (distant metastases), 7 (local recurrence), and 20 (local recurrence) months. Six patients are alive at 6, 9, 9, 18, 23, and 36 months. Three patients underwent revision of failed spinal stabilization.

Esophagus

The esophagus is rarely involved by direct extension from a primary lung cancer. Invasion is usually due to subcarinal nodal metastases. Superficial invasion may be treated by resection of the primary tumor and limited excision of the muscular wall. Rarely has en bloc pulmonary resection and esophagectomy been reported. In seven patients with esophageal involvement only one survived beyond 5 years (30).

Mediastinum

Extended resection of lung cancers invading mediastinal fat (T_4) is rarely described. Martini and colleagues (20) reviewed a combination of 18 T_3 (invasion of mediastinal pleura) and T_4 (invasion of mediastinal fat) lung cancers with mediastinal invasion. Independent survival of these patients is not documented separately, but included in a group of 58 T_3 patients; a 5-year survival of 36% for patients undergoing complete resection was reported.

Meta-analysis of 23 series included 618 patients who underwent extended resection of T_4 carcinomas that invaded the trachea, carina, heart, great vessels, or vertebral bodies. Median and 5-year survivals were 19 months and 32% (Figure 3). The exponential decay in the risk of death is composed of an early rapidly declining component and thereafter a slowly decreasing risk (Figure 4). This

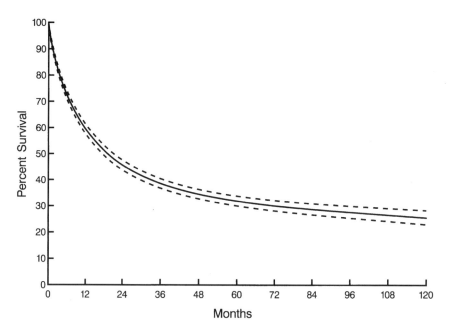

FIGURE 3 Survival after extended resection of T_4 lung cancers with tracheal, carinal, left atrial, aortic, vena caval, or vertebral body invasion. Meta-analysis of 618 patients included in 23 series. Median survival is 19 months (95% CI, 16–23).

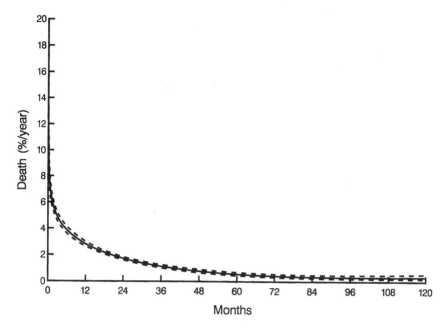

FIGURE 4 Instantaneous risk of death (hazard function) after extended resection of T_4 lung cancers with tracheal, carinal, left atrial, aortic, vena caval, and vertebral body invasion.

reflects the two major causes of death in patients undergoing extended resections: early death that is the result of postoperative complications and late death from recurrent lung cancer.

Satellite Nodule in the Same Lobe

The presence of a satellite nodule in the same lobe as the primary lung cancer was recently defined as T_4. It is estimated that 5% of resected patients will have intralobar satellite metastases and that survival for these patients at 5 years in 29.6% (31). Five-year survival was similar for $T_4N_0M_0$ (67.1%) and $T_4N_1M_0$ (61.4%), but significantly worse for $T_4N_2M_0$ (0%). Yoshino and colleagues (32) reported that survival was good for the infrequent patient with $T_4N_0M_0$ and $T_4N_1M_0$ ipsilateral intrapulmonary metastases, but poor for the more common $T_4N_2M_0$ and $T_4N_3M_0$ patients. Since extended resections are generally not required for $T_4N_0M_0$ and $T_4N_1M_0$ lung cancers with satellite nodules and because there is a potential for prolonged 5-year survival, it is questionable whether these patients should be included in stage IIIB.

Malignant Pleural Effusion

Pleural dissemination of bronchogenic carcinoma and malignant pleural effusion is perhaps the greatest obstacle preventing extended resections in patients with T_4 carcinomas. Median survival of these patients is 6 months or less. There are no long-term survivors with standard palliation. Of 15 patients treated by pulmonary resection, pleural stripping, and intrapleural infusion of chemotherapy or sclerotherapy, no patient survived 3 years (33). Survival was much worse in six patients requiring pleuropneumonectomy (mean survival 8 months). These results influenced Watanabe and colleagues (33) to recommend limited resection and pleurectomy as palliation for pleural disease found at thoracotomy.

Of 20 patients with non–small cell lung cancer and malignant pleural effusion, 10 received systemic chemotherapy and survived a median of 12 months (longest survivor, 21 months) (34). Of four patients undergoing resection, there was one operative death and three long-term survivors at 23 months and 23 and 59 months (postoperative chemotherapy). Six patients received preoperative chemotherapy and pleuropneumonectomy for a median survival of 24 months. Reyes and colleagues (34) recommend that patients should first be treated with systemic chemotherapy. In the few patients who respond and have surgically amenable disease, these authors suggest pulmonary resection and pleurectomy.

Patients discovered at thoracotomy to have T_4 disease because of malignant pleural involvement may have the best prognosis in this IIIB subgroup. A 5-year survival of 14% for 43 of these patients has been reported (35). A 25% 5-year survival was seen in patients receiving intrapleural IL-2 following surgery.

N3 Nodal Metastases

Although mediastinal lymphadenectomy including contralateral nodes has been proposed in the resection of lung cancers, this has not been suggested for known N_3 nodal metastases. The value of lymphadenectomy as a therapeutic modality has not been proven in lung cancer and extended resections of N_3 disease must be considered experimental.

INDUCTION THERAPY AND RESECTION

Downstaging of locally advanced lung cancer by induction chemotherapy or chemoradiotherapy has allowed resection of selected patients with improved results. Albain and colleagues (36) reported similar survival in both stage IIIA and stage IIIB patients treated with two cycles of cisplatin and etoposide and 45 Gy of concurrent radiation. For stage IIIB patients median survival was 17 months and 3-year survival was 24%. Early analysis showed no difference between T_4 and N_3 patients: median and 2-year survival was 27 months and 53% for T_4 and 13 months and 25% for N_3 ($p = .09$) (37). However, long-term follow-up has demonstrated an improved survival for $T_4N_0M_0$ patients when compared to N_2 and N_3 patients; 6-year survival was 49% for T_4 and 18% for N_2 and N_3 (p = .02) (38). If the stage IIIB group is composed principally of T_4 patients, survival will be excellent and similar to stage IIIA (39). If there is a predominance of N_3 patients, survival will be worse than stage IIIA (40).

Twenty-three T_4 patients underwent a combination of induction therapy and extended operations (41). Twenty-six percent of these patients experienced a major postoperative complication and 9%, postoperative death. Three-year survival was 54%. Rendina and colleagues (42) treated 57 patients with unresectable T_4 lung cancers with induction chemotherapy followed by resection. Survival at 4 years was 19.5% for all patients and 31% for those who were completely resected.

CONCLUSIONS

Stage IIIB is a heterogeneous group of locally advanced T_4 or N_3 lung cancers. Treatment is palliative for the majority of patients and ranges from supportive care to chemoradiotherapy. However, in certain patients, surgery is beneficial and may be curative. Patients with $T_4N_0M_0$ tumors invading the distal trachea, carina, left atrium, aorta, superior vena cava, or vertebral bodies may be surgical candidates. Extended resections of these T_4 lung cancers have potential for cure if no mediastinal lymph node metastases (N_2 or N_3) occur and if resection is complete. Increased postoperative mortality exists and extends beyond 30 days as evidenced by a 30-day mortality of 8% and a 90-day mortality of 18%. Improved palliation (median survival 19 months) and cure (31% 5-year survival) are possible in patients who meet the criteria, who undergo extended resection, and who are followed by physicians in facilities with special interests in extended resections. The use of induction therapy and surgery in these T_4 patients may further increase survival.

Extended resections are contraindicated in patients with T_4 lung cancers associated with malignant pleural effusions. Unfortunately, these patients have the worst prognosis. If surgical palliation is an option, only pulmonary resection with pleurectomy and not pleuropneumonectomy should be considered. In contrast, lung cancers with the best prognosis are those T_4 tumors diagnosed because of a satellite tumor nodule within the same lobe. Since extended resections are usually not required, operative mortality is not increased. Five-year survival in patients with satellite intralobar tumor nodules without mediastinal nodal metastases is comparable to survival of resected stage I and II lung cancers. These two extremes of T_4 lung cancers, malignant pleural effusion and satellite intralobar tumor nodules, are not generally considered for extended resections. It is debatable that the definition of T_4 should include these entities.

Currently, extended resections are not indicated in N_3 lung cancers. The use of induction therapy and surgery in this stage IIIB subgroup remains investigational. Thus far, compared to its use in T_4 lung cancer, inferior results have been reported.

REFERENCES

1. Clinical practice guidelines for the treatment of unresectable non–small cell lung cancer. J Clin Oncol 1997; 15:2996–3018.
2. Mountain CF. Revisions in the international system for staging lung cancer. Chest 1997; 111:1710–1717.
3. Naruke T, Goya T, Tsuchiya R, Suemasu K. Prognosis and survival in resected lung carcinoma based on the new international staging system. J Thorac Cardiovasc Surg 1988; 96:440–447.
4. Jensik RJ, Faber P, Kittle F, Miley RW, Thatcher WC, El-Baz N. Survival in patients undergoing tracheal sleeve pneumonectomy for bronchogenic carcinoma. J Thorac Cardiovasc Surg 1982; 84:489–496.
5. Fujimura S, Kondo T, Imai T, Imai T, Yamauchi A, Handa M, Okabe T, Nakada T. Prognostic evaluation of tracheobronchial reconstruction for bronchogenic carcinoma. J Thorac Cardiovasc Surg 1985; 90:161–166.
6. Faber LP. Results of surgical treatment of stage III lung carcinoma with carinal proximity. The role of sleeve lobectomy versus sleeve pneumonectomy. Surg Clin North Am 1987; 67:1001–1014.
7. Deslauriers J, Beaulieu M, McClish A. Tracheal sleeve pneumonectomy. In: Shields TW, ed. General Thoracic Surgery, 3rd ed. Philadelphia: Lea & Febiger, 1989:382–387.
8. Tsuchiya R, Goya T, Naruke T, Suemasu K. Resection of tracheal carina for lung cancer. Procedure, complications and mortality. J Thorac Cardiovasc Surg 1990; 99:779–787.
9. Vogt-Moykopf I, Meyer G. Naunheim K, Rau G, Branscheid D. Bronchoplastic techniques for lung resection. In: Baue AE, Geha AS, Hammond GL, Laks H, Naunheim KS, eds. Glenn's Thoracic and Cardiovascular Surgery, 5th ed. Norwalk, CT: Appleton & Lange 1991:403–417.
10. Mathisen DJ, Grillo HC. Carinal resection for bronchogenic carcinoma. J Thorac Cardiovasc Surg 1991; 102:16–23.
11. Roviaro GC, Varoli F, Rebuffat C, Scalambra SM, Vergani C, Sibilla E, Palmarini L, Pezzuoli G. Tracheal sleeve pneumonectomy for bronchogenic carcinoma. J Thorac Cardiovasc Surg 1994; 107:13–18.
12. Dartevelle P Macchiarini P. Techniques of pneumonectomy: sleeve pneumonectomy. Chest Surg Clin North Am 1999; 9:407–417.
13. Dartevelle PG, Khalife J, Chapelier A, Marzelle J, Navajas M, Levasseur P, Rojas A, Cerrina J. Tracheal sleeve pneumonectomy for bronchogenic carcinoma: report of 55 cases. Ann Thorac Surg 1988; 46:68–72.
14. Tsuchiya R, Asamura H, Kondo H, Goya T, Naruke T. Extended resection of the left atrium, great vessels, or both for lung cancer. Ann Thorac Surg 1994; 57:960–965.
15. Macchiarini P, Dartevelle P. Extended resections for lung cancer. In: Roth JA, Cox

JD, Hong WK, eds. Lung Cancer, 2nd ed. Malden, MA: Blackwell Science, 1998: 135–161.

16. Shirakusa T, Kimura M. Partial atrial resection in advanced lung carcinoma with and without cardiopulmonary bypass. Thorax 1991; 46:484–487.

17. Shirakusa T, Kawahara K, Iwasaki A, Okabayashi K, Shiraishi T, Yoneda S, Yoshinaga Y, Matsuzoe D, Watanabe K. Extended operation for T₄ lung carcinoma. Ann Thorac Cardiovasc Surg 1998; 4:110–118.

18. Ricci C, Rendina EA, Venuta F, Ciriaco PP, De Giacomo T, Fadda GH. Reconstruction of the pulmonary artery in patients with lung cancer. Ann Thorac Surg 1994; 57:627–633.

19. Nakahara K, Ohno K, Mastumura A, Hirose H, Mastuda H, Nakano S, Shirakura, Kawashima Y. Extended operations for lung cancer invading the aortic arch and superior vena cava. J Thorac Cardiovasc Surg 1989; 97:428–433.

20. Martini N, Yellin A, Ginsberg RJ, Bains MS, Burt ME, McCormack PM, Rusch VW. Management of non–small cell carcinoma with direct mediastinal involvement. Ann Thorac Surg 1994; 58:1447–1451.

21. Klepetko W, Wisser W, Birsan T, Mares P, Taghavi S, Kupilik N, Wolner E. T₄ lung tumors with infiltration of the thoracic aorta: Is an operation reasonable? Ann Thorac Surg 1999; 67:340–344.

22. Piccione W Jr., Faber LP, Warren WH. Superior vena caval reconstruction using autologous pericardium. Ann Thorac Surg 1990; 50:417–419.

23. Dartevelle P, Chapelier A, Navajas M, Levasseur P, Rojas A, Khalife J, Lafontaine E, Merlier M. Replacement of the superior vena cava with polytetrafluoroethylene grafts combined with resection of mediastinal-pulmonary malignant tumors. J Thorac Cardiovasc Surg 1987; 94:361–366.

24. Inoue H, Shohtsu A, Koide S, Ogawa J, Inoue H. Resection of the superior vena cava for primary lung cancer: 5 years' survival. Ann Thorac Surg 1990; 50:661–662.

25. Roberts JR, Abbott PS, Smythe WR, Bavaria JE. Resection of a pulmonary malignancy invading the intrapericardial inferior vena cava. Ann Thorac Surg 1998; 65:263–265.

26. DeMeester TR, Albertucci M, Dawson PJ, Montner SM. Management of tumor adherence to the vertebral column. J Thorac Cardiovasc Surg 1989; 97:373–378.

27. Dartevelle PG, Missenard G, Macchiarini P, Chapelier A. Invited commentary to Grunewald D, Mazel C, Girard P, Berthiot G, Dromer C, Baldeyrou P. Total vertebrectomy for en bloc resection of lung cancer invading the spine. Ann Thorac Surg 1996; 61:723–726.

28. Grunewald D, Mazel C, Baldeyrou P, Girard P. En bloc resection of lung cancer invading the spine. Ann Thorac Surg 1996; 61:1874–1880.

29. York JE, Walsh GL, Lang FF, Putnam JB, McCutcheon IE, Swisher SG, Komaki R, Gokaslan ZL. Combined chest wall resection with vertebrectomy and spinal reconstruction for the treatment of pancoast tumors. J Neurosurg 1999; 91:74–80.

30. Burt ME, Pomerantz AH, Bains MS, McCormack PM, Kaiser LR, Hilaris BS, Martini N. Results of surgical treatment of stage III lung cancer invading the mediastinum. Surg Clin North Am 1987; 67:987–1000.

31. Okada M, Tsubota N, Yoshimura M, Miyamoto Y, Nakai R. Evaluation of TMN

classification for lung carcinoma with ipsilateral intrapulmonary metastasis. Ann Thorac Surg 1999; 68:326–331.

32. Yoshino I, Nakanishi R, Osaki T, Hasuda S, Taga S, Takenoyama M, Yoshimatsu T, Yasumoto K. Postoperative prognosis in patients with non-small cell lung cancer with synchronous ipsilateral pulmonary metastasis. Ann Thorac Surg 1997; 64:809–813.

33. Watanabe Y, Shimizu J, Oda M, Hayashi Y, Tatsuzawa Y, Watanabe S, Urayama H, Iwa T. Results of surgical treatment in patients with stage IIIB non–small cell cancer. Thorac Cardiovasc Surg 1991; 39:50–54.

34. Reyes L, Parvez Z, Regal A, Takita H. Neoadjuvant chemotherapy and operations in the treatment of lung cancer with pleural effusion. J Thorac Cardiovasc Surg 1991; 101:946–947.

35. Ishida T, Kohdono S, Hamatake M, Fukuyama Y, Tateishi M, Sugimachi K, Murayama S, Murakami J, Yasumoto K. Malignant pleurisy and intrathoracic dissemination in carcinoma of the lung: diagnostic, therapeutic and prognostic implications. Int Surg 1995; 80:70–74.

36. Albain KS, Rusch VW, Crowley JJ, Rice TW, Turrisi AT III, Weick JK, Lonchyna VA, Presant CA, McKenna RJ, Gandara DR, Fosmire H, Taylor SA, Stelzer KJ, Beasley KR, Livingston RB. Concurrent cisplatin/etoposide plus chest radiotherapy for stages IIIA (N_2) and IIIB non–small cell lung cancer: Mature results of Southwest Oncology Group phase II study 8805. J Clin Oncol 1995; 13:1880–1892.

37. Rusch VW, Albain KS, Crowley JJ, Rice TW, Lonchyna V, McKenna R Jr, Stelzer K, Livingston RB. Neoadjuvant therapy: a novel and effective treatment for stage IIIB non–small cell lung cancer. Southwest Oncology Group. Ann Thorac Surg 1994; 58:290–295.

38. Albain KS, Rusch VW, Crowley JJ, Rice TW, Turrisi AT III, Weick JK, Lonchyna VA, Presant CA, McKenna RJ, Gandara DR, Fosmire H, Taylor SA, Stelzer KJ, Beasley KR, Livingston RB. Long-term survival after concurrent cisplatin/etoposide plus chest radiotherapy followed by surgery in bulky, stages IIIA (N_2) and IIIB non–small cell lung cancer: 6-year outcomes from Southwest Oncology Group study 8805. Proc ASCO 1999; 18:467a.

39. Rice TW, Adelstein DJ, Koka A, Tefft M, Kirby TJ, Van Kirk MA, Taylor M, Olencki TE, Peereboom D, Budd GT. Accelerated induction therapy and resection for poor prognosis stage III non–small cell lung carcinoma. Ann Thorac Surg 1995; 60:586–592.

40. Rice TW, Adelstein DJ, Ciezki JP, Becker ME, Rybicki LA, Farver CF, Larto MA, Blackstone EH. Short-course induction chemoradiotherapy with paclitaxel in stage III non–small cell lung cancer. Ann Thorac Surg 1998; 66:1909–1914.

41. Macchiarini P, Chapelier AR, Monnet I, Vannetzel JM, Rebischung JL, Cerrina J, Parquin F, Ladurie FL, Lenot B, Dartevelle PG. Extended operations after induction therapy for stage IIIB (T_4) non-small cell lung cancer. Ann Thorac Surg 1994; 57: 966–973.

42. Rendina EA, Venuta F, De Giacomo T, Ciccone AM, Ruvolo G, Coloni GF, Ricci C. Induction chemotherapy for T_4 centrally located non-small cell lung cancer. J Thorac Cardiovasc Surg 1999; 117:225–233.

16

Extended Resections in Stage IIIB NSCLC: Con

Richard I. Inculet
London Health Sciences Centre, London, Ontario, Canada

INTRODUCTION

Lung cancer is the leading cause of cancer death in men and women, having overtaken the mortality of breast cancer. The National Cancer Institute, in their Cancer Statistics Review of 1973 to 1996, report a 27.8% overall increase in the incidence of lung cancer, with a 123.0% increase for women alone. The treatment of lung cancer remains a top priority in clinical and basic oncology research priorities, as the volume of patients diagnosed yearly contributes to an overwhelming burden on the health care system.

The greatest clinical advance in lung cancer management has been the recent refinement of the staging of lung cancer and the increasing ability, through new technologies, to determine the pretreatment clinical stage.

Lung cancer staging was devised to (1) apply stage-dependent treatment strategies, (2) develop and trial new treatments, and (3) predict clinical outcome. Recently, the International System for Staging Lung Cancer was revised (1). Two large databases of patients treated for primary lung cancer were combined for a total of 5319 patients and modifications in the staging system were derived from the survival data. Stage IIIB non–small cell lung cancer is at present defined as some combination of a T_4 primary tumor or an N_3 lymph node.

A T_4 lesion directly invades the mediastinum, heart, great vessels, trachea, esophagus, vertebral body, or carina, and/or is associated with a malignant pleural or pericardial effusion. Satellite tumor nodules within the ipsilateral primary-tumor lobe of the lung also represent a T_4 stage.

An N_3 node is defined as a confirmed metastasis to contralateral mediastinal or hilar lymph nodes or ipsilateral or contralateral scalene nodes.

When Mountain reported the survival results of the patient database used to validate his lung cancer staging, patients with stage IIIB lung cancer (T_4, N_{0-2}, M_O) had 5 year survival of 6–8% (1). The presence of N_3 disease was associated with a 5-year survival of 3%. The difference in survival between these two stage IIIB subgroups, however, was not statistically significant.

Stage IIIB lung cancer has a poor prognosis. Whereas surgery is the treatment of choice for stages I, II, and some IIIA disease, it is not currently the recommended standard of care for stage IIIB disease. Is there a role for extended resection for stage IIIB lung cancer? The thoracic surgeon is frequently faced with this dilemma at the time of thoracotomy. Often despite preoperative staging investigations and imaging, it is only during surgical exploration that direct involvement of extrapulmonary structures is encountered. The decision for the surgeon to decline the resection or to attempt to proceed with a technically challenging resection is difficult. Unfortunately, there is no level I or II evidence today to support this decision. With the evidence we have, to justify extended resection, it is best to look separately at the subgroups of stage IIIB lung cancer.

T_4 TUMORS

Malignant Pleural or Pericardial Effusion

The presence of a cytologically positive malignant effusion may indicate the shedding of tumor cells, either from the primary tumor site or from metastatic deposits within the pleural or pericardial space, resulting in a disruption of pleural or pericardial fluid flow dynamics. There is no extended resection that could possibly encompass a malignant pericardial effusion. Intrapleural malignancy could theoretically be surgically extirpated with a radical extrapleural pneumonectomy. Malignant mesothelioma is a somewhat comparable situation in that there may be malignant involvement of the pleural/pericardial space with effusion. Sugarbaker et al. have repopularized extrapleural pneumonectomy with adjuvant therapy for specific histological subtypes of mesothelioma, with improvement of an otherwise dismal prognosis (2). Mesothelioma, however, is a primary pleural cancer in contrast to a primary non–small cell lung cancer that has invaded into or metastasized to the pleural space. Has there been any reported experience supporting radical extrapleural pneumonectomy for non–small lung cancer with malignant effusion? Several authors have anecdotal experiences of one case with survivals less than 1 year. Watanabe et al. (3) described no long-term survivors among patients with malignant pleural effusion who underwent pleuropneumonectomy. Yokoi and Miyazawa (4) reported a single 5-year survivor of adenocarcinoma of the lung with carcinomatous pleuritis who was treated with pleuropneumonectomy and postoperative adjuvant chemotherapy. Shirakusa et al. (5), in a 10-year review of resected T_4 lung cancer, recommended against surgery for malignant effusion. Although the operative mortality of extrapleural pneumonectomy is decreasing in experienced hands (3.8%) (1), the results do not justify this radical surgery for malignant effusions, secondary to primary lung cancer.

Satellite Lung Cancer Nodules

The presence of satellite tumor nodules may or may not be recognized until after the pulmonary resection is completed, and the pathologist has examined the specimen. Deslauriers et al. reviewed 84 patients who underwent resection of a primary lung cancer accompanied by satellite nodules (6). Five-year survival rates were 21.6% as compared to 44% in 1021 patients resected without satellite nodules. Although satellite tumor nodules appears to confer a worse prognosis, they should not preclude resection.

Heart, Great Vessels, Vertebral Body, Esophagus

The direct invasion of a primary lung cancer into the aorta, vena cava, or atrium has been traditionally associated with an extremely poor prognosis. Technically challenging, the affected mediastinal structure can often be resected and there are numerous case reports and series describing successful operative resection and reconstruction. However, technical success does not necessarily translate into improvement in survival.

Martini et al. published a large retrospective review of surgically resected T_3 and T_4 lung cancer including specifically 44 non–small cell, T_4 N_{0-1}, lung cancer patients (7). Eighteen percent had a complete resection, resulting in a 12% 5-year overall survival. Eleven patients received induction chemotherapy or radiotherapy. An earlier study from the same center described 225 non–small cell lung cancer patients resected for T_3/T_4 tumors with many having N_2 disease or multiple sites of mediastinal involvement (8). Only 22% were able to undergo complete resection with a 5-year survival of 9%. The author concluded that "the resectability and long term survival in patients with T_4 tumors are dismally low." Incomplete resection did not provide a survival advantage. Tsuchiya et al. reported a series of 101 patients with T_4 tumors, invading atrium or great vessels (9). Surgical resection conferred a 13% 5-year survival. In contrast, Watanabe et al. published a 25% 5-year survival rate in 83 stage IIIB resected patients (3). Bergeron et al. had 103 patients who underwent extended resection and a 23%

5-year survival (10). Incomplete resection and N_2 disease were associated with poorer results. These survival figures are also fairly consistent with those reported in the numerous Japanese case series reports. The mortality associated with extended pulmonary resection ranges from 3.3% to 12%.

In summary, surgical resection only of T_4 tumors does not provide a remarkable survival advantage, with case series generally reporting 5-year survivals of 15% or less. Poor prognostic factors include combined T_4 and N_3 disease, incomplete resection, and direct invasion into multiple structures.

N₃ DISEASE

Surgical excision of N_3 disease requires access to the contralateral mediastinal lymph nodes, or ipsilateral and/or contralateral scalene nodes. Contralateral mediastinal lymph node excision can be accomplished via median sternotomy or thoracoscopy. Scalene node excision requires a modified neck dissection. Both are technically feasible. However, once again there is no level I or II evidence that radical N_3 node dissection alters survival. The American College Surgical Oncology Group (ACSOG) is just now undertaking a randomized prospective trial looking at lymph node sampling versus ipsilateral radical node dissection in clinical N_0 patients. No recommendation can be made at this time for radical lymph node excision of N_3 nodes until such time that properly designed clinical trials are completed.

INDUCTION THERAPY

Because surgery alone has been relatively ineffective, several investigators have initiated studies utilizing induction therapies in an attempt to downstage stage IIIB tumors and hopefully modify resectability and outcome.

Rendina et al. enrolled 57 T_4 patients into an induction chemotherapy trial (11). Sixty-three percent were able to undergo complete resection with a 4-year survival of 30.5% compared to an overall survival of 19.5%. Stamatis et al. reported 56 patients with stage IIIB disease who received induction chemoradiotherapy (12). Thirty-four patients went on to surgery. Forty-eight percent of these had a complete resection, with impressive 5-year survivals of 37.5% (T_4, N_{0-1}), 31% (T_{1-2}, N_3), and 23% (T_{3-4}, N_3). Patients who had incomplete resection or no surgery did not survive past 24 months.

A Southwest Oncology Group prospective trial addressed the question of feasibility of neoadjuvant therapy of stage IIIA and IIIB non–small cell lung cancer (13). There were 51 eligible stage IIIB patients who received induction chemoradiotherapy. Of this group, only 40 patients were eligible for surgery, and 38 subsequently went on to thoracotomy. The 2-year overall survival for 51 patients was 39%, 53% for patients with T_4 tumors, and 25% for those with N_3

disease. The latter two were not significantly different. Three-year survival data for the entire 51 patients was reported later as 24% (14). Unfortunately, subsequent 5-year follow-up data that might support the persistence of the treatment effect has not been reported.

SUMMARY

Stage IIIB non–small cell lung cancer is an advanced stage of lung cancer with a poor prognosis. Radical surgical excision plays no role in patients with malignant pleural or pericardial effusions. Patients who have T_4 disease based only on the presence of satellite tumor nodules within the same lobe are candidates for surgical resection.

If a primary lung cancer is found to be directly invading mediastinal structures, resection alone is of little benefit. Early evidence suggests that induction therapy of stage IIIB tumors followed by complete resection may improve survival, but there are no randomized prospective clinical trials to confirm this. Therefore, routine resection of T_4 disease with or without induction therapy has no role outside of well-designed clinical trials established to answer this question.

The effectiveness of radical mediastinal node dissection of N_3 nodes is not supported by any strong evidence at this time and cannot be recommended.

REFERENCES

1. Mountain CF. Revisions in the International System for Staging Lung Cancer. Chest 1997; 111:1710–1717.
2. Sugarbaker DJ, Flores RM, Jaklitsch MT, Richards WG, Strauss GM, Corson JM, DeCamp MM Jr, Swanson SJ, Bueno R, Lukanich JM, Baldini EH, Mentzer SJ. Resection margins, extrapleural nodal status and cell type determine postoperative long-term survival in trimodality therapy of malignant pleural mesothelioma: results in 183 patients. J Thorac Cardiovasc Surg 1999; 117:54–63.
3. Watanabe Y, Shimizu J, Oda M, Hayashi Y, Tatsuzawa Y, Watanabe S, Urayama H, Iwa T. Results of surgical treatment in patients with stage IIIB non–small cell lung cancer. J Thorac Cardiovasc Surg 1991; 39:50–54.
4. Yokoi K, Miyazawa N. Pleuropneumonectomy and postoperative adjuvant chemotherapy for carcinomatous pleuritis in primary lung cancer: a case report of long-term survival. Eur J Cardiothorac Surg 1996; 10:141–143.
5. Shirakusa T, Kawahara K, Iwasaki A, Okabayashi K, Shiraishi T, Yoneda S, Yoshinaga Y, Matsuzoe D, Watanabe K. Extended operation for T_4 lung carcinoma. Ann Thorac Cardiovasc Surg 1998; 4:110–118.
6. Deslauriers J, Brisson J, Cartier R, Fournier M, Gagnon D, Piraux M, Beaulieu M. Carcinoma of the lung: evaluation of satellite nodules as a factor influencing prognosis after resection. J Thorac Cardiovasc Surg 1989; 97:504–512.
7. Martini N, Yellin A, Ginsberg RJ, Bains MS, Burt ME, McCormack PM, Rusch

VW. Management of non–small cell lung cancer with direct mediastinal involvement. Ann Thorac Surg 1994; 58:1447–1451.

8. Burt ME, Pomerantz AH, Bains MS, McCormack PM, Kaiser LR, Hilaris BS, Martini N. Results of surgical treatment of stage III lung cancer invading the mediastinum. Surg Clin North Am 1987; 67:987–1000.

9. Tsuchiya R, Asamura H, Kondo H, Goya T, Naruke T. Extended resection of the left atrium, great vessels, or both for lung cancer. Ann Thorac Surg 1994; 57:960–965.

10. Bergeron P, Martelet JP, Casanova P, Rudondy P, Nazet J, Nenric A, Puisais-Hee A, Longefait H. Justifications and benefits of exploratory thoracotomy in stage IIIB bronchopulmonary cancer. Ann Chir 1990; 44:662–669.

11. Rendina EA, Venuta F, De Giacomo T, Ciccone AM, Ruvolo G, Coloni GF, Ricci C. Induction chemotherapy for T_4 centrally located non–small cell lung cancer. J Thorac Cardiovasc Surg 1999; 117:225–233.

12. Stamatis G, Eberhardt W, Stuben G, Bildat S, Dahler O, Hillejan L. Preoperative chemoradiotherapy and surgery for selected non-small cell lung cancer IIIB subgroups: long-term results. Ann Thorac Surg 1999; 68:1144–1149.

13. Rusch VW, Albain KS, Crowley JJ, Rice TW, Lonchyna V, McKenna Jr. R, Stelzer K, Livingston RB, and the Southwest Oncology Group. Neoadjuvant therapy: a novel and effective treatment for stage IIIB non–small cell lung cancer. Ann Thorac Surg 1994; 58:290–295.

14. Albain KS, Rusch VW, Crowley JJ, Rice TW, Turrisi AT 3rd, Weick JK, Lonchyna VA, Presant CA, McKenna RJ, Gandara DR, et al. Concurrent cisplatin/etoposide plus chest radiotherapy followed by surgery for stages IIIA (N_2) and IIIB non–small-cell lung cancer: mature results of Southwest Oncology Group phase II study 8805. J Clin Oncol 1995; 13:1880–1892.

17

NSCLC: Value of Three-Dimensional Conformal Radiotherapy: Pro

Mary V. Graham

Phelps County Regional Medical Center, Rolla, Missouri

INTRODUCTION

Radiation therapy remains an integral component of therapy for lung cancer. The potential benefits of three-dimensional radiation therapy (3DRT) for lung cancer [primarily non–small cell lung cancer (NSCLC)] include (1) better definition and localization of the tumor target, (2) improved ability to assess and potentially reduce normal tissue toxicity, and (3) increased tumoricidal doses of radiation to the tumor target(s) resulting in improved local control translating into improved survival (1). This chapter will review the progress in achieving these goals and discuss why 3DRT is essential for optimal definitive radiation therapy for lung cancer. However, if the goal of therapy is simply palliation, or relief of symptoms, then less expensive and time-intensive therapy is indicated. If the goal is long-term survival with the absence of morbidity, then 3DRT is clearly the treatment of choice.

BACKGROUND

The "standard of care" for the dose, volume, and beam arrangements for the treatment of NSCLC was established by the Radiation Therapy Oncology

Group (RTOG) dose-escalation trial 7301 (2). In this study, 375 patients were randomly assigned to receive either 40 Gy in 4 weeks with a 2-week break (split course), 40 Gy in 4 weeks, 50 Gy in 5 weeks, or 60 Gy in 6 weeks. The complete and partial response rates (as assessed clinically and radiographically) were 48% in patients treated with 40 Gy, 53% in those treated with 50 Gy, and 56% in those receiving 60 Gy. The incidence of local failure (also evaluated clinically) was lower in patients treated with 60 Gy (33%) than in those receiving 50 Gy (39%) or 40 Gy (44–49%). In this protocol, large volumes of the chest and regional lymphatics were included in the treatment volume. The electively irradiated areas included both hila, bilateral regions of the upper mediastinum, bilateral supraclavicular areas, and 5–8 cm below the carina of the inferior mediastinum. Despite a modest improvement in survival with higher doses at 3 years, by 5 years the overall survival was approximately 5% in all arms.

There are several problems with using the "standard" radiation technique in the twenty-first century. They include:

1. Defining targets and portals of therapy using plain radiographs (simulation films) is difficult and inaccurate. Computerized tomography (CT) and often other modern imaging technologies, such as magnetic resonance imaging (MRI) or positron emission tomography (PET), are critical to achieving accurate diagnoses and tumor target definition. Trying to "translate" accurate tumor targets from diagnostic images to simulation films is often inaccurate. There may be significant errors or need for an added margin to account for error when using standard diagnostic imaging and conventional simulation to delineate portals. Dillman and associates reported that a retrospective quality control review identified 23% of cases in which portal films failed to completely encompass the tumor, even when diagnostic scans were available to the treating radiation oncologist (4). Because of the difficulties in defining targets, large fields have been used, purportedly to encompass "subclinical disease" and treat "electively irradiated regions." One might critically propose that "electively irradiated regions" are used to compensate for the inability of clinicians to accurately define what needs to be treated. The cost of this is undesirable toxicity.

2. Treatment planning with standard techniques is anteropostero (AP/PA) ports to spinal cord tolerance (conservatively estimated) and oblique ports (which questionably encompass the tumor) to the tolerance dose. It is difficult, if not impossible, for planners to use better angles to treat and encompass the tumor without the use of 3D techniques.

3. Assessing the sequelae of radiation therapy (especially pneumonitis, symptomatic fibrosis, and/or esophagitis) prior to their development, based upon the dose distributions from traditional treatment planning, has been near impossible. Side effects of standard techniques have been not insignificant. It is highly

desirable to reduce the negative sequelae of radiation therapy to the chest during the treatment of lung cancers. This is not possible without better assessment (offered by 3DRT) of where the tumor is, and what the costs of treatment are (i.e., assessment of the risks).

4. Increasing radiation therapy dose is not safely possible using standard techniques. In the RTOG protocol 8311, using standard target delineation and portals, doses were escalated to 79.2 Gy (at 1.2 Gy twice daily) (8). No significant beneficial effect was seen for doses greater than 69.6 Gy. The reasons for this have never been fully elucidated, although a higher incidence of high-grade pneumonitis was seen in the higher-dose arms of the study. This may suggest that indiscriminate dose escalation, without knowledge of dose and volume effects to the surrounding lungs, may have a deleterious effect on survival. It is well known that the lungs are exquisitely sensitive to the damaging effects of radiation resulting in a significant chance for injury, including acute pneumonitis and symptomatic pulmonary fibrosis (9,10). What is less well understood or quantitated is the impact of radiation lung damage on long-term survival.

In the early 1990s, the results of several large randomized trials reported increased survival with the addition of chemotherapy (4–6). Each of these trials utilized conventional radiation therapy and delivered 40–50 Gy to the elective nodal regions and 60–65 Gy to the gross disease. Despite the modest improvement demonstrated in these trials, there remains much room for improvement. Long-term survival is still only 8–14% (4,6). Le Chevalier and co-workers (5) reported a decreased metastatic rate with chemotherapy, but both arms had a "histological" local control rate of only 15–17% when evaluated by bronchoscopy and biopsy at 3 months and 10% at 2 years after completion of therapy. These results are considerably lower than the local control rates of 40–60% reported by clinical evaluation (2,3). In addition, lung cancers are usually quite large at presentation. It is the norm to have bulky tumors measuring greater than 2–5 cm. From basic principles advocated by Fletcher, it is thought that doses up to 100 Gy may be necessary to sterilize the size of tumors frequently treated in bronchogenic carcinoma (7).

THREE-DIMENSIONAL RADIATION THERAPY PLANNING FOR NSCLC

To realize the full potential of 3DRT, all components of such planning must be utilized. Tumor and target definition using full three-dimensional volume techniques, virtual simulation, 3D dose calculation, and dose-volume histogram plan evaluation are all critical components of successful 3D therapy for NSCLC.

DEFINING THE TARGET: ACQUISITION, IMMOBILIZATION, VIEWS, AND DISPLAYS

The initiation of 3D radiotherapy is accomplished with the aquisition of a computerized tomographic (CT) data set. The thoracic data set must include not only the entire volume of the tumor, but also the complete lung volume, the entire volumes of the brachial plexi (base of neck), the heart, and the liver. Organs not included in their entirety may potentially be inadvertently treated (when noncoplanar beams are utilized and regions not scanned or contoured are irradiated via the entrance or exit of beams), and/or the volumetric analysis and dose-volume evaluation (DVHs) are meaningless due to lack of the full-volume information of the organ.

After the CT images are obtained, the identification of targets and normal anatomy is performed. This step, called image segmentation, "divides" the CT data set into parts so that anatomical objects of interest and tumor volumes are identified. The skin or external contour can be identified automatically by thresholding and edge-detection algorithms. Contoured normal anatomical structures include the brachial plexi (labeled ipsilateral and contralateral), the total lung volume (the volume of both lungs together), heart (from its base to the level of the base of the aorta), esophagus (in its entirety from larynx to gastroesophageal junction), and liver.

ICRU 50–defined tumor and treatment targets should be utilized (11). The gross tumor volume (GTV) includes all identifiable gross tumor (Figure 1). It should include the primary tumor and any identifiable nodal involvement. However, CT data are not perfectly accurate in the identification of lung cancer and staging (12–15). Other imaging modalities, such as magnetic resonance imaging (MRI), endoscopic ultrasound, and/or positron emission tomography (PET), may be important in identifying the GTV. It should include all primary disease (as identified on the "lung windows" of the CT images), the grossly identifiable regional lymph nodes, such as those abnormally enlarged on CT (short axis greater than 1 cm) (15), those that are mediastinoscopy positive, and possibly those with abnormal metabolic activity identified on PET scanning. If different areas of gross disease are treated to different dose levels, it is useful to subdivide these into separate targets at the time of target delineation. The clinical target volume (CTV) is that anatomical region(s) thought to harbor subclinical or microscopic disease (Figure 2). Because of failure to reach consensus on the exact location of the CTV, the RTOG in its initial dose escalation trial defined the CTV = GTV.

Planning target volumes (PTV) are three-dimensional growth margins around the GTV and/or CTV to account for daily setup variations and patient motion. Because of physiological motion in the chest, the volume of the PTV may be significantly larger than the GTV. Recently several authors

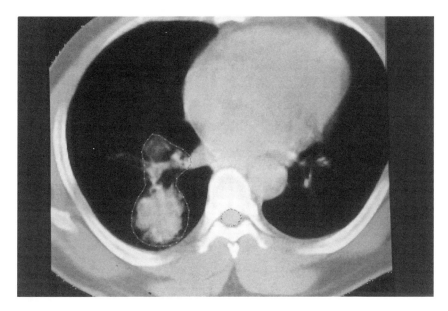

FIGURE 1   Axial CT slice demonstrating the outline of the gross tumor volume (GTV).

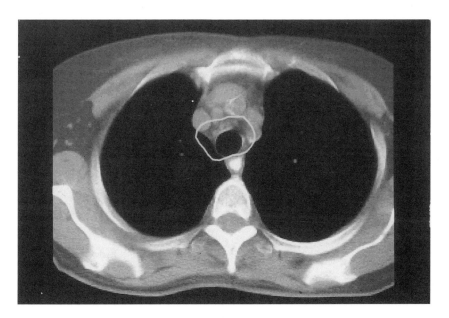

FIGURE 2   Axial CT slice showing the outline of the mediastinum, the anatomical region thought to harbor microscopic disease (the clinical target volume, CTV).

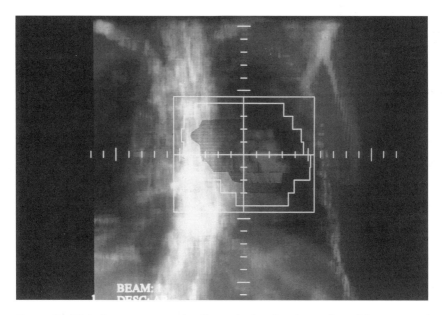

FIGURE 3   Digitally reconstructed radiograph showing the outline of the target volume and the surrounding conformal radiation field.

demonstrated that breath holding can reproducibly "immobilize" targets and lungs between CT scans and presumably treatment sessions (16). Theoretically the volume of irradiated lung could be reduced, PTV margins reduced, and targets better localized during treatment with such a device. Such clinical experience and the measured therapeutic gain from such an approach are expected to be forthcoming.

After the CT data are segmented, a 3D model of the patient is produced and displayed for treatment planning. Organs and targets may be displayed as wire frames, solid surfaces, or with various degrees of opacification (Figure 3). It is important that the 3D images be reviewed prior to planning or treatment plan acceptance to assure that organs were contoured correctly, in their entirety and without image corruption.

VIRTUAL SIMULATION

Virtual simulation begins after all targets and normal anatomy are contoured and treatment planning begins (17–20). The objectives of virtual simulation are to design the treatment apertures (portals) and the beam directions (gantry, collimator, and table angles). In most 3D systems, the simulation of the beam arrangement is performed on the 3D model of the patient. One approach is the development of "class solutions," i.e., a four- or five-field approach with beams AP/PA to spinal cord tolerance and then off-cord oblique fields to the desired tumor dose. This approach is often a good starting point and allows the planner to assess target coverage and irradiation to the lungs and other organs to assess the acceptability of this initial plan. The second approach is for an experienced planner to utilize the beam's-eye view and develop a unique individualized beam arrangement avoiding specific normal organs, such as lungs or esophagus (21). Ideally, treatment angles are found that "separate" the tumor from surrounding normal structures; i.e., the beam is angled to treat just the target volume and miss the normal structure(s). Figure 4 shows a beam's-eye view of a field defined with multileaf collimation around a target volume.

The virtual simulator records and reports all the necessary simulation data including beam names, energy of beams, table, gantry and collimator positions, isocenter location, and any beam modifiers. The display of such data is often facilitated by multiple images and views of the plan (Figure 5, A and B). Axial, coronal, and sagittal displays, as well as room-view display and an opaque view of the patient's skin and the surface appearance of the entrance portal, are often useful in evaluating the virtual simulation process.

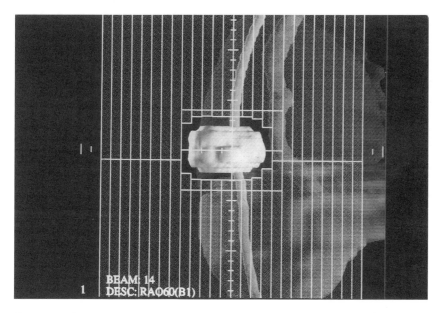

FIGURE 4   Beam's-eye view of the gross target volume demonstrating the multileaf collimation creating the conformal radiotherapy field surrounding the target.

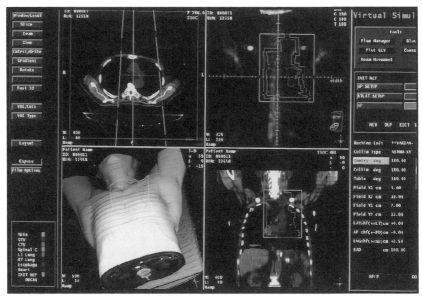

(A)

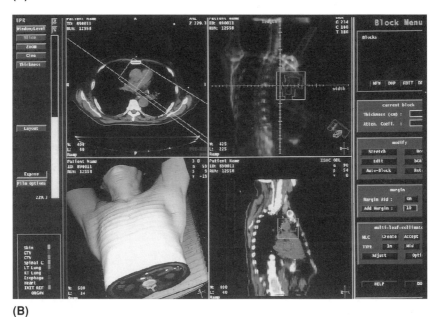

(B)

FIGURE 5   CT simulation can be used to display various images of the target and surrounding anatomy: (A) anterior view; (B) oblique view.

DOSE CALCULATION

Technically, in some systems it may be difficult to separate the process of virtual simulation and dose calculation, so the process of dose calculation and subsequent beam angle and shape readjustment is usually an integral part of the 3D treatment planning. The dose is calculated and displayed on the 3D model. Isodose displays are usually color-coded and can be isodose "nets" or wire frames or color wash displays of dose (Figure 6). Dose may be calculated with a variety of algorithms. It is imperative for the planners and evaluators to understand the strengths and weaknesses of their particular system's dose calculation algorithm (22–29). There may be significant differences in target coverage and normal organ partial volume irradiation depending on whether heterogeneity corrections are applied, or on the specific calculation algorithm. In the future it is expected that Monte Carlo simulations will be the preferred method for 3DRT dose computation. As the price/performance ratio of computer workstations continues to decrease, this type of dose calculation may be practical in the near future.

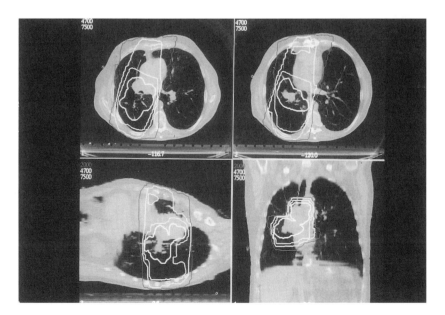

FIGURE 6   Examples of isodose displays showing the "isodose map" of radiation dose around the target.

PLAN OPTIMIZATION AND EVALUATION

The optimization of a treatment plan currently involves an iterative approach and allows for modification of the beam direction, beam shape, beam weights, and beam modifiers. Rapid calculation and recalculation and display of dose distributions enable the planner to make incremental improvements in plans.

The "optimal" plan must achieve the following goals:

1.   The tumor target(s) must be treated to sufficiently high (prescription) dose. For most 3D institutions, this is typically 70 Gy or greater. While in the past the uniformity of dose across the tumor was thought to be a desirable goal, this has recently been called into question. Theoretical models suggest that even partial target volume irradiation may result in improved outcome (30). Prior to 3D treatment systems and accurate dose calculation algorithms, there was little way to test this hypothesis. Graham and co-workers presented preliminary clinical data for NSCLC patients suggesting that maximum tumor target doses of greater than 79 Gy resulted in improved survival for patient with low volume tumors (GTV less than 70–113 ml) (31).

2.   The volume of irradiated lung must be kept sufficiently low. Experience with what constitutes acceptable levels of lung irradiation is presented later in this chapter.

3.   Radiation dose to other nearby organs, such as esophagus, heart, and brachial plexi, must also be kept minimal. There is little clinical data on what the partial volume tolerance doses for these organs are using 3D data.

The development of dose-volume histograms (DVHs) has greatly facilitated the objective plan evaluation and the consolidation of vast amounts of data depicted in the isodose displays (32). While at present nothing has replaced the isodose display and room view displays for the spatial dose information, DVHs allow a planner to rapidly assess the adequacy, uniformity, and target dose coverage, as well as the potential tolerability of nonuniform normal organ radiation treatment. Each contoured target and organ has a separate DVH. Many systems will automatically report specific dose statistics from the DVH such as minimum, mean, and maximum doses with the structure and the percent of the organ exceeding various threshold dose levels. Typical DVHs depict dose on the x-axis and volume (in absolute or percentage) on the y-axis. Traditionally DVHs of normal organs and targets are depicted in a cumulative fashion. In Figure 5, 22% of the total lung volume received in excess of 20 Gy.

It is anticipated that in the future, optimization of plans will be more automated. This will require a greater amount of clinical outcomes to be related to DVH data. But as this becomes more available, specific parameters upon which to optimize a plan could be utilized. Computerized optimization utilizing normal tissue complication probability (NTCP), tumor control probability (TCP), and

DVHs and "inverse" planning is used in intensity-modulated radiation therapy (IMRT). At the time of this writing, there has been little published information on IMRT for lung cancer. This is probably because of two reasons: (1) concern about the respiratory movement during treatment and resultant intensity-modulated calculations not reproducibly produced during treatment, and (2) heterogeneity factors (most important in the lungs) not reproducibly accounted for in some intensity-modulated systems. Pilot planning studies have been reported by Derycke and co-workers (33). The authors reported that certain class solutions utilizing specific TCP and NTCP parameters could be used to optimize lung plans using IMRT for stage III NSCLC patients.

Other approaches to optimization of treatment planning include: (1) a database of previously designed successful (or acceptable) treatment plans could be used to establish a rule-based computer system and used as a template to match the current needs of a given plan; this type of artificial intelligence has not been used very much thus far (34); (2) utilization of radiation beams that avoid specific normal structures (35); or (3) various algebraic methods or objective functions for treatment plan optimization (36–40).

Unfortunately each of these approaches suffers from serious drawbacks. There is a significant lack of correlation of 3D dose-volume data with clinical outcomes. Even if good dose-volume data become available, it is unclear how to combine all the DVH data from the various targets and normal organs into a single "goodness" of plan. Jain and co-workers attempted to develop a figure of merit (FOM) approach to the evaluation of plans (41–43). Unfortunately, neither the FOM approach nor the inverse calculation techniques can take into account such factors as patient preferences, patient desire to minimize complications or maintain quality of life, institutional standards or practices, or specific physician beliefs and opinions regarding goals and desired outcomes for a given patient.

SO WHAT HAS BEEN ACHIEVED BY 3DRT FOR LUNG CANCER?

Treatment Planning Studies

Early studies with 3DRT were computer-simulated studies comparing 3D with conventional 2D treatment plans for lung cancer (28,44–46). In each of these studies, the authors demonstrated the improvement in treatment planning by dose escalation, reduction in dose to surrounding organs, or both. The authors concluded that 3D planning potentially improved tumor target delineation and target volume coverage (28,46). It appeared that traditional beam arrangements were inadequate or potentially harmful (in terms of normal lung irradiation effects) in the delivery of target doses greater than 70 Gy (45,46).

Assessment of Normal Tissue Toxicity

The development of acute pneumonitis is an undesirable and potentially very debilitating or even fatal complication after radiation therapy to the chest. The doses of radiation that cause either acute radiation pneumonitis or chronic radiation fibrosis have only been partially characterized, and the volume effects of radiation therapy on the lung are incompletely understood. Emami and co-workers gathered data of available literature and published initial estimates of partial volume lung tolerance (44). The data showed normal tissue tolerance doses for a 5% (TD5/5) and 50% (TD50/5) chance of a complication occurring by 5 years of uniform irradiation of one-third, two-thirds, and whole lung. The TD50/5 for whole lung was 17.5 Gy, for two-thirds of the lung was 30 Gy, and for one-third of the lung was 45 Gy.

Martel and co-workers retrospectively reviewed the 3D DVHs for the lungs of 21 patients with Hodgkin's disease and 42 lung cancer patients with the development of acute pneumonitis (47). The authors reported a reasonable prediction for low versus high risk for the development of pneumonitis by dividing the patients into risk groups based upon the calculation of the effective volume (V_{eff}) of the total lung volume (both lungs together). There were differences in the mean lung dose between patients with complications versus no complications for both groups of patients. Patients without the development of acute pneumonitis had mean lung doses of 18–21 Gy (average doses) versus 24–26.1 Gy (average doses) for patient with acute pneumonitis. A study by Oetzel and co-workers showed good correlation for the pneumonitis risk estimations with observed complication rates for ipsilateral lung DVHs, but not paired lungs (or total lung volume) (48). Mean lung doses differed somewhat for patients with and without complications (23.8 Gy vs. 20.1 Gy). Marks and co-workers found the total lung NTCP was the single best predictor for pulmonary symptoms after irradiation (49). The V30 (lung volume receiving ≥30 Gy) was also a strong predictor. Graham et al. reported the single best predictor of acute pneumonitis was the V_{20} (volume of total lung receiving ≥20 Gy), although on univariate analysis, both V_{eff} and total lung mean dose also correlated with acute pneumonitis (50). Kwa et al. pooled the data from five institutions (University of Michigan, University of Heidelberg, Washington University, Duke University, and Netherlands Cancer Institute) for a total of 540 patients (51). Mean lung dose was the only dosimetric parameter collected. Increasing mean lung dose correlated well with the increasing pneumonitis rate.

Others have attempted to evaluate local radiation damage and dose-response relationship to the overall volumetric function of the lung (52,53). Change in perfusion and ventilation pre- and postirradiation was examined and a dose effect for local changes determined. Boersma et al. reported "overall response parameter" as a mean reduction in perfusion over the total lung correlated with the incidence of pneumonitis (54). Marks investigated whether functional DVHs (fDVHs) resulted in better predictions of pneumonitis (53). These f DVHs were based on pretreatment SPECT perfusion data, and were used to take into account local lung function in the design of the optimal treatment plan. Unfortunately, there appeared to be too many confounding factors, such as patients with very severe PFTs improving after radiation therapy, and the functional DVHs did not result in an improved ability to predict pneumonitis. Further studies at Duke University with biochemical markers such as TGF-β showed elevated levels related to increased pulmonary symptoms, though this could not be related to dose or volume dependence, nor when compared with NTCPs or V_{30} was this a strong predictive factor for the development of pneumonitis (45,55). Another factor not accounted for in the models is the indication that the lower lobes of the lungs, or dependent lung bases, are more radiosensitive than the upper lobes (50,56). However, this may simply be a volume effect in that irradiation of lower-lobe tumors results in greater volume of lung irradiation (50).

Graham and co-workers reported the correlation between the V_{20} and actuarial incidence of $\geq$grade 2 pneumonitis to be very strong ($p = 0.001$) (50). When the V_{20} was <22%, the incidence of pneumonitis was 0. When the V_{20} was 22–31%, 32–40%, and >40%, the actuarial incidence of grade 2 pneumonitis was 7%, 13%, and 19%, respectively. Graham et al. reported the severity of pneumonitis to also be related to the V_{20} (50).

V_{20} (%)	Grade 2 (%)	Grade 3–5 (%)
<22	0	0
22–31	7	0
32–40	13	5 (1 fatal)
>40	19	23 (3 fatal)

Graham et al. also reported a very close relationship between the V_{20}, V_{eff}, and mean lung dose. They reported that based on the Washington University data, the V_{20} was the single best predictor of acute pneumonitis on multivariate analysis (50).

Results of Clinical Trials

The results of single-institution 3D clinical trials for NSCLC are shown in Table 1 (57–60). Because these were early trials before significant dose escalation, the doses treated ranged from 60 to 74 Gy. These reports thus represent the results of more standard doses, but with special technical support, such as beam's-eye view or 3D dose calculation. One can see that the results appear somewhat better

TABLE 1   Results of Clinical Trials for NSCLC using 3DRT

Institution	No. of patients	Dose (Gy)	Survival			
			Median (mo)	1 yr (%)	2 yr (%)	3 yr (%)
University of Michigan (57)	88	>60	15	—	37	15
University of Chicago (58)	37	60–70	19.5	75	37	—
Memorial Sloan-Kettering (59)	45	64–72	16	—	33	—
Washington University (60)	126	60–74	21.5	57	43	29

than those from the large chemoradiation trials of the early 1990s. Of course, one must be cautious about drawing conclusions from the emerging single-institution trials (58–61).

Dose-Escalation Trials

The University of Michigan began its phase I dose-escalation trial in 1992 (62). The trial was designed to dose-escalate different patient populations based on their calculated risk of pneumonitis. The V_{eff} parameter was chosen to stratify the patients for their risk of pneumonitis. The risk groups were as follows: the lowest risk group had a V_{eff} of <0.20 Gy. The intermediate risk groups had a V_{eff} of 0.20–0.25 Gy, 0.25–0.31 Gy, 0.31–0.40 Gy. The highest risk group had a V_{eff} of >0.40 Gy. These authors have recently updated their results (63). Of 56 evaluable patients, grade 2 radiation pneumonitis (RP) occurred in five patients and grade 3 RP in only one patient. Other toxicity encountered has been ≥grade 3 esophagitis in two patients. Two patients developed exsanguinating hemorrhages (both patients had tumors surrounding the main pulmonary artery). Currently, in the lowest-risk group (V_{eff} ≤ 12%), the administered doses have been as high as 102.9 Gy. So far, no cases of isolated failures in clinically uninvolved nodal regions (purposely not irradiated) have been found. Of the initial 10 patients treated with ≥84 Gy, there was biopsy-proven residual disease or locally recurrent disease in three patients, and complete histological response in three patients on follow-up bronchoscopy (62).

The Memorial Sloan-Kettering Cancer Center reported, using dose-volume histogram analysis, that grade 3 or higher toxicity occurred in 38% of patients receiving ≥25 Gy to >30% of their lung volume versus 4% of patients with ≤30% of their lung volume receiving ≥25 Gy. Pneumonitis was also correlated with the NTCP. Their dose-escalation protocol is based upon a single dose-escalation schema, but limits who may enter the protocol to an NTCP of ≤20% (59).

The Radiation Therapy Oncology Group (RTOG) dose escalation trial for NSCLC patients stratifies the patients for risk of pneumonitis based on the pre-treatment plan V_{20}. The risk groups are <25%, 25–37%, and >37% (64). Patients in the low-risk group have been successfully dose-escalated so far to 90.3 Gy without the development of high-grade acute pneumonitis.

Each of the above trials has eliminated elective nodal irradiation in an attempt to reduce pulmonary toxicity. This decision was based on the recognition that most failures in lung cancer are at the site of gross disease. Indeed, Hazuka et al. (57) found no difference in local progression-free survival or survival between large-volume treatment (i.e., inclusion of the contralateral hilar or supraclavicular lymph nodes) and small-volume treatment (i.e., exclusion of these elective nodal sites). Similarly, Robinow et al. reported no failures in 101 patients in whom the radiographically uninvolved contralateral hilum was purposely not irradiated (65). It is hoped that in this era of combined-modality therapy, chemotherapy will reduce the recurrence of microscopic disease in the regional lymphatics. It is also recognized that even though the mediastinum is not targeted for the prescription dose, it receives some dose. Clearly portions of the mediastinum and ipsilateral hilum receive varying doses of the entry or exit or scatter dose, depending on their proximity to the gross tumor. However, it has been very difficult to quantitate this dose. The issue of elective nodal irradiation is extremely controversial and the results of the ongoing trials are imperative to establish the practice as standard of care. In addition, after the maximum tolerated dose or doses for NSCLC are established, further trials comparing 3D therapy to conventional doses and volumes may be necessary to establish a therapeutic advantage. Moreover, this strategy will need to be integrated with chemotherapy. Recently Socinski et al. reported a dose-escalation trial using 3D computer-assisted planning techniques from 60 to 74 Gy in patients receiving induction carboplatin (C) and paclitaxel (P) and concurrent weekly C/P. Of these patients, 97% (31/32) completed therapy to 74 Gy as planned. The grade 3/4 esophagitis rate overall was relatively low at only 11%. Moreover, Socinski et al. found a promising median survival of 26 months and 3-year survival of 47%. Further escalation of the RT dose in the context of chemotherapy will need to be explored (66). Only in this way will the true value and efficacy of 3D therapy for lung cancer be confirmed.

SUMMARY

3DRT for lung cancer has emerged as an important component of therapy for lung cancer. Results of single institutions have provided parameters upon which to evaluate the risk of acute pneumonitis and thereby stratify patients for dose-escalation studies. Planners using 3D planning for NSCLC can use these parameters to assess and reduce (by iterative planning) the lung complication rates in patients. Further clinical correlations for esophagus, heart, soft tissue, and late pulmonary sequelae are needed. The value of dose escalation with combined-modality therapy remains to be established. It is anticipated that more sophisticated, user-friendly computer-assisted or optimized 3D radiation treatment will be used for the treatment of lung cancer in the future. It is only through the use of such sophisticated treatment that improvements in the radiation therapy for lung cancer will be achieved.

REFERENCES

1. Lichter AS. Three-dimensional conformal radiation therapy: a testable hypothesis. Int J Radiat Oncol Biol Phys 1991; 21:853–855.
2. Perez CA, Pajak TF, Rubin P, et al. Long-term observations of the patterns of failure in patients with unresectable non-oat cell carcinoma of the lung treated with definitive radiotherapy: report by the Radiation Therapy Oncology Group. Cancer 1987; 59:1874–1881.
3. Perez CA, Stanley K, Rubin P, et al. Impact of irradiation technique and tumor extent in tumor control and survival of patients with unresectable non-oat cell carcinoma of the lung: report by the Radiation Therapy Oncology Group. Cancer 1982; 50: 1091–1099.
4. Dillman RO, Seagren SL, Propert KJ, et al. A randomized trial of induction chemotherapy plus high-dose radiation versus radiation alone in stage III non–small-cell lung cancer. N Engl J Med 1990; 323:940–945.
5. Le Chevalier T, Arriagada R, Quoix E, et al. Radiotherapy alone versus combined chemotherapy and radiotherapy in nonresectable non-small-cell lung cancer: first analysis of a randomized trial in 353 patients. J Natl Cancer Inst 1991; 83:417.
6. Sause W, Scott C, Taylor S, et al. Radiation Therapy Oncology Group (RTOG) 8808 and Eastern Cooperative Oncology Group (ECOG) 4588: preliminary results of a phase III trial in regionally advanced unresectable non-small-cell lung cancer. J Natl Cancer Inst 1995; 87:198.
7. Fletcher G. Clinical dose-response curves of human malignant epithelial tumours. Br J Radiol 1973; 46:1.
8. Cox J, Axarnia N, Byhardt R, et al. A randomized phase I/II trial of hyperfractionated radiation therapy with total doses of 60.0 Gy to 79.2 Gy. Possible survival benefit with ≥69.6 Gy in favorable patients with Radiation Therapy Oncology Group stage III non–small-cell lung carcinoma: report of Radiation Therapy Oncology Group 8311. J Clin Oncol 1990; 8:1543.
9. Maasilta P. Radiation-induced lung injury. From the chest physician's point of view. Lung Cancer 1991; 7:367.
10. Roberts CM, Foulcher E, Saunders JJ, et al. Radiation pneumonitis: a possible lymphocyte-mediated hypersensitivity reaction. Ann Intern Med 1993; 118(9): 696.
11. International Commission on Radiation Units and Measurements. Report No. 50: Prescribing, Recording, and Reporting Photon Beam Therapy. Bethesda, MD: International Commission on Radiation Units and Measurements, 1993.
12. Venuta F, Rendina EA, Ciriaca P, et al. Computed tomography to stage for preopera-

tive assessment of T_3 and T_4 bronchogenic carcinoma. Eur J Cardiothoracic Surg 1992; 6(5):238.

13. Dales RE, Stark RM, Raman S. Computed tomography to stage lung cancer. Approaching a controversy using meta-analysis. Am Rev Respir Dis 1990; 141(5): 1096.

14. Platt JF, Glazer GM, Orringer MB, et al. Radiologic evaluation of the subcarinal lymph nodes: a comparative study. AJR 1988; 151(2):279.

15. McCloud TC, Bourgouin PM, Breeberg RW, et al. Bronchogenic carcinoma: analysis of staging in the mediastinum with CT by correlative lymph node mapping and sampling. Radiology 1992; 182:319.

16. Ramsey CR, Scaperoth D, Arwood D, et al. Clinical efficacy of respiratory gated conformal radiation therapy. Med Dosimetry 1999; 24(2):115.

17. Lichter AS, Sandler HM, Robertson JM, et al. Clinical experience with three-dimensional treatment planning. Semin Radiat Oncol 1992; 2:257.

18. Sailer SL, Chaney EL, Rosenman JG, et al. Treatment planning at the University of North Carolina at Chapel Hill. Semin Radiat Oncol 1992; 2:267.

19. Sherouse GW, Chaney EL. The portable virtual simulator. Int J Radiat Oncol Biol Phys 1991; 21:475.

20. Cullip TJ, Symon JR, Rosenman JG, et al. Digitally reconstructed fluoroscopy and other interactive volume visualizations in 3-D treatment planning. Int J Radiat Oncol Biol Phys 1993; 27:145.

21. Fraass BA, McShan DL, Weeks KJ. 3-D treatment planning III: complete beam's-eye-view planning capabilities. In: Bruinvis IAD, van Kleffens F, Wittkamper FW, eds. The Use of Computers in Radiotherapy. Amsterdam: North-Holland, 1987:193.

22. Rosen IJ, Lane RG, Morrill SM, et al. Treatment plan optimization using linear programming. Med Phys 1991; 18:141.

23. Gokhale P, Hussein Ema. Determination of beam orientation in radiotherapy planning. Med Phys 1994; 21(3):393.

24. Starkschall G. A constrained least-squares optimization method for external beam radiation therapy treatment planning. Med Phys 1984; 11:659.

25. Bortfield TR, Boyer AL. The exponential radon transform and projection filtering in radiotherapy planning. Int J Imaging Syst Technol 1995; 6:62.

26. Gustafsson A, Lind BK, Brahme A. A generalized pencil beams algorithm for optimization of radiation therapy. Med Phys 1994; 21:343.

27. Powlis D, Altschuler MD, Censor Y, et al. Semi-automated radiotherapy treatment planning with a mathematical model to satisfy treatment goals. Int J Radiat Oncol Biol Phys 1989; 16:271.

28. Llacer J. Inverse radiation treatment planning using the dynamically penalized likelihood method. Med Phys 1997; 24:1751.

29. Cho PS, Lee S, Marks RJ, et al. Optimization of intensity modulated beams for volume constraints using two methods: cost function minimization and projections onto convex sets. Med Phys 1998; 25:435.

30. Deasey TO. Tumor control probability models for nonuniform dose distributions. 5th International Conference on Dose, Time and Fractionation in Radiation Oncology, Madison, WI, 1997:65.

31. Graham MV, Purdy JA, Harms W, et al. Survival and prognostic factors of non–

small cell lung cancer (NSCLC) patients treated with definitive three-dimensional (3D) radiation therapy. Int J Radiat Oncol Biol Phys 1998; 42:166.

32. Drzymala RE, Mohan R, Brewster L, et al. Dose-volume histograms. Int J Radiat Oncol Biol Phys 1991; 21:71.

33. Derycke S, DeGersem WRT, VanDuyse BB, et al. Conformal radiotherapy of stage III non–small cell lung cancer: a class solution involving non-coplanar intensity-modulated beams. Int J Radiat Oncol Biol Phys 1998; 41:771.

34. Kalet IJ, Jacky JP. Knowledge-based computer simulation for radiation therapy planning. In: Bruinvis AD, vander Biessen PH, van Kleffens, HF, Wittkamper FW, eds. Proceeding of the 19th International Conference on the Use of Computers in Radiation Therapy. Amsterdam: Elsevier Science Publishers, 1987:553.

35. Chen GTY, Spelbring DR, Pelizzari CA, et al. The use of beam's eye view volumetrics in the selection of non-coplanar ports. Int J Radiat Oncol Biol Phys 1992; 23:153.

36. Lyman JT, Wolbarst AB. Optimization of radiation therapy III: a method of assessing complication probabilities from dose-volume histograms. Int J Radiat Oncol Biol Phys 1987; 13:103.

37. Kutcher GJ, Burman C. Calculation of complication probability factors for non-uniform normal tissue radiation: the effective volume method. Int J Radiat Oncol Biol Phys 1989; 1:1623.

38. Mohan R, Mageras GS, Baldwin B, et al. Clinically relevant optimization of 3D conformal treatments. Med Phys 1992; 19:933.

39. Kallman P, Lind BK, Brahme A. An algorithm for maximizing the probability of complication-free tumour control in radiation therapy. Phys Med Biol 1992; 37:871.

40. Niemierko A, Urie M, Goitein M. Optimization of 3D radiation therapy with both physical and biological end points and constraints. Int J Radiat Oncol Biol Phys 1992; 23:99.

41. Jain NL, Kahn MG, Drzymala RE, et al. Objective evaluation of 3D radiation treatment plans: a decision-analytic tool incorporating treatment preferences of radiation oncologists. Int J Radiat Oncol Biol Phys 1993; 26:321.

42. Graham MV, Jain NJ, Kahn MG, et al. Evaluation of an objective plan-evaluation model in the three dimensional treatment of non–small cell lung cancer. Int J Radiat Oncol Biol Phys 1996; 34:469–74.

43. Graham MV, Jain NJ, Kahn MG, et al. Objective plan evaluation using a score function tool. Front Radiat Ther Oncol 1996; 29:81–85.

44. Emami BE, Lyman J, Brown A, et al. Tolerance of normal tissues to therapeutic irradiation. Int J Radiat Oncol Biol Phys 1991; 21:109.

45. Armstrong JG, Burman C, Leibel S, et al. Three-dimensional conformal radiation therapy may improve the therapeutic ratio of high dose radiation therapy for lung cancer. Int J Radiat Oncol Biol Phys 1993; 26:685.

46. Graham MV, Mathews JW, Harms WB, et al. 3-Dimensional radiation treatment Planning study for patients with carcinoma of the lung. Int J Radiat Oncol Biol Phys 1994; 29:1105–1117.

47. Martel MK, Ten Haken RK, Hazuka MB, et al. Dose-volume histogram and 3-D treatment planning evaluation of patients with pneumonitis. Int J Radiat Oncol Biol Phys 1994; 28(3):575.

48. Oetzel D, Schraube P, Hensley F, et al. Estimation of pneumonitis risk in three-dimensional treatment planning using dose-volume histogram analysis. Int J Radiat Oncol Biol Phys 1995; 33:455.

49. Marks LB, Munley M, Bentel G, et al. Physical and biological predictors of changes in whole-lung function following thoracic irradiation. Int J Radiat Oncol Biol Phys 1997; 39:563.

50. Graham MV, Purdy JA, Emami BE, et al. Clinical dose volume histogram analysis for pneumonitis after 3D treatment for non-small cell lung cancer (NSCLC). Int J Radiat Oncol Biol Phys 1999; 45(2):323–329.

51. Kwa S, Lebesque J, Theuws J, et al. Radiation pneumonitis as a function of mean dose: an analysis of pooled data of 540 patients. Int J Radiat Oncol Biol Phys 1998; 42:1.

52. Boersma LJ, Damen EMF, de Boer RW, et al. A new method to determine dose-effect relations for local lung-function changes using correlated SPECT and CT data. Radiother Oncol 1993; 29(2):110.

53. Marks LB, Munley MT, Spencer DP, et al. Quantification of radiation-induced regional lung injury with perfusion imaging. Int J Radiat Oncol Biol Phys 1997; 38(2): 399.

54. Boersma LJ, Damen EM, deBoer RW, et al. Estimation of overall pulmonary function after irradiation using dose-effect relations for local functional injury. Radiother Oncol 1995; 36:15.

55. Anscher MS, Kong FM, Andrews K, et al. Plasma transforming growth factor beta 1 as a predictor of radiation pneumonitis. Int J Radiat Oncol Biol Phys 1998; 41: 1029.

56. Liao ZX, Travis EL, Tucker SL. Damage and morbidity from pneumonitis after irradiation of partial volumes of mouse lung. Int J Radiat Oncol Biol Phys 1995; 32:1359.

57. Hazuka MB, Turrisi AT, Lutz ST, et al. Results of high-dose thoracic irradiation incorporating beam's eye view display in non–small cell lung carcinoma: a retrospective multivariate analysis. Int J Radiat Oncol Biol Phys 1993; 27:273.

58. Sibley GS, Mundt AJ, Shapiro C, et al. The treatment of stage III non–small cell lung cancer using high dose conformal radiotherapy. Int J Radiat Oncol Biol Phys 1995; 33:1001.

59. Armstrong J, Zelefsky M, Burt M, et al. Promising survival with 3-dimensional conformal radiation therapy for non–small cell lung cancer. Proc Am Soc Clin Oncol 1994; 13:651.

60. Graham MV, Purdy JA, Harms WB, et al. Survival and prognostic factors of non–small cell lung cancer (NSCLC) patients treated with definitive three-dimensional (3D) radiation therapy. Int J Radiat Oncol Biol Phys 1998; 42(1):166.

61. Graham MV, Purdy JA, Emami BE, et al. Preliminary results of a prospective trial using three dimensional radiotherapy for lung cancer. Int J Radiat Oncol Biol Phys 1995; 33:993–1000.

62. Robertson JM, Ten Haken RK, Hazuka MB, et al. Dose escalation for non-small cell lung cancer using conformal radiation therapy. Int J Radiat Oncol Biol Phys 1997; 37:1079.

63. Hayman J, Martel M, Ten Haken R, Todd R, Turrisi A, Lichter A. Dose escalation

in non-small cell lung cancer (NSCLC) using conformal 3 dimensional radiation therapy (C3DRT): update of a phase I trial. Proc ASCO 1999; 18:459.

64. Graham MV. Predicting radiation response (editorial). Int J Radiat Oncol Biol Phys 1997; 39:561.

65. Robinow JS, Shaw EG, Eagan RT, Lee RL, Creagan ET, Frytak S, et al. Results of combination chemotherapy and thoracic radiation therapy for unresectable non–small cell cancer of the lung. Int J Radiat Oncol Biol Phys 1989; 17:1203–1210.

66. Socinski MA, Halle J, Schell MJ, Clark J, Limentani S, Mitchell W, Fraser R, Rosenman JA. Induction (I) and concurrent (C) carboplatin/paclitaxel (C/P) with dose-escalated thoracic conformal radiotherapy (TCRT) in stage IIIA/B non–small cell lung cancer (NSCLC): A phase I/II trial. Proc ASCO 2000; 19:496a.

18

NSCLC: Value of Three-Dimensional Conformal Radiotherapy: Con

Eli Glatstein

University of Pennsylvania Medical Center, Philadelphia, Pennsylvania

Biology is King, Patient selection is Queen, Technical maneuvers are the Prince and Princess. Occasionally the Prince or Princess tries to usurp the throne; they almost always fail to overcome the powerful forces of the King and Queen.

—Blake Cady, *Archives of Surgery*, 1997

INTRODUCTION

The truly astonishing aspect of radiation oncology is simply that radiation is effective in the treatment of cancer. A priori, there is no reason to have anticipated such an outcome. However, because radiation oncology is a physical solution to what is truly a biological problem of cancer, there are limitations on just how effective it can be. It is unequivocally a major treatment modality, but it should not be seen as ''the answer'' to the biological problem; rather, it should be seen as a component of the answer.

NEW TECHNOLOGIES

With the optimization of the linear accelerator, essentially completed by the mid-1980s, it became apparent that there was no need for a linear accelerator to have x-ray energies greater than approximately 20–25 MeV strength. Higher energies and greater penetration in tissue would simply not be of any further major advantage to patients. Hence, in the latter part of the 1980s and in the 1990s, the emphasis has been on new technologies, rather than increasing the energy of the beam. These new technologies represent the logical conclusion of the introduction of the computer into our lives, and radiotherapy simply represents one pathway.

Without question, there are benefits from some of these high-tech solutions. Clearly they accelerate the process of treatment and significantly improve patient throughput. In addition, developments like the multileaf collimator make it much easier physically for therapists to carry out their routine functions. They are not required to lift heavy blocks; when there are multiple fields to treat, they do not have to go back and forth into the room to change fields. Rather, the radiation field can be adjusted directly from the control station. These high-tech solutions are here to stay and they will be exploited in radiation therapy and in lung cancer. Yet, these advances pale in comparison to the advent of megavoltage radiation, which resulted in a dramatic improvement in the results of treatment compared to orthovoltage that had been used up to that time. The reason for this improvement was that, for the first time, megavoltage equipment allowed significant doses of radiation to be delivered with less side scattering to deep-seated neoplasms. Thus, the current ''high-tech'' innovations need to be seen and identified as a refinement of a technology that has already been in existence, rather than a ''breakthrough.''

A multileaf collimator is a device for automatically shaping the beam and allowing flexibility in that shape. When it is used with a fixed beam, its basic function is that of a customized block. Ultimately, the leaves that do the shaping will alter their position as the beam arcs around the tumor. Perhaps that may result in some enhanced value, but when the beam is actually fixed, the same effects can be achieved by individually fabricated blocks.

3-D TREATMENT PLANNING

There is no doubt that there are individual patients who will benefit from three-dimensional (3-D) treatment planning, multileaf collimation and intensity-modulated radiation therapy. However, there is a manic euphoria within our field that is building momentum about the *presumed* impact of 3-D treatment planning and conformal therapy on patient outcome. Clearly, these developments are here to stay and there will be improvements in selected patients, largely by allowing noncoplanar fields to be introduced relatively easily into the treatment plan for greater conformality. What we should not lose sight of is the fact that 3-D treatment planning is based on a series of 2-D images. A stack of 2-D CT scans has been available for almost 20 years. The 3-D planning does not represent new data; what is new is the reconstructed image and the relatively fast and easy way to add noncoplanar fields and achieve an integrated dose. In the past, radiation oncologists were required to view all the sections and try to integrate the stack in their minds to come up with the third dimension for planning.

A wide variety of papers written in recent years show treatment plans based on 3-D treatment planning that appear superior to conventional radiation therapy. The real question is: Will this really have an impact on patient outcome? We need clear documentation of an improvement in outcome, especially survival. Prior trials in medical oncology have shown that hematopoietic growth factors allow for greater cumulative doses of chemotherapy, but fail to document any improvement in survival. The presumption that more is somehow better should not go unchallenged.

It is entirely appropriate to investigate the hypothesis that improvements in x-ray dose distribution can lead to an improvement in outcome in patients who have cancer, including lung cancer. The mere act of delivering an increased dose to a defined target does not necessarily mean that an improved outcome will result. We have data from another era that demonstrate that in lung cancer, among others, postoperative radiotherapy following a "curative" surgical resection results in significantly improved local control without achieving any significant gain in survival (1). Presumably this phenomenon was due to the presence of undetectable micrometastatic lesions that ultimately determine the survival of patients who have lung carcinoma.

Recently, in the era of adjuvant or neoadjuvant chemotherapy, the issue of the impact of improved local control upon survival has resurfaced for lung and breast cancers (2,3). These new studies suggest a statistically significant improvement in survival resulting from the delivery of radiation therapy in conjunction with chemotherapy. These gains appear to be real, but nonetheless they are modest. They are consistent with the degree of absolute gain achieved by adjuvant chemotherapy in breast cancer. We need to acknowledge these gains, but not overstate them. A patient who could be cured by conventional radiation therapy techniques is not about to be cured twice by new technologies.

Clearly, reducing normal tissue effects is a major consideration and potential benefit of 3-D conformal radiotherapy. On the other hand, the development of improved imaging has made target volume definition vastly more precise than it was 25 years ago. This in turn has made for better targeted treatment and less morbidity. In addition, in today's world, most radiation oncologists have the advantage of being able to select from a range of three or four photon energies, as well a half-dozen electron energies. This has permitted a degree of patient customization that was inconceivable 30 years ago. These two developments have markedly decreased the risks of major long-term radiation injuries to major organs and tissues *prior* to the development of 3-D conformal radiotherapy. It is astonishing to interview graduating trainees in radiation oncology and realize that few have seen more than a handful of cases of radiation pneumonitis or chronic enteritis during their training. Many have not had to admit a patient to the hospital for a severe acute or chronic radiation injury and are inexperienced in treating these problems. One has to be concerned whether they will recognize such problems when they do occur or simply have a reaction of denial; the latter response is not uncommon if a patient develops a symptom complex that one has not previously recognized as part of a discrete diagnostic entity.

Most lung cancer patients have serious underlying cardiopulmonary restrictions due to the long-term effects of cigarette smoking, or other pulmonary processes, or a prior surgical resection. Pulmonary function is a major limitation on what any modality can accomplish in the treatment of lung cancer. Exposing larger volumes of normal tissue, albeit to more modest doses of radiation, may further compromise lung function. In some patients, this may result in a worse functional outcome than completely wiping out a smaller volume with conventional radiation. In addition, as we increase the doses to the target volume to 90–100 Gy, there will be times when the vasculature or bronchial cartilage will necrose after such high doses. Indeed, in the phase I dose escalation study for lung cancer at the University of Michigan, two of 48 patients developed exsanguinating hemorrhages (4). Likewise, phrenic nerves that are coincidentally irradiated to doses greater than 7500 cGy can be expected to manifest a finite probability of paralysis after some years.

LONG-TERM EFFECTS OF RADIOTHERAPY

The sine qua non for long-term effects of radiation therapy on normal tissues is slow, but progressive cell loss. One can predict that if portions of the heart receive high radiation doses and the patient lives several years, (a) cardiac muscle cells will drop out, and (b) local areas of ventricular or atrial aneurysm will ultimately develop and prove extremely difficult to correct surgically as a result of the prior treatment. If a high dose of radiation coincides with the location of the atrioventricular node within the heart, a variety of challenging arrhythmias ultimately result. While these may be risks worth taking in lung cancer, we have to be aware of them before we conclude that normal tissue tolerance has been underestimated. Perhaps the biggest improvements from conformal and intensity-modulated treatment will be in children (5,6), owing to the critical problem of radiation effects on growing tissues.

Conformality of external radiation has much appeal, but brachytherapy in some patients may do just as well in selected situations. In fact, it may be better in that the falloff in dose peripheral to the target volume will spare normal tissues far better than any modulated radiation plan. This also proves to be the case for protons, where the combination of a Bragg peak, the absence of an exit dose, and a major reduction in the entrance dose relative to the target dose promise a major gain in therapeutic ratio.

There is no way in which a new advantage can be obtained without paying some price. A major potential clinical disadvantage of intensity modulation treatment or conformal therapy has been largely neglected to date. We all agree that it is desirable to minimize tumor doses to normal tissues outside of target volumes in a radiation portal. But the principle of conformal treatment is to use multiple fields to achieve the desired dose within the target volume by spreading more modest doses of radiation therapy over a much larger volume of normal tissues peripheral to the target volume. While this may be advantageous from a functional point of view, it is well documented that more modest doses of radiation therapy to normal tissues are associated with a paradoxically higher rate of mutagenesis and oncogenesis (7).

It is true that we see a relatively low risk of secondary cancers in most patients treated with radiotherapy. However, this has resulted from two different factors: (1) higher doses of radiation actually eliminate cells that are otherwise destined to manifest oncogenic mutations, and (2) there is still a major death rate during the years of latency within our patient population, usually due to progressive tumor outside our fields, but nonetheless effectively decreasing the number of patients at risk for long-term observation. There is a need to be sensitive to any detectable increase in tumor induction that appears to result from exposing an increased volume of normal tissues to modest radiation doses.

IMPROVED IMAGING

It is obvious that improved imaging is critical to any effort in radiation therapy because optimal radiation therapy is so dependent upon accurate targeting. In today's world, we are able to aim beams with astonishing precision. The variance and range of reproducibility are quite remarkable. On the other hand, there are major limitations in our ability to aim at a clinical target accurately. Most extracranial structures, including tumors, are moving frequently due to normal physiological function. The larynx moves when one swallows. We know today that even prostates move, and so do any tumors that are contained therein. Clearly, a mass in the lung will move vertically with respiration, while one close to the heart may be affected more horizontally by cardiac contraction. The degree of movement may vary, but generally these movements exceed the limits of reproducibility with which we can deliver our beams.

While the lung is an enticing area for intensity-modulated radiation therapy (IMRT), inverse treatment planning to a target that moves (as much as the lungs do) should send up a red flag to therapeutic enthusiasts. The process of IMRT with inverse treatment planning integrates information from a large number of beams, treating in effect pixel by pixel. The plans that look so impressive on paper are only a snapshot in time. Motion will throw those calculations off significantly. Fractionation will compensate to some degree, but the thorax and upper abdomen are not ideal targets for IMRT at present, owing to the significant impact of movement. While it is certainly possible to link actual beam-on time to some of these physiological motions, such as respiration or cardiac contraction, the gating system would have to be truly excellent to negate this dosimetric issue. Even if successful, that is nothing more than another refinement to what is already done on a daily basis. There are still instances in which patients will have unanticipated movements. Patients cough, sneeze, scratch, or do something else to make the target move with respect to the prior centering of the beam. These events can and do occur despite the best efforts at immobilization. If the movements are observed, the treatment can be interrupted. Surely there are mechanical devices that can be developed for this purpose that will prove to be faster and more sensitive than the human eye. Nonetheless, it is essential that radiation oncologists not lose sight of the obvious fact that the world of virtual reality is not reality.

Radiation treatments are planned with great care. When a patient is simulated, it is assumed that everything will be carried out exactly as planned. Isodose distributions and dose–volume histograms are reviewed with inherent assumptions about the superimposition of the isodose curves over the treatment volumes with respect to the localization of the tumor *on paper*. The reality is that sometimes patients move, that sometimes fields are not centered optimally, that sometimes patients are slightly rotated, that sometimes a variety of physiological and spontaneous motions introduce artifacts into the treatment plan.

These are obvious physiological limitations on the process of carrying out radiation therapy, and they represent a critical portion of reality that must not be overlooked. Nonetheless, the most overwhelming aspect of our reality check is simply that we do not know the exact extent of a cancer's infiltration. Cancer is an infiltrating biological process. While we may see a mass with radiological imaging, its true extent often exceeds the resolving power of our imaging technologies. Clearly, we cannot see the neoplastic microscopic extensions that come off that mass and infiltrate or spread into adjacent tissues or nodal regions. It should be acknowledged that microscopic residual disease is the key reason for which radiation oncologists recommend radiation therapy postresection, after the surgeon has "got it all." It is for that reason that we typically treat elective nodal regions (e.g., mediastinum) in lung cancer. However, 3-D conformal dose-escalation trials for NSCLC focus the beams on the gross tumor volume (GTV) only and exclude elective nodal regions. This "strategy" is applied purely out of necessity, as it is impossible to safely escalate doses to the prior traditionally larger treatment volumes. The impact of this strategy has not yet been well studied. This leap of faith is of particular concern in lung cancer, where the risk of microscopic disease (outside of the GTV) is known to be high. The "advantage" of 3-D radiotherapy, improved conformality of treatment, may ultimately be its greatest disadvantage, in that microscopic disease outside of the GTV will not be adequately treated.

The ability to determine the accurate target volumes based on CT or MRI is modest at best. In lung cancer, there are studies that compare the extent of disease utilizing these imaging techniques to the extent of involvement defined by the gold standard of surgical resection with microscopic evaluation. The specificity ranged only from 50% to 60% and the sensitivity was low (8–10). More recently, PET scanning has been suggested as a "better" tool for staging accurately (11), but this has yet to be confirmed. It follows logically that we have to be concerned that, for every patient who may benefit to some unknown degree from an increase in dose, there is another whose survival may be compromised by decreasing the target volume. This leads to a prediction that radiation oncologists may ultimately resort to excessive pride in figures of local control rather than the crucial endpoint of survival. Indeed, we must be concerned with progressively smaller margins around the target volume. Reducing the margin around the tumor volume in this fashion means that there is a genuine uncertainty introduced regarding the issue of what is the true dose at the periphery of the target, even if we neglect the major issue of movement.

RADIATION TOLERANCE

The concept of "radiation tolerance" is based on a probability of injury over time. It is not unusual among patients who have been cured to discover significant injury at 10 years that was not recognized at 5 years, and morbidities at 15 years that were not appreciated at 10 years. This recognition process is further complicated today by an analytical process utilizing actuarial projection. Looking at populations of patients plotted on an actuarial curve has become standard, with publications resulting as soon as the magic 5-year mark has been reached, and sometimes earlier. Assuming a relatively constant accrual of patients, that would imply that the median period of follow-up is not 5 years, but roughly about 2.5 years. This is simply not long enough to conclude that the limits of normal tissue tolerance have been identified. To reach that conclusion, one has to have a minimum period of follow-up of 5 years for *all* patients, and preferably longer. Radiation is not metabolized; once radiation has been administered, it cannot be removed. A study to redefine tissue tolerance is not a 5-year commitment; it is a commitment of 20 years to accumulate the numbers needed and adequate follow-up on them.

The enthusiasm for going to higher doses is ultimately based upon a dose-response curve. The critical question is: How steep is that radiation dose-response curve? Most of the clinical information is based on retrospective data, typically without regard to tumor size, fractionation, and a variety of other variables. Thus, the clinical data are actually subject to a variety of interpretations. Likewise, cell survival curves represent in vitro assessments, but do not necessarily take into account a variety of factors that are known to be important clinically. It is obvious that size of the tumor mass is an important factor. Histological subtype also seems to be important in dose response. Unequivocally, the concentration of oxygen, as well as a variety of other nutrients, is important in the expression of a dose-response curve in tissue culture. Cell kinetic factors appear to be involved as part of the process of redistribution. It is hard to conceive that DNA repair systems are not somehow involved. Many papers have analyzed molecular markers to correlate them to response as well. There must be a variety of other unknown factors that have yet to be recognized, but will ultimately be established to be important. These various factors may be able to account for the enormous heterogeneity that exists among patients and their varied response to treatment. If each of these elements could be factored out of the dose-response curve, then the remainder of what we call "cellular radiosensitivity" that persists after the removal of these factors would leave a curve representing the true impact of radiation dose alone, which would likely be considerably flatter than our usual preconception.

It is critical that radiation therapy acknowledge the importance of physics and technology as we enter the twenty-first century. On the other hand, it is clear that the major gains in the next century will not be obtained by fine-tuning dosimetry. The major gains to be achieved will be obtained through biological investigation and biological developments. How higher doses of radiation can help if the tumor cells are capable of repairing radiation-induced damage remains unclear. It would seem more logical that we have to learn how to manipulate the behavior and response of both malignant and normal cells.

CANCER A BIOLOGICAL PROBLEM

We must not lose sight of the fact that cancer is a biological problem. Future gains will be achieved through biological breakthroughs, such as radioactive antibodies or gene therapy, or some other development, such as radiosensitizers or radioprotectors. It is worth noting that if we had an effective radiosensitizer with a modest sensitizing enhancement ratio of 1.4, it would have more impact on our local tumor control figures than all the high-tech solutions that are presently ongoing. Even so, that would only help us in the issue of local control; the biggest gains in the future are to be made by dealing with cells that we cannot identify at present, typically out of the field of irradiation.

It should also be emphasized that a biological solution in any of these areas would ultimately result in a reduction in cost for both patients and institutions. It is absolutely astonishing to recognize how much spatial, economic, and manpower resources have become consumed by today's high-tech dosimetric solutions. In many departments of radiation oncology, biology receives only lip service today. That cannot be true if we are to survive and grow as a field in the twenty-first century.

Three-dimensional treatment planning and conformal radiation therapy, with or without intensity modulation, are here to stay. This work should continue, but it needs to be tested to determine what we have achieved. We should not simply assume that these technologies are making outcomes better because the treatment plan looks better on paper or a higher tumor dose is achieved. These gains need to be tested prospectively. Although some have said verbally that randomizing patients to 3-D would be immoral, I strongly disagree; "more" should not be assumed to be "better." It is hard to assess these putative gains by retrospective comparisons as there has been a remarkable stage migration resulting from improved screening and diagnostic maneuvers.

It is true that the megavoltage techniques were not prospectively randomized compared to orthovoltage. The reason is that there were no comparable treatment schema that could be developed at the target level owing to the remarkable difference in depth dose characteristics and in skin tolerance with those two modalities. It is fair to ask why such studies should be carried out today. The answer is that the gains are unclear in quantitative terms, the new technologies are quite expensive, and reimbursement schemes today are determined by third-party and federal bureaucrats, unlike the 1960s. As these high-tech solutions are expensive, they remain a major issue simply in terms of who will pay for them. If we cannot show an unequivocal gain with convincing evidence that these technologies result in better survival, then we can realistically expect that our hospital administrators will harbor a backlash if we ask them to spend money on future purchases. Today's economic marketplace has become, in a word, "Darwinian."

Finally, there is also a global problem evolving within radiation oncology in that the field is unknowingly painting itself into a corner. We are being perceived more and more as super technicians and less and less as physicians. It is essential that we be vigilant that our enthusiasm for high-tech is focused and balanced toward the solution of medical problems, and not simply high-tech for its own sake.

REFERENCES

1. Lung Cancer Study Group. Effects of postoperative mediastinal radiation on completely resected stage I and stage II epidermoid cancer of the lung. N Engl J Med 1986; 315:1377–1381.
2. Schaake-Koning C, Van Den Bogaert W, Dalesio O, et al. Effects of concomitant cisplatin and radiotherapy on inoperable non–small cell lung cancer. N Engl J Med 1992; 326:524–530.

3. Overgaard M, Hansen PS, Overgaard J, et al. Postoperative radiotherapy in high risk premenopausal women to receive adjuvant chemotherapy. N Engl J Med 1997; 337:949–955.
4. Robertson JM, Ten Haken RK, Hazuka MB, et al. Dose escalation for non–small cell lung cancer using conformal radiation therapy. Int J Radiat Oncol Biol Phys 1997; 37:1079.
5. Smith ME, McPeak EM, Donaldson SS. The advantages of three-dimensional conformal radiotherapy for the treatment of childhood cancer. Radiat Res 1998; 150: S170–S177.
6. Loeffler JS, Kooy HM, Tarbell NJ. The emergence of conformal radiotherapy: special implications for pediatric neuro-oncology. Int J Radiat Oncol Biol Phys 1999; 44:237–238.
7. Upton AC. The dose response relation in radiation induced cancer. Cancer Res 1961; 21:717–729.
8. McCloud TC, Bourgouin PM, et al. Bronchogenic carcinoma: analysis of staging in the mediastinum with CT by correlative lymph node mapping and sampling. Radiology 1992; 182:319–323.
9. McKenna RJ Jr, Libshitz HI, et al. Roentgenographic evaluation of mediastinal nodes for preoperative assessment in lung cancer. Chest 1985; 88:206–210.
10. Webb WR, Gatsonis C, et al. CT and MR imaging in staging non–small cell bronchogenic carcinoma: report of the radiologic diagnostic oncology group. Radiology 1991; 178:705–713.
11. Vansteenkiste JF, Stroobants SG, et al. Mediastinal lymph node staging with FDG-PET scan in patients with potentially operable non–small cell lung cancer: a prospective analysis of 50 cases. Chest 1997; 112:1480–1486.

19

Evolving Role of Chemotherapy in Stage IV NSCLC

Desmond N. Carney

Mater Hospital and University College Dublin, Dublin, Ireland

INTRODUCTION

Non–small cell lung cancer (NSCLC), including adenocarcinoma, squamous cell carcinoma, and large cell carcinoma, accounts for 75% of all newly diagnosed cases of lung cancer (1). At the time of diagnosis, approximately 70% of patients will have either locally advanced inoperable disease or distant metastatic disease. In the United States it is estimated that 127,500 patients developed NSCLC in 1997. Of these, only 38,250 (30%) were candidates for a curative resection. Another 30% of patients had locally advanced disease and the remaining 51,000 patients (40%) had confirmed metastases at diagnosis.

If 50% of patients who undergo a curative resection relapse within 5 years, as currently occurs, then of the 127,000 newly diagnosed patients with NSCLC in a given year in the United States, 108,375 (or 85%) of all cases of NSCLC are potential candidates for systemic chemotherapy.

For many, the question continues to be asked: Is chemotherapy worthwhile in advanced NSCLC, in particular for recurrent or stage IV metastatic disease?

Patients with inoperable NSCLC consist of two major subsets whose treatment approaches are different. For those fit patients with locally advanced inoper-

309

able NSCLC, combined-modality therapy of chemotherapy and radiation therapy is now considered the appropriate standard of care. Among such patients, combined-modality therapy can yield a median survival of 14–18 months with a 5-year survival approaching 10% (2).

While combined-modality therapy should be considered for suitable patients with locally advanced lung cancer, numerous studies are still required to consider the best chemotherapy regimen to be combined with radiation therapy. Moreover, studies are needed to define the optimal radiation dose, volume, and fractionation schedule for radiation therapy; and the proper integration of radiation therapy with chemotherapy (concurrent vs. sequential vs. both) for potentially curative treatment needs to be defined. In addition, the best means of integrating the newer therapeutic agents active in NSCLC with radiation still needs detailed studies.

The outcome for patients with stage IV metastatic NSCLC, while improving, remains pessimistic. The median survival time without chemotherapy is 4–6 months; it improves to 6–12 months in randomized trials using both older and newer chemotherapeutic regimens. However, cures are almost never achieved. For such patients best supportive care, palliative radiation therapy, and chemotherapy, alone or in combination, are the most commonly used treatments.

Until recent years, for many the question repeatedly raised was whether chemotherapy was indicated or clinically worthwhile in stage IV metastatic disease.

In this chapter the issues of chemotherapy and metastatic NSCLC will be addressed with specific reference to its effectiveness in inducing a remission, its impact on quality of life, and its impact on survival in treated patients.

CHEMOTHERAPY FOR ADVANCED NSCLC

Until approximately 5 years ago, most of the data on the use of chemotherapy in stage IV NSCLC patients was based on the analysis of multiple clinical trials containing numerous two- and three-drug combinations of older active agents in NSCLC, specifically cisplatin, carboplatin, vinca alkyloids, etoposide, etc. (3,4) (Table 1). The analysis of individual trials, some positive, some negative, led to major controversy regarding the proper role, if any, of chemotherapy in stage IV metastatic disease. In 1995, a meta-analysis of 52 randomized trials of almost 10,000 patients showed that compared to palliative radiation or best supportive care, the results for cisplatin-containing chemotherapy regimens favored chemotherapy in all comparisons and reached conventional levels of significance when used with radiation and best supportive care compared to either modality alone (5). Of note, an analysis of studies using long-term alkylating agents tended to show a negative impact of chemotherapy. This study changed the views of many and indicated that chemotherapy, particularly when it incorporated cisplatin, had

TABLE 1 Active Single
Agents in Non–Small Cell
Lung Cancer

Cisplatin
Carboplatin
Docetaxel
Etoposide
Gemcitabine
Irinotecan
Ifosfamide
Mitomycin C
Paclitaxel
Vindesine
Vinorelbine
Vinblastine

a role in the treatment of advanced-stage NSCLC. In addition, at that time, many studies of chemotherapy in advanced NSCLC clearly demonstrated that despite objective response rates of only 20–30%, many more patients (60–70%) demonstrated a significant improvement in disabling symptoms including cough, pain, hemoptysis, dyspnea, etc. (6).

These and other studies and the development of many new agents with significant activity in the treatment of NSCLC have led to a new optimism and an explosion in clinical trials in the treatment of inoperable NSCLC including patients with stage IV metastatic disease.

PROGNOSTIC VARIABLES IN ADVANCED-STAGE NSCLC

As in all cancers, several important prognostic factors dictate treatment decisions:

1. The likelihood of an individual person to benefit from systemic chemotherapy
2. The likelihood of an individual person to tolerate chemotherapy without a deterioration in quality of life or survival due to its toxicity and side effects

Numerous studies have addressed the issue of prognostic factors in advanced-stage inoperable NSCLC patients who participated in clinical trials. In considering the outcome of these studies, it is important to remember that the stage IV patients included in these trials were themselves a highly select group of patients, in that they met the strict eligibility criteria for entrance into these trials. Thus, many patients with stage IV NSCLC were not included in these trials (and thus not subject to analysis) for a variety of reasons, including advanced age, poor performance status, significant comorbid medical illnesses, the presence of brain metastases, etc., or treatment-limiting abnormalities of hepatic or renal function.

The majority of studies have clearly indicated that patients with an ECOG performance status of 0 or 1 were more likely to tolerate chemotherapy better or have a more prolonged survival than those with performance status of 2 or worse (4). Other prognostic variables identified included weight loss, anorexia, laboratory data including initial hemoglobin level, albumin level, and lactate dehydrogenase. Such prognostic variables are common to many cancers. The impact of such prognostic variables has been clearly demonstrated in several recent studies of a more detailed analysis of prognostic variables in large cohorts of patients with advanced NSCLC who received chemotherapy. In the study of Paesmans et al., the prognostic factors for survival were reported on all eligible patients ($n = 1052$) with advanced NSCLC registered onto one of seven trials conducted by EORTC over a decade (7). The median survival of all patients was 29 weeks, and with a median follow-up duration of 10 years, the actuarial 5-year survival rate was 1.5%. In this study, factors predictive of short survival included poor performance status, disseminated disease, an elevated neutrophil count at diagnosis, age greater than 60, weight loss, and the presence of bone, skin, or hepatic metastases. Albain et al. analyzed 2531 patients entered into the SWOG extensive NSCLC database from 1974 to 1988 (8). In this study, the authors identified similar prognostic variables associated with a favorable outcome including good performance status (ECOG 0-1), single metastatic sites, normal LDH, normal alkaline phosphatase, a baseline hemoglobin level greater than 11.0 g/dl, and minimal weight loss.

The importance of these two major assessments of prognostic variables for outcome in advanced NSCLC is that subgroups of patients could be identified who are likely to respond and benefit from chemotherapy. Conversely, and of equal importance, it was possible to identify patients not likely to respond to chemotherapy either in the classic manner (complete response/partial response) or by improvement in quality of life.

In the study of Paesmans et al. (Table 2), using variables such as gender, disease extent, performance status, weight loss, and initial white cell count, four sets of patients could be identified with median survival times ranging from 14 to 60+ weeks, 1-year survival ranging from 10 to 53%, and 2-year survival ranging from 2 to 27%. In a similar manner, in the retrospective analysis of Albain et al., the authors also identified a subset of patients with variable prognosis. Based on performance status, hemoglobin level, age, and LDH level, patients could be subdivided into three groups with the median survival ranging from 3.0

TABLE 2 Prognostic Factors
for Survival in Advanced-Stage
Non–Small Cell Lung Cancer

Group	MST (weeks)	1-year survival (%)
I	60	53
II	38	38
III	26	21
IV	14	10

Source: Paesmans et al. (7). See text
for details.

to 7.6 months, 1-year survival ranging from 6 to 27%, and 2-year survival ranging from 1 to 8% (Table 3).

Jiroutek evaluated data from 1960 patients with advanced NSCLC treated with cisplatin-based chemotherapy over five consecutive ECOG trials from 1981 to 1992 to define prognostic factors affecting survival (9). In this analysis, the median age of patients was 60.7 years (19–82 years); 86% of patients had an ECOG performance status of 0–1. The overall median survival was 6.5 months for all patients. Factors associated with a significantly poor outcome included performance status greater than 1, presence of metastatic symptoms, male gender, a reduced appetite, and the presence of bone and liver metastases. (See Table 4.)

While many of the studies of prognostic variables report on the impact of individual factors and survival, only one recent report evaluated the importance

TABLE 3 Outcome of Different Prognostic Groups
($n = 904$)

Group	No. of patients	Median survival (mo)	1-year survival (%)
1. PS 0–1 HB ≥ 11.0 Age ≥ 47 years	410	7.6	27
2. Others	277	5.1	16
3. PS 2–4 LDH ≥ normal	217	3.0	6

Source: Adapted from Albain et al. (8).

TABLE 4   Precursive Partitioning Analysis

	MS (mo) Appetite	
	Intact (n)	Decreased (n)
PS 0		
Female	12.58 (111)	8.54 (15)
Male	9.86 (219)	6.74 (50)
PS 1		
Female	7.77 (214)	6.95 (102)
Male	6.70 (421)	5.00 (224)
PS 2		
Female	5.31 (24)	2.30 (27)
Male	4.30 (64)	3.43 (100)

of performance status in patients with advanced NSCLC undergoing treatment with combination chemotherapy with "newer agents."

In the preliminary report of ECOG study E1594 by Johnson et al. a randomized trial of four different combination-chemotherapy regimens in patients with confirmed stage IIIB/IV NSCLC, the unexplained toxicity observed in patients with performance status 2 led to the cessation of accrual of these patients into the trial (10). Although the number of patients with performance status 2 was small ($n = 64$), the low response rates (6–17%) and median survival (1.9–7.9 months) observed did not justify the excess toxicity.

Studies of prognostic variables in patients with advanced-stage NSCLC undergoing chemotherapy clearly demonstrate the importance of including such information as stratification variables in clinical trials in this disease. Failure to do so may lead to unintended treatment imbalances and, consequently, a misinterpretation of the outcome of trials either in favor of a specific treatment strategy or, conversely, against a specific treatment. It is clear that outside of defined clinical trials, the use of these prognostic variables may enable us to select patients for whom chemotherapy is an appropriate option or identify patients for whom chemotherapy would not likely to be a major benefit and indeed may give rise to unacceptable toxicity.

"NEW" AGENTS IN ADVANCED NSCLC

Since the mid-1990s the availability of a substantial number of chemotherapeutic drugs demonstrating reasonable activity both as single agents and in combination regimens has increased the optimism and enthusiasm for the treatment of advanced-stage inoperable NSCLC (11). These agents include paclitaxel, docetaxel, navelbine (Vinorelbine), gemcitabine, and irinotecan. As single agents, each has shown activity in the phase II trials in previously untreated patients with NSCLC and, in some cases, has also exhibited activity in patients who have failed prior chemotherapy. Now, with the development of these new agents with demonstrated response rates of 20–25% (rates observed in the past mainly with cisplatin-based combination chemotherapy), NSCLC is no longer considered a drug-resistant tumor, but rather a cancer that is modestly sensitive to chemotherapy.

We will briefly overview the reported activity of these new compounds both as single agents and in combination trials of two or more cytotoxic compounds.

Gemcitabine

Gemcitabine (difluorordeoxycytidine), an analog of deoxycytidine, is a pyrimdine antimetabolite (12). It is active in a variety of murine solid tumors and leukemias, in addition to human xenografts. Gemcitabine has been studied as a single agent in more than 500 previously untreated patients with advanced-stage NSCLC, including a substantial number of patients with stage IV disease. As a single agent gemcitabine yields a response rate of 20% with a median survival time of approximately 9 months. In one randomized study of 299 symptomatic patients with advanced or metastatic NSCLC, gemcitabine was compared to best supportive care (13). The overall response rate for gemcitabine was 17%. No difference in median survival (24.4 weeks vs. 25.5 weeks) was observed. However, control of symptoms and improvement in patients assessed on symptom scale favored the gemcitabine arm.

The combination of gemcitabine and cisplatin has been evaluated in at least seven studies involving more than 300 patients (12). In these studies cisplatin was administered as a single dose on either day 1, 2, or 15 (five studies) or weekly times three (two studies). The overall response rates ranged from 28 to 54% with a median survival time ranging from 8.4 to 15.4 months. The difference in survival time observed between trials could be explained by the small number of patients in each study (usually less than 50) and the varying entry criteria and prognostic variables, particularly stage and performance status of these patients in each trial.

Two studies have compared gemcitabine as a single agent to the combination cisplatin/etoposide (14,15). In one study of 50 patients there were no differences in response rates (19% for gemcitabine vs. 21% for the combination), time to progression (8.8 vs. 8.5 months), or median survival (37 weeks vs. 48 weeks).

Manegold et al. compared gemcitabine to etoposide/cisplatin in 130 patients. There were no obvious differences between the two arms' response rate, time to progression, and median survival. Both of these trials confirmed the activity of gemcitabine as a single agent; and in both studies hematological and nonhematological toxicity were substantially less for the gemcitabine treatment arms.

There have been several randomized studies of the combination of gemcitabine/cisplatin versus other regimens including cisplatin/etoposide, MIC (mitomycin/ifosfamide/cisplatin), and single-agent cisplatin (15–17). These randomized studies have involved large numbers of patients. In all three studies, there was a trend for a higher response rate for the gemcitabine/cisplatin combination with response rates observed for this combination ranging from 31 to 41%. The median survival for all gemcitabine/cisplatin arms in these three studies was consistent at 8.7, 8.6, and 9.1 months, respectively. In the trial comparing gemcitabine/cisplatin to single-agent cisplatin, a significant survival advantage was noted for the combination. In the other two combination trials, survival rates were not statistically different.

More recently, several phase II trials of double and triplet combination of gemcitabine with other agents active in NSCLC (carboplatin, taxenes, Vinorelbine, etc.) have been reported (12,18–20). But the number of patients in these studies is relatively small, and it is too soon to say whether any of these combinations will prove superior to gemcitabine/cisplatin or indeed single-agent therapy alone when survival is used as the main endpoint of the treatment.

Paclitaxel

Paclitaxel is a novel cytotoxic agent that exerts its antitumor activity by inducing excessive polymerization of tubulin, thereby interfering with normal mitotic function. In numerous phase II studies of patients with advanced NSCLC, paclitaxel has shown reproducible response rates of 20% or more (21–24). Earlier studies utilized paclitaxel as a 24-hr infusion; more recent studies have used shorter infusion times (3 or 1 hr), demonstrated similar activity, and clearly offered an economic advantage by avoiding hospitalization necessitated by the more prolonged infusion. In addition, myelosuppression was less pronounced. Although a clear dose-response relationship has not been demonstrated, it appears that the best response rates were observed at doses of 200–225 mg/m^2 with 3-hr infusion schedule.

The activity of paclitaxel in NSCLC has been confirmed by a phase III study comparing paclitaxel at 200mg/m^2 over 3 hr every 3 weeks to best supportive care. The survival advantage of the single-agent paclitaxel treatment (6.8 months vs. 4.8 months) was significantly in favor of paclitaxel (22).

Numerous studies have been made of paclitaxel in combination with other agents, in particular carboplatin and cisplatin (21,25–30). Phase II studies of paclitaxel/cisplatin cited response rates ranging from 35 to 47%. Dose-limiting toxicity for this combination was peripheral neuropathy and appeared both dose-related and cumulative. The combination of paclitaxel/carboplatin has also been evaluated in numerous phase II trials. Because little response difference was observed between 24-hr infusion and the shorter 3-hr infusion, most studies now utilize the 3-hr infusion. With the shorter, more convenient infusion time, less myelosuppresion is observed while there also appears to be a myeloprotective effect of paclitaxel on carboplatin-associated thrombocytopenia with the combination of paclitaxel and carboplatin. In numerous studies, response rates ranging from 12 to 63% have been observed with 1-year survivals ranging from 32 to 55%.

Several recent phase III studies have compared paclitaxel alone or in combination with cisplatin to other active regimens in NSCLC. The phase III comparative study of high-dose cisplatin versus cisplatin/paclitaxel reported by Gatzemeier et al. involved more than 400 patients with advanced NSCLC (28). While the overall response rates favored the paclitaxel arm (26% vs. 17%), there were no significant differences in median survival (35 vs. 37 weeks) or 1-year survival (35 vs. 32 weeks). An ECOG study compared the standard combination cisplatin/etoposide to two different cisplatin/paclitaxel (24-hr) iterations, one giving the higher dose (250 mg/m^2) with G-CSF support, the other using a lower dose (135 mg/m^2) without G-CSF (26). While higher response rates were observed in the paclitaxel arms, there were no significant differences in response rates or survival between the low (135 mg/m^2) and high (250 mg/m^2) paclitaxel arms. The cisplatin/paclitaxel arms were associated with a significantly higher response rate (32% vs. 12%) and a superior median survival compared to cisplatin/etoposide. The EORTC study compared paclitaxel/cisplatin to a combination of teniposide and cisplatin. While the paclitaxel arm yielded a superior response rate, there was no survival advantage for either arm of the study. However, hematological toxicity was greater in the cisplatin/teniposide arm (29).

In the study of Belani et al. (27) comparing cisplatin/etoposide to paclitaxel (225 mg/m^2/3 hr) and carboplatin (AUC 6), the response rate again favored the paclitaxel arm (23% vs. 15%). However, the median and 1-year survival rates were marginally lower in the paclitaxel arm.

In a randomized study of paclitaxel with either carboplatin or cisplatin no significant differences were observed between either arm of the study. For many in North America, the combination of carboplatin/paclitaxel has evolved into a standard regimen for the treatment of advanced-stage NSCLC (30).

It is clear that paclitaxel is one of the more active agents in NSCLC. In many studies, however, the increased response rates observed with this agent, either alone or in combination, does not always translate into improved median or 1-year survival. Like many of the newer agents, the best way to use this drug (i.e., dose, schedule) and the optimal combination with other agents remain to be determined.

Docetaxel

Docetaxel (31–41) is a semisynthetic taxane with a similar mechanism of action and range of antitumor activity as paclitaxel. In phase II trials of more than 150 patients the overall response rate observed was 27% (24–39%) with a median response duration of 2 months (31–35). In these studies the median survival for all patients enrolled was 9.2 months, and 1- and 2-year survival rates were 39% and 20%, respectively. In these studies the majority of patients had an excellent performance status (ECOG 0–1 83%) and the predominant cell type was adeno-carcinoma.

In several phase II studies of patients previously platinum-exposed, the overall response rate ranged from 16 to 22% with a median survival ranging from 7 to 11 months among almost 170 patients (39). Two separate phase III studies, one comparing docetaxel at either 75 mg/m^2 or 100 mg/m^2 to vinorelbine or ifosfamide, the other comparing the same two doses to BSC, have demonstrated a survival benefit for salvage treatment with docetaxel (39a, 39b).

In many of these phase II studies, doses of either 60, 75, or 100 mg/m^2 of docetaxel were evaluated, but no clear dose-response effect emerged. The major toxicity remains hematological. The use of corticosteroids has led to a reduction in the frequency of fluid retention and skin rashes.

Recent studies have reported the efficacy of combining docetaxel and cis-platin in advanced-stage NSCLC (36–38). In studies of more than 100 patients, a response rate of 38% with a median survival of 10 months was observed, results not too dissimilar from those with single-agent docetaxel, questioning to what extent cisplatin contributes to the responses observed. Many other ongoing studies are evaluating docetaxel with the other agents known to be active in NSCLC (40,41). The proven efficacy of this agent as a single compound in both untreated and previously treated patients with advanced disease encourages its continued evaluation in NSCLC. One ongoing phase III trial compares cisplatin/docetaxel and carboplatin/docetaxel to Vinorelbine/cisplatin; another gives a fixed dose of carboplatin (AUC 6) and randomizes patients to either docetaxel (75 mg/m^2) or paclitaxel (225 m/gm^2).

Navelbine (Vinorelbine)

Vinorelbine (42–48) is a semisynthetic vinca alkaloid that has been extensively evaluated in NSCLC. Like other vinca alkaloids it inhibits microtubule assembly. In almost 13 studies of more than 1000 patients, the single-agent response rate overall is 14%, with a median response duration of 14–34 weeks, a median sur-vival of 27–40 weeks, and 1-year survival of approximately 25% (42). In the elderly ($\geq$70 years), single-agent Vinorelbine has proven superior to BSC in terms of both survival and quality of life (42a). In a large number of phase I/II studies Vinorelbine has been evaluated with other agents in NSCLC. In studies of Vinorelbine and cisplatin in almost 1500 patients, response rates of 26–52% have been observed with a median survival time ranging from 26 to 55 weeks (42,43). In three randomized trials, the combination Vinorelbine/cisplatin was compared to either single-agent cisplatin, single-agent Vinorelbine, or Vindesine/

cisplatin (44–47). Overall, the response rate of 30–45% was higher for the new-agent combination arm, with median and 1-year survival superior in the Vinorelbine combinations, confirming the efficacy of Vinorelbine in the management of NSCLC and its improved activity when combined with cisplatin. This combination has yielded acceptable toxicity in a disease where the main goal of treatment still remains symptom palliation and life prolongation.

INVESTIGATIONAL AGENTS (49–52)

Topoisomerase 1 Inhibitors

The campothecins are a family of natural products that exert their antitumor activity through inhibition of the enzyme topoisomerase 1. The two agents irinotecan and topotecan have both been evaluated in small numbers of patients with advanced NSCLC. In studies of greater than 150 patients, responses to irinotecan were observed in 32–41% of patients. The dose-limiting toxicity was major leukopenia and diarrhea. In one study of 72 patients the median survival for stage IV patients was 40 weeks (49,50). Combination weekly cisplatin and irinotecan has yielded a median survival of 47 weeks (50a). A phase III study of cisplatin/irinotecan versus cisplatin/Vindesine versus single-agent irinotecan has demonstrated an improved response rate for the new-agent combination, with a trend toward improved survial. Ongoing trials are evaluating the role of irinotecan with other agents in the treatment of this disease.

Topotecan has also been evaluated in a small number of patients. Responses ranging from 0 to 25% have been reported (51,52). In one trial of a small number of patients, a partial response rate of 36% was noted in five of 14 patients with squamous cell histology. The responses to topotecan may also be schedule dependent; higher response rates have been observed when this agent is given over 5 days.

TIRAPAZAMINE

Tirapazamine (53) is a new bioreductive anticancer agent with specific activity toward cells at low oxygen tension. Under hypoxic conditions, this agent is activated to a toxic free radical and produces a tumor-specific potentiation of cell kill by cisplatin. The drug is inactive until metabolized to a damaging radical, which only occurs at oxygen tensions lower than those within normal cells but well within the range found in solid tumors such as lung cancer, head and neck cancer, etc. In clinical trials with cisplatin and tirapazamine, both response rate and survival times of patients with advanced NSCLC were significantly increased when the combination of drugs was compared to cisplatin alone.

TREATMENT FOR ADVANCED STAGE IV
NSCLC: SUMMARY

We have reviewed the response rates observed with many chemotherapeutic regimens in the treatment of inoperable NSCLC. It is difficult to draw consistent conclusions, but the following can be stated with some conviction.

1.   In selected patients, chemotherapy and particularly cisplatin-based chemotherapy has proven superior to best supportive care in terms of survival and quality of life.

2.   There is no standard chemotherapy regimen or combination of drugs for advanced NSCLC. In an evaluation of numerous phase II and phase III trials of the ''newer agents,'' it is clear that no drug has demonstrated superior activity in terms of response rate, median survival, or overall survival, either as a single agent or in combination with cisplatin or carboplatin. Thus the selection of a particular regimen will be dictated by the ease of administration, the toxicity associated with the regimen, the presence or absence of comorbid medical conditions, and the cost of the agent. An example of this tenet is the recently completed SWOG trial of two of the ''newer agents'' combined with cisplatin and carboplatin (54). In over 400 patients, the combination of Vinorelbine/cisplatin (C/V) was compared to combination paclitaxel/carboplatin (T/C). Both arms yielded an identical response rate (27%), median survival (8 months), and 1-year survival (37%). While the median survival time of 8 months was inferior to that reported in numerous phase II/III trials, without question these results more accurately reflect what would happen in the general community, where selection procedures for treatment are likely less stringent. Of note, while the toxicity profile was different for each regimen with more nausea and vomiting for the C/V arm and fourfold increase in sensory neuropathy for T/C, a significant difference in cost existed, according to the investigators, between the regimens favoring the cisplatin/Vinorelbine arm of the study.

3.   There is a general agreement that the ''old standards,'' e.g., etoposide, ifosfamide, and mitomycin, have now been replaced and sidelined by combinations of the newer agents with cisplatin/carboplatin, etc. However, in the few randomized studies comparing old versus new, while higher response rates were frequently observed for the newer agents, this observation did not always translate into improved survival. (Tables 5 and 6).

SHOULD ALL PATIENTS WITH STAGE IV NSCLC
RECEIVE CHEMOTHERAPY?

The data presented above indicate that we have made modest advances in the treatment of NSCLC with systemic chemotherapy. While numerous phase II/III trials look highly promising in terms of response rates and 1-year survival com-

TABLE 5 Randomized Trial of "Newer" Chemotherapy Agents in Advanced Non–Small Cell Lung Cancer

	Patients	RR%	MS	1 yr
Cisplatin[a]	218	10%	6.0 mo	16%
Cisplatin/Vinorelbine[a]	214	25%	7.0 mo	35%
Cisplatin[b]	154	10%	32 wk	28%
Cisplatin/Gemcitabine[b]	155	32%	39 wk	39%
Cisplatin[c]	205	17%	37 wk	32%
Cisplatin/paclitaxel[c]	202	26%	35 wk	35%
Cisplatin[d]	219	14%	28 wk	21%
Cisplatin/tirapazamine[d]	218	28%	35 wk	33%

Source:
[a] Wozniak et al. (44).
[b] Sandler et al. (18).
[c] Gatzemeier et al. (28).
[d] Von Pawel et al. (53a).

TABLE 6 Randomized Trial of "Old" Versus "New" Combinations of Chemotherapy in Non–Small Cell Lung Cancer

	Patients	RR%	MS (mo)	1 yr %
Cisplatin/paclitaxel (135 mg/m^2)[a]	189	27	9.6	37
Cisplatin/paclitaxel (250 mg/m^2)[a]	191	32	10	39
Cisplatin/etoposide[a]	194	12	7.7	32
Cisplatin/paclitaxel[b]	155	44	9.4	41
Cisplatin/teniposide[b]	157	30	9.7	43
Cisplatin/etoposide[c]	179	15	39 wk	37
Carboplatin/paclitaxel[c]	190	23	33 wk	32
Cisplatin/gemcitabine[d]	155	38	37 wk	33
Cisplatin/mitomycin C/ifosfamide[d]	152	26	39 wk	34

Source:
[a] Bonomi et al. (26).
[b] Giaccone et al. (29).
[c] Belani et al. (27).
[d] Crino et al. (17).

pared to historical controls, these data have not always been confirmed by randomized comparative trials. Moreover, as we take these studies into multicenter randomized trials, with less stringent patient entry criteria, the median survivals expected (i.e., 10–12 months) consistently drop to 8–10 months, a marginal improvement over historical data.

It must be remembered that with current standards of treatment, patients with stage IV NSCLC have incurable disease. The primary goal of treatment is to palliate symptoms, improve quality of life, and, if possible, improve survival with acceptable treatment side effects. Responses can be observed by improvement in symptoms (60–70% of patients) and by clinically or radiologically detected means (20–30% of patients). Responses ideally should be of meaningful duration with acceptable toxicity. If we treat patients with advanced NSCLC with our current chemotherapy regimens, a modest gain of 2–4 months in survival is expected. While we as physicians might have certain criteria for determining "effective" chemotherapy, a recent report by Silvestri et al. based on interviews of patients with lung cancer attempted to determine how these patients would value the tradeoff between a survival benefit of 2–4 months with chemotherapy and its expected toxicities (55). The study involved 81 patients who had received cisplatin-based chemotherapy for inoperable NSCLC. As one might have expected, patients' willingness to accept chemotherapy for the treatment of this disease showed wide variation. Some patients would accept chemotherapy for survival advantage of 1 week, while others would not choose chemotherapy even for a survival benefit of more than 2 years. Many patients, however, would not choose chemotherapy for its likely survival benefit of 3 months alone, but would if quality of life were improved. It is clear from this study that patients should be fully informed as to the likely benefit of chemotherapy for metastatic NSCLC, including survival advantage and effects on quality of life. This openness might help clarify the situation when chemotherapy is being considered for patients with advanced-stage disease.

It is the author's view that the percentage of patients with metastatic NSCLC who should receive combination chemotherapy and who are likely to benefit probably represents only 25–33% of all patients with stage IV disease. Patients with significant comorbid medical conditions and those with a performance status worse than ECOG 1 appear not to tolerate the newer chemotherapy combinations and have a significant rate of toxicity with no significant quality-of-life benefit. It is also clear from a review of the numerous prognostic factors outlined that while patients with good performance status and single or limited sites of metastatic disease benefit from chemotherapy, the efficacy of chemotherapy in patients with large-volume metastatic disease or metastatic disease in multiple sites remains questionable. Clearly each patient needs to be considered based on his or her individual needs and expectations.

The impact of current chemotherapy regimens on survival in patients with metastatic NSCLC is small with a median survival advantage of 2–3 months but with no chance of cure. These figures have encouraged some of argue that chemotherapy should be offered to all patients with advanced disease, while others remain unconvinced. By using strict selection criteria based on prognostic factors, we can identify patients who are likely to benefit in a meaningful way from chemotherapy. In addition, we should be able to discuss openly with these patients the likely benefits and risk from chemotherapy so that they become part of the treatment and decision-making process.

REFERENCES

1. Ginsberg RJ, Kris MG, Armstrong JG. Cancer in the lung. In: DeVita VT, Hellman S, Rosenberg SA, eds. Cancer: Principles and Practice of Oncology, 4th ed. Philadelphia: JB Lippincott, 1993:673–723.
2. Ruchdeschel JD. Combined modality therapy for non-small cell lung cancer. Semin Oncol 1977; 24:429–439.
3. Ramanathan RK, Belani CP. Chemotherapy for advanced stage non-small cell lung cancer. Past present future. Semin Oncol 1977; 24:440–454.
4. Shepherd F, Carney DN. Treatment of non–small cell lung cancer—chemotherapy. In: Hansen HH, ed. IASLC Textbook of Lung Cancer. London: Martin Dunitz, 1999: 213–242.
5. Non–small Cell Lung Cancer Collaborative Group. Chemotherapy in non-small cell lung cancer: a meta-analysis using updated data on individual patients from 52 randomized clinical trials. Br Med J 1995; 311:899–909.
6. Ellis PA, Smith IE, Hardy JR, et al. Symptom relief with MVP (mitomycin C, vinblastine and cisplatin) chemotherapy in advanced non–small cell lung cancer. Br J Cancer 1995; 71:366–370.
7. Paesmans M, Sculier JP, Libert P, et al. Prognostic factors for survival in advanced non–small-cell lung cancer: univariate and multivariate analysis including recursive partitioning and amalgamation algorithms in 1,052 patients. J. Clin Oncol 1995; 13: 1221–1230.
8. Albain S, Crowley J, LeBlanc M, Livingston B. Survival determinants in extensive-stage non–small-cell lung cancer: the southwest oncology group experience. J Clin Oncol 1991; 9:1618–1626.
9. Liroutek M, Johnson D, Blum D, et al. Prognostic factors in advanced non–small-cell lung cancer: analysis of ECOG trials from 1981–1992. Proc. ASCO 1998; 17: 1774 (abstr).
10. Johnson DH, Zhu J, Schiller J, et al. E1594. A randomised phase III trial in metastatic non–small cell lung cancer. Outcome of PS 2 patients. Proc ASCO 1999; 18:1779 (abstr).
11. Carney DN. New agents in the management of advanced non–small cell lung cancer. Semin Oncol 1998; 25(4):83–88.
12. Sandler A, Ehinger DS. Gemcitabine; single agent and combination therapy in non–small cell lung cancer. Oncologist 1999; 4(3):241–252.
13. Anderson H, Cottier B, Nicolson M, et al. Phase III study of gemcitabine versus best supportive care in advanced non–small cell lung cancer. Lung Cancer 1997; 8(suppl 1):9a.

14. Perng RP, Chen YM, Ming-Liu, et al. Gemcitabine versus the combination of cisplatin and etoposide in patients with inoperable non–small cell lung cancer in a phase II randomised study. J Clin Oncol 1997; 15:2097–2102.
15. Manegold T, Bergman B, Chemaissani A, et al. Single-agent gemcitabine versus cisplatin-etoposide: early results of a randomised phase II study in locally advanced or metastatic non-small cell lung cancer. Ann Oncol 1997; 8:525–529.
16. Cardenal F, Lopez-Cabrerizo MP, Anton A, et al. Randomised phase III study of gemcitabine-cisplatin versus etoposide-cisplatin in the treatment of locally advanced or metastatic non-small cell lung cancer. J Clin Oncol 1999; 17:12–18.
17. Crino L, Conte P, De Marinis F, et al. A randomised trial of gemcitabine versus mitomycin, ifosfamide, and cisplatin in advanced non–small cell lung cancer. A multicenter phase II study. Proc Am Soc Clin Oncol 1998; 17:455a.
18. Sandler A, Nemunaitis J, Denham C, et al. Phase III study of cisplatin (C) with or without gemcitabine (G) in patients with advanced non–small cell lung cancer (NSCLC). Proc ASCO 1998; 17:454a (abstr 1747).
19. Iaffaioli RV, Tortoriello A, Facchini G, et al. Phase I–II study of gemcitabine and carboplatin in stage IIIB–IV non–small-cell lung cancer. J Clin Oncol 1999; 17:921–926.
20. Giaccone G, Smit E, Laan D, et al. Phase I/II study of paclitaxel and gemcitabine in advanced non-small cell lung cancer (NSCLC). Proc Am Soc Clin Oncol 1998; 17:486a.
21. Langer G, Ehinger DS. The burgeoning role of paclitaxel in advanced pulmonary malignancy. Oncologist 1998; (3)2:67–85.
22. Socinski MA. Single agent paclitaxel in the treatment of advanced non–Small Cell lung cancer. Oncologist 1999; 4(5):408–416.
23. Greco FA, Hainsworth JD. Paclitaxel-based therapy in non–small-cell lung cancer: improved third generation chemotherapy. Ann Oncol 1999; 10(5):563–567.
24. Rowinsky EK, Donehower RC. Paclitaxel (Taxol). N Engl J Med 1995; 332:1004–1014.
25. Bonomi P, Kim J, Kugler J, et al. Comparison of survival for stage IIIB versus stage IV non–small cell lung cancer (NSCLC) patients with etoposide-cisplatin versus taxol-cisplatin. An Eastern Cooperative Oncology Goup (ECOG) trial. Proc Am Soc Clin Oncol 1997; 16:454a.
26. Bonomi P, Kim K, Chang A, et al. Phase III trial comparing etoposide (E) cisplatin (C) versus Taxol (T) with cisplatin-G-CSF (G) versus Taxol-cisplatin in advanced non–small cell lung cancer. An Eastern Cooperative Oncology Group (ECOG) trial. Proc Am Soc Clin Oncol 1996; 15:382a.
27. Belani CP, Natale RB, Lee JS, et al. Randomised phase III trial comparing cisplatin/etoposide verus carboplatin/paclitaxel in advanced and metastatic non–small cell lung cancer (NSCLC). Proc Am Soc Clin Oncol 1998; 17:455a.
28. Gatzemeier U, Von Pawel J, Gottfried M, Tenveldegp M, Mattson K, DEMarinas F, Harper P, et al. Phase III comparative study of high-dose cisplatin (HD-Cis) versus a combination of paclitaxel (TAX) and cisplatin (CIS) in patients with advanced non–small cell lung cancer (NSCLC). Proc ASCO 1998; 17:454a (abstr 1748).
29. Giaccone G, Splinter T, Postmus P, et al. Paclitaxel-cisplatin versus teniposide cisplatin in advanced non–small cell lung cancer. Proc Am Soc Clin Oncol 1996; 15:373 (abstr 1109).

30. Macha HN, Gatzemeier U, Betticher DC, et al. Randomized multicenter trial comparing paclitaxel/carboplatin versus paclitaxel/cisplatin in advanced non–small cell lung cancer. Proc ASCO, 1998; 17 (abstr 1789), p 465a.

31. Ornstein DC, Rigas JR. Taxotere: clinical trials in non–small cell lung cancer. Oncologist 1998; 3:86–93.

32. Von Hoff DD. The taxoids: same roots, different drugs. Semin Oncol 1997; 24(suppl 13):10–13.

33. Francis P, Rigas JR, Kris MG, et al. Phase II trial of docetaxel in patients with stage III and IV non–small cell lung cancer. J Clin Oncol 1994; 12:1232–1237.

34. Fossella FV, Lee JS, Murphy WK, et al. Phase II study of docetaxel for recurrent or metastatic non–small cell lung cancer. J Clin Oncol 1994; 12:1238–1244.

35. Cerny T, Kaplan S, Pavlidis N, et al. Docetaxel (Taxotere) is active in non small cell lung cancer: a phase II trial of the EORTC Early Clinical Trials Group (ECTG). Br J Cancer 1994; 70:384–387.

36. Mattson K, Saarinen A, Jekunen A. Combination treatment with docetaxel (Taxotere) and platinum compounds for non–small cell lung cancer. Semin Oncol 1997; 24(suppl 14):5–8.

37. Millward MJ, Zalcbery J, Bishop JF, et al. Phase I trial of docetaxel and cisplatin in previously untreated patients with advanced solid tumours. J Clin Oncol 1997; 15:1071–1079.

38. Pronk LC, Schellens JHM, Planting AST, et al. Phase I and pharmacolgic study of docetaxel and cisplatin in patients with advanced solid tumours. J Clin Oncol 1997; 15:1071–1079.

39. Gandara DR, Vokes E, Green M, et al. Multicenter trial of docetaxel (Taxotere) in platinum-treated non–small cell lung cancer (NSCLC): confirmation of prolonged survival. Lung Cancer 1997; 18:21a.

39a. Fossella F, DeVore R, Kerr R, et al. Phase III trial of docetaxel 100 mg/m^2 or 75 mg/m^2 vs. vinorelbine/ifosfamide for non–small cell lung cancer (NSCLC) previously treated with platinum-based chemotherapy. Proc Am Soc Clin Oncol 1999; 18:460a (abstr 1776).

39b. Shepherd F, Ramlau R, Mattson K, et al. Randomized study of taxotere versus best supportive care in non–small cell lung cancer patients previously treated with platinum-containing chemotherapy. Proc Am Soc Clin Oncol 1999; 18:463a (abstr 1784).

40. Georgoulias V, Kourousis C, Androulakis N, et al. Docetaxel (Taxotere) and gemcitabine in the treatment of non-small cell lung cancer: preliminary results. Semin Oncol 1997; 24(suppl 14):22–25.

41. Georgoulias V, Kourousis C, Androulakis N, et al. Docetaxel (Taxotere) and vinorelbine in the treatment of non–small cell lung cancer. Semin Oncol 1997; 24(suppl 14):9–14.

42. Gralla R, Harper P, Johnson S, Delgado FM. Vinorelbine (Navelbine) in the treatment of non–small cell lung cancer: studies with single agent therapy and in combination with cisplatin. Ann Oncol 1999; 10(5):541–545.

42a. Elderly Lung Cancer Vinorelbine Italian Study Group. Effects of vinorelbine on quality of life and survival of elderly patients with advanced non–small cell lung cancer. J Natl Cancer Inst 1999; 91:2774.

43. Gralla R, Harper P, Johnson S, Delgado FM. Vinorelbine (Nabvelbine) in the treatment of non–small cell lung cancer: recent developments in combination chemotherapy and radiotherapy. Ann Oncol 1999; 10(5):547–551.

44. Wozniak AJ, Crowley JJ, Balcerzak GR, et al. Randomized phase III trial of cisplatin (CDDP) vs. CDDP plus navelbine in treatment of advanced non–small cell lung cancer (NSCLC): report of a Southwest Oncology Group study (SWOG-9308). Proc Am Soc Clin Oncol 1996; 15:374 (abstr 1110).

45. Depierre A, Chestang C, Quoix E, et al. Vinorelbine versus vinorelbine plus cisplatin in advanced non-small cell lung cancer: a randomized trial. Ann Oncol 1994; 5:37–42.

46. Gil Deza E, Balbiani L, Coppola F, et al. Phase II study of navelbine (NVB)0 vs NVB plus cisplatin in non–small cell lung cancer stage III or IV. Proc Am Soc Clin Oncol 1996; 15:394 (abstr 1193).

47. Le Chevalier T, Brisgand D, Douillard JY, et al. Randomized study of vinorelbine and cisplatin versus vinorelbine alone versus vendesine and cisplatin in advanced non–small cell lung cancer: results of a European multicenter trial including 612 patients. J Clin Oncol 1994; 12:360–367.

48. Smith TJ, Hillner BE, Neighbors DM, McSorley PA, Le Chevalier T. Economic evaluation of a randomized clinical trial comparing vinorelbine, vinorelbine plus cisplatin an vestine plus cisplatin fro non-small cell lung cancer. J Clin Oncol 1995; 13:2166–2173.

49. Fukuoka M, Niitani H, Sizuki A, et al. A phase II study of CPT-11, a new derivative of camptothecin, for previously treated non–small cell lung cancer. J Clin Oncol 1992; 10:16–20.

50. Asakawa M, Fujiti A, Fukuoka M, Niitanitt, Taguchi T. Phase II study of CPT-11, a new comptothecin derivative in previously untreated non–small cell lung cancer. Lung Cancer 1991; 7:125–129 (abstr 465).

50a. Masuda N, Fukuoka M, Negoro S, et al. Randomized trial comparing cisplatin and irinotecan versus cisplatin and vindesine versus irinotecan alone in advanced non–small cell lung cancer, a multicenter phase III study. Proc Am Soc Clin Oncol 1999; 18:459a (abstr 1774).

51. Perez-Solar R, Fossela F, Glisson BS, et al. Phase II study of topotecan in patients with advanced non–small cell lung cancer not treated previously with chemotherapy. J Clin Oncol 1996; 14:503–513.

52. Lynch T, Kalish L, Strauss G, et al. Phase II study of topotecan in non–small cell lung cancer. J Clin Oncol 1994; 12:347–352.

53. Wouters BG, Wang LH, Martin M, Brown J. Tirapazamine: a new drug producing tumour specific enhancement of platinum-based chemotherapy in non–small cell lung cancer. Ann Oncol 1999; 10(5):529–533.

53a. Von Pawel J, von Roemeling R, et al. Survival benefit from tirapazamine and cis-platin in advanced non–small cell lung cancer (NSCLC) patients: final results from the international phase III CATAPULT I trial. Proc Am Soc Clin Oncol 1998; 17:454a.

54. Kelly K, Crowley J. Bunn PA et al. A randomized phase III trial of paclitaxel/carboplatin versus vinorelbine cisplatin in untreated advanced non small cell lung cancer. Proc ASCO 1999; 18:1777a.

55. Silvestri G, Pritchard R, Welch HG. Preferences for chemotherapy in patients with advanced non–small cell lung cancer: descriptive study based on scripted interviews. Br Med J 1999; 317:771–775.

20

Chemotherapy Dose Intensification: Is There a Benefit in NSCLC?

**Primo N. Lara, Jr., Derick Lau, and
David R. Gandara**
University of California Davis Cancer Center, Sacramento, California

INTRODUCTION

In preclinical models, a majority of chemotherapeutic agents demonstrate relatively steep dose-response curves against human malignancy, including non–small cell lung cancer (NSCLC). While dose response quantitates the relationship between drug dose and the degree of tumor cell kill in in vitro systems, dose intensity (DI) refers to drug dose administered per unit of time, and can be readily applied to clinical trials of cancer chemotherapy. To standardize terminology, DI is typically described in $mg/m^2/week$, regardless of the actual schedule of administration. DI can be achieved by either increasing the dose of the agent per unit of time (dose escalation) or reducing the time interval between treatments (dose density) (1). Theoretical advantages to dose density include compression of the time to tumor regrowth between drug exposures and utility with chemotherapeutic agents characterized by less steep dose-response relationships (2). Another concept, the "threshold dose," refers to the dose level below which there is little or no antitumor activity, and is an integral component of dose-response relationships.

327

Although chemotherapy DI remains a potentially important strategy in the therapeutic approach to a number of malignancies, establishing ''proof of principle'' in patient studies has proven to be difficult. The hypothesis that relative drug resistance can be overcome by simply increasing dose remains largely speculative, especially in NSCLC. This chapter will review preclinical and clinical data regarding this ''more is better'' concept in NSCLC, as well as dose-schedule interactions, focusing on platinum compounds and new chemotherapeutic agents now commonly used in the therapeutic approach to NSCLC.

PLATINUM COMPOUNDS (CISPLATIN AND CARBOPLATIN)

Of chemotherapeutic agents with clinical activity in NSCLC, cisplatin has had by far the greatest impact. A number of randomized clinical trials and meta-analyses support the conclusion that platinum-based chemotherapy improves survival, symptom control, and quality of life compared to best supportive care alone in stage IV disease, and that platinum-containing combined-modality approaches result in superior survival compared to radiotherapy or surgery alone in stage III patients (3–9). In an analysis of over 2000 patients with advanced NSCLC treated on trials of the Southwest Oncology Group (SWOG), cisplatin therapy proved to be an independent prognostic variable predicting improved survival (10). Until recently, it was unclear whether combination-chemotherapy regimens in advanced NSCLC were superior to cisplatin or carboplatin alone in terms of survival. While previous cooperative group trials in EORTC, SWOG, and ECOG showed increased response rates with the addition of etoposide, mitomycin C, or other chemotherapeutic agents to a platinum compound, in none of these studies was survival improved compared to single-agent cisplatin or carboplatin (11–13). Nevertheless, the objective response rate to single-agent platinum compounds in cooperative group trials is relatively low, and clinical resistance emerges within a few months of initiation of therapy in most patients with advanced NSCLC.

The importance of cisplatin DI in the treatment of NSCLC has been controversial. In vitro, cisplatin demonstrates a steep dose-response relationship in NSCLC (14). A review of clinical studies investigating single-agent cisplatin in advanced NSCLC suggests that if regimens are standardized for projected DI, response rate increases as projected DI increases from 20 mg/m^2/week or less (equivalent to 60 mg/m^2 every 3–4 weeks) to the level of approximately 30–40 mg/m^2/week (i.e., 100–120 mg/m^2 every 3–4 weeks or higher) (15). However, early attempts to achieve these higher levels of cisplatin DI were accompanied by an unacceptable level of nephrotoxicity (16). Further clinical investigation of cisplatin DI was possible only after the introduction of hypertonic saline as a vehicle for preserving renal function in patients receiving high-dose cisplatin (17).

After these observations, Gandara et al. developed a pharmacokinetically designed high-dose cisplatin (HDP) regimen delivering 200 mg/m^2 (or a projected DI of 50 mg/m^2/week) in a divided dose schedule as 100 mg/m^2 in 3% saline on days 1 and 8 of a 28-day schedule (18). Following phase I and phase II trials demonstrating encouraging results in advanced NSCLC, this HDP regimen, with or without mitomycin C (HDP-M), was evaluated in a phase III comparison (SWOG 8738) versus "standard dose" cisplatin (SDP) at 50 mg/m^2 on days 1 and 8 (11). Although progressive disease occurred almost twice as frequently in the SDP arm ($p < 0.05$), confirmed response rates and updated survival data were similar for SDP and HDP (Table 1). In a third arm of HDP plus mitomycin C, the response rate was significantly higher ($p < 0.05$), but survival time was no longer. The results of this study do not substantiate a clinically significant dose-response effect for cisplatin in advanced NSCLC above a dose level of 100 mg/m^2 in a 4-week cycle (a planned DI of 25 mg/m^2/week). However, it is important to point out that this study did not address cisplatin dose response below this level. Even the SDP regimen tested in this SWOG trial would be considered "high dose" by many criteria.

Other randomized studies have also failed to demonstrate the clinical significance of cisplatin DI in advanced NSCLC (19,20). A recent trial of the Spanish Lung Cancer Group in advanced NSCLC compared a dose-intense arm (cisplatin 35 mg/m^2 and etoposide 200 mg/m^2 days 1–3 every 4 weeks) or to a dose-dense arm (same regimen every 3 weeks with rhGM-CSF support). This trial demonstrated that although dose intensification of cisplatin-etoposide was feasible, there was no apparent improvement in patient outcome (21). This same group addressed the issue of preoperative cisplatin DI in stage III disease, randomizing 83 patients to either 100 mg/m^2 or 50 mg/m^2 in combination with mitomycin and ifosfamide for three cycles prior to surgical resection (22). There were no significant differences in complete resection rates, pathological response, or overall survival. Finally, a meta-analysis by Donnadieu et al. reviewed the relationship

TABLE 1 Phase III Evaluation of Cisplatin Dose Intensity in Stage IV NSCLC

	Standard-dose cisplatin ($n = 105$)	High-dose cisplatin ($n = 108$)	High-dose cisplatin plus mitomycin C ($n = 110$)
Complete response	0 (0%)	3 (3%)	4 (4%)
Response rate (CR + PR)	13 (12%)	15 (14%)	29 (27%)
Progressive disease	60 (57%)	41 (38%)	37 (33%)
Median survival (months)	6.9	6.0	7.2
1-year survival	24%	22%	24%

of cisplatin dose to response rate in NSCLC (23). Of almost 2000 patients treated with cisplatin-based chemotherapy, those receiving a dose of $\geq$100 mg/m^2 had a significantly higher response rate, 34%, than those patients receiving lower dose regimens (<70 mg/m^2), 28%, p = 0.005. Based on these observations, a cisplatin dose of 70–100 mg/m^2 given in a conventional schedule in combination with other active chemotherapeutic agents is reasonable, with no evidence that higher dose levels improve therapeutic efficacy.

While DI of carboplatin in NSCLC has been less well studied, extrapolation from the cisplatin database cited above appears appropriate. Although toxicity profiles of these two platinum compounds vary substantially, the mechanism of action is identical. The ratio of relative platinum equivalents based on platinum-DNA adducts for cisplatin compared to carboplatin is 4:1, or a carboplatin dose of 400 mg/m^2 being considered comparable to 100 mg/m^2 of cisplatin (11). Of note, early trials of carboplatin in NSCLC and other tumor types administered carboplatin on a standard mg/m^2 basis, as would be done with other chemotherapeutic agents. With recognition of the importance of renal excretion of carboplatin, recent trials have changed to dosing based on calculated area under the concentration-versus-time curve (AUC) (24). AUC dosing of carboplatin thus avoids underdosing patients with normal renal function, and minimizes overdosing those with renal compromise. Some trials have attempted dose escalation of carboplatin to an AUC of 7.5 or above in combination with paclitaxel as shown later in Table 3. A retrospective estimation of carboplatin exposure by AUC of patients receiving carboplatin at doses of 320 mg/m^2 or 400 mg/m^2 on ECOG 1583 suggested a trend toward improved survival for patients whose projected AUCs exceeded 5.9 mg/ml/min by the Chatelut formula (24a). But there is no randomized literature confirming that dose intensification of carboplatin adds to efficacy in NSCLC, and it is clear that higher doses clearly increase overlapping myelosuppression in many combination regimens. As a result, carboplatin at an AUC of 5–6 has become an accepted standard in most combination regimens where carboplatin is substituted for cisplatin.

TAXANES (PACLITAXEL AND DOCETAXEL)

Paclitaxel

Taxanes are among the most active agents in NSCLC. Paclitaxel is the prototype of the class and has been extensively evaluated in NSCLC. Preclinical studies suggest that the antitumor activity of paclitaxel is dose- and schedule-dependent (25,26). Early clinical data suggested that paclitaxel may exhibit a significant dose-response relationship in NSCLC (27). However, the optimal dose of paclitaxel remains under study and is highly interrelated to the schedule of administration. Initial clinical trials administered paclitaxel over 24 hr in an attempt to

TABLE 2   Representative Phase II Trials of Single-Agent Paclitaxel in NSCLC

Author	Paclitaxel dose (mg/m^2)	Infusion time (hr)	Number of patients	Response Rate (%)	Median survival (mo)
Johnson (31)	250	24	24	21	5.7
Murphy (32)	200	24	25	24	9.5
Gatzemeier (33)	225	3	50	24	9.5
Alberola (34)	210	3	47	24	NR*
Ranson (35)	200	3	21	19	NR
Millward (36)	175	3	51	10	6.5

* NR: not reported.

ameliorate hypersensitivity reactions (28). Subsequent clinical investigations lengthened the infusion time to 96 hr, or shortened it to 1 or 3 hr. Although the optimal schedule remains to be defined, for practical reasons most oncologists now deliver paclitaxel as a 3-hr infusion every 21 days. A recent development has been the administration of attenuated doses of paclitaxel on a dose-dense weekly schedule, resulting in comparable or higher delivered dose intensity (29,30). Toxicities vary depending on the length of paclitaxel infusion, with increased myelosuppression seen with longer infusion schedules ($\geq$24 hr) and dose-limiting neurotoxicity with the shorter infusions times (1–3 hr).

Phase II trials of single-agent paclitaxel in advanced NSCLC report response rates of approximately 10–30%, median survival times of 6–9 months, and 1 year survival rates of 30–40% (Table 2). Within these dose ranges, there is no clear evidence of a dose-response effect. Rather, these studies suggest a significant level of single-agent activity for paclitaxel at or above 175 mg/m^2. Paclitaxel has been studied in combination, most commonly with platinum compounds, either cisplatin or carboplatin. Table 3 summarizes several dose-

TABLE 3   Representative Phase II Trials of Paclitaxel and Carboplatin in NSCLC

Author	Paclitaxel dose (mg/m^2), infusion time	Carboplatin dose (AUC)	Number of patients	Response rate (%)	Median survival (mo)
Langer (37)	135–215, 24 hr	7.5	54	64	12
Johnson (38)	135–175, 24 hr	6	51	27	9
Belani (39)	135–225, 24 hr	5–11	26	50	NR*
Vafai (40)	150–250, 3 hr	6	27	63	NR
Langer (41)	135–280, 1 hr	7.5	22	55	NR

* NR: not reported.

escalation studies of paclitaxel in combination with carboplatin. These studies demonstrated uniformly high response rates, with a suggestion that activity improved at or above the level of 175 mg/m^2, but the concomitant use of carboplatin confounds interpretation of dose-response effects of paclitaxel. Unfortunately, survival, a more important outcome, was not uniformly reported in these trials.

The most important study of paclitaxel DI is a large phase III Eastern Cooperative Oncology Group (ECOG) trial reported by Bonomi and others (42). This trial compared two different doses of paclitaxel given in a 24-hr infusion in combination with cisplatin to the ECOG standard of cisplatin and etoposide (PE). A total of 560 patients were randomized to cisplatin and paclitaxel at 135 mg/m^2 or 250 mg/m^2 plus G-CSF or to PE. The taxane-containing arms in this trial were found to be superior to PE in terms of response (29% vs. 12%) and median survival (10 vs. 7.7 months). The high-dose paclitaxel arm did not result in significantly improved efficacy compared to the lower-dose paclitaxel combination. However, toxicity was greatly increased. In particular, severe neutropenia and death from febrile neutropenia were increased in the high-dose arm. Even more important, over 40% of patients receiving high-dose paclitaxel and cisplatin developed severe peripheral neuropathy. Based on these results, paclitaxel as a 24-hr infusion in NSCLC appears to exhibit no clinically important dose-response efficacy between 135 mg/m^2 and 225 mg/m^2. However, there is a steep dose-response relationship for toxicity.

Several other trials suggest that there may be a threshold dose for paclitaxel efficacy in NSCLC in combination with a platinum compound. The results of a study by Kosmidis et al. support the belief that the threshold dose for efficacy for paclitaxel in NSCLC is a minimum of 175 mg/m^2 given as a 3-hr infusion every 3 weeks (43). In this randomized phase II trial, patients with advanced NSCLC received paclitaxel at either 175 mg/m^2 or 225 mg/m^2 plus carboplatin at an AUC of 6. Time to progression was significantly longer in patients receiving the higher dose of paclitaxel (6.4 vs. 4.3 months, $p = 0.04$). Response rates, median survival, and 1-year survival were also greater with the higher-dose regimen, but did not reach statistical significance owing to the relatively small numbers of patients ($p = 0.1$). Nevertheless, these results are consistent with other data showing that there may be an inferior outcome with paclitaxel at a dose of 175 mg/m^2/3 hr when given with a platinum compound on a 3-week schedule. A phase III trial by Gatzemeier et al. randomized patients to cisplatin alone or cisplatin with paclitaxel at 175 mg/m^2 as a 3-hr infusion (44). Although the response rate was clearly higher in the combination arm, there was no increase in the median survival or 1-year survival over single-agent cisplatin in this study. Similarly, a randomized trial conducted by the European Organization for Research and Treatment of Cancer (EORTC) (45) reported that paclitaxel at a dose of 175 mg/m^2 as a 3-hr infusion plus cisplatin resulted in a higher response rate (41%) than a regimen of teniposide plus cisplatin (28%), but survival was not improved. Most ongoing cooperative group studies in NSCLC (ECOG, SWOG, CALGB) investigating paclitaxel and carboplatin have adopted regimens with a paclitaxel dose of 225 mg/m^2 over 3 hr, repeated every 3 weeks.

Weekly infusion schedules of paclitaxel increase DI by increasing dose density, thus increasing the exposure time of dividing tumor cells to the anticancer effects of paclitaxel (46–48). At weekly doses $\leq$100 mg/m^2, hematological toxicity is mild, even in heavily pretreated patients. In some dose-dense weekly schedules of paclitaxel, however, substantial neurotoxicity has been observed, probably related to relatively high peak plasma concentrations and high cumulative dose. Chang et al. reported that paclitaxel at 50–100 mg/m^2 as a 1-hr infusion weekly for 3 weeks out of 4 was active and well tolerated in metastatic breast and NSCLC (49). Maximum tolerated dose (MTD) has not been reached at 100 mg/m^2. However, response rate was not clearly related to the dose level in this phase I trial. In comparison, Akerley et al. administered weekly paclitaxel at 175 mg/m^2 over 3 hr for 6 weeks of an 8-week cycle. In the first 30 patients treated, delivered DI was 83% in cycle 1, 75% in cycle 2, 58% in cycle 3, and 50% in cycles 4 and 5. The development of grade II/III neuropathy in later cycles precluded delivery of the planned dose intensity. There were 14 responders in 25 evaluable patients for an overall response rate of 56%. Median duration of response and 1-year survival were 6.5 months and 53%, respectively. A phase II trial of paclitaxel 150 mg/m^2/wk $\times$ 6 every 8 weeks conducted by CALGB yielded a response rate of 39% and median survival of 10 months in 36 evaluable patients (49a). Although there have been no randomized phase III trials comparing weekly versus every-3-week regimens of paclitaxel in NSCLC, dose-dense (and therefore dose-intense) weekly schedules are clearly active, with acceptable toxicity profiles at levels at or below 100 mg/m^2/week.

Docetaxel

Docetaxel is a newer taxane that exhibits activity in both platinum-naive and platinum-refractory patients with NSCLC. Although antitumor activity of docetaxel is dose-dependent in vitro, schedule dependency is less apparent. In contrast to wide variability in paclitaxel infusion duration, clinical trials of docetaxel have uniformly utilized a 1-hr infusion. No formal dose intensification studies of docetaxel have been conducted in NSCLC. However, phase II trials of single-agent docetaxel at dose levels of 60–100 mg/m^2 every 3 weeks have been conducted (Table 4). These studies suggest that as docetaxel dose is escalated, there is at best a modest increase in response rate, but no appreciable impact on overall survival. Furthermore, dose-limiting toxicities of neutropenia, neuropathy, and fluid accumulation are clearly dose-related, compromising the therapeutic index of this agent at high dose levels. An additional consideration in docetaxel dosing is the reported interpatient differences in pharmacokinetics due to variability in

TABLE 4 Examples of Single-Agent Docetaxel Trials in
Previously Untreated NSCLC

Author	Docetaxel	n	Response rate (%)	Survival (mo)
Kunitoh (56)	60	75	19	10
Miller (57)	75	20	25	14
Fossella (58)	100	39	33	13
Cerny (59)	100	43	23	11
Latreille (60)	100	45	25	10
Francis (61)	100	29	38	7

plasma levels of alpha-1 acid glycoprotein, a ubiquitous acute-phase protein. Recent studies have combined docetaxel with cisplatin or carboplatin (50–53). Docetaxel dose levels have ranged from 75 to 100 mg/m^2, with increased myelosuppression at the higher dose levels.

A phase I trial of a dose-dense approach using docetaxel administered weekly for 6 consecutive weeks followed by a 2-week rest period demonstrated marked alteration in docetaxel's toxicity profile. Myelosuppression was uncommon while fatigue and asthenia became the dose-limiting toxicities. The recommended phase II dose was 30–36 mg/m^2/week (54). The efficacy of this novel dose-intensified schedule needs to be confirmed in ongoing trials.

Docetaxel appears to be one of the most active chemotherapeutic agents in second-line therapy of NSCLC (Table 5). Fossella et al. reported the results of a phase III trial randomizing NSCLC patients previously treated with platinum to docetaxel (100 mg/m^2 vs. 75 mg/m^2 every 3 weeks) or vinorelbine/ifosfamide (55). The overall response rate was similar between the two docetaxel arms (12% vs. 8%), and significantly better compared to the vinorelbine/ifosfamide arm. Median survival was approximately 5.6 months in all three arms, but 1-year sur-

TABLE 5 Examples of Single-Agent Docetaxel Trials in Previously Treated
NSCLC

Author	Docetaxel dose (mg/m^2)	Number of patients	Response rate (%)	Median survival (mo)
Gandara (62)	100	80	15	7
Fossella (63)	100	44	21	10
Alexopoulos (64)	100	60	25	8

vival favored the 75 mg/m^2 arm of docetaxel (32%), compared to 100 mg/m^2 (21%), or vinorelbine/ifosfamide (19%). When results were censored for effects of subsequent chemotherapy, 1-year survival was superior in both docetaxel arms. Toxicity was increased in the 100 mg/m^2 arm. The results of this trial do not support docetaxel dose escalation above 75 mg/m^2 in previously treated patients with NSCLC.

In summary, there is no definite evidence of a clinically significant dose-response relationship with taxanes in NSCLC. Rather, the data are more consistent with a threshold effect for efficacy, a modest dose-response curve, and a subsequent plateau in antitumor activity. The dose-response curve for toxicity, however, continues to rise with increasing dose, outweighing potential benefit. One exception may be dose-dense approaches of weekly taxane administration, although this requires confirmation in the phase III setting.

GEMCITABINE

Gemcitabine is a novel nucleoside analog of cytarabine that possesses single-agent activity in NSCLC superior to that seen with platinum compounds. Dose intensification of gemcitabine has been of particular interest in view of the demonstrated activity of high-dose cytosine arabinoside in refractory acute leukemia. After initial clinical trials investigating alternative schedules, most studies in NSCLC have delivered gemcitabine weekly for 3 out of every 4 weeks. When gemcitabine was administered on this schedule to pretreated patients, the MTD was 790 mg/m^2.

In chemonaive patients, gemcitabine administered on this weekly ×3 schedule has been generally well tolerated, with grade III/IV neutropenia and thrombocytopenia observed in approximately 25% and 5% of patients, respectively. Table 6 summarizes examples of the largest phase I/II trials in chemonaive patients with NSCLC treated with single-agent gemcitabine.

TABLE 6 Examples of Early-Phase Trials of Single-Agent Gemcitabine Given on Days 1, 8, and 15 of a 28-Day Cycle in Previously Untreated NSCLC

Author	Gemcitabine dose (mg/m^2/week)	Number of patients	Response rate (%)	Median survival (mo)
Fossella (65)	1000–2800	32	25	10.5
Abratt (66)	1000–1250	76	20	9.2
Gatzemeier (67)	1250	151	22	9.4
Anderson (68)	800–1000	79	20	7.0
Takada (69)	1000–1250	73	26	NR*

* NR: not reported.

A recent analysis of trials of single-agent gemcitabine at starting doses of 800–1250 mg/m^2 weekly concluded that optimal therapeutic effects were achieved at doses of 1000 mg/m^2 or more (70). Patients who received a median dose of 700 mg/m^2 or less had a response rate of 3%, while higher doses yielded a response rate of approximately 20%. These data also suggest a plateau in efficacy, with no further benefit at dose levels above 1200 mg/m^2/week.

Other schedules of gemcitabine have been investigated. In an early phase I trial, gemcitabine given every other week yielded no antitumor activity despite an MTD of 4660 mg/m^2, equivalent to a delivered DI of 2330 mg/m^2/week (71). Other schedules (twice weekly, daily over 5 days) reported increased toxicity, despite a very low delivered DI of gemcitabine (72). For example, dose-limiting toxicity with the twice-weekly schedule was thrombocytopenia, with an MTD of 65 mg/m^2 or a delivered DI of 130 mg/m^2/week. With the daily $\times$ 5 regimen, dose-limiting toxicity consisted of flu-like symptoms, with an MTD of only 12 mg/m^2/day. Clearly, further attempts at dose intensification of gemcitabine must carefully consider the schedule-dependent toxicity of this agent.

In view of the central role of cisplatin in the therapy of NSCLC, gemcitabine/cisplatin combinations have been extensively studied. Preclinical data suggest that the combination was synergistic in vitro, likely related to inhibition of repair of cisplatin-induced damage by gemcitabine (73). Activity of the gemcitabine-cisplatin combinations is schedule dependent in preclinical models. Simultaneous treatment with both agents resulted in synergism only if the exposure duration exceeded 4 hr. Sequential administration (gemcitabine prior to cisplatin or vice versa) also resulted in synergism, but with increased toxicity in in vivo models. To explore these preclinical observations in patients with NSCLC, phase I/II trials of gemcitabine-cisplatin have been performed (Table 7). Although all these trials delivered gemcitabine on the standard weekly schedule for 3 weeks, the cisplatin schedule was highly variable. In aggregate, these combi-

TABLE 7 Phase I/II Trials of Gemcitabine-Cisplatin in Advanced NSCLC

Author	Gemcitabine dose (mg/m^2) on days 1, 8, 15	Cisplatin (mg/m^2), schedule (days)	Number of patients	Response rate (%)	Median survival (Mo)
Shepherd (74)	1000–1800	30 (d 1, 8, 15)	47	30	6
Steward (75)	1000	100 (d 15)	43	42	10
Crino (76)	1000	100 (d 2)	48	54	15
Sandler (77)	1000	100 (d 1)	27	37	8.4
Abratt (78)	1000	100 (d 15)	50	48	13

nations of gemcitabine-cisplatin yielded response rates and survival times in NSCLC that were higher than expected for either agent alone.

In some trials, dose-limiting myelosuppression (particularly thrombocytopenia) reduced the planned DI and appeared to be related to the timing of cisplatin administration in individual combinations. In the Sandler trial, only 27% of the intended gemcitabine dose was delivered in the first cycle. In a recent analysis of these studies, schedules where cisplatin is delivered on day 15 followed by a 2-week rest period (Abratt and Steward trials) were reported to optimize DI and provide the longest median duration of exposure to gemcitabine (79).

Since day 15 gemcitabine is commonly omitted due to thrombocytopenia in weekly $\times$ 3 regimens, a modified schedule of gemcitabine given on days 1 and 8 of a 21-day cycle has been incorporated into recent studies of gemcitabine-platinum combinations. The Spanish Lung Cancer Group randomized patients with advanced NSCLC to 21-day cycles of cisplatin (100 mg/m^2 on day 1) and either gemcitabine at 1250 mg/m^2 (days 1 and 8) or etoposide (100 mg/m^2 days 1–3) (80). Grade III/IV thrombocytopenia occurred in only 20% of patients compared to 25–50% in trials of the traditional day 1, 8, 15 regimens. There was a significantly higher overall response rate for the gemcitabine/cisplatin regimen (48%) versus etoposide/cisplatin (22%). Therefore, the day 1 and 8 gemcitabine schedule in combination with cisplatin appears to retain clinical activity while reducing dose-limiting hematological toxicity, thus increasing delivery of the planned DI. Similar observations have been made in recent studies combining gemcitabine with carboplatin (81). In particular, a trial by Carrato et al. demonstrated reduced toxicity, improved dose delivery, and equivalent efficacy of carboplatin with day 1 and 8 gemcitabine every 21 days compared to day 1, 8, 15 dosing every 28 days (82). In this study, the median dose per week of gemcitabine was 1130 mg on the every-3-week schedule and 980 mg on the every-4-week regimen.

VINORELBINE

Vinorelbine is a semisynthetic vinca alkaloid that demonstrates superior antitumor activity in vitro compared to older compounds in its drug class. Several clinical trials have reported single-agent activity against previously untreated patients with NSCLC at a dose level of 30 mg/m^2/week (Table 8).

In the two large phase III trials in which single-agent vinorelbine has been compared with other chemotherapy regimens (85,86), the response rate to vinorelbine was 12–14% with a median survival of approximately 7 months. There have been no formal dose-intensification studies of single-agent vinorelbine beyond the MTD of 30 mg/m^2/week because of dose-limiting neutropenia (87). In other tumor types, pilot studies of vinorelbine dose escalation in combination with hemopoietic growth factors have been reported (88). As a second-line agent,

TABLE 8 Examples of Trials Using Weekly Single-Agent Vinorelbine in
Advanced NSCLC

Author	Dose (mg/m^2)	Number of patients	Response rate (%)	Median survival (mo)
LeChevalier (85)	30	206	14	7.4
Depierre (83)	30	70	33	8
O'Rourke (86)	30	143	12	7
Furuse (84)	25	80	29	9

vinorelbine possess little or no antitumor efficacy at dose levels of 20–25 mg/
m^2/week as summarized in Table 9. A single study by Santoro reports a response
rate of 20% but patients were not well characterized with regard to response
status to primary chemotherapy.

Vinorelbine/platinum combinations have been evaluated in a number of
studies, but do not provide definitive information regarding vinorelbine dose response. In a phase I–II trial of vinorelbine/carboplatin (AUC 7), responses were
first observed at a vinorelbine dose of 15 mg/m^2/week (93). In combination with
cisplatin, vinorelbine given at 25–30 mg/m^2/week has been shown to result in
superior response rates and survival times compared to either cisplatin alone or
a vindesine/cisplatin regimen (94,95). Although caution must be taken in comparing these trials, the results are very similar, whether the 25 mg/m^2/week dose
was used, as in the Wozniak study, or 30 mg/m^2/week, as employed in the Le
Chevalier trial. Substantial reductions and omissions in vinorelbine dosing were
required in both studies. More recently, day 1 and 8 regimens of vinorelbine in
combination with either cisplatin or carboplatin have been evaluated, deleting
day 15 vinorelbine and shortening the cycle to 21 days.

TABLE 9 Single-Agent Vinorelbine as Second-Line
Therapy for NSCLC

Author	Vinorelbine dose (mg/m^2/wk)	Number of patients	Response rate (%)
Rinaldi (89)	20	18	0
Pronzato (90)	25	15	0
Santoro (91)	30	10	20
Fossella (92)	30	87	1

IRINOTECAN

Irinotecan hydrochloride is a semisynthetic camptothecin derivative that inhibits DNA topoisomerase I and demonstrates impressive single-agent activity in NSCLC. In three representative phase II trials using irinotecan at a dose of 100 mg/m²/week (96–98), the overall response rate ranged from 15 to 34% with a median survival of 6–7 months. A European trial administered the agent at a dose of 350 mg/m² once every 3 weeks, similar to the dose schedule used for colorectal cancer (99). This schedule represents a modest increase in planned DI from 100 mg/m²/week to 116 mg/m²/week. Despite this increase, the response rate (36%) was similar to the weekly regimen employed by Japanese and North American investigators. Because of preclinical tumor models that demonstrated therapeutic synergy with the irinotecan plus cisplatin, several phase I/II trials of this combination are now being conducted (100).

HIGH-DOSE CHEMOTHERAPY WITH AUTOLOGOUS BONE MARROW (ABMT) OR STEM CELL TRANSPLANTATION (SCT)

Advances in technology for bone marrow transplantation enabled investigations into applying this approach to solid tumors such as NSCLC and small cell lung cancer. Although high-dose chemotherapy with ABMT or SCT has resulted in long-term survival in advanced Hodgkin's disease, non-Hodgkin's lymphoma, and multiple myeloma, its efficacy remains highly controversial in most solid tumors such as breast cancer. NSCLC represents an older male population of current or previous smokers with a high incidence of underlying chronic obstructive pulmonary or cardiovascular disease. Pilot studies of high-dose chemotherapy in advanced NSCLC have generally been accompanied by equally high rates of treatment-related morbidity and no long-term survival.

An example of this approach in advanced NSCLC was reported by Socinski and Shea where carboplatin was escalated in combination with paclitaxel 250 mg/m² over 24 hr with SCT and filgastrim support. A carboplatin MTD of AUC 18 was identified (101). In this trial, six of seven patients had major responses. Dose-limiting toxicities included severe, transient nephrogenic diabetes insipidus and prolonged neutropenia lasting over 2 weeks. Other serious toxicities included neurotoxicity, diarrhea, and mucositis. A phase II CALGB trial is ongoing to test the efficacy of this approach using the 3-hr infusion schedule of paclitaxel at 250 mg/m² in combination with carboplatin at an AUC of 18. Another phase II study mounted at Fox Chase Cancer Center failed to show any obvious advantage: 10 patients with bulky IIIA NSCLC or potentially resectable III NSCLC underwent mobilization with etoposide 2 gm/m² and G-CSF followed by two cycles of carboplatin (AUC 12–16) and paclitaxel (250 mg/m²) with stem cell and G-CSF support. Only one pCR was observed at surgery. Median time to progression was 57 weeks and median survival 124 weeks (102). Until the emergence of convincing efficacy data for high-dose therapy with stem cell support in NSCLC, this approach must still be considered investigational.

CONCLUSION

The concept of DI is based on the kinetics of cancer cell growth and the steep dose-response curves observed with many chemotherapeutic agents in vitro. Whether or not this concept translates into tangible clinical benefit in NSCLC remains unproven. In fact, based on currently available literature, there is very little evidence to support arbitrary dose intensification of chemotherapeutic agents above dose levels recognized to be effective in NSCLC. Most clinical studies performed to date suggest that chemotherapeutic efficacy reaches a plateau beyond which further dose escalation only adds to toxicity. Of equal importance is recognition of the threshold dose concept. This is especially true when considering multidrug regimens, which inherently require dose reduction of all agents in the regimen to avoid overlapping toxicity. Despite the ongoing discovery of active new chemotherapeutic agents, it has been difficult to demonstrate the superiority of three-drug regimens over two drug regimens in the treatment of NSCLC and other human malignancies. To a large extent, these results may reflect the threshold dose concept. Finally, several new classes of novel nonchemotherapeutic antineoplastic agents now in development possess unique mechanisms of action that target tumor cell populations that are classically resistant to standard chemotherapy. Since these agents are likely to be used in combination with currently available chemotherapy, it is quite likely that future advances in NSCLC will result not from the principles of DI but from the principles of drug diversity.

REFERENCES

1. Hryniuk WM, Levine MN. Analysis of dose intensity for adjuvant chemotherapy trials in stage II breast cancer. J Clin Oncol 1986; 4:1162–1170.
2. Norton L. Conceptual basis for advances in the systemic drug therapy of breast cancer. Semin Oncol 1997; 24(4)(suppl 11):S11-2–S11-12.
3. Rapp E, Pater JL, Willan A, et al. Chemotherapy can prolong survival in patients with advanced non–small-cell lung cancer—report of a Canadian multicenter randomized trial. J Clin Oncol 1988; 6:633–641.
4. Cartei G, Cartes F, Cantone A, et al. Cisplatin-cyclophosphamide-mitomycin combination chemotherapy with supportive care versus supportive care alone for treatment of metastatic non–small-cell lung cancer. J Natl Cancer Inst 1993; 85:794–800.
5. Non–Small Cell Lung Cancer Collaborative Group. Chemotherapy in non–small

cell lung cancer: a meta analysis using updated data on individual patients from 52 randomized clinical trials. Br Med J 1995; 311:899–909.

6. Sause WT, Scott C, Taylor S, et al. Radiation Therapy Oncology Group (RTOG) 8808 and Easter Cooperative Oncology Group (ECOG) 4588: preliminary results of a phase III trial in regionally advanced, unresectable non–small cell lung cancer. J Natl Cancer Inst 1995; 87:198–205.

7. Dillman RO, Seagren SL, Propert KJ, Guerra J, Eaton WL, Perry MC, et al. A randomized trial of induction chemotherapy plus high-dose radiation versus radiation alone in stage III non–small-cell lung cancer. N Engl J Med 1990; 323: 940–945.

8. Rosell R, Gómez-Codina J, Camps C, et al. A randomized trial comparing preoperative chemotherapy plus surgery with surgery alone in patients with non–small-cell lung cancer. N Engl J Med 1994; 330:153–158.

9. Roth J, Fosella F, Komaki R, et al. A randomized trial comparing peri-operative chemotherapy plus surgery alone in resectable stage IIIA non–small cell lung cancer. J Natl Cancer Inst 1994; 86:673–680.

10. Albain KS, Crowley JS, LeBlanc MM., et al. Survival determinants in extensive stage non–small cell lung cancer: the Southwest Oncology Group experience. J Clin Oncol 1991; 9:1618–1626.

11. Gandara DR, Crowley J, Livingston RB, Perez EA, Miller TP, Weiss G, et al. Evaluation of cisplatin dose intensity in metastatic non–small cell lung cancer: a phase III study of the Southwest Oncology Group. J Clin Oncol 1993; 11:873–878.

12. Gandara DR, Wold HG, Perez EA, Deisseroth A, Doroshow J, Meyers F, et al. Cisplatin dose intensity in non–small cell lung cancer: phase II results of a day 1 and 8 high dose regimen. J Natl Cancer Inst 1989; 81:790–794.

13. Klastersky J, Sculier JP, Bureau G, Libert P, Ravez P, Vandermoten G, Thiriaux J, Lecomte J, Cordier R, Dabouis G, et al. Cisplatin versus cisplatin plus etoposide in the treatment of advanced non–small-cell lung cancer. J Clin Oncol 1989; 7(8): 1087–1092.

14. Perez EA, Poitras MC, Gandara DR. In vitro cytotoxicity of cisplatin and carboplatin in non–small cell lung cancer cell lines. Proc Am Assoc Cancer Res 1991; 32:408.

15. Gandara DR, Wold HG, Perez EA, Deisseroth A, Doroshow J, Meyers F, et al. Cisplatin dose intensity in non–small cell lung cancer: phase II results of a day 1 and 8 high dose regimen. J Natl Cancer Inst 1989; 81:790–794.

16. Ozols RF, Behrens BS, Ostchega Y, Young RC. High dose cisplatin and high dose carboplatin in refractory ovarian cancer. Cancer Treat Rev 1985; 12:59–65.

17. Litterst CL. Alterations in the toxicity of *cis*-dichlorodiammineplatinum-II and tissue localization of platinum as a function of NaCl concentration in the vehicle of administration. Toxicol Appl Pharmacol 1981; 61:99–108.

18. Gandara DR, DeGregorio MW, Wold HJ, et al. High-dose cisplatin in hypertonic saline: reduced toxicity of a modified dose schedule and correlation with plasma pharmacokinetics. A Northern California Oncology Group pilot study in non–small cell lung cancer. J Clin Oncol 1986; 4:1787–1793.

19. Klastersky J, Sculier JP, Ravez P, Libert P, Michel J, Vandermoten G, Rocmans

P, Bonduelle Y, Mairesse M, Michiels T, et al. A randomized study comparing a high and a standard dose of cisplatin in combination with etoposide in the treatment of advanced non–small-cell lung carcinoma. J Clin Oncol 1986; 4(12):1780–1786.

20.   Sculier JP, Klastersky J, Giner V, Bureau G, Thiriaux J, Dabouis G, Efremidis A, Ries F, Berchier MC, Sergysels R, et al. Phase II randomized trial comparing high-dose cisplatin with moderate-dose cisplatin and carboplatin in patients with advanced non–small-cell lung cancer. J Clin Oncol 1994; 12(2):353–359.

21.   Font A, Moyano AJ, Puerto JM, et al. Increasing dose intensity of cisplatin-etoposide in advanced nonsmall cell lung carcinoma: a phase III randomized trial of the Spanish Lung Cancer Group. Cancer 1999; 85(4):855–863.

22.   Felip E, Rosell R, Moreno I, et al. Spanish lung cancer group randomized trial of preoperative chemotherapy (cisplatin either 100 mg/m^2 or 50 mg/m^2) in state IIIA (N$_2$) non–small cell lung cancer (NSCLC). Proc ASCO 1998; 17:1740.

23.   Donnadieu N, Paesmans M, Sculier JP. Chemotherapy of non–small cell lung cancer according to disease extent: a meta-analysis of the literature. Lung Cancer 1991; 7:243–252.

24.   Calvert AH, Newell DR, Gumbrell LA, et al. Carboplatin dosage: prospective evaluation of a simple formula based on renal function. J Clin Oncol 1989; 7(11):1748–1756.

24a. Belani CP, Kim K, Bonomi P, et al. Retrospective estimation of carboplatin exposure by Calverts and Chatelut's formulae and correlation with pharmacodynamic effects in metastatic non-small cell lung cancer (NSCLC). Proc Am Soc Clin Oncol 1996; 15:A-1119.

25.   Rowinsky ED. The taxanes: dosing and scheduling considerations. Oncology 1997; 11(3)(suppl 2):7–19.

26.   Arbuck SG, Canetta R, Onetto N, et al. Current dosage and scheduling issues in the development of paclitaxel (Taxol). Semin Oncol 1993; 4(suppl 3):31–39.

27.   Hainsworth JD, Thompson DS, Greco FA. Paclitaxel by 1 hour infusion: an active drug in metastatic non–small cell lung cancer. J Clin Oncol 1995; 13:1609–1614.

28.   Rowinsky EK, Donehower RC. Paclitaxel (Taxol). N Engl J Med 1995; 332:1004–1014.

29.   Akerley W. Phase I/II trial of weekly paclitaxel in patients with advanced lung cancer. Semin Oncol 1996; 23(suppl 16):55–58.

30.   Loffler TM, Freund W, Lipke J, et al. Schedule and dose-intensified paclitaxel as a weekly 1-hour infusion in pretreated solid tumors: results of a phase I/II trial. Semin Oncol 1996; 23(suppl 16):32–34.

31.   Johnson D, Chang AY, Ettinger DS. Taxol (paclitaxel) in the treatment of lung cancer: the Eastern Cooperative Oncology Group experience. Ann Oncol 1994; 5(Suppl 6):S45–50.

32.   Murphy WK, Fossella FV, Winn RJ, et al. Phase II study of taxol in patients with untreated advanced non-small cell lung cancer. J Natl Cancer Inst 1993; 85(5): 384–388.

33.   Gatzemeier U, Heckmayer M, Neuhauss R., et al. Chemotherapy of advanced inoperable non-small lung cancer with paclitaxel: a phase II trial. Semin Oncol 1995; 22(suppl 15):24–28.

34.   Alberola V, Rosell R, Gonzales-Larriba JL, et al. Single agent Taxol, 3 hour infu-

sion in untreated advanced non–small cell lung cancer. Ann Oncol 1995; 6:49–52.

35. Ranson MR, Jayson G, Perkins S, et al. Single agent paclitaxel in advanced non small cell lung cancer: single center phase II study using a 3-hour administration schedule. Semin Oncol 1997; 24(4)(suppl 12):S12-6–S12-9.

36. Millward MJ, Bishop JF, Friedlander M, et al. Phase II trial of a 3-hour infusion of paclitaxel in previously untreated patients with advanced non-small cell lung cancer. J Clin Oncol 1996; 14:142–148.

37. Langer CJ, Leighton JC, Comis RL, et al. Paclitaxel and carboplatin in combination in the treatment of advanced non-small cell lung cancer: a phase II toxicity, response, and survival analysis. J Clin Oncol 1995; 13:1860–1870.

38. Johnson DH, Paul DM, Handle K, et al. Paclitaxel and carboplatin in advanced non–small cell lung cancer: a phase II trial. J Clin Oncol 1996; 14:2054–2060.

39. Belani CP, Aisner J, Hiponia D, et al. Paclitaxel and carboplatin with and without filgrastim support in patients with metastatic non small cell lung cancer. Semin Oncol 1995; 22(suppl 5):7–12.

40. Vafai D, Israel V, Zaretsky S, et al. Phase I/II trial of combination carboplatin and Taxol in non–small cell lung cancer. Proc ASCO 1995; 11:1067.

41. Langer C, Kaplan R, Rosvold E, et al. Paclitaxel by 1 hour infusion combined with carboplatin in advanced non small cell lung carcinoma. Proc ASCO 1996; 12:1200.

42. Bonomi P, Kim K, Kusler J, Johnson D. Cisplatin/etoposide vs paclitaxel/cisplatin/G-CSF vs paclitaxel/cisplatin in non–small-cell lung cancer. Oncology (Huntingt) 1997; 11(4)(suppl 3):9–10.

43. Kosmidis PA, Mylonakis N, Skarios D, et al. A multicenter randomized trial of paclitaxel (175 mg/m^2) plus carboplatin versus paclitaxel (225 mg/m^2) plus carboplatin (6AUC) in advanced non–small cell lung cancer (NSCLC). Proc ASCO 1999; 18:1785.

44. Gatzemeier U, von Pawel J, et al. Phase III comparative study of high dose cisplatin (HD-cis) versus a combination of paclitaxel (TAX) and cisplatin (CIS) in patients with advanced non–small cell lung cancer. Proc ASCO 1998; 17:454a.

45. Giacconne G, Manegold C, Rosell R, et al. An update on European randomized studies in non–small cell lung cancer. Semin Oncol 1998; 25(4)(suppl 6):11–17.

46. Fennelly D, Aghajanian C, Shapiro F, et al. Phase I and pharmacologic study of paclitaxel administered weekly in patients with relapsed ovarian cancer. J Clin Oncol 1994; 12:2682–2686.

47. Klaassen U, Wilke H, Strumberg D, et al. Phase I study with a weekly 1 hour infusion of paclitaxel in heavily pretreated patients with metastatic breast and ovarian cancer. Eur J Cancer 1996; 32A:547–549.

48. Akerley W, Choy H, Safran H, et al. Weekly paclitaxel in patients with advanced lung cancer: preliminary data from a phase II trial. Semin Oncol 1997; 24(suppl 12):S12-10–S12-13.

49. Chang A, Boros L, Asbury R, et al. Weekly moderate dose paclitaxel in stage IV non–small cell lung cancer. Proc ASCO 1998; 14:1806.

49a. Akerley W, Herndon J, Egorin M, Lyss M, et al. CALGB: phase II trial of weekly paclitaxel for advanced non–small cell lung cancer (NSCLC). Proc Am Soc Clin Oncol 1999; 18:A-1783.

50. Millward MJ, Zalcberg J, Bishop JF, et al. Phase I trial of docetaxel and cisplatin in previously untreated patients with advanced non–small cell lung cancer. J Clin Oncol 1997; 15:750–758.
51. Cole JT, Gralla RJ, Marquez CB, et al. Phase I–II study of cisplatin and docetaxel in non-small cell lung cancer. Proc ASCO 1995; 14:357.
52. Le Chevalier T, Belli L, Monnier A, et al. Phase II study of docetaxel (Taxotere) and cisplatin in patients with advanced non small cell lung cancer. Proc ASCO 1995; 14:1059.
53. Mattson K, Saarinen A, Jekunen A, et al. Combination treatment with docetaxel and platinum compounds for non–small cell lung cancer. Semin Oncol 1997; 24: S14-5–S14-8.
54. Hainsworth J, Burris H, Erland J, et al. Phase I trial of docetaxel administered by weekly infusion in patients with advanced refractory cancer. J Clin Oncol 1998; 16:2164–2168.
55. Fossella FV, Devore R, Kerr R, et al. Phase III trial of docetaxel 100 mg/m^2 or 75 mg/m^2 vs. vinorelbine/ifosfamide for non–small cell lung cancer (NSCLC) previously treated with platinum based chemotherapy (PBC). Proc ASCO 1999; 18: 1776.
56. Kunitoh H, Watanabe K, Onoshi T, et al. Phase II trial of docetaxel in previously untreated advanced non–small cell lung cancer: a Japanese cooperative study. J Clin Oncol 1996; 14:1649–1655.
57. Miller VA, Rigas JR, Francis PA, et al. Phase II trial of a 75 mng/m^2 dose of docetaxel with prednisone premedication for patients with advanced non–small cell lung cancer. Cancer 1995; 74:968–972.
58. Fossella FV, Lee JS, Murphy WK, et al. Phase II study of docetaxel for recurrent or metastatic non-small cell lung cancer. J Clin Oncol 1994; 16:1238–1244.
59. Cerny T, Kaplan S, Pavlidis N, et al. Docetaxel (Taxotere) is active in non–small cell lung cancer: a phase II trial of the EORTC Early Clinical Trials Group. Br J Cancer 1994; 70:384–387.
60. Latreille J, Laberge F, Gelmon K, et al. Docetaxel has moderate activity in patients with advanced non–small cell lung cancer. Anti Cancer Treatment, Sixth International Congress, 1996; 76.
61. Francis P, Rigas JR, Kris MG, et al. Phase II trial of docetaxel in patients with stage III and IV non–small cell lung cancer. J Clin Oncol 1994; 12:1232–1237.
62. Gandara DR, Vokes E, Green M, et al. Docetaxel (Taxotere) in platinum-treated non–small cell lung cancer: confirmation of prolonged survival in a multicenter trial. Proc ASCO 1997; 16:1632.
63. Fossella FV, Lee JS, Shin DM, et al. Phase II study of docetaxel for advanced or metastatic platinum-refractory non–small cell lung cancer. J Clin Oncol 1995; 13: 645–651.
64. Alexopolous K, Kouroussis C, Androulakis N, et al. Docetaxel and granulocyte colony stimulating factor in patients with advanced non–small cell lung cancer previously treated with platinum based chemotherapy: a multicenter phase II trial. Cancer Chemother Pharmacol 1999; 43:257–262.
65. Fossella FV, Lippman SM, Tarasoff P, et al. Phase I/II study of gemcitabine, an

active agent for advanced non–small-cell lung cancer (NSCLC). Proc ASCO 1995; 14:1144.

66. Abratt RP, Bezwoda WR, Falkson G, et al. Efficacy and safety profile of gemcitabine in non–small cell lung cancer: a phase II study. J Clin Oncol 1994; 12:1535–1540.

67. Gatzemeier U, Shepherd FA, le Chevalier T, et al. Activity of gemcitabine in patients with non–small cell lung cancer: a multicentre, extended phase II study. Eur J Cancer 1996; 32:243–248.

68. Anderson H, Lund B, Bach F, et al. Single agent activity of weekly gemcitabine in advanced non–small-cell lung cancer: a phase II study. J Clin Oncol 1994; 12: 1821–1826.

69. Takada M, Negoro S, Kudo S, et al. Activity of gemcitabine in non–small-cell lung cancer: results of the Japan gemcitabine group (A) phase II study. Cancer Chemother Pharmacol 1998; 41(3):217–222.

70. Shepherd FA. Phase II trials of single agent activity of gemcitabine in patients with advanced non–small cell lung cancer: an overview. Anti Cancer Drugs 1995; 6(suppl 6):19–25.

71. Vermorken JB, Quatalla JP, Hatty SR, et al. Phase I study of gemcitabine using once every two weeks schedule. Br J Cancer 1997; 76:1489–1493.

72. Kaye SB. Gemcitabine: current status of phase I and II trials. J Clin Oncol 1994; 112:1527–1531.

73. Peters GJ, Bergman AM, Ruiz van Haperen VW, et al. Interaction between cisplatin and gemcitabine in vitro and in vivo. Semin Oncol 1995; 22(4)(suppl 11):72–79.

74. Shepherd FA, Burkes R, Cormier Y, et al. Phase I dose escalation trial of gemcitabine and cisplatin for advanced non-small cell lung cancer: usefulness of mathematical modeling to determine maximum tolerated dose. J Clin Oncol 1996; 14:1656–1662.

75. Steward WP, Dunlop DJ, Dabouis G, et al. Phase I/II study of gemcitabine and cisplatin in non–small cell lung cancer: preliminary results. Semin Oncol 1996; 5: 43–47.

76. Crino L, Scagliotti G, Marangolo M, et al. Cisplatin-gemcitabine combination in advanced non–small cell lung cancer: a phase II study. J Clin Oncol 1997; 15: 297–303.

77. Sandler AB, Ansari R, McClean J, et al. Gemcitabine plus cisplatin in non–small cell lung cancer (NSCLC): a phase II study. Eur J Cancer 1995; 131A:S225.

78. Abratt RP, Bezwoda WR, Goedhals L, et al. Weekly gemcitabine with monthly cisplatin: effective chemotherapy for advanced non–small cell lung cancer. J Clin Oncol 1997; 15:744–749.

79. Abratt RP, Sandler A, Crino L, et al. Combined cisplatin and gemcitabine for non–small cell lung cancer: influence of scheduling on toxicity and drug delivery. Semin Oncol 1998; 25(suppl 9):35–43.

80. Rosell R, Tonato M, Sandler A. The activity of gemcitabine plus cisplatin in randomized trials in untreated patients with advanced non–small cell lung cancer. Semin Oncol 1998; 25(suppl 9):27–34.

81. Langer CJ, Calvert P, Ozols RF. Gemcitabine and carboplatin in combination: phase I and phase II studies. Semin Oncol 1998; 25(4)(suppl 9):51–54.

82. Carrato A, Alberola V, Massuti B, et al. Combination of gemcitabine (GEM) and carboplatin (carbo) as first line treatment in non–small cell lung cancer (NSCLC). Ann Oncol 1998; 9:89.
83. Depierre A, Lemaire E, Dabouis G, et al. A phase II study of Navelbine (vinorelbine) in the treatment of non–small cell lung cancer. Am J Clin Oncol 1991; 14: 115–119.
84. Furuse K, Kubota K, Kawahara M, et al. A phase II study of vinorelbine, a new derivative of vinca alkaloid, for previously untreated advanced non–small cell lung cancer. Japan Vinorelbine Lung Cancer Study Group. Lung Cancer 1994; 11:385–391.
85. LeChevalier T, Brisgand D, Douillard JY, et al. Randomized study of vinorelbine and cisplatin versus vindensine and cisplatin versus vinorelbine alone in advanced non–small cell lung cancer: results of a European multicenter trial including 612 patients. J Clin Oncol 1994; 12:360–367.
86. O'Rourke M, Crawford J, Schiller J, et al. Survival advantage for patients with stage IV NSCLC treated with single agent Navelbine in a randomized controlled trial. Proc ASCO 1991; 13:1147.
87. Mathe G, Reizenstein P. Phase I pharmacologic study of a new vinca alkaloid: Navelbine. Cancer Lett 1985; 27:285–293.
88. Livingston RB, Ellis GK, Gralow JR, et al. Dose-intensive vinorelbine with concurrent granulocyte colony-stimulating factor support in paclitaxel-refractory metastatic breast cancer. J Clin Oncol 1997; 15(4):1395–1400.
89. Rinaldi M, Della GM, Venturo I, et al. Vinorelbine as single agent in the treatment of advanced non–small cell lung cancer. Proc ASCO 1994; 13:360.
90. Pronzato P, Landucci M, Vaira P, et al. Failure of vinorelbine to produce response in pre-treated non–small cell lung cancer patients. AntiCancer Res 1994; 14:1413–1416.
91. Santoro A, Maiorino L, Santoro M. Second line with vinorelbine in the weekly monotherapy for the treatment of advanced non small cell lung cancer. Lung Cancer 1994; 11:130.
92. Fossella FV, Devore R, Kerr R, et al. Phase III trial of docetaxel 100 mg/m^2 or 75 mg/m^2 vs. vinorelbine/ifosfamide for non small cell lung cancer (NSCLC) previously treated with platinum based chemotherapy (PBC). Proc ASCO 1999; 18: 1776.
93. Garst J, Crawford J, O'Rourke, et al. Vinorelbine (NVB) and carboplatin (C) for the treatment of patients with advanced non–small cell lung cancer (NSCLC): a phase II response, toxicity and survival study. Proc ASCO 1996; 15:1233.
94. Wozniak AJ, Crowley JJ, Balcerzak SP, et al. Randomized trial comparing cisplatin with cisplatin plus vinorelbine in the treatment of advanced non–small-cell lung cancer: a Southwest Oncology Group study. J Clin Oncol 1998; 16(7):2459–2465.
95. Le Chevalier T, Brisgand D, Douillard JY, et al. Randomized study of vinorelbine and cisplatin versus vindesine and cisplatin versus vinorelbine alone in advanced non–small-cell lung cancer: results of a European multicenter trial including 612 patients. J Clin Oncol 1994; 12(2):360–367.
96. Negoro S, Fukuoka M, Niitani H, et al. A phase II study of CPT-11, a new deriva-

tive of camptothecin, in patients with primary lung cancer: CPT11 Cooperative Study Group. Gan To Kagaku Ryobo 1991; 18:1013–1019.

97. Fukuoka M, Niitani H, Suzuki A, et al. A phase II study of CPT-11, a new derivative of camptothecin, for previously untreated non–small cell lung cancer. J Clin Oncol 1992; 10:16–20.

98. Baker L, Khan R, Lynch T, et al. Phase II study of irinotecan (CPT-11) in advanced non–small cell lung cancer. Proc ASCO 1997; 16:1658.

99. Douillard J, Ibrahim N, Riviere A, et al. Phase II study of CPT-11 (irinotecan) in non small cell lung cancer. Proc ASCO 1995; 14:1118.

100. Devore R, Johnson D, Crawford J, et al. Irinotecan plus cisplatin in patients with advanced non–small cell lung cancer. Oncology 1998; 12(8)(suppl 6):79–83.

101. Socinski MA, Shea TC. High dose therapy with carboplatin and paclitaxel in non small cell lung cancer. Semi Oncol 1997; 24(suppl 12):S12-45–S12-51.

102. Schilder RJ, Goldberg M, Millenson M, et al. Phase II trial of induction high-dose chemotherapy followed by surgical resection and radiation therapy for patients with marginally resectable non–small cell lung cancer of the lung. Lung Cancer 2000; 27:37–45.

21

Chemoprevention of Lung Cancer

Daniel D. Karp
Harvard Medical School, Boston, Massachusetts

Mark D. Bergman
Beth Israel Deaconess Medical Center, Boston, Massachusetts

INTRODUCTION AND CURRENT PERSPECTIVE

The American Cancer Society estimated there would be 164,100 cases of lung cancer in the United States in 2000 with approximately 156,900 deaths (1). These figures represent the continued decline in overall lung cancer mortality that began to occur over the last decade. While this decline has occurred in men, death rates appear to have stabilized, but not decreased, for women. At many levels of government, tobacco is recognized as an addictive drug warranting regulation by the Federal Drug Administration (FDA) (2). Approximately 46.3 million individuals—26% of U.S. adults—smoke, and approximately 45 million are former smokers (3). While studies indicate that approximately 70% of smokers state they "want" to quit, only 2.5% succeed (4). Despite programs such as the Community Intervention Trial for Smoking Cessation (COMMIT), addiction to tobacco remains a major health problem. Twenty percent of long-term survivors of lung cancer are now conservatively estimated to have a risk of developing second primary cancers, and former smokers now comprise at least half of newly diagnosed cases of lung cancer (3).

Even if all persons stopped using tobacco now, the legacy of decades of smoking and other environmental and occupational risk factors in older adults would continue to produce huge numbers of new cases of lung cancer worldwide (5). Therefore, elimination of tobacco use as primary prevention of lung cancer remains a crucial intervention for teenagers and young adults. Furthermore, the risk of second primary tumors for people cured of primary cancers of the lung or head and neck remains high and does not seem to be effectively improved by smoking cessation alone (6). Consequently, new prevention strategies must be developed (7). Lung cancer death rates among the neighborhoods of Boston range from 25 to 60 per 100,000 with a mean value of 42.8 (8). Overall U.S. cancer death rates also have a wide state-to-state variation.

According to the National Cancer Institute Surveillance Epidemiology and End Results data (www.seer.gov), Utah has the lowest rate (119 per 100,000), and the Midwest farming states range from 145–160, whereas many of the eastern industrial states have consistently higher death rates. The highest mortality rates are observed in Louisiana, Delaware, Kentucky, Maine, and West Virginia (8a). Lung cancer death rates appear to vary markedly as well even within regions. These estimates are clearly subject to limitations and also are affected by differences in median age, ethnic variability, and relative smoking rates. Nevertheless, these state-to-state differences are striking and suggest that if we can identify those groups at highest risk and help effect changes in behavior and environmental exposure, we can produce meaningful decreases in the number of people dying from lung cancer. For example, Utah, with the lowest incidence of lung cancer mortality, is next to Nevada, one of the states with the highest incidence. Figure 1 shows lung cancer estimated death rates per 100,000 population. Because lung cancer accounts for approximately 30% of U.S. cancer deaths annually, effective interventions in lung cancer prevention could significantly reduce the number of people dying from cancer in this country.

Hong et al. reported in 1990 that isotretinoin (13-*cis* retinoic acid) could prevent second primary tumors (SPTs) in patients with previously treated squamous cell carcinoma of the head and neck (9). Since that time, it has been hoped that similar strategies could reduce the incidence of lung cancer in current smokers, former smokers, and those with a previously treated aerodigestive-tract malignancy. In that regard, SPTs must be distinguished from a recurrence of a previously treated cancer. Hong has categorized SPTs as new cancers (1) separated from the original tumor by 2 cm of normal epithelium, or (2) consisting of a different histological type, or (3) recurring more than 5 years after the original cancer. Metachronous tumors are those that occur more than 6 months after the original tumor, whereas synchronous cancers are those diagnosed within 6 months of the original cancer (9). These distinctions are pivotal in chemoprevention research. SPTs after prior treatment of lung cancer occur with relatively constant frequency (i.e., 3–4% per year in a high-risk cohort) and are felt to result from a field defect (see below) rather than being treatment related.

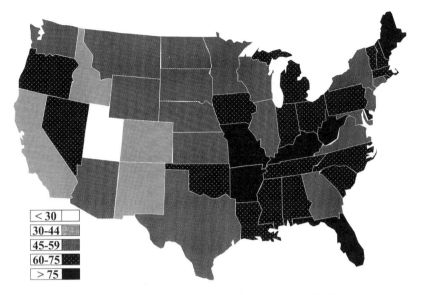

FIGURE 1   Lung cancer mortality per 100,000 population (ACS estimates 1999).

In this chapter, we focus on recent developments and current chemoprevention research strategies for lung cancer as well as treatment of carcinoma in situ.

As far back as 1922, Mori reported that a diet low in fat-soluble vitamin A resulted in squamous metaplasia in the trachea and larynx of experimental animals (10). Since that time, there have been numerous studies and publications questioning or proposing a link between vitamin intake and risk of developing lung cancer. While appealing, this link is still unproven. Nevertheless, vitamins and other dietary supplements make up a billion-dollar health food industry supported by millions of people seeking to prevent not only cancer, but the aging process in general.

Slaughter and colleagues beginning in 1944, introduced the concept of the multiplicity of cancer origin (11,12)—the so-called "field cancerization" concept. In 1953, they reported that 88 of 783 (11.2%) patients with oral cancer had two or more independent squamous cell carcinomas. Slaughter also found that abnormal and hyperplastic—often atypical—epithelium surrounded virtually all oral cancers for varying distances (13). In 1956, Auerbach et al. reported epithelial changes in the lungs of 41 patients with bronchogenic cancer not present in the lungs of nonsmokers: hyperplasia, loss of cilia, and atypical cells. The authors defined carcinoma in situ as the presence of all three of these abnormalities (14). These two landmark studies were the first to suggest that, rather than being an isolated event, lung cancer is the end result of a series of genetic defects that accumulate in the bronchial tree following long-term exposure to tobacco and other carcinogens. Sporn coined the term ''chemoprevention'' in the mid-1970s, thereby defining an entirely new area of cancer research. Chemoprevention is the attempt to ''arrest or reverse pre-malignant cells during their progression to invasive malignancy, using physiologic mechanisms that are not toxic'' (15). He further expanded this concept to develop interventions to retard the promotional events that make up the dynamic multistep process of carcinogenesis.

MULTISTEP CARCINOGENESIS

It is now widely accepted that a sequence of oncogene activation events is required for the development of an invasive lung cancer cell. This mechanism of malignant tumors arising from a multistep process of sequential chromosomal loss has been worked out in detail for colon cancer by Vogelstein et al. (16). Although the process of suppressor gene loss and oncogene activation in bronchogenic cancer is less well understood, it appears that multiple genetic mutations are also involved in lung cancer development (17–23). These mutations seem to be irreversible and remain silent until additional genetic alterations occur that further promote neoplastic development. Thus, lung cancer development requires the accumulation of multiple genetics alterations over a prolonged period of time. Furthermore, it appears that abnormalities in p53 and mutations of K-ras occur relatively early in the development of lung cancer (24) (see Figure 2).

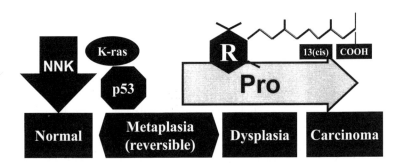

NNK = initiation by NNK and other Nicotine metabolites.
Pro = promotional events following early oncogene
activation that lead to invasive carcinoma.

FIGURE 2 Chemoprevention: using Retinoids and other agents to attempt to slow the promotional events that lead from dysplasia to carcinoma. NNK = initiation by NNK and other nicotine metabolites. Pro = promotional events following early oncogene activation that lead to invasive carcinoma.

The protein encoded by the p53 gene is a key element in regulating the cell cycle and apoptosis, particularly in response to cellular damage. The chromosomal region where p53 resides (17p13) is frequently deleted in lung cancer,and the remaining allele has undergone mutational inactivation in 50–70% of lung cancers (25). Inhibition of the tumor-promoting activity of ras genes, by antagonists of the cellular enzyme farnesyl protein transferase (an enzyme required for ras genes to transform cells), represents a rational attempt to utilize newly gained knowledge of how transforming proteins operate, to create novel anticancer agents (26).

MOLECULAR EPIDEMIOLOGY: FINDING SUBJECTS AT INCREASED RISK FOR CANCER

The triad of lung cancer causation is shown in Figure 3. The causal pathway initiated by smoking includes a long list of factors: duration of smoking, depth of inhalation, chronic obstructive lung disease, and deposition of particulate matter. A second branch of the pathway includes chronic inflammation, release of proteolytic enzymes, release of oxygen radicals, and macrophage secretion of polypeptide growth factors (27). Genetic susceptibility makes up the third component (28). Knudson, in 1985, hypothesized that certain individuals have increased susceptibility to development of cancer based on the loss or mutation of a single gene, which then makes it more likely that they could suffer a ''second hit'' as a result of carcinogen exposure or some other mutational stimulus (29). This hypothesis connects sporadic and familial cancers and has a broad range of appli-

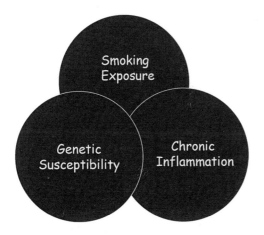

FIGURE 3 Triad of lung cancer causation.

cability for both basic and clinical research. Because only 10–15% of smokers ultimately develop lung cancer, it is this group who could most benefit from chemoprevention (30); consequently, a variety of tests and models have been investigated to predict those at greatest risk for the development of lung cancer.

Krontiris et al. reported an association of variability in the HRAS1 minisatellite locus and the risk of several epithelial cancers, including lung cancer (31). A recently completed Eastern Cooperative Oncology Group (ECOG) study (E3Y92) has expanded this observation by testing for the presence of such genetic polymorphisms in siblings with cancer to better define the concept of ''cancer families.''

The majority of chemical carcinogens require metabolic activation before they interact with cellular macromolecules and initiate tumor development. It has thus been hypothesized that an individual's risk of developing lung cancer may be based on genetic polymorphisms in carcinogen-metabolizing pathways. For example, as mentioned above, although cigarette smoking is the main cause of lung cancer, not all smokers develop malignant lung tumors. It was previously shown that individuals whose P450 cytochrome system (CYP2D6) metabolized the drug debrisoquine slowly were at higher risk of development of lung cancer (32). However, recent studies by Shaw et al. (33) and Kivisto et al. (34) have not confirmed this observation. Altered phenotypes and genotypes in other metabolizing enzymes (e.g., CYP1A1 and CYP2E1) have also been associated with tobacco-smoke-induced lung cancer and other cancers; however, other studies have shown no association (35,36). Nevertheless, the concept of individual variation in susceptibility to carcinogens is potentially of great importance and merits further evaluation.

SPECIFIC CHEMOPREVENTIVE AGENTS

For a drug to be effective as a chemopreventive agent, it should retard or reverse the long, multistep process of carcinogenesis—from metaplasia (a premalignant state) to dysplasia (further cellular disorder), to carcinoma in situ, to finally an invasive tumor, i.e., cancer (37). See Figure 2.

Vitamin A and Dietary Intake

A statistical decrease in the risk of lung cancer has been associated with increased consumption of green or yellow vegetables or carotenoids in 14 of 15 retrospective diet studies. Furthermore, decreased serum retinol levels have been correlated with an increased risk of cancer (38). There is still no compelling evidence to date, however, that a diet supplemented with vitamin A will prevent lung cancer, although one study using retinyl palmitate has suggested a potential benefit [see Pastorino et al. (76)].

The Retinoids

Retinoids, derivatives of vitamin A, are critical for epithelial differentiation, normal vision, and reproduction. Natural and synthetic retinoids given at pharmacological doses can restore regulation of differentiation in vitro, so they were a natural choice for early studies (39). Retinoids are potent regulators of gene expression (40,41) and work through an elaborate system that consists of a family of cytoplasmic retinoic acid–binding proteins as well as intranuclear retinoic acid receptors (42).

The family of retinoid nuclear receptors consists of two main types—RAR and RXR—each with at least three subtypes: alpha, beta, gamma. RAR-α, RAR-β, and RAR-γ have been localized to chromosomes 17q21.1, 3p24, and 12q13, respectively, whereas RXR-α, RXR-β, and RXR-γ have been localized to chromosomes 9q34.3, 6p21.3, and 1q22-23 (24). The nuclear retinoid receptors are homologous to the steroid/thyroid hormone family (43). Structurally, RARs have three separate domains: a transcription-activating domain, a DNA-binding domain, and a hormone-binding domain together with a hinge region (Figure 4).

Once a retinoid reaches the cytoplasm, it enters or is transported to the nucleus where it binds to the hormone-binding domain of either the RARs or RXRs. These ligand-receptor complexes then bind to DNA as either homo- or heterodimers and inhibit protein kinase C, modulate growth of premalignant cells, and suppress evolution of premalignancy to overt neoplasia. In particular, abnormality or loss of detectable RAR-β has been associated with lung cancer and lung cancer cell lines (44,45) and a majority of oral premalignant lesions responding

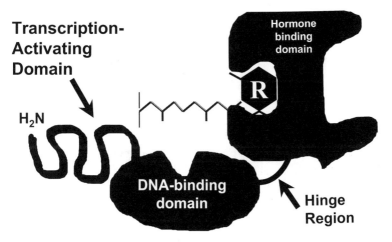

FIGURE 4   Retinoid receptor structure. RARs have three separate domains.

clinically to 13cRA treatment have been shown to have an increase in the RAR-β level (46).

The retinoid receptors do not appear to bind directly to 4-HPR (all *trans*-4-hydroxyphenyl retinamide) and it is therefore termed a ''prodrug,'' whereas 9-*cis* and other retinoids bind to both RAR and RXR (47) (Figure 5).

The startling discovery that all *trans*-retinoic acid can induce differentiation and clinical remission in patients with acute promyelocytic leukemia was a major milestone in the quest for a more biologically based approach to the prevention and treatment of malignant disease (48) (Figure 6). Etretinate is a second-generation compound and the Arotinoids LGD 1069 and Tazarotene, third-generation agents, have been modified in the ring structure to provide more differentiation and gene regulation activity (47). Future work with these and other synthetically derived retinoids should yield new agents that can specifically restore the regulation of differentiation in vivo in premalignant pulmonary tissues.

Carotenoids

Beta-carotene is a dimer of the active moiety retinol that is plentiful in green and yellow vegetables (Figure 7). It appeared to have an advantage over preformed vitamin A and was a popular agent for clinical trials over the past decade. However, recent reports from three large studies have not shown benefits in chemoprevention of lung cancer and two have even suggested that overall death rate and deaths from lung cancer are higher in smokers who take pharmacological doses of beta-carotene. The Alpha Tocopherol Beta Carotene (ATBC) Study was

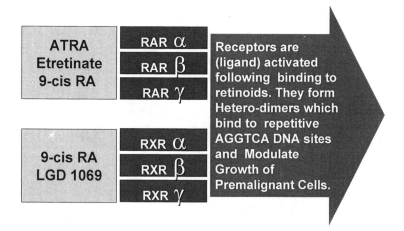

FIGURE 5 Retinoic acid receptor binding and mechanism of action.

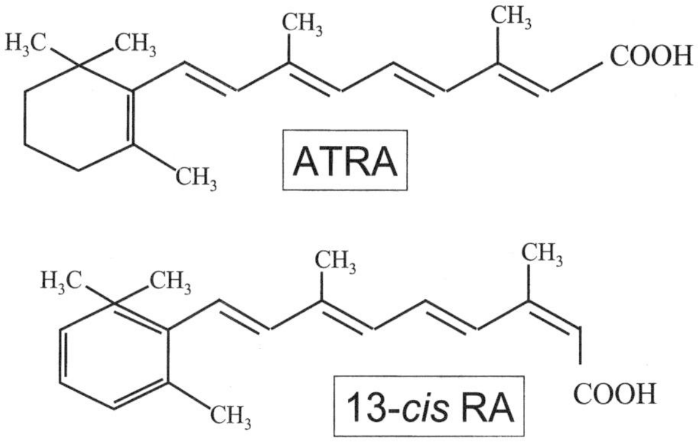

FIGURE 6 All *trans*-retinoic acid (ATRA) and isotretinoin (13-*cis* RA) are both in clinical use.

carried out on 29,133 male Finnish smokers. Those participants who took 20 mg of beta-carotene developed 18% more lung cancers and had 8% more deaths than those ATBC participants who did not (49). The Physician's Health Study was a randomized 2 × 2 factorial trial that accrued 22,070 U.S. male physicians aged 40–84 years. Eleven percent of the participants were smokers when recruited to the study and 51% had smoked at some time in their life. Participants took either beta-carotene 50 mg every other day or a placebo and 325 mg of aspirin or a placebo on alternate days. This study showed no benefit or harm from beta-carotene regarding cancer or cardiovascular events (Figure 8).

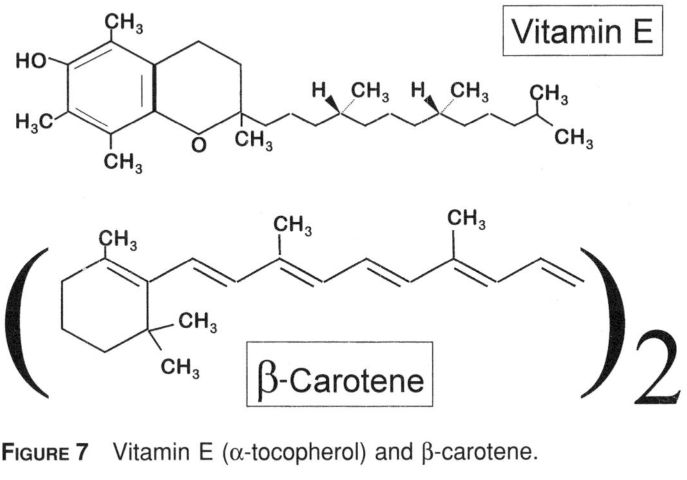

FIGURE 7 Vitamin E (α-tocopherol) and β-carotene.

STUDY	SIZE	DRUGS	RESULT
A.T.B.C. Study; NEJM'94	**29,133** Male Finnish smokers	β-Carotene 20mg and α Tocopherol	Higher rates of Lung CA & Deaths 18% and 8%
C.A.R.E.T. Beta Carotene And Retinol Evaluaton Trial	**18,314** 14,254 smokers, and 4,060 asbestos workers	β-Carotene 30mg and Vit.E 25,000 IU	Higher rates of Lung CA (388) & Deaths (974) 28% and 17%
Physicians' Health Study'82 C. Hennekens	**22,071** Males 11% current and 51% former smokers; age40-84	β-Carotene 50mg QOD and Aspirin 325mg	44% decrease in Myocardial Infarct (ASA)
Women's Health Study J. Buring, Sc.D.	**40,000** Professional Women aged ≥ 45	Vit.E. 600 IU & Aspirin 100mg	**Ongoing** (β Carotene stopped)

FIGURE 8 Placebo-controlled studies have shown no β-carotene benefit for smokers.

The Beta Carotene and Retinol Efficacy Trial (CARET) study involved 18,314 smokers, former smokers, or aerospace workers exposed to asbestos. It was terminated in January 1996 after a planned interim analysis showed a 28% higher rate of lung cancer and 17% higher overall death rate in those participants taking beta-carotene. The participants were notified to stop taking their study medications and obtain follow-up and a physical examination. The dose of beta-carotene in that study was 30 mg/day, which is equivalent to 50,000 IU of vitamin A, or about five medium-sized carrots. Other trials using beta-carotene were halted. The ongoing Women's Health Study is continuing using vitamin E and aspirin only. Although it is disappointing that beta-carotene demonstrated no benefits for those participants, these important studies have shown the unquestionable importance of placebo-controlled studies in chemoprevention research. Many individuals have been taking beta-carotene on the premise that it could not be harmful. The ATBC and CARET studies suggest the opposite. Smokers should not take beta-carotene supplements. They should stop smoking.

In a recent randomized, placebo-controlled trial in subjects with documented histories of occupational asbestos exposure, McLarty et al. (50) reported on the efficacy of combination therapy with β-carotene (50 mg) and retinol (25,000 IU) given on alternate days. Despite a median treatment duration of 5 years, no significant reduction in sputum atypia was seen.

N-Acetylcysteine (NAC)

Cigarette smoke contains dozens of carcinogens: benzene, benzo(apyrene), NNK [4-(methylnitrosamino)-1-(3-pyridyl)-1butanone], crotonaldehyde, epoxides, free radicals, and peroxides. It has been estimated that each puff of smoke contains 1016 oxidant molecules, a level that can overwhelm the glutathione detoxification system (GSH) (51). Of note, oxidant exposure can rapidly activate K-ras oncogene DNA (52). N-Acetyl cysteine (NAC) (Figure 9) is an aminothiol precursor of reduced GSH that has been used since the early 1960s as a mucolytic agent (53). When taken orally, NAC is rapidly absorbed, deacetylated, and incorporated into intra- and extracellular GSH stores (54). It is highly effective in ameliorating acetaminophen hepatotoxicity and is safe when given in doses of 30 g daily for several days (55). NAC detoxifies reactive electrophiles and free radicals through reduction of oxygen species and by conversion to cysteine, which supports GSH biosynthesis and acts directly as an antioxidant or as substrate in the GSH redox cycle. In vitro, NAC decreases carcinogen-induced DNA damage and inhibits type IV collagenases as well as chemotaxis, invasion, and metastasis by some malignant cells (56).

Conaway et al. (57) recently reported on the chemopreventive potential of NAC along with three other agents (fumaric acid, retinamide and β-carotene) in preventing NNK-induced lung tumors in A/J mice. Although none of these agents effectively reduced tumor incidence or multiplicity, both NAC and β-carotene significantly retarded the malignant progression of adenomas to adenocarcinomas. The European Organization for Research and Treatment of Cancer (EORTC) studied NAC at a dose of 600 mg daily as well as vitamin A in the form of retinyl palmitate (300,000 IU) in a 2 × 2 factorial design. Side effects of NAC were very low, with 86% of participants taking NAC alone reporting essentially no toxicity (58). Final results of this study have been disappointing,

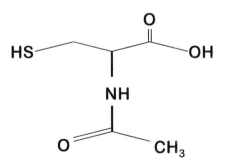

FIGURE 9 N-Acetyl cysteine (NAC) was used in the "Euroscan" study.

with no advantage for NAC, retinyl palmitate (RP), or the combination versus no intervention, and no difference in the incidence of second primary tumors (59).

Vitamin E (α-Tocopherol)

Vitamin E is a naturally occurring antioxidant (Figure 7). Epidemiological and dietary studies have suggested that there is an inverse relationship between vitamin E intake and the incidence of lung cancer (60). Data from Dimery et al. suggested that the toxicity of high-dose 13-*cis*-retinoic acid could be ameliorated when α-tocopherol was given concurrently, without affecting the retinoid's plasma concentration (61). Furthermore, preliminary evidence indicates that α-tocopherol (1200 IU/day), when given with 13-*cis*-retinoic acid (100 mg/m²/day) and interferon-alpha (3 MU/m²), exerts a protective effect on advanced premalignant oral lesions by modulating p53 and Ki-67 expression (62). However, no data on toxicity were reported. It remains to be determined what role, if any, α-tocopherol has on its own or as a modulator of retinoid toxicity, and whether similar effects on gene expression (e.g., p53 and Ki-67) are observed in pulmonary lesions.

Selenium

Selenium, an essential trace element, was first associated with cancer protection in the 1960s (63), and epidemiological evidence suggests that selenium plays a major role in preventing the development of human cancers (64) (see Figure 10).

A randomized controlled trial by Clark et al. (65) with 1312 patients suggested that selenium supplementation (200 μg/day), in the form of a brewers' yeast tablet, was associated with a reduction in the risk of developing lung cancer. The original primary endpoint was to evaluate the effect of selenium supplementation on the risk of developing nonmelanoma skin cancers (no protection was observed). Further analysis of the data, however, revealed a significant (39%) reduction in cancer incidence (77 vs. 119 in controls) and a 48% reduction in mortality (29 deaths vs. 57 in controls). Despite this observation, other randomized trials have not shown a similar degree of protection against cancer. Whether this inconsistency is the result of the dose or form of selenium, or the specific cancers studied, is unclear (66). Proposed mechanisms of selenomethionine activity include stimulation of glutathione peroxidase, alterations in carcinogen metabolism, production of cytotoxic metabolites, and inhibition of protein synthesis (Table 1).

Further randomized studies are needed to confirm these results before public health recommendations regarding selenium supplementation can be made. A large, phase III, randomized, placebo-controlled Intergroup trial opened in October 2000.

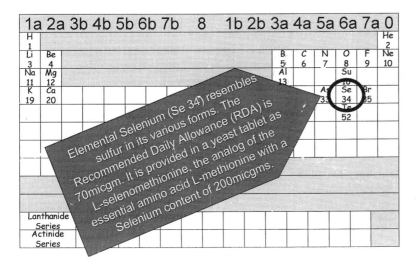

1a	2a	3b	4b	5b	6b	7b		8			1b	2b	3a	4a	5a	6a	7a	0
H 1																		He 2
Li 3	Be 4												B 5	C 6	N 7	O 8	F 9	Ne 10
Na 11	Mg 12												Al 13			Su		
K 19	Ca 20														As 33	Se 34 Te 52	Br 35	

Elemental Selenium (Se 34) resembles sulfur in its various forms. The Recommended Daily Allowance (RDA) is 70micgm. It is provided in a yeast tablet as L-selenomethionine, the analog of the essential amino acid L-methionine with a Selenium content of 200micgms.

FIGURE 10   Selenium 34 shares some properties with sulfur.

Isothiocyanates

Isothiocyanates such as phenethyl isothiocyanate (PEITC) and benzyl isothiocyanate (BITC) occur in conjugated form in a wide variety of cruciferous vegetables and are released during chewing by the enzyme myrosinase. As described by Hecht (67), isothiocyanates prevent tumors in a number of rat tissues including lung, mammary gland, esophagus, liver, small intestine, colon, and bladder. Both NNK and benzo(a)pyrene (BaP) exert their deleterious effects by enhanced formation of DNA adducts after metabolic activation. This is presumably followed by multiple genetic alterations in oncogenes and tumor suppressor genes resulting in carcinogenesis. BITC inhibits BaP-induced lung tumorigenesis in mice, whereas PEITC inhibits NNK-induced lung tumors in rats and mice. They must be present at the time of carcinogen exposure to be effective, however, and thus

TABLE 1   L-Selenomethionine: Proposed Mechanism(s)

Stimulation of glutathione peroxidase thereby lowering tissue peroxides
Alterations in carcinogen metabolism
Production of cytotoxic selenium metabolites
Inhibition of protein synthesis
Inhibition of specific enzymes
Stimulation of apoptosis

would be most likely to confer benefit when incorporated into a daily nutrition program that begins early in life. Notably, in smokers who consumed a diet supplemented with watercress, which contains substantial amounts of a PEITC precursor, decreased metabolic activation of NNK resulted in increased excretion of its two metabolites: NNAL and NNAL-gluc (67).

Other Agents

Chalcones are synthetic open-chain flavanoids. They are stilbene derivatives that bind to steroid receptors and have some structural similarity to tamoxifen. Another agent, myoinositol, is a nontoxic phytate derivative that has been used clinically to treat diabetic neuropathy. Both chalcones and myoinositol inhibit NNK pulmonary adenoma formation in female A/J mice (68,69). Wattenberg et al. (70) recently reported on the chemoprevention of lung tumors by aerosolized budesonide, a synthetic glucocorticoid. Female A/J mice were treated for 1 min six times a week, 1 week after three oral administrations of BaP. Treated animals developed 80–90% fewer pulmonary adenomas than controls, who received sham aerosolizations with either H_2O or ethanol. Of note was a partial (50%) reduction in tumor incidence in controls compared to animals who received BaP without aerosolization, which is consistent with the known association of elevated glucocorticoid levels (presumably from the stress of the aerosolization technique), low body weight (as noted in this study), and reduced tumorigenesis (71,72). Yang et al. (73) showed that administration of black tea polyphenols inhibited NNK-induced bronchiolar cell proliferation as well as progression of adenoma to adenocarcinoma in A/J mice. Once again, treated animals had lower body weights, which may have influenced these observations. Other studies in mice suggest that antagonists of the autocrine growth factors gastrin-releasing peptide (74) and vasoactive intestinal peptide (75) may prevent lung carcinogenesis. These and other novel inhibitors of pulmonary tumor formation (e.g., epidermal growth factor receptor inhibitors, farnesyl transferase inhibitors, and metalloproteinase inhibitors) hold promise for new interventions in prevention of lung cancer.

PREVENTING SPTS IN PATIENTS AT RISK

At present, there is no standard chemoprevention therapy, nor is there an FDA-approved agent for the prevention of lung cancer or development of SPTs. In the original high-dose placebo-controlled 13cRA study of Hong et al. in head and neck cancer, with approximately 50 participants in each arm, three lung cancers developed in the control group whereas none developed in the treatment group (9). In 1993 Pastorino et al. reported a study of 307 patients with resected stage I non–small cell lung cancer who were randomized to receive 300,000 units of retinol palmitate daily or placebo for 12 months (76). After a median follow-up of 46 months, 51 SPTs developed in 47 patients. There were 18 SPTs in the treatment arm and 29 in the control arm. The overall estimated survival rate at 5 years was 62% versus 54% ($p = 0.44$). The Intergroup Study 91025 randomized patients with stage I ($T_1N_0M_0$ or $T_2N_0M_0$) resected non–small cell lung cancer to 13 cRA (30 mg daily $\times$ 5 years) versus placebo. This study, which concluded in 1997, was coordinated by the M. D. Anderson Cancer Center and included participation by the Cancer and Acute Leukemia Group B (CALGB), community CCOPs, ECOG, the North Central Group (NCCTG), and the Southwest Group (SWOG). Accrual of 1295 randomized patients was completed in April 1997, at which time a planned blinded interim analysis did not meet early stopping criteria (77). A total of 226 cases have reached the study endpoints (73 new primaries and 153 relapses). Already, valuable lessons have been learned from this study. The involvement of a group of active and committed thoracic surgeons as well as medical and radiation oncologists proved crucial to the successful accrual engendered by this ambitious study. Patients were highly motivated to enter and maintained a high rate of compliance. To date, yearly endpoint analysis has been consistent with the Lung Tumor Cooperative Group findings of 2–3% new SPTs per year in such a group (78). However, the actual number of recurrences and SPTs in such a large, carefully staged patient group will be a valuable by-product of this study. Those with stage I NSCLC had an even distribution of SPTs and metastatic recurrences of the original primary, while in those with stage II NSCLC the ratio was $1:2$ (77). To date, cRA has not yielded a reduction in SPTs or a change in survival rate; those on cRA who continue to smoke had an increased risk of SPTs. The EORTC Chemoprevention Study in Lung Cancer (EUROSCAN, EORTC #08871) began in March 1988 and completed accrual in January 1994. Patients with curative treatment for T_1, T_2, or T_3, N_0 squamous cancer of the oral cavity and larynx, or resected non–small cell lung cancer, were randomized in a 2×2 factorial design to receive retinol palmitate (PO 150,000–300,000 IU/day for 12–24 months) and/or N-acetylcysteine (NAC) (PO 600 mg/day for 24 months). This study reported on 2592 participantss (60% with head and neck cancer and 40% with lung cancer). After a median follow-up of 49 months, 916 patients were reported with an event (recurrence, second primary tumor, or death). No statistically significant difference was observed in overall survival or event-free survival between patients who received retinyl palmitate and patients who did not.

INTERMEDIATE ENDPOINTS

Multiple intermediate endpoints have been employed in chemoprevention research to identify useful new strategies. These include oncogene activation, presence of micronuclei, assays of DNA ploidy, biochemical measures such as levels of ornithine decarboxylase, prostaglandin synthetase, and blood group antigens. Exfoliated cells can now be analyzed for the presence of bronchial metaplasia. However, changes in such biomarkers have not been validated to be associated with decreased risk of developing lung cancer. Nevertheless, these important surrogates are of key importance in providing information rapidly and allowing studies with reduced sample size (80).

CLINICAL TRIALS OF CHEMOPREVENTIVE AGENTS

Lee et al. reported the results of a prospective trial of the use of isotretinoin in 86 heavy smokers (81). The authors attempted to confirm the results of an earlier uncontrolled French trial that reported that etretinate (25 mg/day for 6 months) could produce a decline in extent of squamous metaplasia in the bronchial epithelium of smokers (82). Participants were taken from an original group of 152 smokers who were found on bronchoscopy to have frank dysplasia or metaplasia in greater than 15% of the biopsy sections examined (metaplasia index). They then received either isotretinoin (1.0 mg/kg) or placebo for 6 months and were reevaluated carefully with bronchoscopic biopsies from six separate sites. Interestingly, a large number of participants in both groups stopped smoking during the study and the metaplasia index decreased over time in 54% of the treatment group and 59% of the control group. Although this was termed a "negative" study, it did document that a placebo-controlled study with a bronchoscopically determined intermediate endpoint is feasible in lung cancer chemoprevention trials. It also demonstrated that high-risk patients who had not (yet) developed lung cancer could be recruited successfully to such trials. Smoking cessation can be associated with a sizable decrease in the degree of bronchial metaplasia over a 6-month period. It is also quite possible that markers other than metaplasia index will emerge that are more useful in future studies.

OTHER STUDIES

The NCI Early Detection Branch is conducting a 16-year, 74,000-participant randomized screening trial for prostate, lung, colorectal, and ovarian cancer, the PLCO trial, to assess whether studies such as flexible sigmoidoscopy, chest x-ray, digital rectal examination, serum PSA, CA 125, and transvaginal ultrasound can reduce cancer mortality in men and women aged 60–74 (83). ECOG is evaluating immunostaining of induced sputum specimens, shed antigens, and the presence of growth factor elevation in bronchial lavage fluid for the early detection of second primary lung cancers in patients with curatively respected stage I non–small cell lung cancer. Hopefully, these and other studies will yield a wealth of important information for the screening and prevention of lung cancer.

CARCINOMA IN SITU

Carcinoma in situ (Tis) is also known as stage 0 non–small cell lung cancer and denotes microscopic squamous cell carcinoma, usually discovered during the course of bronchoscopy. The in situ designation refers to squamous cell type only and ordinarily does not apply to the other histological forms of lung cancer. Occult lung cancer (Tx), on the other hand, denotes a patient whose sputum or bronchial washings contain malignant cells although tumor is not visualized on imaging studies or by bronchoscopy (84). The usual scenario consists of a smoker with a negative chest x-ray and no other evidence of disease who is being evaluated for a productive cough or hemoptysis. Histologically, in situ squamous carcinoma ranges from thickening, erythema, and loss of the normal bronchial mucosal longitudinal ridges to ulceration and full-thickness atypia of the squamous epithelium (85). The multistage model assumes that atypical squamous metaplasia and dysplasia precede the development of in situ carcinoma, which in turn evolves to invasive cancer (86). Frost and co-workers showed that cancer developed in approximately 12% of individuals with moderate atypia and 37% of those with severe atypia (87). Therefore, careful pathological evaluation is the key to proper treatment of these lesions.

Surgery

Carcinoma in situ and occult lung cancers are noninvasive by definition and, if localized, should be curable with surgical resection. A useful practice guideline algorithm has recently been published by Cameron et al. (88). Any patient with a positive sputum cytology should have a full medical history and complete physical examination, including a careful otolaryngology evaluation to rule out the possibility of a lesion in the oral cavity, larynx, pharynx, or hypopharynx. Additional studies include a chest x-ray, serum chemistries, a CT scan of the chest and upper abdomen, and pulmonary function tests. Selective bronchoscopy with brushings and washings of the individual lobes should be the next step. If a localized unequivocally malignant area is identified, lobectomy or pneumonectomy would then be a curative approach to the problem. If any question remains regarding the degree of dysplasia, a waiting period followed by repeat bronchoscopy may be a valuable maneuver. During this period the patient should absolutely refrain from smoking. In the event that no localizing cytology is obtained, the patient should stop smoking and have careful follow-up with history and physical examination, repeat bronchoscopy, and radiographic imaging. A 6–12-week interval is a reasonable standard. If a specific lesion is identified later, surgery can still hopefully provide long-term successful treatment.

Photodynamic Therapy (PDT)

PDT [see review by Edell and Cortese (89)] has been used for both advanced and early superficial lung cancer since 1980. PDT involves a photosensitizing agent (e.g., hematoporphyrin derivatives), which, when exposed to light of the proper wavelength, forms toxic oxygen radicals that result in cell death. PDT appears to be an alternative to surgical resection in some patients with localized bronchogenic carcinoma. A bronchoscopically fitted laser light source can be used to visualize and ablate localized tumor. This technique has the advantage of preserving lung tissue in a population of patients who often have compromised pulmonary function and are at high risk for multiple cancers. However, such an approach requires close follow-up and if PDT is unsuccessful, patients will require surgical "salvage" and continued surveillance for second primary cancers.

Chemopreventive Therapy

Patients with carcinoma in situ have probably accumulated a sequence of oncogene activation events and other mutational stimuli (see above). Therefore, a single agent such as vitamin-based therapy may not be adequate. It will probably require a more aggressive approach comprising a combination of agents that inhibit different phases of the carcinogenesis process. This is also true of long-term survivors of small cell cancer, who have an alarming rate of second primary non–small cell cancers. Discussions are underway to study (90) small cell cancer survivors using combination therapy with agents such as retinoids, vitamin E, and N-acetylcysteine.

CONCLUSIONS AND CONSIDERATIONS FOR THE FUTURE

Chemoprevention is a new discipline and yet has made important strides over the last decade. A coalition of patients, health professionals, researchers, and governmental staff now exists to promote increased research and intervention programs nationally. Several large studies have finished accrual and provide valuable insights. It is imperative that practicing oncologists seek out and support programs for their high-risk patients. Beta-carotene has been shown in two large studies to increase the overall death rate as well as risk of developing cancer in active smokers by a mechanism that is unknown at this time. This experience with beta-carotene has stimulated multiple researchers to investigate this paradox and has taught us that uncontrolled use of health food supplements should be avoided in smokers until it is clear that a particular agent is beneficial. Health professionals must increase efforts to eliminate tobacco use in our citizens— especially the young ones, who can benefit most. Smoking cessation alone appears to be capable of reversing metaplasia in some individuals. Studies with retinoids and retinyl palmitate have suggested benefits in preventing second primary cancers. Patients with a long history of smoking, strong family history, and/or extensive occupational or environmental exposures should be urged to take advantage of chemoprevention protocols when available. In the meantime, a diet containing proper amounts of cruciferous vegetables and fruits is an important health practice that should be encouraged early in life since many dietary components must be present at the time of carcinogen exposure to confer benefit.

An impressive catalog of intermediate markers and activated oncogenes is now available to provide surrogate endpoints for new research. New techniques such as phototherapy may soon add a new dimension to the diagnosis and conservative therapy for very-early-stage and in situ lung cancer. Such advances, while important, are very costly. Finally, new classes of agents such as the triterpenoids are showing potent activity with regard to differentiation, proliferation, and inflammation. These remarkable new substances are the result of rational molecular drug design and promise to expand our capabilities even further in the near future (91).

Patient care costs have proven to be a substantial barrier to the performance of chemoprevention studies in some settings. Nurses, dedicated support staff, and data managers are necessary to ensure a high level of patient compliance and data accuracy in chemoprevention programs. Physicians, health plan administrators and payers, and representatives of the pharmaceutical industry and governmental agencies must form partnerships to take chemoprevention to the next level of success. As our country approached the twentieth century, lung cancer was a rare disease. As we plan programs in the twenty-first century, we have an increasing number of powerful tools to diagnose, prevent, and treat lung cancer. If we employ all the tools at our disposal, we may be able to make a great impact on this lethal hundred-year epidemic of lung cancer and benefit our patients in a meaningful way.

REFERENCES

1. Greenlee RT, Murray T, Bolder S, et al. Cancer Statistics 2000. CA Cancer J Clin 2000; 50:7–33.
2. ''President's message to teenage smokers.'' Boston Herald, Aug 22, 1996, p 1.
3. Strauss G, DeCamp M, Dibiccaro E, Richars W, Harpoie D, Healey E, Sugarbaker D. Lung cancer diagnosis is being made with increasing frequency in former cigarette smokers! Proc Am Soc Clin Oncol 1995; 14:362.
4. Major professional organizations join forces in fight against tobacco addiction. Reuters Health Information News Service, June 25, 1996.
5. Garfinkel L, Stellman SD. Smoking and lung cancer in women: findings in a prospective study. Cancer Res 1988; 48:6951–6955.
6. Karp DD, Vaughan CW, Willet B, Heeren T, DiMartino NA, Vincent ME, Picardi ME, Hong, WK. Long term survival following induction chemotherapy for squamous cell carcinoma of the head and neck: a ten year follow-up. In: Salmon SE, ed. Adjuvant Therapy of Cancer V. Orlando, FL: Grune & Stratton, 1987:119–128.
7. Brown CC, Kessler LG. Projections of lung cancer mortality in the United States, 1985–2025. J Natl Cancer Inst 1988; 80:43–51.
8. Lung cancer death rates in Boston from 1994–1996. Boston Globe, Nov 10, 1998; 255(133):1.
8a. Ries LA, Wingo PA, Miller DS, et al. The annual report to the nation on the status

of cancer 1973–1997, with a special section on colorectal cancer. Cancer 2000; 88(10):2398–2424.

9. Hong WK, Lippman SM, Itri LM, Karp DD, Lee JS, Byers RM, Schantz SP, Kramer AM, Lotan R, Peters LJ. Prevention of second primary tumors with isotretinoin in squamous-cell carcinoma of the head and neck. N Engl J Med 1990; 323:795–801.

10. Mori S. The changes in the para-ocular glands which follow the administration of diet low in fat soluble A; with note of the effects of the same diets on the salivary glands and the mucosa of the larynx and trachea. Johns Hopkins Hosp Bull 1922; 33:357–359.

11. Slaughter, DP. The multiplicity of origin of malignant tumors; collective review, Int Abstr Surg 1944; 79:89–98.

12. Slaughter DP. Multicentric origin of intraoral carcinoma. Surgery 1946; 20:133–146.

13. Slaughter DP, Southwick HW, Smejkal W. "Field cancerization" in oral stratified squamous epithelium. Clinical implications of multicentric origin. Cancer 1953; 6: 963–968.

14. Auerbach O, Patrick TG, Stout AP, et al. The anatomical approach to the study of smoking and bronchogenic carcinoma: a preliminary report of forty-one cases. Cancer 1956; 9:76–83.

15. Sporn MB, Dunlop NM, Newton DL, Smith JM. Prevention of chemical carcinogenesis by vitamin A and its synthetic analogs (retinoids). Fed Proc 1976; 35:1332–1338.

16. Vogelstein B, Fearon ER, Hamilton SR, Kern SE, Preisinger AC, Leppert M, Nakamua Y, White R, Smits AM, Bos JL. Genetic alterations during colorectal tumor development. N Engl J Med. 1988; 319:525–535.

17. Huber MH, Lee JS, Hong WK. Chemoprevention of lung cancer. Semin Oncol 1993; 20(2):128–141.

18. Westra WH, Slebos RJ, Offerhaus GJ, Goodman, SN, Evers SG, Kensler TW, Askin FB, Rodenhuis S, Hruban RH. K-ras oncogene activation in lung adenocarcinomas from former smokers: evidence that K-ras mutations are an early and irreversible event in the development of adenocarcinoma of the lung. Cancer 1993; 72:432–438.

19. Johnson BE. The role of MYC, JUN, and FOS oncolgenes in human lung cancer. In: Pass HI, Mitchell JB, Johnson DH, Turrisi AT, eds. Lung Cancer: Principles and Practice. Philadelphia: Lippincott-Raven, 1996:83–98.

20. Morkve O, Halvorsen OJ, Stangeland L, Gulsvik A, Laerum OD, Mrkve O. Quantitation of biological markers (p53, c-myc, Ki-67, and DNA ploidy) by multiparameter flow cytometry in non–small cell lung cancer. Int J Cancer 1992; 52:851–855.

21. Vogt PK, Bos TJ. Jun: oncogenes and transcription factors. Adv Cancer Res 1990; 55:1–35.

22. Angel P, Karin M. The role of Jun, Fos, and the AP-1 complex in cell proliferation and transformation. Biochim Biophys Acta 1991; 1072:129–157.

23. Distel RJ, Spiegelman BM. Protooncogene c-fos as a transcription factor. Adv Cancer Res 1990; 55:37–55.

24. Hong WK, Lippman SM, Hittelman WN, Lotan R Retinoid chemoprevention of aerodigestive cancer: from basic research to the clinic. Clin Cancer Res 1995; 1: 677–686.

25. Greenblatt MS, Bennett WP, Hollstein M, Harris CC. Mutations in the p53 tumor suppressor gene: clues to cancer etiology and molecular pathogenesis. Cancer Res 1994; 54:4855–4878.
26. Gibbs JB, Oliff A, Kohl NE Farnesyltransferase inhibitors: ras research yields a potential cancer therapeutic. Cell 1994; 77:175–178.
27. Islam SS, Schottenfeld D. Declining FEV_1 and chronic productive cough in cigarette smokers: a 25-year prospective study of lung cancer incidence in Tecumseh, Michigan. Cancer Epidemiol Biomarkers Prev 1994; 3:289–298.
28. Schottenfeld D. Epidemiology of lung cancer. In: Pass HI, Mitchell JB, Johnson DH, Turrisi AT, eds. Lung Cancer: Principles and Practice. Philadelphia: Lippincott-Raven, 1996:305–321.
29. Knudson AG. Hereditary cancer, oncogenes, and anti-oncogenes. Cancer Res 1985; 45:1437–1443.
30. Mattson ME, Pollack ES, Cullen JW. What are the odds that smoking will kill you? Am J Public Health 1987; 77:425–431.
31. Krontiris TG, Devlin B, Karp DD Robert NJ, Risch N. An association between the risk of cancer and mutations in the HRAS1 minisatellite locus. N Engl J Med 1993; 329:517–523.
32. Speirs CJ, Murray S, Davies DS, Biola Mabadeje AF, Boobis AR. Debrisoquine oxidation phenotype and susceptibility to lung cancer. Br J Clin Pharmacol 1990; 29:101–109.
33. Shaw GL, Falk RT, Frame JN, Weiffenbach B, Nesbitt JC, Pass HI, Caporaso NE, Moir DT, Tucker MA Genetic polymorphism of CYP2D6 and lung cancer risk. Cancer Epidemiol Biomarkers Prev 1998; 7(3):215–219.
34. Kivisto KT, Griese EU, Stuven T, Fritz P, Friedel G, Kroemer HK, Zanger UM. Analysis of CYP2D6 expression in human lung: implications for the association between CYP2D6 activity and susceptibility to lung cancer. Pharmacogenetics 1997; 7(4):295–302.
35. Raunio H, Husgafvel-Pursiainen K, Anttila S, Hietanen E, Hirvonen A, Pelkonen O. Diagnosis of polymorphisms in carcinogen-activating and inactivating enzymes and cancer susceptibility—a review. Gene 1995; 159(1):113–121.
36. Hirvonen A. Genetic factors in individual responses to environmental exposures. Occup Environ Med 1995; 37(1):37–43.
37. Sporn MB. Carcinogenesis and cancer—different perspectives on the same disease. Cancer Res 1991; 51:6215–6218.
38. Willett WM, MacMahon B. Diet and cancer: an overview. N Engl J Med 1984; 310:697–703.
39. Smith MA, Parkinson DR, Cheson BD, Friedman, MA Retinoids in cancer therapy. J Clin Oncol 1992; 10:839–864.
40. Borden EC, Lotan R, Levens D, Young CW, Waxman S. Differentiation therapy of cancer: laboratory and clinical investigations. Cancer Res 1993; 53:4109–4115.
41. Gudas L. Hu L. The regulation and gene expression by retinoids in normal and tumorigenic epithelial cells. Proc Annu Meet Am Assoc Cancer Res 1993; 34:588–589.
42. Kitamura M, Shirasawa T, Mitarai T, Muramatsu T, Maruyama N. A retinoid responsive cytokine gene, MK is preferentially expressed in the proximal tubules of the kidney and human tumor cell lines. Am J Pathol 1993; 142(2):425–431.

43. Wagner H, Ruckdeschel JC. Screening, early detection, and early intervention strategies for lung cancer. Cancer Control, J Moffitt Cancer Center 1995; 6(2):493–502.

44. Gebert JF, Moghal N, Frangioni JV, Sugarbaker DJ, Neel BG. High frequency of retinoic acid receptor beta abnormalities in human lung cancer. Oncogene 1991; 6: 1859–1868.

45. Lotan R, Sozzi G, Ro J, Lee JS, Pastorino U, Pilotti S, Kurie J, Hong WK, Xu XC. Selective suppression of retinoic acid receptor b (RAR-b) expression in squamous metaplasia and in non–small cell lung cancers (NSCLC) compared to normal bronchial epithelium. Proc Am Soc Clin Oncol 1995; 14:165.

46. Lotan R, Xu XC, Lippman SM, Ro JY, Lee JS, Lee JJ, Hong WK. Suppression of retinoic acid receptor in premalignant oral lesions and its upregulation by isotretinoin. N Engl J Med 1995; 332:1405–1410.

47. Lippman SM, Heyman RA, Kurie JM, Benner SE, Hong WK. Reinoids and chemoprevention: clinical and basic studies. J Cell Biochem 1995; (suppl 22):1–10.

48. Huang M, Ye Y, Chen S, Chai JR, LU JX, Zhoa L, Gu LJ, Wang ZY. Use of all-*trans*-retinoic acid in the treatment of acute promyelocytic leukemia. Blood 1988; 72:567–572.

49. Alpha-Tocopherol, Beta Carotene Cancer Prevention Study Group. The effect of vitamin E and beta carotene on the incidence of lung cancer and other cancers in male smokers. N Engl J Med 1994; 330:1029–1035.

50. McLarty JW, Holiday DB, Girard WM, Yanagihara RH, Kummet TD, Greenberg SD. Beta-carotene, vitamin A, and lung cancer chemoprevention: results of an intermediate endpoint study. Am J Clin Nutr 1995; 62(6 suppl):1431S–1438S.

51. van Zandwijk N. *N*-Acetylcystene (NAC) and glutathione (GSH): antioxidant and chemopreventive properties, with special reference to lung cancer. J Cell Biochem 1995; (supplement 22):24–32.

52. Cochrane CG. Cellular injury by oxidants. Am J Med 1991; 91:23–30.

53. Webb WR. Clinical evaluation of a new mucolytic agent acetyl cysteine. J Thorac Cardiovasc Surg 1962; 44:330–343.

54. Meister A, Anderson M. Glutathione. Annu Rev Biochem 1983; 52:711–760.

55. Miller LF, Rumack BH. Clinical safety of high oral doses of acetylcysteine. Semin Oncol 1983; 10(suppl 1):76–85.

56. De Flora S, Cesarone CF, Balansky RM, Albini A, D'Agostini, F, Bennicelli C, Bagnasco M, Camoirano A, Scatolini L, Rovida A, Izzotti A. Chemopreventive properties and mechanisms of *N*-acytelcysteine. The experimental background. J Cell Biochem 1995; (suppl 22):33–41.

57. Conaway CC, Jiao D, Kelloff GJ, Steele VE, Rivenson A, Chung FL. Chemopreventive potential of fumaric acid, *N*-acetylcysteine, *N*-(4-hydroxyphenyl) retinamide and β-carotene for tobacco-nitrosamine induced lung tumors in A/J mice. Cancer Lett 1998; 124:85–93.

58. van Zandwijk N, Pastorino U, de Vries N, Dalesio O. EUROSCAN: the European Organization for Research and Treatment of Cancer (EORTC): chemoprevention study in lung cancer. Lung Cancer 1993; 9:351–356.

59. van Zandwijk N, Dalesio O, Pastorino U, et al. EUROSCAN, a randomized trial of vitamin A and *N*-acetylcysteine in patients with head and neck or lung cancer. J Natl Cancer Inst 2000; 92(12):977–986.

60. Menkes MS, Constock GW, Vuilleumier JP, et al. Serum beta carotene, vitamin A and E, and selenium and the risk of lung cancer. N Engl J Med 1986; 315:1250–1254.

61. Dimery I, Shirinian M, Heyne K, Lippman S, Fritsche H, Guillory C, Fossella F, Shin D, Hong WK. Reduction in toxicity of high-dose 13-*cis*-retinoic acid (13-cRA) with a tocopherol (AT). Proc Am Soc Clin Oncol 1992; 11:399.

62. Shin DM, Mao L, Papadimitrakopoulou V, El-Naggar A, Clayman G, Shin HJ, Lee JS, Lippman SM, Gillenwater A, Hittelman WN, Hong WK Modulation of biomarkers with biochemoprevention therapy in advanced premalignant lesions in the upper aerodigestive tract. Proc ASCO 1997; 16:A1557.

63. Shamberger RJ, Frost DV. Possible protective effect of selenium against human cancer. Can Med Assoc J 1969; 100:682.

64. van den Brandt PA, Goldbohm RA, van't Veer P, Bode P, Dorant E, Hermus RJJ, Sturmans F. A prospective cohort study on selenium status and the risk of lung cancer. Cancer Res 1993; 53:4860–4865.

65. Clark LC, Combs GF Jr, Turnbull BW, Slate EH, Chalker DK, Chow J, Davis LS, Glover RA, Graham GF, Gross EG, Krongrad A, Lesher JL Jr, Park HK, Sanders BB Jr, Smith CL, Taylor JR. Effects of selenium supplementation for cancer prevention in patients with carcinoma of the skin. A randomized controlled trial. Nutritional Prevention of Cancer Study Group. JAMA 1996; 276(24):1957–1963.

66. Blot WJ, Li JY, Taylor PR, Guo W, Dawsey S, Wang GQ, Yang CS, Zheng SF, Gail M, Li GY. Nutrition intervention trials in Linxian, China: supplementation with specific vitamin/mineral combinations, cancer incidence, and disease-specific mortality in the general population. J Natl Cancer Inst 1993; 85(18):1483–1492.

67. Hecht SS. Chemoprevention of lung cancer by isothiocyanates. Adv Exp Med Biol 1996;401:1–11.

68. Estenser RD, Wattenberg LW. Studies of the chemopreventive effects of myo-inositol on benzo[a]pyrene induced neoplasia of the lung and forestomach of female A/J mice. Carcinogenesis 1993; 14:1975–1977.

69. Wattenberg L. Chalcones, *myo*-inositol and other novel inhibitors of pulmonary carcinogenesis. J Cellular Biochem 1995; (suppl 22):162–168.

70. Wattenberg LW, Wiedmann TS, Estensen RD, Zimmerman CL, Steele VE, Kelloff GJ. Chemoprevention of pulmonary carcinogenesis by aerosolized budesonide in female A/J mice. Cancer Res 1997; 57(24):5489–5492.

71. Nelson JF, Karelus K, Bergman MD, Felicio LS. Neuroendocrine involvement in aging: evidence from studies of reproductive aging and caloric restriction. Neurobiol Aging 1995; 16(5):837–843.

72. Weindruch R. Dietary restriction, tumors, and aging in rodents. J Gerontol 1989; 44(6):67–71.

73. Yang G, Wang ZY, Kim S, Liao J, Seril DN, Chen X, Smith TJ, Yang CS. Characterization of early pulmonary hyperproliferation and tumor progression and their inhibition by black tea in a 4-(methylnitrosamino)-1-(3-pyridyl)-1-butanone-induced lung tumorigenesis model with A/J mice. Cancer Res 1997; 57(10):1889–1894.

74. Marquez C, Treston A, You L, Jakowlew S, Rice P, Malkinson A, Moody T. Chemoprevention of lung adenomas by BW2258U89. Proc Am Assoc Cancer Res 1996; 7:270.

75. Moody T, You L, Jakowlew S, Rice P, Malkinson A. Chemoprevention of lung adenomas by a VIP receptor antagonist. Proc Am Assoc Cancer Res 1996; 7:364.

76. Pastorino U, Infante M, Maioli M, et al. Adjuvant treatment of stage I lung cancer with high-dose vitamin A. J Clin Oncol 1993; 11(7):1216–1222.

77. Lippman SM, Lee JJ, Karp DD, Vokes EE, Benner SE, Goodman GE, Kardinal C, Winn RJ, Roth JA, Hong WK. Phase-III intergroup trial of 13-*cis*-retinoic acid to prevent second primary tumors in stage-I non–small cell lung cancer (NSCLC): interim report of NCI #I91-0001. Proc ASCO 1998; 17:A1753.

78. Thomas P, Rubinstein L, and the Lung Cancer Study Group. Cancer recurrence after resection: T_1N_0 non–small cell lung cancer. Ann Thorac Surg 1990; 49:242–246.

79. Kirkpatrick A, EORTC Central Office. Personal communication.

80. Huber MH, Lippman SM. Chemoprevention strategies. In: Pass HI, Mitchell JB, Johnson DH, Turrisi AT, eds. Lung Cancer: Principles and Practice. Philadelphia: Lippincott-Raven, 1996:351–358.

81. Lee JS, Lippman SM, Benner SE, Lee JJ, Ro JY, Lukeman JM, Morice RC, Peters EJ, Pang AC, Fritsche HA Jr. Randomized placebo-controlled trial of isotretinoin in chemoprevention of bronchial squamous metaplasia. J Clin Oncol 1994; 12:937–945.

82. Misset JL, Mathe G, Santelli G, Gouveia J, Homasson JP, Sudre MC, Gaget H. Regression of bronchial epidermoid metaplasia in heavy smokers with etretinate treatment. Cancer Detect Prev 1986; 9:167–170.

83. Current clinical trials: oncology. National Cancer Institute PDQ 1996; 3(3):199.

84. Beahrs OH, Henson DE, Hutter RVP, Kennedy BJ, eds. Handbook for Staging of Cancer. American Joint Committee on Cancer. Philadelphia: JB Lippincott, 1993: 129–136.

85. Travis WD, Linder J, Machay B. Classification, histology, cytology, and electron microscopy. In: Pass HI, Mitchell JB, Johnson DH, Turrisi AT, eds. Lung Cancer: Principles and Practice. Philadelphia: Lippincott-Raven, 1996:361–395.

86. Melamed MR, Zaman MB, Flehinger BH, Martini N. Radiologically occult in situ and incipient invasive epidermoid lung cancer: detection by sputum cytology in a survey of asymptomatic cigarette smokers. Am J Surg Pathol 1977; 1:5–16.

87. Frost JK, Ball WC Jr, Levin ML, Tockman MS, Erozan YS, Gupta PK, Eggleston JC, Pressman NJ, Donithan MP, Kimball AW Jr. Sputum cytopathology: use and potential in monitoring the workplace environment by screening for biological effects of exposure. J Occup Med 1986; 28(8):692–703.

88. Cameron R, Fringer J, Taylor C, Gilden R, Figlin RA. Practice guidelines for non–small cell lung cancer. Cancer J from Sci Am May/June 1996; 2(3A suppl):S69–S77.

89. Edell ES, Cortese DA. Photodynamic therapy. Its use in the management of broncho-genic carcinoma. Clin Chest Med 1995; 16(3):455–463.

90. Winn R. Personal communication.

91. Suh N, Wang Y, Honda T, et al. A novel synthetic oleanane triterpenoid, 2-cyano-3,12-dioxoolean-1,9-dien-28-oic acid, with potent differentiating, antiproliferative, and anti-inflammatory activity. Cancer Res 1999; 59(2):336–341.

22

Supportive Care in Thoracic Oncology: Perioperative Pulmonary Concerns

Earl King

Fox Chase Cancer Center, Philadelphia, Pennsylvania

INTRODUCTION

Surgical resection offers a patient presenting with non–small cell carcinoma the greatest potential for long-term survival. However, the bulk of patients presenting with lung cancer may not be surgical candidates owing to distant disease or are medically inoperable on the basis of significant lung limitation preoperatively or predicted insufficient lung function postoperatively. Other significant medical comorbidities may render the patient inoperable. Unfortunately, tobacco use not only contributes to the risk of developing lung cancer but also contributes greatly to the comorbidities rendering a patient medically inoperable. This chapter will focus on issues facing the multidisciplinary team in evaluating a patient for potential pulmonary resection from the perspective of a respiratory physician.

As respiratory physicians we are asked to evaluate patients preoperatively to identify risk factors that will portend a poor outcome and modify those risk factors that can be altered to improve outcomes. Goals of the preoperative visit can be outlined as follows.

1. Identify those patients with prohibitive risk to surgery (severely compromised lung function that will result in a respiratory death or respiratory cripple)
2. Modify risk factors to improve patient outcome (smoking cessation, antianginals, antihypertensives)
3. Initiate maximal bronchodilator therapy, instruct patient on proper usage to improve lung function (increase ventilatory reserve and gas exchange peripostoperatively)
4. Delineate those patients who will need additional testing prior to surgery (history/ECG evidence suggesting a patient would benefit from further cardiac evaluation/risk stratification/intervention)
5. Identify those patients who will benefit from surgery (staging confirms that the malignancy is confined to site of proposed resection)
6. Identify those patients who may benefit from increased postoperative interventions (increased attention to pulmonary toilet in those with limited perioperative ventilatory reserve)
7. Assess need for postoperative supplemental oxygen use long term (prepare patient and family for use of oxygen systems)
8. Educate patients and their families regarding postoperative function and expected symptoms (dyspnea with excessive activity)

RISK FACTORS

Risk factors that contribute to perioperative morality and morbidity include the following and will be discussed individually.

Extent of resection
Pulmonary dysfunction
Active smoking
Cardiac disease
Obesity
Age
Poor postoperative pain control

Extent of Resection

Historically the greater the extent of resection the higher the mortality, with the pneumonectomy rate being at least twice that of lobectomy (6.9% and 2.9%, respectively) (1). Segmental resection, though less desirable as a cancer operation, may offer long-term control of the malignancy with an acceptable operative mortality of 1.4% for those with severely compromised lung function (1). The largest series of patients undergoing pulmonary resection collected prospectively has reported operative mortalities of 4.97% for pneumonectomies, 0.39% for lobectomies, and 0.13% for segmental resections (2).

Pulmonary

Complications

With pulmonary resection a portion of an organ crucial to survival is removed. Surgical manipulation of the ventilatory apparatus and pulmonary parenchyma along with the anesthetic and postoperative pain control requirements set the stage for postoperative pulmonary complications. Complications include secretion retention (preoperative bronchitis, smoking, insufficient cough to generate sheering force due to pain, limited respiratory reserve), atelectasis (contributing to shunt fraction with resultant hypoxemia, ventilation/perfusion imbalance creating hypoxemia and hypercapnia, and increased work of breathing secondary to reduced lung compliance), and pneumonia from endogenous flora or nosocomial flora. The above contribute to the increased requirements for aggressive pulmonary toilet and bronchoscopy. More serious complications include respiratory failure necessitating invasive or noninvasive ventilatory support. Postpneumonectomy syndrome (3) and respiratory insufficiency are the most feared complications. Subcutaneous emphysema and air leak as a result of nonanatomical resection generally do not increase mortality but may contribute to increased patient discomfort and increased length of stay. Other complications occur less frequently but may contribute to substantial morbidity and mortality. They include stump dehiscence (4,5), empyema (6), lobar torsion and gangrene (7), pulmonary artery disruption, pulmonary vein thrombosis, bronchial artery disruption, and infarction of tissue (8–10). Recurrent laryngeal nerve dysfunction or postoperative vocal cord dysfunction will significantly impair cough effectiveness, contributing to the need for more aggressive pulmonary toilet support to prevent secretion retention.

Physiological Alterations of Thoracic Surgery

Prior to a discussion on pulmonary functional evaluation for thoracic resection, a discussion regarding the physiological alterations as a result of thoracic surgery is warranted. Much has been written on this subject but the core of observations predate modern anesthetic and surgical techniques.

Mucociliary transport is depressed and interrupted immediately postoperatively secondary to inhalational anesthetics (11); the other factor, tobacco smoke, impairs mucociliary transport pre- and postoperatively (11). Inhaled beta-agonists may facilitate ciliary function even in the absence of demonstrable airflow obstruction.

Cough force is reduced to <30% of preoperative levels and may only increase to >50% by day 7 postoperative (11). Stein (12) noted that a reduction in maximal expiratory flow is a predictor of postoperative pulmonary complications due to an ineffective cough. The patient with a severe restrictive ventilatory defect, however, will be able to generate sufficient airflow to clear secretions. This finding, coupled with the knowledge that cough force is necessary to generate airflow of sufficient sheer velocity to purge the airways of secretions, is the most relevant demand on aggressive and timely postoperative pain management and pulmonary toilet.

Lung compliance is significantly reduced as a result of imperfect reexpansion of remaining parenchyma within the resected and nonresected lobes, secondary to bruising of the parenchyma, loss of sigh secondary to narcotics, and shallow breathing as a result of the respiratory center's attempt to minimize the work of breathing (13–21).

Chest wall compliance decreases to $<50\%$ of the preoperative measurements whether or not lung parenchyma is resected. As a result of diminished lung and chest wall compliance, the work of breathing may be elevated to $>140\%$ of the preoperative levels. In a patient with marginal cardiac or respiratory reserve this may cause outright ventilatory failure even though predicted postoperative lung function may be adequate for sedentary existence (13–21).

As a result of the operation there is a reduction in the measured capacities (TLC, VC, FRC) and volumes (TV, ERV) with the end result being a higher ventilatory rate to preserve minute ventilation (14–22). Despite the preservation of minute ventilation this is an inefficient method of breathing owing to an increase in work of breathing and dead space ventilation with subsequent hypercapnia. The most important capacity affected is the functional residual capacity [FRC, volume of gas remaining in the lungs and airways at the end of tidal expiration; composite of expiratory reserve volume (ERV) and residual volume (RV)]. FRC reflects small airway patency and alveolar volume. The closing volume (CV) is a lung volume above the RV in which the dependent lung zones do not ventilate. When the CV is greater than FRC, atelectasis occurs in the dependent lung zones during tidal breathing. Hypoxemia occurs as a result of venous admixture created by shunt of capillary blood through atelectatic lung and ventilation perfusion inequality in surrounding parenchyma. The reduction in FRC occurs immediately with the induction of the anesthesia and is further compromised by the surgery and altered ventilatory pattern afterward (23,24).

Pulmonary Functional Evaluation

A pulmonary-specific history and examination in addition to a general medical history and examination is mandatory to uncover potential problems in the patient undergoing resection. Missing the presence of obstructive sleep apnea could create not only an airway problem for the anesthesiologist but also a potential catastrophe with increasing upper-airway compromise postoperatively. In general, a profile of daily living activities is useful to determine exercise tolerance, and a dyspnea assessment is useful to help remind patients and their families postoperatively that things were not normal preoperatively if they had significant limitation prior to surgery. Tobacco history and counseling is useful and may result in termination of smoking long term. Assessment of current symptoms may uncover areas to focus treatment efforts to optimize perioperative and postoperative function. Previous pulmonary problems are addressed as well (i.e., prior intubation for COPD exacerbation), which should heighten the vigilance of the postoperative care givers.

A plethora of tests, procedures, and indices have been advocated to determine the physiological operability of lung cancer patients. The core of information regarding outcomes (death, survival) has been collected over decades with updated reevaluation and refinement. In general they include measurements of pulmonary function (timed flows, volumes and capacities, diffusion), arterial blood gases and saturation, quantitation of ventilation and perfusion, exercise testing to determine maximum oxygen uptake, and predictors of outcome based on manipulation of the test results. While evaluating the patient who requires a resection several caveats must be kept in mind. First, the cancer patient does not have a static malignancy (doubling time of malignancy with certain cell types that are more likely to metastasize) and therefore the evaluation has to proceed with urgency. Second, an objectiveness to new complaints has to be maintained as an initial stage I patient may suddenly become a stage IV patient by virtue of discovering distant disease based on a new complaint. Third, in evaluating a patient for a "simple lobectomy" preparation and planning for a more extensive resection has to be anticipated with the potential of operative findings requiring a pneumonectomy. Finally, lung cancer resection offers the greatest potential for the longest disease-free survival and postoperative complications are not always predictable (i.e., DVT/PE, aspiration). Therefore, a certain acceptance of risk on behalf of the patient and surgeon has to occur in an otherwise fatal disease.

All patients undergoing lung resection should have preoperative pulmonary function tests. Postoperative complaints of dyspnea are frequent enough that a rational assessment of postoperative function can be predicted and the patient can be advised in advance of what to expect. Most patients with lung cancer have signs and symptoms of airflow limitation and emphysema. It is in these patients that a detailed assessment is often needed (25).

A significant contribution to the knowledge base present today regarding quantitation of loss of function came from the era of tuberculosis surgery (26–35). Observations made then have been better refined and detailed. A reasonable assessment of loss of function (conversely postoperative function) can be estimated with the knowledge that each segment of lung removed contributes roughly 1/19 of total lung function (total of 19 segments, with the superior segments of the lower lobes being larger); therefore, removing the right middle lobe will contribute to loss of 2/19 (10.5%) of total lung function (i.e., FEV_1, DLCO, VO_2

max). Unfortunately, lung function in patients with lung cancer is seldom uniform owing to airflow limitation and emphysema. Addition of quantitative perfusion lung scanning allows a more accurate partitioning of lung function participating in gas exchange after surgery (2,33–43).

Prior to the use of quantitative perfusion scanning bronchospirometry was used to partition lung function for pneumonectomy. Original tests were done by Jacobaeus (44) with a double-lumen rigid bronchoscope until Carlens (45) developed a flexible double-lumen catheter, the forerunner of today's double-lumen tube. Despite accurate assessments with this method (46), considerable skill was needed in placing these tubes, the patient discomfort was excessive, and it was a limited utility for pneumonectomy assessment alone. Other means of partitioning lung function were developed. A noninvasive means of partitioning lung function was advocated by the lateral position test, which establishes the FRC by having the patient perform spirometry in the right and left decubitus position (47–49). Again this test only allows partitioning of lung function to right and left lung and therefore is limited to assessment for pneumonectomy. In patients with obstructive lung disease this method may be unreliable (50,51).

Guidelines for limiting complications and death related to pneumonectomy were originally outlined in 1955 by Gaensler et al. (26) based upon maximum breathing capacity (now known as maximum voluntary ventilation) and forced vital capacity. Current opinion focuses on the predicted postoperative lung function, the simplest being spirometry. Olsen (52) used a minimum FEV_1 as a cutoff based on the work of Segall (53). He demonstrated that hypercapnia was more likely to occur with lung function less than 800 ml. In 1986 Gass and Olsen (33) introduced the concept of using the percent of predicted FEV_1, which considers the anthropometrics of the patient. The value proposed for a cutoff was a FEV_1 30% of predicted. Since then Markos has advocated using a cutoff of a FEV_1 of 40% of predicted as it pertains to a pneumonectomy. Spirometry and lung volumes test the airways and the bellows function of the ventilatory apparatus and should not be used to predict outcomes unrelated to their measurements, such as aspiration pneumonia, ischemic cardiac complications, and thromboembolism.

Diffusion capacity (DLCO) is a sensitive, but nonspecific test for pulmonary and cardiac disease. It measures the available alveolar-capillary surface area for gas diffusion, alveolar membrane integrity, and the capillary blood volume in the pulmonary parenchyma. The DLCO reflects vascular capacitance of the pulmonary parenchyma; it has been shown to be an independent predictor of risk of mortality after major lung resections and the percent of predicted DLCO has been associated with cardiovascular morbidity (54–59). A preoperative DLCO of 60% is considered adequate for pneumonectomy. A predicted postoperative DLCO of <40% indicates an increased risk for pneumonectomy. With lesser resections it is generally accepted that a DLCO >35% of predicted, postoperatively, is adequate although multiple authors have extended the cutoff especially if the FEV_1 is adequate.

The preoperative diffusion capacity in conjunction with quantitative perfusion can be used to help estimate the likelihood of oxygen requirements postoperatively. In general, regardless of the extent of resection, a patient with a predicted postoperative DLCO > 50% of predicted (ppo DLCO %pred) does not require oxygen. The finding of a ppo DLCO %pred < 35% often predicts the need for oxygen either continuously or with sustained exertion. Between 35 and 50% of predicted DLCO a large "gray zone" exists and to some extent the better the FEV_1 the less likely a patient will need oxygen. Owens (57) studied patients with obstructive lung disease and correlated exercise oxyhemoglobin desaturation with measurements of DLCO and FEV_1 and found a better correlation with the former.

Arterial blood gas analysis is included in predicting risk after thoracic resections (60–69). Currently there are no objective data to specify a cutoff value to prohibit resection. Preoperative hypoxemia may be secondary to a severe mismatch of ventilation and perfusion (partially obstructed bronchus with perfusion to the involved region requiring resection). Hypercapnia ($PaCO_2 > 45$) is uncommon when the FEV_1 is >1 L and unpredictable when the FEV_1 is less than 1 L. When hypercapnia is present with what appears to be adequate lung function, a careful search for muscle weakness and its potential cause is of great importance. Obstructive sleep apnea and/or obesity hypoventilation must be considered.

Exercise testing has been used to assess the need for pulmonary rehabilitation by delineating the cause of the dyspnea and by assessing the presence of suspected or known ischemic cardiac disease. Not surprisingly, this has been applied in the selection of marginal candidates for lung resection (70–81). With exercise a progressive increase in muscle oxygen consumption (VO_2) occurs with an increase in cardiac output and work performed. The maximum oxygen uptake (VO_2 max) or aerobic capacity occurs when increasing the workload does not lead to an increase in oxygen consumption (82,83). As a general rule the cardiovascular system determines the limits of oxygen consumption since the pulmonary vascular bed expands and ventilation increases to maintain adequate gas exchange. VO_2 max can be expressed in units of L/min or related to body mass, ml/kg/min. Bollinger (84) found a cutoff value of 60% of predicted VO_2 max as a single best indicator of postoperative complications after lung resection and the only deaths in his series occurred in patients with less than this measured value. Morice (73) identified preoperative high-risk criteria for lung resection (ppo $FEV_1 < 33\%$, $PaCO_2 > 45$, and preoperative $FEV_1 < 40\%$) and offered surgery to patients if VO_2 peak was > 50% of maximum predicted with no mortality in his series. The later study included patients undergoing limited resections and has no relevance to the patient requiring a pneumonectomy.

Interviewing the patient in detail can identify the potential maximum oxygen consumption based on the work of Myers et al. (85). Oxygen consumption at rest in a 40-year-old, 70-kg man is approximately 3.5 ml/kg/min or 1 MET (metabolic equivalent). Walking slowly on the level would lead to a VO_2 of 10.5 ml/kg/min (3 METs) and walking 4 miles in one hour or washing a car requires a VO_2 of 17.5 ml/kg/min (5 METs). Jogging slowly, rapidly walking up a flight of stairs, or moving heavy furniture leads to a VO_2 of 28 ml/kg/min (8 METs). The above findings give some credence to surgeons taking their patients for a walk preoperatively prior to more modern exercise regimens.

Smoking

Patients who continue to actively smoke up to the time of surgery will have an increase in postoperative pulmonary morbidity including secretion retention, atelectasis, and pneumonia. Studies by Carrel et al. (86), Laszlo et al. (87), and Wightman (88) clearly demonstrate an increase in the above complications in those who smoke. The effect of nicotine and elevated carbon monoxide (tachycardia, decreased oxygen-carrying capacity) (89,90) contribute also to an increased cardiovascular morbidity. The presence of decreased ciliary function (11) and an increase in tracheobronchial bacterial pathogen burden, along with poor oral hygiene, contribute to the respiratory complications encountered.

Smoking cessation programs have to be multifaceted including behavioral and pharmacological (88) therapies with encouragement by the thoracic surgeon and pulmonary specialist. Secondhand smoke must be strongly discouraged. For the patient with severely limited lung function a period of smoking cessation coupled with an intensive course of bronchodilator therapy must precede resection by at least 2 weeks. Unfortunately, the full benefit of prolonged smoking cessation cannot be realized in the lung cancer patient owing to the time constraints of rapid therapy. The primary-care provider can initiate such programs as the patient is undergoing preliminary evaluations.

Cardiovascular Conditions

Cardiovascular complications (56,57,69) after lung resection occur with an overall incidence of 25% (81,91–94). These include arrhythmias, myocardial infarction, right heart failure, and cardiogenic pulmonary edema. The patient for pulmonary resection is frequently old, smokes, and has significant underlying airflow obstruction. Therefore, the limitation imposed by preexisting obstructive lung disease impairs the assessment for risk from significant underlying coronary disease. Further cardiovascular risk assessment should be considered in patients with risk factors of advanced age and prior vascular events (ischemic neurological events, claudication). Patients with unstable coronary syndromes, untreated or uncontrolled rhythm disturbances, and poorly compensated congestive heart failure should not undergo surgery (95) until maximally treated either medically or by mechanical intervention. On occasion in patients needing urgent coronary revascularization, combining coronary artery bypass with resection of a pulmonary malignancy is feasible. In those patients with severe aortic/mitral stenosis, valvuloplasty may be a temporizing measure to allow pulmonary resection first, followed at a later date by valve replacement or repair.

Obesity

The obese patient presenting for pulmonary resection is disadvantaged from a surgical, anesthetic, cardiopulmonary, and nursing standpoint. The operative procedure may be technically more difficult and postoperative wound healing may be delayed. Airway management is more difficult secondary to redundant tissues of the upper airway creating a more difficult intubation sequence (96,97). Furthermore, with obesity there is a more rapid oxyhemoglobin desaturation secondary to a lower FRC (alveolar oxygen stores) and an elevated closing volume so that during spontaneous breathing there is closure of basilar/dependent lung units and subsequent severe V/Q mismatch (15). Upper-airway closure secondary to preexisting obstructive sleep apnea may worsen postoperatively as a result of pain control requirements creating the potential for further derangement of gas exchange. Postoperative ambulation and mobilization is more difficult for the obese patient contributing to the already increased risk of deep vein thrombosis and thromboemboli (98).

Age

With advanced age there is an increase in other serious medical illnesses that contribute to poor postoperative outcomes (99–101). From a pulmonary standpoint there is a predictable decrement in FEV_1 and maximum voluntary ventilation along with a decrease in cough force. The chest wall compliance decreases with aging and there is an increase in the closing volume and residual volume, which creates an increase in the alveolar arterial oxygen gradient.

Pain Control

Pain after thoracic surgery is severe and prevents the patient from participating in his or her bronchial hygiene and normal ventilatory pattern. As a result of the skin incision, muscle interruption, pleural violation, and costovertebral strain (and the occasional rib resection/fracture), the pattern of breathing after thoracotomy is frequently one that minimizes pain. The pattern of breathing is one of active expiration, expiratory muscle contraction (splinting), and limited inspiration with an ineffective cough. As a result there is secretion retention, atelectasis, potential for pneumonia, increased ventilation perfusion inequality, hypoxemia, increased work of breathing, and the possibility of respiratory failure.

Options for pain control include cryoanalgesia, intrapleural regional analgesia, epidural narcotic/anesthetic, intercostal nerve blocks, patient-controlled analgesia, and intravenous narcotic administration. Cryoanalgesia provides effective long-term intercostal nerve block with the major potential side effects of dysesthesias and long-term intercostal muscle paralysis (102–105). Epidural opioid administration with either morphine or fentanyl with or without a local anesthetic such as bupivacaine is the most commonly utilized method of pain control (106–109). The major side effects of respiratory depression are easily managed with a decrease in the infusion rate and/or naloxone. Urinary retention is prevented with bladder intubation at time of surgery and pruritus is controlled with small doses of naloxone or antihistamines. With effective epidural opioid administration there is an increase in expiratory flows, vital capacity, and FRC (110). Intrapleural regional analgesia is accomplished by placing a catheter percutaneously into the thorax positioned between the visceral and parietal pleural surface (111,112). A local anesthetic is then infused into the pleural space. Failures are due to a runoff of the anesthetic via the chest tube, dilution of the anesthetic by blood or fluid, and partitioning of the anesthetic secondary to loculations (113).

SUMMARY

Preoperative evaluation of the thoracic cancer patient is valuable in assessing what risk factors can be modified to decrease postoperative morbidity and mortality. Smoking cessation can be initiated at the primary-care delivery site and supplemented upon referral to the thoracic surgeon and respiratory physician. Frequently, marginal candidates for resection due to ventilatory limitations can be rescued with intensive bronchodilator therapy and smoking cessation. An assessment of postoperative function can be estimated with readily available tests of lung function in conjunction with radionuclide scanning. The patient and family can be educated on the potential life-style changes that may occur as a result of thoracic resection, namely the potential need for oxygen use. Pain relief is of paramount importance not only for patient comfort but also for effective pulmonary toileting. Effective relief of pain can be achieved in a variety of fashions and each institution may have its favored method.

REFERENCES

1. Ginsberg RJ, Hill LD, Egan RT, et al. Modern thirty day operative mortality for surgical resection in lung cancer. J Thorac Cardiovasc Surg 1983; 86:654–658.
2. Miller JI. Physiologic evaluation of pulmonary function in the candidate for lung resection. J Thorac Cardiovasc Surg 1993; 105:347–352.
3. Zeldin RA, Normandin D, Landtwing D, Peters RM. Postpneumonectomy pulmonary edema. J Thorac Cardiovasc Surg 1984; 87:359–365.

4. Vester SR, Faber LP, Kittle F, Warren WH, Jensik RJ. Bronchopleural fistula after stapled closure of bronchus. Ann Thorac Surg 1991; 52:1253–1258.
5. Hankins JR, Miller JE, Attar S, et al. Bronchopleural fistula. Thirteen-year experience with 77 cases. J Thorac Cardiovasc Surg 1978; 176:755–762.
6. Shamji FM, Ginsberg RJ, Cooper JD, et al. Open window thoracostomy in the management of postpneumonectomy empyema with or without bronchopleural fistula. J Thorac Cardiovasc Surg 1983; 86:818–822.
7. Kucich VA, Villarreal JR, Schwartz DB. Left upper lobe torsion following lower lobe resection. Early recognition of a rare complication. Chest 1989; 95:1146–1147.
8. Nagasaki F. Complications of surgery in treatment of carcinoma of the lung. Chest 1982; 82:25–29.
9. Busch E, Verazin G, Antkowiak JG, et al. Pulmonary complications in patients undergoing thoracotomy for lung carcinoma. Chest 1994; 105:760–766.
10. Downey RJ. Perioperative care of the patient undergoing lung resection. In: Alfred P Fishman, Pulmonary Diseases and Disorders, 3rd edition, New York: McGraw-Hill, 1998. Chapter 104, 1649–1660.
11. Gamdu G. Postoperative impairment of mucous transport in the lung. Am Rev Respir Dis 1976; 114:673–675.
12. Stein M, Cassara EL. Preoperative pulmonary evaluation and therapy for surgery patients. JAMA 1970; 211:787–790.
13. Peters R, Wallons H, Howe T. Total compliance and work of breathing after thoracotomy. J Thorac Cardiovasc Surg 1969; 57:348.
14. Bolton J, Weiman D. Physiology of lung resection. Clin Chest Med 1993; 14:293–303.
15. Sabanathan S, Eng J, Mearns A. Alterations in respiratory mechanics following thoractomy. JR Coll Surg Edinb 1990; 35:144–150.
16. Bremer JL. The fate of the remaining lung tissue after lobectomy or pneumonectomy. J Thorac Surg 1936; 6:336.
17. Smith TC, Cook FD, Dekornfeld TJ, et al. Pulmonary function in the immediate postoperative period. J Thorac Cardiovasc Surg 1960; 39:788.
18. Woodruff W, Merkel CG, Wright GW. Decisions in thoracic surgery as influenced by the knowledge of pulmonary physiology. J Thorac Surg 1953; 26:156.
19. Brownlee WE, Allbritten FF Jr. The significance of the lung-thorax compliance in ventilation during thoracic surgery. J Thorac Surg 1956; 32:454.
20. Martin FE, Stead WW. Physiologic studies following thoracic surgery. III. Ventilatory studies in the immediate postoperative period. J Thorac Surg 1953; 25:417.
21. Birath G, Crafoord C, Rudstrom P. Pulmonary function after pneumonectomy and lobectomy. J Thorac Surg 1947; 16:492.
22. Birath G. Lung function after pneumonectomy in man. Clin Sci 1965; 29:59–72.
23. Rehder K, Cameron PD, Krayer S. New dimensions of the respiratory system. Anaesthesiology 1985; 62:230–233.
24. Hendenstierna G, Tokics L, Standberg A, et al. Correlation of gas exchange impairment to development of atelectasis during anaesthesia and muscle paralysis. Acta Anaesth Scand 1986; 30:183–191.
25. Marshall MC, Olsen GN. The physiologic evaluation of the lung resection candidate. Clin Chest Med 1993; 14:305–320.

26. Gaensler EA, Cugell DW, Lindgren T, et al. The role of pulmonary insufficiency in mortality and invalidism following surgery for pulmonary tuberculosis. J Thorac Surg 1955; 29:163–187.

27. Mittman C. Assessment of operative risk in thoracic surgery. Am Rev Respir Dis 1961; 84:197–207.

28. Lockwood P. Lung function test results and the risk of post-thoracotomy complications. Respiration 1973; 30:529–542.

29. Boushy SF, Billig DM, North LB, Helgason A. Clinical course related to preoperative and postoperative pulmonary function in patients with bronchogenic carcinoma. Chest 1961; 59:383–391.

30. Boysen PG, Block AJ, Moulder PV. Relationship between preoperative pulmonary function tests and complications after thoracotomy. Surg Gynecol Obstet 1981; 152:813–815.

31. Block AJ, Olsen GN. Preoperative pulmonary function testing. JAMA 1976; 235: 257–258.

32. Miller JI. Pulmonary function test criteria for operability and pulmonary resection. Surg Gynecol Obstet 1981; 153:893–895.

33. Gass GD, Olsen GN. Preoperative pulmonary function testing to predict postoperative morbidity and mortality. Chest 1986; 89:127–135.

34. Markos J. Preoperative assessment as a predictor or mortality and morbidity after lung resection. Am Rev Respir Dis 1989; 139:902–910.

35. Kristersson S, Lindell S, Svanberg L. Prediction of pulmonary function loss due to pneumonectomy using ^{133}Xe-radiospirometry. Chest 1972; 62:696–698.

36. Olsen, GN, Block AJ, Tobias JA. Prediction of post-pneumonectomy pulmonary function using quantitative macroaggregate lung scanning. Chest 1974; 66: 13–16.

37. Boysen PG, Block AJ, Olsen GN, Moulder PV, et al. Prospective evaluation for pneumonectomy using the [99m]technetium quantitative perfusion lung scan. Chest 1977; 72:422–425.

38. Boysen PG, Harris JO, Block AJ, Olsen GN. Prospective evaluation for pneumonectomy using perfusion scanning. Follow-up beyond one year. Chest 1981; 80: 163–166.

39. Bria WF, Kanarek DJ, Kazemi H. Prediction of post-operative pulmonary function following thoracic operations. J Thorac Cardiovasc Surg 1983; 86:186–192.

40. Ali MK, Ewer MS, Atallah MR, et al. Regional and overall pulmonary function changes in lung cancer: correlations with tumor stage, extent of pulmonary resection, and patient survival. J Thorac Cardiovasc Surg 1983; 86:1–8.

41. Wernly JA. Clinical value of quantitative ventilation-perfusion lung scans in the surgical management of bronchogenic carcinoma. J Thorac Cardiovasc Surg 1980; 80:535–543.

42. Ali MK. Predicting loss of pulmonary function after pulmonary resection for bronchogenic carcinoma. Chest 1980; 7:337–341.

43. Zeiher BG. Predicting post-operative pulmonary function in patients undergoing lung resection. Chest 1995; 108:68–72.

44. Jacobaeus HC. A bronchospirometric study on the ability of the human lungs to substitute for one another. Acta Med Scand 1940; 105(3):193–210.

45. Carlens E. A new flexible double lumen catheter for bronchospirometry. J Thorac Surg 1949; 18:742–746.

46. Neuhaus H, Cerniack NS. A bronchospirometric method of estimating the effect of pneumonectomy on the maximum breathing capacity. J Thorac Cardiovasc Surg 1968; 55:144–148.

47. Bergan F. A simple method for determination of the relative function of the right and left lung. Acta Chir Scand 1960; 253(suppl). 58.

48. Marion JM, Alderson PO, Lefrak SS, et al. Unilateral lung function. Chest 1976; 69:5.

49. Walkup RH, Vossel LD, Griffin JP, Proctor RJ. Prediction of postoperative pulmonary function with the lateral position test: a prospective study. Chest 1980; 77: 24–27.

50. Jay SJ, Stonehill RB, Kiblani SO, Norton J. Variability of the lateral position test in normal subjects. Am Rev Respir Dis 1980; 121:165–168.

51. Schoonover GA, Olson GN, Habibian MR, Edwards DG, Spurrier P. Lateral position test and quantitative lung scan in the preoperative evaluation for lung resection. Chest 1984; 86:854–859.

52. Olsen GN. Pulmonary function evaluations of the lung resection candidate: a prospective study. Am Rev Respir Dis 1975; 111:379–387.

53. Segall J. Ventilatory capacity in chronic bronchitis in relation to carbon dioxide retention. Scand J Respir Dis 1966; 47:215–219.

54. Weinberger SE. Use and interpretation of the single-breath diffusing capacity. Chest 1980; 78(3):483–488.

55. Owens GR. The diffusing capacity as a predictor of arterial oxygen desaturation during exercise in patients with chronic obstructive pulmonary disease. N Engl J Med 1984; 310:1218–1221.

56. Ferguson MK, Little L, Rizzo L, et al. Diffusing capacity predicts morbidity and mortality after pulmonary resection. J Thorac Cardiovasc Surg 1988; 96:894–900.

57. Markos J, Mullan BP, Hillman DR, et al. Pre-operative assessment as a predictor of mortality and morbidity after lung resection. Am Rev Respir Dis 1989; 139: 902–910.

58. Menna Barreto SS, McClean PA, Szalai JP, Zamel N. Reduction of lung diffusion for carbon monoxide in patients with lung carcinoma. Chest 1993; 103:1142–1146.

59. Ferguson MK. Optimizing selection of patients for major lung resection. J Thorac Cardiovasc Surg 1995; 109:275–283.

60. Stein M, Koota GM, Simon M, Frank HA. Pulmonary evaluation of surgical patients. JAMA 1962; 181:765–770.

61. Keagy BA, Lores ME, Starek PJ, et al. Elective pulmonary lobectomy: factors associated with morbidity and operative mortality. Ann Surg 1985; 40:349–352.

62. Kristersson S, Lindell SE, Svanberg L. Prediction of pulmonary function loss due to pneumonectomy using ^{133}Xe-radiospirometry. Chest 1972; 62:694–698.

63. Boushy SF, Billig DM, North LB, Helgason AH. Clinical course related to preoperative and postoperative pulmonary function in patients with bronchogenic carcinoma. Chest 1972; 59:383–391.

64. Kearney DJ, Lee TH, Reilly JJ, et al. Assessment of operative risk in patients under-

going lung resection. Importance of predicted pulmonary function. Chest 1994; 105:753–759.

65. VanNostrand D, Kjelsberg MO, Humphrey EW. Preresectional evaluation of risk from pneumonectomy. Surg Gynecol Obstet 1968; 127:306–312.

66. Milledge JS, Nunn JF. Criteria of fitness for anesthesia in patients with chronic obstructive lung disease. Br Med J 1975; 3:670–673.

67. Zibrak J. Indications for pulmonary function testing. Ann Intern Med 1990; 112: 763–771.

68. Tisi GM. Preoperative evaluation of pulmonary function. Am Rev Respir Dis 1979; 119:293–310.

69. Burrows B. Chronic obstructive pulmonary disease: interrelationships of pulmonary function data. Am Rev Respir Dis 1965; 91:861–868.

70. Weber K, Janicki J, McElroy P, Reddy H. Concepts and applications of cardiopulmonary exercise testing. Chest 1988; 93:843–847.

71. Schraufnagel DE, Rivington RN, Pardy RL. Exercise testing in evaluation of patients for lung resection. Am Rev Respir Dis 1982; 125:605–606.

72. Smith TP, Kinasewitz GT, Tucker WY, et al. Exercise capacity as a predictor of postthoracotomy morbidity. Am Rev Respir Dis 1984; 129:730–734.

73. Bechard D, Wetstein L. Assessment of exercise oxygen consumption as preoperative criterion for lung resection. Ann Thorac Surg 1987; 44:344–349.

74. Miyoshi S, Nakahara K, Ohno K, et al. Exercise tolerance test in lung cancer patients: the relationship between exercise capacity and post-thoracotomy hospital mortality. Ann Thorac Surg 1987; 44:487–490.

75. Olsen GN, Weiman DS, Bolton JWR, et al. Submaximal invasive exercise testing and quantitative lung scanning in the evaluation for tolerance of lung resection. Chest 1989; 55:267–273.

76. Morice RC, Peters EJ, Ryan MB, et al. Exercise testing in the evaluation of patients at high risk for complications from lung resection. Chest 1992; 101:356–361.

77. Holden DA, Rice TW, Stelmach K, Meeker DP. Exercise testing, 6-min. walk, and stair climb in the evaluation of patients at high risk for lung resection. Chest 1992; 102:1774–1779.

78. Nakagawa K, Nakahara K, Miyoshi S, Kawashima Y. Oxygen transport during incremental exercise load as a predictor of operative risk in lung cancer patients. Chest 1992; 101:1369–1375.

79. Dales RE. Preoperative prediction of pulmonary complications following thoracic surgery. Chest 1993; 104:155–159.

80. Walsh GL. Resection of lung cancer is justified in high risk patients selected by exercise oxygen consumption. Ann Thorac Surg 1994; 58:704–711.

81. Pate P. Preoperative assessment of the high risk patient for lung resection. Ann Thorac Surg 1996; 61:1494–1500.

82. Morice RC. Redefining the lowest exercise peak oxygen consumption acceptable for lung resection of high risk patients. Chest 1996; 110(suppl):161S.

83. Wait J. Cardiopulmonary stress testing. A review of non-invasive approaches. Chest 1996; 90:504–510.

84. Bollinger CT. Exercise capacity as a predictor of post-operative complications in lung resection candidates. Am J Respir Crit Care Med 1995; 151:1472–1480.

85. Myers J, Do D, Herbert W, et al. A nomogram to predict exercise capacity from a specific activity questionnaire and clinical data. Am J Cardiol 1994; 73:591–596.
86. Carrel T, et al. Preoperative assessment of the likelihood of infection of the lower respiratory tract after cardiac surgery. J Thorac Cardiovasc Surg 1991; 39: 85–88.
87. Laszlo G, et al. The diagnosis and prophylaxis of pulmonary complications of surgical operation. Br J Surg 1973; 60:129–134.
88. Wightman JAK. A prospective survey of the incidence of postoperative pulmonary complications. Br J Surg 1968; 55:85.
89. Stromskag KE, Minor B, Steen PA, et al. Side effects and complications related to intrapleural analgesia: an update. Acta Anaesthesiol Scand 1990; 34:473.
90. Pearce AC, Jones RM, et al. Smoking and anesthesia: preoperative abstinence and perioperative morbidity. Anesthesiology 1984; 61:576.
91. Eagle KA, et al. Guidelines for perioperative cardiovascular evaluation for noncardiac surgery. Report of the American College of Cardiology/American Heart Association Task Force on Practice Guidelines. Circulation 1996; 93:1278.
92. Keagy BA, Schorlemmer GR, Murray GF, et al. Correlation of preoperative pulmonary function testing with clinical course in patients after pneumonectomy. Ann Thorac Surg 1983; 36:253.
93. Patel RL, Townsend ER, Fountain SW, et al. Elective pneumonectomy: factors associated with morbidity and operative mortality. Ann Thorac Surg 1992; 54:84.
94. Pierce RJ. Preoperative risk evaluation for lung cancer resection: predicted postoperative product as a predictor of surgical mortality. Am J Respir Crit Care Med 1994; 947–55.
95. American Thoracic Society. Comprehensive outpatient management of COPD. Am J Respir Crit Care Med 1995; 152:84–96.
96. Wahi R, McMurtrey MS, DeCaro LF, et al. Determinates of perioperative morbidity and mortality after pneumonectomy. Ann Thorac Surg 1989; 48:33.
97. Wilson SL, Mantena NR, Hulverson JD, et al. Effects of atropine, glycopyrrolate, and cimetidine on gastric secretions in morbidly obese patients. Anesth Analg 1981; 60:37.
98. Rocke DA, Murray WB, Rout CC, et al. Relative risk analysis of factors associated with difficult intubation in obstetric anesthesia. Anesthesiology 1992; 77:67.
99. Pasulka PS, Bistrian BR, Benotti PN, et al. The risks of surgery in obese patients. Ann Intern Med 1986; 104:540.
100. Djokovic JL, Hedley-Whyte J, et al. Prediction of outcome of surgery and anesthesia in patients over 80. JAMA 1979; 242:2301.
101. Dripps RD, et al. Postoperative atelectasis and pneumonia: diagnosis, etiology and management based upon 1,240 cases of upper abdominal surgery. Ann Surg 1946; 124:94.
102. Hallen B. Computerized anesthesia record keeping. Acta Anal Scand 1973; 52(suppl):47.
103. Katz J. Cryoanalgesia for post-thoracotomy pain. Ann Thorac Surg 1989; 48:5.
104. Muller LC, Salzer GM, Ransmayr G, et al. Intraoperative cryoanalgesia for postthoracotomy pain relief. Ann Thorac Surg 1989; 48:15.
105. Maiwand MO, Makey AR, Reed A, et al. Cryoanalgesia after thoracotomy. Im-

provement of technique and review of 600 cases. J Thorac Cardiovasc Surg 1986; 92:291.

106. Rooney S, Jain S, McCormack P, et al. A comparison of pulmonary function tests for postthoracotomy pain using cryoanalgesia and transcutaneous nerve stimulation. Ann Thorac Surg 1986; 41:204.

107. Behar M, Magora F, Olshwang D, et al. Epidural morphine in the treatment of pain. Lancet 1979; 1:527.

108. Shulman MS, Sandler AN, Bradley JW, et al. Post-thoracotomy pain and pulmonary function following epidural and systemic morphine. Anesthesiology 1984; 61: 569–575.

109. Rawal N, Sjostrand U, Dahlstrom B, et al. Postoperative pain relief by epidural morphine. Anesth Analg 1981; 60:726.

110. Bromage PH, Camporesi E, Leslie J, et al. Epidural narcotics for postoperative analgesia. Anesth Analg 1980; 59:473.

111. Torda TA, Pybus DA, et al. Clinical experience with epidural morphine. Anaesth Intensive Care 1981; 9:129–134.

112. Ferrante FM, Chan VW, Arthur GR, et al. Intrapleural analgesia after thoracotomy. Anesth Analg 1991; 72:105.

113. Scheinin B, Lindgren L, Rosenberg PH, et al. Treatment of post-thoracotomy pain with intermittent instillations of intrapleural bupivocaine. Acta Anaesthesiol Scand 1989; 33:156.

23

Supportive Care in Thoracic Oncology: Chemoradiation Pneumonitis and Esophagitis—Characteristics and Management

Sandra McDonald and Jan Dombrowski
Genesee Hospital, Rochester, New York

Jacqueline Williams and Philip Rubin
University of Rochester Cancer Center, Rochester, New York

INTRODUCTION

Concurrent chemotherapy and radiation is increasingly utilized in patients with both small cell and non–small cell lung cancer, where damage to normal lung and esophagus is unavoidable and dose-limiting. Pulmonary complications resulting from anticancer therapy can range from acute fatal respiratory distress to varying degrees of chronic pulmonary compromise, which can manifest years after the initial cancer therapy. Additionally, in young children, lung and thoracic development can be impaired, augmenting the direct pulmonary sequelae of therapy. Understanding the pathophysiology of radiation/chemotherapy lung injury is essential in planning new directions of treatment where, classically, our efforts to improve survival have been focused on giving higher doses of radiation and drugs, as well as combining therapies.

The clinical syndrome of radiation pneumonitis develops in 5–20% of all irradiated patients (1–3). Factors that can add to the development of radiation pneumonitis include concomitant chemotherapy, previous irradiation, withdrawal of steroids, and postradiation surgery (4). Age and underlying chronic obstructive pulmonary disease do not appear to play a role in the development of radiation pneumonitis.

The list of anticancer drugs known to cause pulmonary toxicity has grown, and it is estimated that 5–10% of patients taking chemotherapy may experience an adverse pulmonary reaction. As multidrug regimens, multimodality therapies, and dose-intensive protocols increase patients' exposure, the potential for treatment-induced toxicity may become even greater. Some agents are more commonly associated with pulmonary complications [e.g., bleomycin, mitomycin, carmustine (BCNU), cytosine arabinoside (Ara-C), interleukin-2, and methotrexate], while others rarely are (5). Factors that increase the incidence and severity of drug toxicity include: concomitant administration of oxygen (bleomycin, BCNU, interleukin-2, Ara-C); radiation therapy (doxorubicin, actinomycin D, cyclophosphamide, methotrexate, bleomycin, mitomycin); route of administration; going above an established cumulative threshold dose (bleomycin, BCNU, chlorambucil); comorbidities (renal dysfunction); and age (the very young and the elderly).

Esophageal complications are a frequent acute side effect of anticancer radiochemotherapy and may be dose-limiting. In the acute phase, the abnormalities created by chemotherapy and radiation are relatively similar. Late complications are rare, but may be severe. Chemotherapy agents such as 5-FU, methotrex-

TABLE 1 Incidence of Acute Esophagitis with Different Treatment Regimens (6–9)

Radiation		Chemotherapy		
Fractionation	Total dose (Gy)	Timing	Type	% Esophagitis > grade III
2 Gy qd	60	Induction	P/Vbl	1.3%
2 Gy qd	60	Concurrent	P/Vbl	6%
1.8 Gy qd	45	Concurrent	P/E	11%
1.5 Gy bid	45	Concurrent	P/E	27%
1.2 Gy bid	69.6	Concurrent	P/E	34%
1.6 Gy bid[a]	73.6	NA	None given	18% acute; 30% late
1.5 Gy tid[b]	54	NA	None given	4%

[a] Concurrent boost 1.25 Gy (6).
[b] CHART (7).
P = cisplatin; Vbl = velban; E = etoposide; NA = not applicable.

ate, and other drugs such as purine antagonists can frequently cause esophagitis. The incidence of moderate to severe esophagitis increases from 1% (with standard radiation) to 34% (with concurrent, hyperfractionated radiation and chemotherapy) (Table 1) (6–9). Concomitant doxorubicin greatly exacerbates the reaction, and some "radiation-recall" esophagitis is commonly observed with doxorubicin-containing regimens given after thoracic radiotherapy. Children are at higher risk of developing later esophageal stricture after receiving doxorubicin with radiation doses of 40 Gy or higher (10). Severe esophageal injury has been seen in patients with HIV with modest doses of irradiation (11,12).

PULMONARY TOXICITY

Radiation

Pathophysiology

The histopathological changes and resultant physiological abnormalities of pulmonary toxicity are relatively similar for both radiation and chemotherapy. However, cytotoxic drugs affect the entire lung, whereas radiation changes are generally confined to the region of the lung that has been radiated.

A large spectrum of histological changes due to radiation has been documented in animals; the data for humans remain incomplete since the discussion on pathophysiological changes reflects in vivo studies on normal, nondiseased lungs. It is likely, however, that even small doses of radiation would result in histological changes in most patients and that preexisting lung disease impacts the effects of both drugs and radiation on the lung.

Histopathological changes of radiation-induced pulmonary toxicity can be divided into four phases (13), based on the time course after radiation and distinct histological and molecular alterations:

Latent Phase. This is the period extending from immediately after irradiation, but prior to the overt appearance of radiation pneumonitis, and ranges from 1 to 3 months. Although no clinical or histological changes at the light microscopic level have been noted during this time, electron microscopic studies (14–16) suggest that damage to the type II pneumocyte and the endothelial cell are closely linked to the development of the pneumonitic process. The type II pneumocyte, which produces surfactant and maintains patent alveoli, has been well studied. After radiation exposure, a rapid decrease in the content of cytoplasmic surfactant-containing lamellar bodies occurs, followed by ultimate sloughing of some of the cells into the alveolar lumen (17,18). Change in the surfactant levels leading to alterations in alveolar surface tension and low compliance is, most likely, a direct result of the radiation on type II cells (15,19,20), although it has been postulated to indirectly result from exudation of plasma proteins (21,22).

Endothelial cell damage results in changes in perfusion and permeability of vessel wall. In the first few days to weeks after irradiation, ultrastructural alterations in the capillary endothelial lining become evident. The cells become pleomorphic, vacuolated, and may slough, producing areas of denuded basement membrane and occlusion of the capillary lumen by debris and thrombi (22–24). These phenomena are dose dependent; scattered changes can be seen at 5 Gy, but lesions become widespread following increasingly lethal doses of irradiation. However, death only occurs during the period when obvious histological damage is noted.

Ongoing research by our group and others (25–28) suggests that cytokine-mediated multicellular interactions, initiating and sustaining the fibrogenic process, take place within hours to days after radiation. Studies by Hallahan et al. (23,29) have demonstrated dose-dependent, increased levels of adhesion molecules (ICAM-1, P-selectin, E-selectin) in mice within hours of irradiation following doses as low as 2 Gy. Such expression was shown, through the use of transgenic knockout models, to be directly related to inflammatory cell infiltration into the irradiated lung. Similarly, we and others have shown an early induction of the proinflammatory cytokine, tumor necrosis factor-alpha (TNFα) (28, 30), and our group has demonstrated subsequently that disruption of the TNF-signaling pathway at the CD40-CD40 ligand leads to reduced pulmonary inflammation (31). It is now generally accepted that the immediate expression of injury after radiation leads to synthesis and secretion of numerous growth and inhibitory factors. This cascade of events continues for weeks to months, during the so-called latent period, and ultimately results in the expression of late effects. Since both radiation and chemotherapy induce similar cytokine responses, there is a suggestion that common molecular mechanisms may be the basis for enhanced late-effect injury following combined-modality approaches. It is therefore conceivable that modulation of growth factors, administration of cytokines or anticytokines, or interference in intercellular signaling pathways may be used to modify the severity of these reactions (32). These will be discussed later.

Pneumonitis.   Depending on the radiation dose, there may be resolution, or the next phase of radiation pneumonitis, with associated clinical symptoms and signs, may develop within 6 months of lung irradiation.

Initially there is exudation of proteinaceous material into the alveoli, leading to impairment of gas exchange. An infiltration of inflammatory cells consisting of macrophages, lymphocytes, and mononuclear cells, as well as desquamation of epithelial cells from the alveolar walls, occurs (14,33), and diffuse alveolar damage is seen. Within a few weeks, the interstitial edema organizes into collagen fibrils, which eventually leads to thickening of the alveolar septa. Depending on the volume of lung parenchyma irradiated, the total dose, and the dose per fraction, these exudative changes can result in the potentially fatal clinical syndrome of acute radiation pneumonitis.

This period is closely associated with the increased expression of chemokines. This increased expression is due, at least in part, to the release of TNFα from type II pneumocytes/endothelial cells/macrophages in the irradiated lung; the chemokines then act in an autocrine/paracrine fashion to stimulate the further release of chemokines from cells including macrophages, epithelial cells, and fibroblasts. Chemokines are a growing superfamily of chemotactic peptides that play a role in the recruitment of inflammatory cells into sites of pulmonary infection or damage. The superfamily has been subdivided into classes based on the organization of the first pair of conserved cysteine motifs and the cell types affected. C × C chemokines, such as interleukin-8 (IL-8), γ-interferon-inducible protein (IP-10), macrophage inflammatory protein (MIP-2), and KC, are primarily responsible for neutrophilic chemotaxis, although IP-10 also targets monocytes and T cells. The CC(β) chemokines, such as *r*egulated on *a*ctivation, *n*ormal *T* cells, *e*xpressed and *s*ecreted (RANTES), monocyte chemoattractant protein (MCP-1), eotaxin, MIP-1α, and MIP-1β, are predominantly chemotactic for monocytes and lymphocytes and have little neutrophilic chemotactic overlap with the C × C chemokines.

Several members of the chemokine superfamily have been shown to induce leukocyte migration both in vitro and in vivo (34,35). For instance, Taub et al. have demonstrated that human T lymphocytes could traffic to the peripheral tissues of said mice in response to the chemokines RANTES, MCP-1, and IP-10 (36,37). MCP-1 is a heparin-binding protein that is a potent agonist for mononuclear leukocytes, and preferentially recruits monocytes and T cells in vitro (38,39). Potential cellular sources of MCP-1 in the lungs include epithelial cells (40,41), endothelial cells (42), fibroblasts (43), and alveolar macrophages (44,45). The chronic expression of this chemokine during the inflammatory cell recruitment and activation phase after thoracic irradiation is believed to contribute to the development of radiation pneumonitis and, ultimately, to late radiation fibrosis.

Intermediate Phase. These changes may resolve in a few weeks to months, if the volume and dose of radiation were below critical levels. Clinical symptoms improve, but the lungs are not totally normal; foci of foamy macrophages may be found in the air spaces, with hyperplasia of type II pneumocytes. Death is uncommon during this phase where there is resolution of the early exudative alveolitis of the pneumonitic process.

Fibrosis. The late lung injury becomes evident 6 months or longer after the radiation injury and is characterized by progressive fibrosis of alveolar septa that become thickened by bundles of elastic fibers. The alveoli collapse and are obliterated by connective tissue. The mechanisms of chronic injury may be related to the effects of radiation on the pulmonary vasculature (endothelial cells) and/or somatic cells. The nature of the triggering event in the pathogenesis of radiation lung fibrosis is unknown.

The classic hypothesis that fibrosis is a connective tissue replacement process following parenchymal cell death is currently being challenged. The recent discoveries of elevated pretreatment plasma levels of transforming growth factor-β1 (TGFβ1) in breast cancer patients with pulmonary complications from bone marrow transplant (46) and elevated pretreatment TNFα levels in leukemia patients who develop a variety of complications when undergoing cyclophosphamide/radiation bone marrow transplant (47) have led to speculation that fibrosis after chemotherapy/irradiation may be due to aberrant early and late cytokine production (48–50). For instance, preliminary clinical and preclinical data suggest that chronic exposure to basic fibroblast growth factor (bFGF) after irradiation can result in increased toxicity due to fibrosis; similar findings also have been observed with TGFβ1 (48,51,52). Transforming growth factor-β1 stimulates fibroblasts and endothelial cells to migrate to sites of injury, where they proliferate and play an important part in wound healing (53,54). TGFβ1 also stimulates fibroblasts to produce extracellular matrix, including the synthesis of collagens I and III and fibronectin. It is implicated in the pathogenesis of chronic hepatitis, idiopathic pulmonary fibrosis, systemic sclerosis, mesangial proliferative glomerulonephritis, and cirrhosis after exposure to carbon tetrachloride. A progressive fibrotic process characterizes these syndromes. More recently, TGFβ1 has been associated with pneumonitis and veno-occlusive disease after chemotherapy-only autologous transplants of breast cancer patients (46,55). Since then, the importance of circulating TGFβ in pulmonary fibrosis after bone marrow transplantation, in pulmonary irradiation for lung cancer, and in murine experimental radiation pneumonitis, has been documented by others (46,48,55,56). In particular, chronically elevated, rather than temporarily elevated, TGFβ1 levels were associated with radiographic radiation fibrosis of patients with lung cancer (48); radiographic radiation fibrosis can also be seen in women receiving breast irradiation who are also given tamoxifen, an antiestrogen that up-regulates active TGFβ expression (57,58). All of these data have led investigators to examine the importance of TGFβ1 expression levels in predicting fibrosis and to look for TGF modulators as potential agents to alleviate late fibrosis.

Volume Factors

Whole Lung Volume.   Young children appear to experience more chronic toxicity at lower doses than older children and adults, because of interference with lung and chest wall function in addition to fibrosis and volume loss. After 20 Gy, mean total lung volumes and diffusing capacity of the lung for carbon monoxide (DLCO) were reduced to 60% of predicted values (59) and restrictive changes have been reported after doses of 11–14 Gy (60,61). In older children and adults, clinically significant lung injury is uncommon following approximately 16–25 Gy in 1.5–2.0-Gy fractions (62,63). Symptomatic pneumonitis occurs in about 15% of patients who receive additional mediastinal irradiation beyond the whole lung therapy (64,65). When the "safe" doses for single versus multiple fractions are compared, there is a clear protective effect of fractionation, similar to what has been seen in animal studies (66,67).

Partial Lung Volume. The impact of partial lung irradiation, used in the vast majority of patients, has been studied to a far lesser degree in comparison to whole lung irradiation. If assessed, subtle changes in radiographs and pulmonary function tests are almost always present. Fifty to 90 percent of patients have radiographic and/or pulmonary function abnormalities following therapy (2,68–70). Mah et al. (68) utilized the endpoint of increase in lung density within the irradiated volume on CT in the posttreatment period. Doses above 30 Gy in 10–15 days to 45–50 Gy in 25–30 days yielded radiographic changes ranging from 30 to 90% (71).

One convenient way of expressing this type of information is the dose-volume histogram (DVH), correlating the shape of the DVH curve with the subsequent development of pulmonary complications. Martel and colleagues (72) have shown that an empirical model can be created that accurately predicts the chances of radiation pneumonitis for lung irradiation in Hodgkin's patients. It is well appreciated that there is a clear separation between whole organ and regional organ tolerance. While regional injury is commonly identifiable within the irradiated field, the impact on whole organ function will depend on the DVH.

To better define partial lung tolerance to irradiation, Marks et al. (3) evaluated several traditional and newer indices of biological function for predicting outcome after radiation therapy. Their results indicate that the percent volume of lung receiving in excess of 30 Gy was the best predictive test for the development of pneumonitis; these findings are similar to those of other authors (73,74). Marks et al. (3) report an incidence of RT-induced symptoms of 44% in their highest-risk-patient quartile when using the percent volume greater than 30 Gy parameter.

The RTOG trial 93-11 is evaluating prospectively whether DVH parameters stratify lung cancer patients into risk groups for pneumonitis (75). This study stratifies the escalating doses based on the percent of the total lung receiving greater than 20 Gy: incidences of high-grade pneumonitis occurred 0–4% with less than 25% lung volume, up to 19–30% pneumonitis with lung volumes greater than 37% receiving 20 Gy.

Chemotherapy

Pathophysiology

In recent years, there has been a proliferation in the number of chemotherapeutic and biological agents responsible for pulmonary toxicity (Table 2). Drug-related

TABLE 2 Anticancer Drugs and Associated Lung and Esophageal Toxicity

Chemotherapy agents	Lung toxicity	Esophageal toxicity	Radiation potentiation lung (L)/ esophagus (E)
Alkylating agents			
Busulphan	+		
Cyclophosphamide	+		
Ifosfamide	+		
Chlorambucil	+		L
Melphalan	+		
Nitrosoureas			
BCNU (carmustine)	+		
Methyl-CCNU (semustine)	+		
CCNU (lomustine)	+		
Antimetabolites			
5-Fluorouracil	+	+	E
Methotrexate	+	+	L/E
Mercaptopurine	+	+	
Azathioprine	+		
Ara-C	+	+	
Edatrexate	+		
Fludarabine	+		
Antitumor antibiotics			
Bleomycin	+	+	L/E
Mitomycin	+	+	L/E
Doxorubicin	+	+	L/E
Actinomycin D	+	+	L
Alkaloids			
Etoposide (VP-16)	+		E
Teniposide (VM26)	+		
Vincristine	+	+	
Vinblastine	+	+	
Vindesine	+		
Miscellaneous			
Procarbazine	+	+	
Taxol	+		L/E
L-Asparaginase	+		
Tamoxifen	+		

pulmonary disease has been found to be the result of toxicity, hypersensitivity, or idiosyncrasy (5). There are multiple recognized mechanisms by which antineoplastic drug-induced lung injury may manifest:

Oxidized lung injury (e.g., bleomycin)
Direct cytotoxic effect on alveolar capillary endothelial cells
Deposition of phospholipid within pulmonary cells, particularly the alveolar macrophage, by amphophilic drugs
Immune-mediated injury
Bronchiolitis obliterans with organizing pneumonitis (BOOP)
Bronchospastic changes (e.g., taxoids)
Pleural effusions
Pulmonary veno-occlusive disease with vasculitis (particularly following high-dose chemotherapy with bone marrow transplantation)
Thromboembolic disease

Toxicity, with a dose response, has been shown for bleomycin, chlorambucil, and the nitrosoureas. Pulmonary damage, likely mediated through allergic mechanisms, is caused by cyclophosphamide, methotrexate, procarbazine, and bleomycin. This mechanism is suggested by the acute onset of the illness, prominent eosinophilia, and, frequently, a pathological picture of granulomatous reaction in the lungs. Lung injury following low-dose bleomycin has been explained by idiosyncrasy, possibly due to genetically impaired drug metabolism. The pathogenesis of bleomycin injury has been studied extensively (76,77). Similar to radiation-induced damage, abnormalities are seen in endothelial and epithelial cells. The initial injury is to the capillary endothelium (78) and its mechanism of cell toxicity appears to include formation of free radicals and lipid peroxidation of phospholipid membranes. This may also be the mechanism by which cyclophosphamide and mitomycin C damage the capillary endothelium (79). Permeability increases, resulting in interstitial edema. Thereafter, swelling and necrosis of type I pneumocytes occur. Hyaline membranes are produced by plasma proteins and fluid enters the alveoli through the denuded epithelium. Type I pneumocytes are then replaced by cuboidal cells, and proliferation of fibroblasts then occurs with resulting fibrosis. Interstitial pneumonitis, either the desquamative type (which appears to be an earlier stage) or the usual type with fibrinous exudation, hyaline membranes, and interstitial fibrosis, is also seen with alkylating agents and nitrosoureas. This may lead to the development of pulmonary fibrosis, characterized by the enhanced production and deposition of collagen and other matrix components. A rare manifestation of cytotoxic drug injury is pulmonary veno-occlusive disease with vasculitis and intimal fibrosis, resulting in pulmonary hypertension, and has been reported with bleomycin, mitomycin (80), and BCNU (81).

Antineoplastic agents more commonly associated with pulmonary toxicity are the following:

Alkylating Agents. Pulmonary toxicity is an infrequent, but potentially lethal, complication and interstitial pneumonitis is the most common lesion. Atypical epithelial proliferation of the distal airways may result from melphalan and busulphan, and acute noncardiogenic pulmonary edema has been described with cyclophosphamide and ifosfamide (5). Interstitial pneumonitis due to cyclophosphamide and ifosfamide does not appear to be dose related (82,83), in contrast to chlorambucil toxicity, which occurs after 2000 mg accumulated dose and at least 6 months of therapy (5,84).

Nitrosoureas. BCNU has been commonly employed as a single agent in the treatment of brain tumors. The clinicopathological features are similar to those with bleomycin; fibrosis predominates. There is a bibasilar reticular pattern on the chest radiograph, but this might be normal. A decrease in diffusion capacity is seen, which may precede all other signs, and there is a restrictive ventilatory defect. The incidence is 20–30% and it is dose related (85,86), but may be as high as 30–50% when a cumulative dose of 1500 mg/m^2 or greater is given. Weinstein et al. (86) have reported that toxicity very rarely occurs when the cumulative dose is <960 mg/m^2. There is an increased risk with preexisting lung disease and tobacco use. In children treated for brain tumors with BCNU and radiation, 35–47% of survivors died of lung fibrosis (87,88). Twelve percent died within 3 years of treatment; however, 24% died of progressive lung fibrosis after a symptom-free interval of 7–12 years. All the long-term survivors had evidence of restrictive disease and small lung volumes. Delayed fibrosis has been seen up to 17 years after the drug was stopped (88). Although BCNU has been most commonly associated with pulmonary fibrosis, pulmonary toxicity has been reported with all other nitrosoureas (89,90).

Antimetabolites. Methotrexate, mercaptopurine, and azathioprine can cause desquamative interstitial pneumonitis and eosinophilic pneumonitis (5). Pulmonary toxicity after methotrexate therapy ranges from 3% in adolescents to 8% in adults. Recovery is common within 10–45 days after discontinuation of therapy, and development of pulmonary fibrosis is unusual (91). There is no dose relationship. Noncardiogenic pulmonary edema has been reported after therapy with cytosine-arabinoside (92,93), where it is dose related (20% frequency with high-dose schedules), and after intrathecal methotrexate, where it is less common (94).

Antitumor Antibiotics. Lung toxicity has been reported with bleomycin, pepleomycin, mitomycin, and neocarzinostatin. Doxorubicin and actinomycin D do not cause pulmonary toxicity by themselves, but have been found to potentiate radiation pneumonitis (95).

Pulmonary complications associated with bleomycin administration are manifested by an interstitial pneumonitis leading to fibrosis that results in substantial morbidity and mortality. On chest x-ray, interstitial infiltrates are visualized as diffuse, reticular densities, while alveolar infiltrates appear as nodular patches. These changes are seen in both lung fields, particularly at the bases. In advanced cases widespread infiltrates are seen, occasionally with lobar consolidation. Sometimes these changes can be confused with lung metastases and CT may be useful in the differentiation. Pulmonary function testing reveals a restrictive ventilatory defect with hypoxia, hypocapnia, and chronic respiratory alkalosis due to impaired diffusion and hyperventilation. Some authors consider a reduced DLCO to be the most sensitive tool for bleomycin toxicity. Alveolar volume and vital capacity are decreased, remaining low for 18–24 weeks before slowly returning to normal. The incidence of interstitial fibrosis from bleomycin has varied in published reports from 2% to 40%. Several variables can increase the risk of toxicity and induce severe symptoms in 35–55% of patients treated (96). These include:

Age: older patients (>70 years) appear to be more susceptible (97)
Dose: cumulative bleomycin dose above 450 U, in which case 10% will experience fibrosis (97)
Radiation therapy to the chest (98,99)
Supplemental oxygen therapy, damaging lung through increased production of oxygen radicals (89)
Renal insufficiency (100)
Other chemotherapeutic agents such as cisplatin or cyclophosphamide (101,102)
Non-Hodgkin's lymphoma
Bolus intravenous infusion

Mitomycin-related pneumonitis is not dose dependent and is fatal in up to 33% of patients; risk factors include anesthesia or treatment with vinblastine. Increased sensitivity to cancer chemotherapy has been noted in infants (103). In the Second National Wilms' Tumor Study, severe hematological, pulmonary, and hepatic toxicity was seen with the use of vincristine, doxorubicin, and actinomycin D in babies under 12 months of age. When drug doses were halved in response to this observation, toxicity was reduced and treatment-related deaths were reduced from 6% to zero (104).

Vinca Alkaloids. Pulmonary toxicity with these agents alone is unusual. It is usually seen in combination with mitomycin therapy, presenting as bronchospasm or interstitial pneumonitis (105).

Combined-Modality Interactions

Radiation-Chemotherapy Interaction

Many antineoplastic agents potentiate the damaging effects of radiation on the lung. Testing effects of commonly used chemotherapeutic agents, Phillips et al. (106) reported actinomycin D, cyclophosphamide, and, to a lesser extent, vincristine enhanced the lethal potential of thoracic irradiation. The effect of actinomycin D was seen if it was given as long as 30 days before, but not when given 30 days after, radiation. Bleomycin given with lung irradiation produces lung toxicity that is greater than when either agent is given alone. This effect appears to be maximal when bleomycin is given concurrently with radiation (107). Although 500 U of bleomycin without radiation can be lethal in 1–2% of patients, as little as 30 U can be fatal when given with radiation. Collis et al. (108) assessed bleomycin-and-radiation-induced lung damage in mice and found enhanced damage from combined treatment with extent of lung damage dependent on schedule, mode of administration, and dose of the drug, but no time-dependent interaction was found. Cyclophosphamide also enhances radiation lung damage, but in contrast to bleomycin, the enhancement has been found to be time dependent (109). Von der Maase et al. (110) assessed various antineoplastic drugs in combination with radiation and found dose-enhancing effects for adriamycin, bleomycin, cyclophosphamide, and mitomycin C at various time points. However, 5-FU, methotrexate, and cisplatin appeared to have no effect on the radiation response at the intervals investigated.

Interferons have been shown to increase radiation cytotoxicity in vitro in a number of studies. Natural human leukocyte interferon [HuIFN-β(Le)] was the first interferon to be combined with radiation therapy in the treatment of small cell lung cancer (111). A potentiation of both antitumor effect and normal tissue toxicity of radiation was observed in this treatment. In laboratory modeling at the University of Rochester Cancer Center, Betaseron (recombinant human interferon betaser, rHuIFN-Bser) appeared less toxic and better tolerated than HuIFN-β(Le) and produced approximately the same potentiation effect in vitro. In a mouse study, enhanced acute toxicity was seen, but a decrease in fibrosis was suggested using endpoints of breathing rate, procollagen III release, and electron microscopy (112). A clinical trial, combining thoracic irradiation with escalating Betaseron doses, demonstrated no increase in pulmonary toxicity, with encouraging tumor responses (113). The mechanisms of these interactions in the lung are not clear, but the therapeutic implications are important.

Chemotherapy-Chemotherapy Interactions

Toxicity is seen at much lower doses than expected when certain drug combinations are used. Synergism is seen with combinations of nitrosoureas and cyclophosphamide (114) and also with bleomycin and cyclophosphamide/vincristine/

doxorubicin/cisplatinum (5,89). Vinca alkaloids appear to cause pulmonary toxicity only in the presence of mitomycin (5,105).

Clinical Presentation

The clinical and radiographic presentations may mimic other pulmonary conditions that can occur in cancer patients; it is therefore important to recognize the potential for drug- or radiation-induced pulmonary injury. Clinical findings, radiological studies, and pulmonary function tests can be nonspecific; however, these represent measurable endpoints with which to quantify toxicity.

Depending on the impact of injury on organ function, the range of respiratory compromise can extend from acute lethal events to degrees of chronic pulmonary morbidity, manifesting years after the initial cancer therapy. The clinical pathological course of lung injury after radiation is dependent upon total dose, volume of lung irradiated, number of fractions, the dose rate, concomitant exposure to systemic agents, and pulmonary surgery following radiation therapy and chemotherapy (4,115,116). Death can ensue if both lungs are irradiated to high doses (8–10 Gy single dose), or if threshold doses of drugs are exceeded. Lower doses of lung irradiation (less than 7 Gy single dose) produce subclinical pathological effects that can be expressed by added insult such as infection, drugs, or surgery (4). There is not a significant difference in the incidence of radiation pneumonitis between the young and the elderly, but pneumonitis tends to be more severe in the latter (117).

During radiation therapy, the larger bronchioles and bronchi may be irritated with resultant cough; however, symptoms of acute radiation pneumonitis usually only become evident within 3–6 months following completion thoracic irradiation with high doses exceeding clinical thresholds and volumes. An accelerated phase of the syndrome develops within a period of days after concomitant insult by drugs. In general, the early onset of symptoms implies a more serious and more protracted clinical course. The severity of symptoms of the acute pneumonitis syndrome is dependent on the degree of pulmonary involvement. There may be low-grade fever and nonspecific respiratory symptoms such as congestion, cough, and fullness in the chest. In more severe cases, dyspnea, pleuritic chest pain, and nonproductive cough may be present. Later, small amounts of sputum, which can be bloodstained, may be produced.

On physical examination, signs of pulmonary involvement are usually minimal or absent. Occasionally moist rales, a pleural friction rub, or evidence of consolidation or effusion may be heard over the area of irradiation. When tolerance doses are exceeded, pneumonitis can be very severe and produce acute respiratory distress, with the patient experiencing spiking temperatures and acute cor pulmonale that can lead to death (118). Patients who survive this phase experience a protracted period of pneumonitis—possibly up to several months. This is the stage at which mortality and most morbidity occurs. Generally the pneumonitic phase with the acute symptoms is relatively short in duration and may be typically managed by approximately 1 mg/kg of prednisone per day for 2–3 weeks, tapered. The acute phase is followed by an intermediate phase when symptoms improve, even though histological changes continue. This progresses to the eventual fibrotic phase.

In contrast to the acute reaction, the permanent changes seen in radiation fibrosis take 6–24 months to evolve, even though histological and biochemical changes are evident sooner. Pulmonary fibrosis develops insidiously in the previously irradiated field, stabilizing after 1 or 2 years. The clinical expression is directly related to the volume of lung parenchyma involved and to the patient's preexisting pulmonary reserves. Most patients with radiation fibrosis are asymptomatic, because of the large functional reserve of the lung. In a few patients, particularly those who have had severe pneumonitis, chronic respiratory failure may be present, characterized by dyspnea on exertion, reduced exercise tolerance, orthopnea, cyanosis, sometimes chronic cor pulmonale, and finger clubbing. In such cases, there may be a continuous symptomatology from the acute to the chronic stage. Symptoms are generally minimal if fibrosis is limited to less than 50% of one lung (119). If the volume increases above this limit, dyspnea may manifest clinically and progressive chronic cor pulmonale leading to right heart failure may occur.

Diagnostic Imaging

Although radiographic abnormalities are always found in the presence of clinical radiation pneumonitis, asymptomatic patients often exhibit radiographic abnormalities. The frequency of detecting these abnormalities depends upon the sensitivity of the radiographic assessment used. Chest radiography may reveal a diffuse infiltrate corresponding to the radiation field. This appears as a result of an acute exudative edema that is initially faint and progresses to homogeneous or patchy air-space consolidation. There frequently is associated volume loss of the affected portion of the lung. Cases of radiographic changes outside treatment portals have been described (120,121), but this phenomenon is rare and has been suggested to represent a hypersensitivity pneumonitis. Symptoms develop earlier than classic radiation pneumonitis (2–4 weeks after completion of therapy) and usually resolve without sequelae. Bronchoalveolar lavage analysis by Morgan and Breit support a suggested immunologically mediated mechanism for what they termed sporadic radiation pneumonitis (122).

While chest radiographs are occasionally abnormal (1), CT scans are more sensitive and detect abnormalities in more than 50% of patients (123). CT studies of the lung used to evaluate for increased lung density have been correlated with radiation effects (68). CT findings demonstrate a well-defined dose-response relationship (124). With radiation fibrosis, chest radiographs have the appearance of linear streaking, radiating from the area of previous pneumonitis, which may extend outside the irradiated region, with concomitant regional contraction, pleural thickening, and tenting of the diaphragm. The hilum or mediastinum may be retracted with a densely contracted lung segment resulting in compensatory hyperinflation of adjacent or contralateral lung tissue. This is usually seen 12 months to 2 years after radiation. CT is currently favored to image regions subjected to radiation therapy (68,125).

Pulmonary Function Tests

No gross abnormalities in lung function occur until 4–8 weeks after completion of a course of radiotherapy, usually coincident with the period of clinical pneumonitis. Restrictive changes gradually develop with volume loss from each of several compartments being equivalent. This persists and progresses with time with little evidence of recovery (21). Gas exchange abnormalities, ranging from 5% to 20%, are synchronous with the changes in lung volumes, but show some tendency toward recovery after 6–12 months. In studies assessing multiple pulmonary parameters, reductions in diffusion capacity are generally most severe (70,126,127). Whole lung irradiation in the dose range of 11–14 Gy has resulted in restrictive changes in lungs of children treated for various malignancies (60,61).

The clinical spectrum of drug-induced pulmonary toxicity varies widely. Some patients are asymptomatic and the diagnosis is suspected only when there is an abnormal chest radiograph or laboratory finding. Three typical clinical patterns of pulmonary toxicity have been described: pneumonitis/fibrosis, acute hypersensitivity, and noncardiogenic pulmonary edema. Drug-induced pneumonitis/fibrosis has a similar clinical presentation to that described after radiotherapy. Drug-related lung injury might present as one or more of multiple clinical syndromes. There may be significant overlap between syndromes clinically and it can occur during treatment with a number of drugs: bleomycin, methotrexate, mitomycin, nitrosoureas, alkylating agents, and vinca alkaloids (79). In most cases, the onset is subacute and the patient presents with the insidious development of low-grade fever, a nonproductive cough, and dyspnea, which is progressively disabling. Late-onset pulmonary fibrosis has been reported many years after discontinuing cyclophosphamide (110) and BCNU (5). Hypersensitivity reactions (induced by methotrexate, procarbazine, or bleomycin) or noncardiogenic pulmonary edema (induced by methotrexate, cytosine arabinoside, ifosfamide, or cyclophosphamide) usually arises within days of beginning treatment (5,79) and is unlikely to result in late-onset pulmonary toxicity. High fever appears to be a common finding with hypersensitivity reaction.

Fever, cough, and shortness of breath are the most common symptoms of pneumonitis. Other indicators include an inability to lie flat. The principal signs of both acute and delayed pneumonopathy are: respiratory rate, signs of pleural effusion or consolidation, rales, rhonchi, bronchial breath sounds, and, in severe cases, cyanosis.

Laboratory Tests of Serum or Blood

Biochemical markers for identifying lung cancer and/or to predict for damaging late radiation effects in lung would provide a valuable tool in patient care, allowing the radiation and/or medical oncologist to determine if treatment is exceeding normal tissue tolerance (19,128). If biochemical markers of tissue damage can be detected in the subclinical phase, prior to the accumulation of significant injury, one could terminate therapy or institute treatment to prevent or attenuate later lesions. An ideal marker should be a simple, reproducible, positive/negative biochemical test; there are a large number of substances whose release potentially may reflect or predict the degree of radiation and/or chemotherapy injury to the lung. Surfactant apoprotein, procollagen type 3, and an increasing number of cytokines, such as TGFB1, and growth factors can be measured in the blood (46,129–131). It is possible that other important factors, such as angiotensin-converting enzyme, blood plasminogen-activating factor, and prostacyclin, may also prove to be good prognostic markers (132). Some of the various factors have been correlated with either acute or delayed radiation pneumonopathy (46,128,129). Significant additional work is required to evaluate the usefulness of such blood level measurements, but they should be considered in any prospective evaluation of toxicity grading.

Prevention and Treatment

Prevention is the optimal goal in the management of patients who are at high risk for pulmonary complications from antineoplastic therapy. Strict attention should be paid to drug doses and cumulative restrictions.

1. *Modification of radiation treatment techniques*.

Fractionation: Significant sparing of damage to normal lung tissue can be achieved by decreasing the dose per fraction (67,133).
Volume of normal lung should be minimized within the radiation field, and particular care should be exercised in the lung bases (134,135).

2. During drug (e.g., bleomycin) therapy, *monitoring of symptoms*/signs, pulmonary function tests, and chest x-rays can aid in detecting problems early and the causative agent can be withdrawn. After withdrawal of bleomycin, early stages of bleomycin-induced pneumonitis have reversed clinically and radiographically (136,137).

3. Currently, *molecular-oriented modes of therapy* are being investigated such as gene therapy. In a recent study, normal human epithelial cells were

transfected with liposomes containing a human manganese superoxide dismutase (MnSOD) transgene-containing plasmid. This enzyme is involved in the reduction of oxygen-free radicals. The athymic nude mice receiving this human MnSOD transgene via intratracheal injection demonstrated detectable transgene levels. Lung sections from treated mice subsequently showed a decrease in acute pulmonary changes of irradiation-induced organizing alveolitis (138).

4. When following survivors of cancer therapy, *vigilant evaluation* of symptoms of respiratory compromise is necessary, and should be anticipated when thoracic irradiation or drugs with known pulmonary toxicity have been used. Chronic cough and/or dyspnea should be further evaluated with pulmonary function tests and chest radiography. In the absence of symptoms, chest x-rays and lung function testing are recommended every 2–5 years. In cases of radiation pneumonitis where corticosteroids have been used, it is important to withdraw steroids very slowly to avoid reactivation. Prophylactic administration of steroids before therapy has no proven use and may actually do more harm than good. Strenuous counseling on the risks of smoking is imperative in these patients, as well as awareness of the risks of general anesthesia, pollution, infection, and aging.

5. *Corticosteroids* play a useful role in relief of symptoms from pneumonitis caused by a variety of drugs and radiation. The usual steroid dose is approximately 1 mg/kg/day for 2–3 weeks with a slow taper of 3–4 weeks or more. If exacerbation of symptoms occurs, higher doses of steroid for a more prolonged period may be needed. Severe symptoms necessitating treatment can be relieved markedly and rapidly by corticosteroids in half the patients; however, prevention or reversal of the fibrotic phase does not occur. Supportive care with bronchodilators, expectorants, antibiotics, bed rest, and oxygen can be beneficial for symptom relief in pneumonitis and fibrosis.

Future Studies

Understanding new molecular mechanisms, involving immediate cytokine release (27) in the initiation of the fibrosis process, opens the door for intervention and protection. Substances, such as targeted cytokines or anti-cytokines, ACE inhibitors (129,132,139), and pentoxifylline (140), that oppose or inhibit fibrosis could be utilized during therapy, resulting in the desired enhanced therapeutic ratio.

ESOPHAGEAL TOXICITY

Pathophysiology

The esophageal mucosa is a rapid-turnover cell system, often representing the dose-limiting, early-responding tissue in the management of thoracic tumors. In the acute phase, the abnormalities created by chemotherapy and radiation are relatively similar.

Chemotherapy agents such as 5-fluorouracil (5-FU), methotrexate, and other drugs, such as purine antagonists, can frequently cause esophagitis (141,142) and, in the case of 5-FU, method of delivery can enhance the effect (Table 2). Additionally, combinations of drugs such as 5-FU and leucovorin may potentiate the esophagitis (143,144). Once-weekly or low-dose protracted infusions produce much less esophagitis as opposed to intensified 5-day continuous-infusion regimens. Esophagitis may develop over 7–14 days after the initiation of treatment, and likely represents damage throughout the reproducing mucosal epithelial cells, leading to inflammation and ulceration (145).

In patients receiving chemotherapy, esophagitis can be a result of the direct effect of drugs on the mucosa, or the indirect effect of myelosuppression. A similar pattern may be seen with radiotherapy, with involvement of symptoms in the second to third week of treatment. Methods of delivery can also have significant effects on the development of esophagitis, as evidenced by the increase in esophagitis seen in hyperfractionated or accelerated fractionation regimens, as opposed to standard once-a-day therapy. In a study by King et al. (6), using accelerated, hyperfractionated techniques for lung cancer, 18% of patients experienced grade III esophagitis, with a 2-year actuarial risk of 30% grade III or greater late toxicity.

In contrast to chemotherapy, radiation produces late effects most commonly in the form of esophageal stricture and/or stenosis. These can lead to symptoms of obstruction, usually developing 4–6 months after treatment, although they can develop as late as 2 years after treatment. The risk of stricture has been variously estimated, and authors such as Emami et al. (146) have estimated the risk of clinical stricture following esophageal radiation as a function of volume and total dose. These authors proposed a 5% risk of stricture at 5 years when approximately one-third of the esophagus has been radiated to a total dose of 60 Gy; a similar rate of stricture development can be seen when 55 Gy is delivered to the entire esophagus. Late pathological changes due to radiation of the esophagus are primarily related to changes in the muscle wall, although mucosal changes may also be observed.

In summary, target cells producing the majority of acute effects are those of the basal epithelial layer of the esophagus. The late effects are predominantly the result of radiation effects on the muscle cells and the infiltration of fibroblasts and inflammatory cells into the muscle wall. Telangiectasia and narrowing of the blood vessels have been reported, but their significance in the production of late effects is controversial (147).

Clinical Syndromes

Radiotherapy and Chemotherapy

The acute effects of either radiation or chemotherapy may develop within the first weeks after the initiation of treatment and consist of substernal burning, along with dysphagia and odynophagia when eating or drinking liquids. Depending upon the severity of symptoms, analgesics may be required, although the symptoms may subside during the course of treatment with more conventional chemo/radiation programs. Radiation stricture/stenosis, however, may present with the sensation of increasing fullness, difficulty passing solids, regurgitation, and other symptoms consistent with obstruction.

Radiographic findings consist of variable segments of esophageal narrowing with multiple discrete ulcers or granular appearance on double-contrast barium swallows (148,149). In the case of stricture, there will be obvious luminal narrowing. Endoscopic findings may be minimal despite symptoms of esophagitis. Mascarenhas et al. (150) reported that 12 of 18 patients with symptoms of esophagitis had endoscopic evidence when evaluated. However, histological changes were confirmed in only eight of those 12 patients.

Chemotherapy-Chemotherapy Interactions

Combinations of drugs may potentiate oral and esophageal mucositis. A good illustration is the potentiation of 5-FU from the addition of leucovorin (143,144). Increased mucositis is also seen with the combination of two mucositis-producing cytotoxic drugs, e.g., methotrexate and 5-FU.

Radiation-Chemotherapy Interactions

In a study of several RTOG lung cancer studies by Byhardt et al. (8), conventional radiotherapy regimens for treatments of non–small cell lung carcinoma produced grade II esophagitis of 12% and grade III toxicity of, approximately, 3%. Single-agent chemotherapy can be anticipated to produce esophagitis at similarly low rates. Although approximately 40% of patients receiving combination chemotherapy develop oral mucositis, the esophagus is affected less frequently (141,142). However, it is clear from multiple studies that the combination of chemotherapy and radiation produces an increased risk of esophagitis. Drugs such as etoposide, cisplatin, 5-FU, actinomycin D, adriamycin, mitomycin, bleomycin, and methotrexate can augment the acute effects of radiation therapy on the esophagus and, in some cases, late effects (151,152). In addition, concurrent radiation and chemotherapy produces a greater incidence of acute and late effects than when treatments are sequential. Umsawasdi et al. (153) noted a higher rate of stricture or fistula development in patients treated initially with chemoradiation than in those treated with two cycles of chemotherapy followed by radiation (30% vs. 2%). In the Byhardt study (8), it was clear that the addition of concurrent chemotherapy produced a higher rate of acute esophagitis than sequential regimens (6% vs. 1%) and that concurrent chemotherapy and hyperfractionation produced the highest rates of severe acute esophagitis (34%). Similar statistics have been confirmed in other chemotherapy regimens, using concurrent chemotherapy with once-a-day or multiple-fraction radiotherapy.

Prevention and Treatment

Prevention

Clearly the simplest way to prevent esophagitis is to minimize exposure to noxious agents.

  In the case of radiation, this may mean designing portals using 3D treatment planning to spare the esophagus (154,155). Dose-volume histograms can provide a useful tool in reducing both the volume and total dose to the esophagus in treatment of thoracic malignancies.

  Similarly, alterations of chemotherapy/radiation protocols (e.g., use of single fractions as opposed to twice-daily fractionation or sequencing of certain drugs) may also provide reduction in esophageal symptoms; this is, of course, presuming equal effect on the primary tumor.

  Other protective strategies may include cytoprotective agents such as amifostine, a radioprotector (156). A randomized trial (n = 146) showed a significant reduction with amifostine in both radiation esophagitis and pneumonitis in patients receiving radiotherapy alone for lung cancer (157). In a smaller randomized trial (n = 68), amifostine ($300mg/m^2$) administered before chemotherapy and daily RT reduced the incidence of acute esophagitis and grade 3 pneumonitis. There was no difference in the rate of complete and partial responses (158). This agent is currently being actively studied by the Radiation Therapy Oncology Group in a randomized trial (± amifostine) in patients receiving intensive chemoradiation for locally advanced non–small cell lung cancer (RTOG 98-01). Prospective quality of life data is being collected in this RTOG trial.

  Finally, patients with medical conditions that are predisposed to increased sensitivity to either radiation or chemotherapy, such as collagen/vascular diseases, ataxia-telangiectasia, or Bloom's syndrome (congenital, telangiectatic erythema), and HIV, may be considered to have relative contraindications to high-dose radiotherapy (11,12).

Treatment

Management of acute esophagitis, whether derived from chemotherapy, radiotherapy, or the combination, is based on the presumptive cause. If these symptoms can be attributed to mucositis, topical agents (e.g., xylocaine) and sucralfate (159) may be of benefit. Analgesics often provide adequate symptom relief. In patients predisposed to gastric reflux, agents such as H_2 blockers, antacids or metoclopramide may be of value in lessening the degree of esophagitis. However, patients may be neutropenic or have other underlying medical conditions that may dispose them to esophagitis. Infection with *Candida*, cytomegalovirus, or herpes simplex virus can be the causative agents of esophagitis; the latter two can be seen in AIDS patients or patients undergoing bone marrow transplantation. While esophagoscopy may provide a definitive answer, this may not be a practical or safe option. Empirical therapy directed toward the presumed causative agent may be indicated.

In the case of late radiation effects, most notably stricture/stenosis, management is primarily through esophageal dilatation, which may be required multiple times (160). O'Rourke et al. (161) reported that in 17 patients who developed benign stricture after radiation alone, the median time between dilatations was 5 months and the median number of dilatations was 2.5.

REFERENCES

1. Polansky SM, Ravin CE, Prosnitz LR. Pulmonary changes after primary radiation for early breast carcinoma. Am J Radiol 1980; 134:101–105.
2. Movsas B, Raffin TA, Epstein AH, Link CJ Jr. Pulmonary radiation injury. Chest 1997; 111:1061–1076.
3. Marks LB, Munley MT, Bentel GC, Zhou SM, Hollis D, Scarfone C, Sibley GS, Kong FM, Jirtle R, Jaszczak R, Coleman RE, Tapson V, Anscher M. Physical and biological predictors of changes in whole-lung function following thoracic irradiation. Int J Radiat Oncol Biol Phys 1997; 39:563–570.
4. Fowler WC, Langer CJ, Curran WJ Jr., Keller SM. Postoperative complications after combined neoadjuvant treatment of lung cancer. Ann Thorac Surg 1993; 55: 986–989.
5. Lehne G, Lote K. Pulmonary toxicity of cytotoxic and immunosuppressive agents. A review. Acta Oncol 1990; 29:113–124.
6. King SC, Acker JC, Kussin PS, Marks LB, Weeks KJ, Leopold KA. High-dose, hyperfractionated, accelerated radiotherapy using a concurrent boost for the treatment of nonsmall cell lung cancer: unusual toxicity and promising early results. Int J Radiat Oncol Biol Phys 1996; 36:593–599.
7. Saunders MI, Rojas A, Lyn BE, Pigott K, Powell M, Goodchild K, Hoskin PJ, Phillips H, Verma N. Experience with dose escalation using CHARTWEL (continuous hyperfractionated accelerated radiotherapy weekend less) in non–small-cell lung cancer. Br J Cancer 1998; 78:1323–1328.
8. Byhardt RW, Scott C, Sause WT, Emami B, Komaki R, Fisher B, Lee JS, Lawton C. Response, toxicity, failure patterns, and survival in five Radiation Therapy Oncology Group (RTOG) trials of sequential and/or concurrent chemotherapy and radiotherapy for locally advanced non–small-cell carcinoma of the lung. Int J Radiat Oncol Biol Phys 1998; 42:469–478.
9. Turrisi AT, Kim K, Blum R, Sause WT, Livingston RB, Komaki R, Wagner H, Aisner S, Johnson DH. Twice-daily compared with once-daily thoracic radiotherapy in limited small-cell lung cancer treated concurrently with cisplatin and etoposide. N Engl J Med 1999; 340:265–271.
10. Mahboubi S, Silber JH. Radiation-induced esophageal strictures in children with cancer. Eur Radiol 1997; 7:119–122.
11. Leigh BR, Lau DH. Severe esophageal toxicity after thoracic irradiation therapy for lung cancer associated with the human immunodeficiency virus: a case report and review of the literature. Am J Clin Oncol 1998; 21:479–481.

12. Costleigh BJ, Miyamoto CT, Micaily B, Brady LW. Heightened sensitivity of the esophagus to radiation in a patient with AIDS. Am J Gastroenterol 1995; 90:812–814.

13. Travis EL, Komaki R. Treatment-related lung damage. In: Lung Cancer: Principles and Practice. Philadelphia: Lippincott-Raven, 1996.

14. Travis EL, Harley RA, Fenn JO, Klobukowski CJ, Hargrove HB. Pathologic changes in the lung following single and multi-fraction irradiation. Int J Radiat Oncol Biol Phys 1977; 2:475–490.

15. Penney DP, Siemann DW, Rubin P, Shapiro DL, Finkelstein J, Cooper RA Jr. Morphologic changes reflecting early and late effects of irradiation of the distal lung of the mouse: a review. Scann Elect Microsc 1982; 413–425.

16. Ward WF, Molteni A, Solliday NH, Jones GE. The relationship between endothelial dysfunction and collagen accumulation in irradiated rat lung. Int J Radiat Oncol Biol Phys 1985; 11:1985–1990.

17. Penney DP, Rubin P. Specific early fine structural changes in the lung irradiation. Int J Radiat Oncol Biol Phys 1977; 2:1123–1132.

18. Penney DP, Shapiro DL, Rubin P, Finkelstein J, Siemann DW. Effects of radiation on the mouse lung and potential induction of radiation pneumonitis. Virchows Arch B 1981; 37:327–336.

19. Rubin P, Siemann DW, Shapiro DL, Finkelstein JN, Penney DP. Surfactant release as an early measure of radiation pneumonitis. Int J Radiat Oncol Biol Phys 1983; 9:1669–1673.

20. Rubin P, Shapiro DL, Finkelstein JN, Penney DP. The early release of surfactant following lung irradiation of alveolar type II cells. Int J Radiat Oncol Biol Phys 1980; 6:75–77.

21. Gross NJ. Experimental radiation pneumonitis. IV. Leakage of circulatory proteins onto the alveolar surface. J Lab Clin Med 1980; 95:19–31.

22. Gross NJ. The pathogenesis of radiation-induced lung damage. Lung 1981; 159:115–125.

23. Hallahan DE, Virudachalam S. Ionizing radiation mediates expression of cell adhesion molecules in distinct histological patterns within the lung. Cancer Res 1997; 57:2096–2099.

24. Phillips TL, Margolis LW. Radiation pathology and the clinical response of lung and esophagus. Front Radiat Ther Oncol 1972; 6:254–273.

25. Rubin P, Finkelstein J, Shapiro D. Molecular biology mechanisms in the radiation induction of pulmonary injury syndromes: interrelationship between the alveolar macrophage and the septal fibroblast. Int J Radiat Oncol Biol Phys 1992; 24:93–101.

26. Finkelstein JN, Johnston CJ, Baggs R, Rubin P. Early alterations in extracellular matrix and transforming growth factor beta gene expression in mouse lung indicative of late radiation fibrosis. Int J Radiat Oncol Biol Phys 1994; 28:621–631.

27. Rubin P, Johnston CJ, Williams JP, McDonald S, Finkelstein JN. A perpetual cascade of cytokines postirradiation leads to pulmonary fibrosis. Int J Radiat Oncol Biol Phys 1995; 33:99–109.

28. Johnston CJ, Piedboeuf B, Rubin P, Williams JP, Baggs R, Finkelstein JN. Early and persistent alterations in the expression of interleukin-1 alpha, interleukin-1 beta

and tumor necrosis factor alpha mRNA levels in fibrosis-resistant and sensitive mice after thoracic irradiation. Radiat Res 1996; 145:762–767.

29. Hallahan DE, Virudachalam S. Intercellular adhesion molecule 1 knockout abrogates radiation induced pulmonary inflammation. Proc Natl Acad Sci USA 1997; 94:6432–6437.

30. Hallahan DE, Spriggs DR, Beckett MA, Kufe DW, Weichselbaum RR. Increased tumor necrosis factor alpha mRNA after cellular exposure to ionizing radiation. Proc Natl Acad Sci USA 1989; 86:10104–10107.

31. Adawi A, Zhang Y, Baggs R, Rubin P, Williams J, Finkelstein J, Phipps RP. Blockade of CD40-CD40 ligand interactions protects against radiation-induced pulmonary inflammation and fibrosis. Clin Immunol Immunopathol 1998; 89:222–230.

32. Rogers DF, Laurent GJ. New ideas on the pathophysiology and treatment of lung disease. Thorax 1998; 53:200–203.

33. Penney DP. Ultrastructural organization of the distal lung and potential target cells of ionizing radiation. Proceedings of the International Conference on New Biology of Lung and Lung Injury and Their Implications for Oncology, Porvoo, Finland, 1987.

34. Haelens A, Wuyts A, Proost P, Struyf S, Opdenakker G, Van Damme J. Leukocyte migration and activation by murine chemokines. Immunobiology 1996; 195:499–521.

35. Negus RP. The chemokines: cytokines that direct leukocyte migration. J Roy Soc Med 1996; 89:312–314.

36. Taub DD. Chemokine-leukocyte interactions. The voodoo that they do so well. Cytokine Growth Factor Rev 1996; 7:355–376.

37. Taub DD, Key ML, Longo DL, Murphy WJ. Chemokine-induced human lymphocyte infiltration and engraftment in huPBL-SCID mice. Methods Enzymol 1997; 287:265–291.

38. Boring L, Gosling J, Chensue SW, Kunkel SL, Farese RV, Jr., Broxmeyer HE, Charo IF. Impaired monocyte migration and reduced type 1 (Th1) cytokine responses in C-C chemokine receptor 2 knockout mice. J Clin Invest 1997; 100:2552–2561.

39. Li FK, Davenport A, Robson RL, Loetscher P, Rothlein R, Williams JD, Topley N. Leukocyte migration across human peritoneal mesothelial cells is dependent on directed chemokine secretion and ICAM-1 expression. Kidney Int 1998; 54:2170–2183.

40. Barrett EG, Johnston C, Oberdoster G, Finkelstein JN. Silica-induced chemokine expression in alveolar type II cells is mediated by TNF-alpha. Am J Physiol 1998; 275:L1110–L1119.

41. Johnston CJ, Finkelstein JN, Oberdorster G, Reynolds SD, Stripp BR. Clara cell secretory protein-deficient mice differ from wild-type mice in inflammatory chemokine expression to oxygen and ozone, but not to endotoxin. Exp Lung Res 1999; 25:7–21.

42. Krishnaswamy G, Kelley J, Yerra L, Smith JK, Chi DS. Human endothelium as a source of multifunctional cytokines: molecular regulation and possible role in human disease. J Interferon Cyt Res 1999; 19:91–104.

43. Hogaboam CM, Steinhauser ML, Chensue SW, Kunkel SL. Novel roles for chemokines and fibroblasts in interstitial fibrosis. Kidney Int 1998; 54:2152–2159.

44. Suga M, Iyonaga K, Ando M. Role of alveolar macrophages in the pathogenesis of idiopathic interstitial pneumonia. Jpn J Thorac Dis 1996; 34:175–180.

45. Cavaillon JM. Cytokines and macrophages. Biomed Pharm 1994; 48:445–453.

46. Anscher MS, Peters WP, Reisenbichler H, et al. Transforming growth factor-β as a predictor of liver and lung fibrosis after autologous bone marrow transplantation for advanced breast cancer. N Engl J Med 1993; 328:1592–1598.

47. Holler E, Kolb HJ, Mittermuller J, Kaul M, Ledderose G, Duell T, Seeber B, Schleuning M, Hintermeier-Knabe R, Ertl B, et al. Modulation of acute graft-versus-host-disease after allogeneic bone marrow transplantation by tumor necrosis factor alpha (TNF alpha) release in the course of pretransplant conditioning: role of conditioning regimens and prophylactic application of a monoclonal antibody neutralizing human TNF alpha (MAK 195F). Blood 1995; 86:890–899.

48. Anscher MS, Murase T, Prescott DM, Marks LB, Reisenbichler H, Bentel GC, Spencer D, Sherouse G, Jirtle RL. Changes in plasma TGF beta levels during pulmonary radiotherapy as a predictor of the risk of developing radiation pneumonitis. Int J Radiat Oncol Biol Phys 1994; 30:671–676.

49. Hallahan DE, Haimovitz-Friedman A, Kufe DW, Fuks Z, Weichselbaum RR. The role of cytokines in radiation oncology. Imp Adv Oncol 1993; 71–80.

50. Neta R. Modulation of radiation damage by cytokines. Stem Cells 1997; 15(suppl 2):87–94.

51. Anscher MS, Kong FM, Marks LB, Bentel GC, Jirtle RL. Changes in plasma transforming growth factor beta during radiotherapy and the risk of symptomatic radiation-induced pneumonitis. Int J Radiat Oncol Biol Phys 1997; 37:253–258.

52. Kraft M, Oussoren Y, Stewart FA, Dorr W, Schultz-Hector S. Radiation-induced changes in transforming growth factor beta and collagen expression in the murine bladder wall and its correlation with bladder function. Radiat Res 1996; 146:619–627.

53. Bernstein EF, Sullivan FJ, Mitchell JB, Salomon GD, Glatstein E. Biology of chronic radiation effect on tissues and wound healing. Clin Plast Surg 1993; 20:435–453.

54. Bernstein EF, Harisiadis L, Salomon G, Norton J, Sollberg S, Uitto J, Glatstein E, Glass J, Talbot T, Russo A, et al. Transforming growth factor-beta improves healing of radiation-impaired wounds. J Invest Dermatol 1991; 97:430–434.

55. Broekelmann TJ, Limper AH, Colby TV, McDonald JA. Transforming growth factor beta 1 is present at sites of extracellular matrix gene expression in human pulmonary fibrosis. Proc Natl Acad Sci USA 1991; 88:6642–6646.

56. Franko AJ, Sharplin J. Development of fibrosis after lung irradiation in relation to inflammation and lung function in a mouse strain prone to fibrosis. Radiat Res 1994; 140:347–355.

57. Butta A, MacLennan K, Flanders KC, Sacks NP, Smith I, McKinna A, Dowsett M, Wakefield LM, Sporn MB, Baum M, et al. Induction of transforming growth factor beta 1 in human breast cancer in vivo following tamoxifen treatment. Cancer Res 1992; 52:4261–4264.

58. Bentzen SM, Skoczylas JZ, Overgaard M, Overgaard J. Radiotherapy-related lung fibrosis enhanced by tamoxifen. J Natl Canc Inst 1996; 88:918–922.
59. Wohl ME, Griscom NT, Traggis DG, Jaffe N. Effects of therapeutic irradiation delivered in early childhood upon subsequent lung function. Pediatrics 1975; 55: 507–516.
60. Benoist MR, Lemerle J, Jean R, Rufin P, Scheinmann P, Paupe J. Effects of pulmonary function of whole lung irradiation for Wilm's tumour in children. Thorax 1982; 37:175–180.
61. Miller RW, Fusner JE, Fink RJ, Murphy TM, Getson PR, Vojtova JA, Reaman GH. Pulmonary function abnormalities in long-term survivors of childhood cancer. Med Pediatr Oncol 1986; 14:202–207.
62. Newton KA, Spittle MF. An analysis of 40 cases treated by total thoracic irradiation. Clin Radiol 1969; 20:19–22.
63. Rab GT, Ivins JC, Childs DS, Jr, Cupps RE, Pritchard DJ. Elective whole lung irradiation in the treatment of osteogenic sarcoma. Cancer 1976; 38:939–942.
64. Fryer CJ, Fitzpatrick PJ, Rider WD, Poon P. Radiation pneumonitis: experience following a large single dose of radiation. Int J Radiat Oncol Biol Phys 1978; 4: 931–936.
65. Carmel RJ, Kaplan HS. Mantle irradiation in Hodgkin's disease. An analysis of technique, tumor eradication, and complications. Cancer 1976; 37:2813–2825.
66. Dubray B, Henry-Amar M, Meerwaldt JH, Noordijk EM, Dixon DO, Cosset JM, Thames HD. Radiation-induced lung damage after thoracic irradiation for Hodgkin's disease: the role of fractionation. Radiother Oncol 1995; 36:211–217.
67. van Rongen E, Travis EL, Thames HD Jr. Repair rate in mouse lung after clinically relevant radiation doses per fraction. Radiat Res 1995; 141:74–78.
68. Mah K, van Dyk J, Keane T, Poon PY. Acute radiation-induced pulmonary damage: a clinical study on the response to fractionated radiation therapy. Int J Radiat Oncol Biol Phys 1987; 13:179–188.
69. Mefferd JM, Donaldson SS, Link MP. Pediatric Hodgkin's disease: pulmonary, cardiac, and thyroid function following combined modality therapy. Int J Radiat Oncol Biol Phys 1989; 16:679–685.
70. Svane G, Rotstein S, Lax I. Influence of radiation therapy on lung tissue in breast cancer patients. CT-assessed density changes 4 years after completion of radiotherapy. Acta Oncol 1995; 34:845–849.
71. Marks LB, Munley MT, Spencer DP, Sherouse GW, Bentel GC, Hoppenworth J, Chew M, Jaszczak RJ, Coleman RE, Prosnitz LR. Quantification of radiation-induced regional lung injury with perfusion imaging. Int J Radiat Oncol Biol Phys 1997; 38:399–409.
72. Martel MK, Ten Haken RK, Hazuka MB, Turrisi AT, Fraass BA, Lichter AS. Dose-volume histogram and 3-D treatment planning evaluation of patients with pneumonitis. Int J Radiat Oncol Biol Phys 1994; 28:575–581.
73. Oetzel D, Schraube P, Hensley F, Sroka-Perez G, Menke M, Flentje M. Estimation of pneumonitis risk in three-dimensional treatment planning using dose-volume histogram analysis. Int J Radiat Oncol Biol Phys 1995; 33:455–460.
74. Graham MV, Jain NL, Kahn MG, Drzymala RE, Purdy JA. Evaluation of an objec-

tive plan-evaluation model in the three-dimensional treatment of nonsmall cell lung cancer. Int J Radiat Oncol Biol Phys 1996; 34:469–474.

75. Graham MV. Predicting radiation response. Int J Radiat Oncol Biol Phys 1997; 39:561–562.

76. Hay J, Shahriar S, Laurent G. Mechanisms of bleomycin-induced lung damage. Arch Toxicol 1991; 65:81–94.

77. Phan SH, Kunkel SL. Lung cytokine production in bleomycin-induced pulmonary fibrosis. Exp Lung Res 1992; 18:29–43.

78. Adamson IY, Bowden DH. The pathogenesis of bleomycin-induced pulmonary fibrosis in mice. Am J Pathol 1974; 77:185–198.

79. Cooper JAD, White DA, Matthay RA. Drug induced pulmonary disease. Part I. Cytotoxic drugs. Am Rev Respir Dis 1986; 133:321–340.

80. McCarthy JT, Staats BA. Pulmonary hypertension, hemolytic anemia, and renal failure. A mitomycin-associated syndrome. Chest 1986; 89:608–611.

81. Lombard CM, Churg A, Winokur S. Pulmonary veno-occlusive disease following therapy for malignant neoplasms. Chest 1987; 92:871–876.

82. Spector JI, Zimbler H, Ross JS. Early-onset cyclophosphamide-induced interstitial pneumonitis. JAMA 1979; 242:2852–2854.

83. Baker W, Fistel SJ, Jones RV, Weiss RB. Interstitial pneumonitis associated with ifosfamide therapy. Cancer 1990; 65:2217–2221.

84. Giles FJ, Smith MP, Goldstone AH. Chlorambucil lung toxicity. Acta Hematol 1990; 83:156–158.

85. Nelson DF, Schoenfeld D, Weinstein AS, Nelson JS, Wasserman T, Goodman RL, Carabell S. A randomized comparison of misonidazole sensitized radiotherapy plus BCNU and radiotherapy plus BCNU for treatment of malignant glioma after surgery; preliminary results of an RTOG study. Int J Radiat Oncol Biol Phys 1983; 9:1143–1151.

86. Weinstein AS, Diener-West M, Nelson DF, Pakuris E. Pulmonary toxicity of carmustine in patients treated for malignant glioma. Cancer Treat Rep 1986; 70:943–946.

87. O'Driscoll BR, Hasleton PS, Taylor PM, Poulter LW, Gattameneni HR, Woodcock AA. Active lung fibrosis up to 17 years after chemotherapy with carmustine (BCNU) in childhood. N Engl J Med 1990; 323:378–382.

88. O'Driscoll BR, Kalra S, Gattamaneni HR, Woodcock AA. Late carmustine lung fibrosis. Age at treatment may influence severity and survival. Chest 1995; 107: 1355–1357.

89. Block M, Lachowiez RM, Rios C, Hirschl S. Pulmonary fibrosis associated with low-dose adjuvant methyl-CCNU. Med Pediatr Oncol 1990; 18:256–260.

90. Massin F, Coudert B, Foucher P, Lombard JN, Reybet-Degat O, Jeannin L, Camus P. Nitrosourea-induced lung diseases. Rev Mal Respir 1992; 9:575–582.

91. van der Veen MJ, Dekker JJ, Dinant HJ, van Soesbergen RM, Bijlsma JW. Fatal pulmonary fibrosis complicating low dose methotrexate therapy for rheumatoid arthritis. J Rheumatol 1995; 22:1766–1768.

92. Jehn U, Goldel N, Rienmuller R, Wilmanns W. Non-cardiogenic pulmonary edema complicating intermediate and high-dose Ara C treatment for relapsed acute leukemia. Med Oncol Tum Pharmacother 1988; 5:41–47.

93. Shearer P, Katz J, Bozeman P, Jenkins J, Laver J, Krance R, Hurwitz C, Mahmoud H, Mirro J. Pulmonary insufficiency complicating therapy with high dose cytosine arabinoside in five pediatric patients with relapsed acute myelogenous leukemia. Cancer 1994; 74:1953–1958.

94. Hamous JE, Guffy MM, Aschenbrener CA. Fatal acute respiratory failure following intrathecal methotrexate administration. Cancer Treat Rep 1983; 67:1025–1026.

95. Verschoore J, Lagrange JL, Boublil JL, Aubanel JM, Blaive B, Pinto J, Namer M. Pulmonary toxicity of a combination of low-dose doxorubicin and irradiation for inoperable lung cancer. Radiother Oncol 1987; 9:281–288.

96. Jules-Elysee K, White DA. Bleomycin-induced pulmonary toxicity. Clin Chest Med 1990; 11:1–20.

97. Comis RL. Bleomycin pulmonary toxicity: current status and future directions. Semin Oncol 1992; 19:64–70.

98. Herrmann G, Hubner K. Fibrosing alveolitis after combined radio- and chemotherapy. A case report. Onkologie 1988; 11:142–144.

99. Molin J, Sogaard PE, Overgaard J. Experimental studies on the radiation-modifying effect of bleomycin in malignant and normal mouse tissue in vivo. Cancer Treat Rep 1981; 65:583–589.

100. Siegel RD, Schiffman FJ. Systemic toxicity following intracavitary administration of bleomycin. Chest 1990; 98:507.

101. Hoyt DG, Lazo JS. Bleomycin and cyclophosphamide increase pulmonary type IV procollagen mRNA in mice. Am J Physiol 1990; 259:L47–L52.

102. Rabinowits M, Souhami L, Gil RA, Andrade CA, Paiva HC. Increased pulmonary toxicity with bleomycin and cisplatin chemotherapy combinations. Am J Clin Oncol 1990; 13:132–138.

103. Jensen BV, Carlsen NL, Nissen NI. Influence of age and duration of follow-up on lung function after combined chemotherapy for Hodgkin's disease. Eur Respir J 1990; 3:1140–1145.

104. Morgan E, Baum E, Breslow N, Takashima J, D'Angio G. Chemotherapy-related toxicity in infants treated according to the Second National Wilms' Tumor Study. J Clin Oncol 1988; 6:51–55.

105. Cooper JA, Zitnik R, Matthay RA. Mechanisms of drug-induced pulmonary disease. Annu Rev Med 1988; 39:395–404.

106. Phillips TL, Wharam MD, Margolis LW. Modification of radiation injury to normal tissues by chemotherapeutic agents. Cancer 1975; 35:1678–1684.

107. Einhorn L, Krause M, Hornback N, Furnas B. Enhanced pulmonary toxicity with bleomycin and radiotherapy in oat cell lung cancer. Cancer 1976; 37:2414–2416.

108. Collis CH, Down JD, Pearson AE, Steel GG. Bleomycin and radiation-induced lung damage in mice. Br J Radiol 1983; 56:21–26.

109. Collis CH, Steel GG. Lung damage in mice from cyclophosphamide and thoracic irradiation: the effect of timing. Int J Radiat Oncol Biol Phys 1983; 9:685–689.

110. von der Maase H, Overgaard J, Vaeth M. Effect of cancer chemotherapeutic drugs on radiation-induced lung damage in mice. Radiother Oncol 1986; 5:245–257.

111. Mattson K, Holsti LR, Niiranen A, Kivisaari L, Iivanainen M, Sovijarvi A, Cantell K. Human leukocyte interferon as part of a combined treatment for previously untreated small cell lung cancer. J Biol Response Modif 1985; 4:8–17.

112. McDonald S, Rubin P, Chang AY, Penney DP, Finkelstein JN, Grossberg S, Feins R, Gregory PK. Pulmonary changes induced by combined mouse beta-interferon (rMuIFN-beta) and irradiation in normal mice—toxic versus protective effects. Radiother Oncol 1993; 26:212–218.

113. McDonald S, Chang AY, Rubin P, Wallenberg J, Kim IS, Sobel S, Smith J, Keng P, Muhs A. Combined Betaseron R (recombinant human interferon beta) and radiation for inoperable non–small cell lung cancer. Int J Radiat Oncol Biol Phys 1993; 27:613–619.

114. Chresta CM, Crook TR, Souhami RL. Depletion of cellular glutathione by N,N'-bis(*trans*-4-hydroxycyclohexyl)-N'-nitrosourea as a determinant of sensitivity of K562 human leukemia cells to 4-hydroperoxycyclophosphamide. Cancer Res 1990; 50:4067–4071.

115. Rusch VW, Benfield JR. Neoadjuvant therapy for lung cancer: a note of caution. Ann Thorac Surg 1993; 55:820–821.

116. Rusch VW, Albain KS, Crowley JJ, Rice TW, Lonchyna V, McKenna R Jr., Livingston RB, Griffin BR, Benfield JR. Surgical resection of stage IIIA and stage IIIB non–small-cell lung cancer after concurrent induction chemoradiotherapy. A Southwest Oncology Group trial. J Thorac Cardiovasc Surg 1993; 105:97–104.

117. Koga K, Kusumoto S, Watanabe K, Nishikawa K, Harada K, Ebihara H. Age factor relevant to the development of radiation pneumonitis in radiotherapy of lung cancer. Int J Radiat Oncol Biol Phys 1988; 14:367–371.

118. Rubin P, Casarett GW. Clinical Radiation Pathology. Philadelphia: WB Saunders, 1968.

119. Rubin P. Radiation toxicology: quantitative radiation pathology for predicting effects. Cancer 1977; 39:729–736.

120. Cohen Y, Gellei B, Robinson E. Bilateral radiation pneumonitis after unilateral lung and mediastinal irradiation. Radiol Clin Biol 1974; 43:465–471.

121. Roberts CM, Foulcher E, Zaunders JJ, Bryant DH, Freund J, Cairns D, Penny R, Morgan GW, Breit SN. Radiation pneumonitis: a possible lymphocyte-mediated hypersensitivity reaction. Ann Intern Med 1993; 118:696–700.

122. Morgan GW, Breit SN. Radiation and the lung: a reevaluation of the mechanisms mediating pulmonary injury. Int J Radiat Oncol Biol Phys 1995; 31:361–369.

123. Mah K, Poon PY, van Dyk J, Keane T, Majesky IF, Rideout DF. Assessment of acute radiation-induced pulmonary changes using computed tomography. J CAT 1986; 10:736–743.

124. Mah K, van Dyk J. Quantitative measurement of changes in human lung density following irradiation. Radiother Oncol 1988; 11:169–179.

125. Libshitz HI. Radiation changes in the lung. Semin Roentgenol 1993; 28:303–320.

126. Marks LB. The pulmonary effects of thoracic irradiation. Oncology 1994; 8:89–106.

127. Boersma LJ, Damen EM, de Boer RW, Muller SH, Valdes Olmos RA, van Zandwijk N, Lebesque JV. Estimation of overall pulmonary function after irradiation using dose-effect relations for local functional injury. Radiother Oncol 1995; 36: 15–23.

128. McDonald S, Rubin P, Constine L, Williams J, Finkelstein J, Smudzin T. Biochemi-

cal markers as predictors for pulmonary effects of radiation. Radiat Oncol Invest 1995; 3:56–63.

129. Ward WF, Lin PJ, Wong PS, Behnia R, Jalali N. Radiation pneumonitis in rats and its modification by the angiotensin-converting enzyme inhibitor captopril evaluated by high-resolution computed tomography. Radiat Res 1993; 135:81–87.

130. O'Brien-Ladner A, Nelson ME, Kimler BF, Wesselius LJ. Release of interleukin-1 by human alveolar macrophages after in vitro irradiation. Radiat Res 1993; 136: 37–41.

131. Thornton SC, Walsh BJ, Bennett S, Robbins JM, Foulcher E, Morgan GW, Penny R, Breit SN. Both in vitro and in vivo irradiation are associated with induction of macrophage-derived fibroblast growth factors. Clin Exp Immunol 1996; 103:67–73.

132. Behnia R, Molteni A, Waters CM, Panos RJ, Ward WF, Schnaper HW, Ts'ao CH. Early markers of ventilator-induced lung injury in rats. Ann Clin Lab Sci 1996; 26:437–450.

133. Dubray B, Henry-Amar M, Meerwaldt JH, Noordijk EM, Dixon DO, Cosset JM, Thames HD. Radiation-induced lung damage after thoracic irradiation for Hodgkin's disease: the role of fractionation. Radiother Oncol 1995; 36:211–217.

134. Shulimzon T, Apter S, Weitzen R, Yellin A, Brenner HJ, Wollner A. Radiation pneumonitis complicating mediastinal radiotherapy postpneumonectomy. Eur Respir J 1996; 9:2697–2699.

135. Travis EL, Liao ZX, Tucker SL. Spatial heterogeneity of the volume effect for radiation pneumonitis in mouse lung. Int J Radiat Oncol Biol Phys 1997; 38:1045–1054.

136. McCrea ES, Diaconis JN, Wade JC, Johnston CA. Bleomycin toxicity simulating metastatic nodules to the lungs. Cancer 1981; 48:1096–1100.

137. White DA, Stover DE. Severe bleomycin-induced pneumonitis. Clinical features and response to corticosteroids. Chest 1984; 86:723–728.

138. Epperly MW, Bray JA, Krager RS, et al. Intratracheal injection of adenovirus containing the human MnSOD transgene protects athymic nude mice from irradiation induced organizing alveolitis. Int J Radiat Oncol Biol Phys 1999; 43(1):169–181.

139. Ward WF, Molteni A, TS'Ao CH, Kim YT, Hinz JM. Radiation pneumotoxicity in rats: modification by inhibitors of angiotensin converting enzyme. Int J Radiat Oncol Biol Phys 1992; 22:623–625.

140. Koh WJ, Stelzer KJ, Peterson LM, Staker BL, Ward WF, Russell KJ, Griffin TW. Effect of pentoxifylline on radiation-induced lung and skin toxicity in rats. Int J Radiat Oncol Biol Phys 1995; 31:71–77.

141. Sonis ST, Sonis AL, Lieberman A. Oral complications in patients receiving treatment for malignancies other than of the head and neck. J Am Dent Assoc 1978; 97:468–472.

142. Dreizen S. Stomatotoxic manifestations of cancer chemotherapy. J Prosthet Dent 1978; 40:650–655.

143. Marini G, Simoncini E, Zaniboni A, Gorni F, Marpicati P, Zambruni A. 5-Fluorouracil and high-dose folinic acid as salvage treatment of advanced breast cancer: an update. Oncology 1987; 44:336–340.

144. Fine S, Erlichman C, Kaizer L, Warr D, Gadalla T. Phase II trial of 5-fluorouracil

and folinic acid in the treatment of advanced breast cancer. Breast Cancer Res Treat 1994; 30:205–209.

145. Herskovic A, Martz K, al-Sarraf M, Leichman L, Brindle J, Vaitkevicius V, Cooper J, Byhardt R, Davis L, Emami B. Combined chemotherapy and radiotherapy compared with radiotherapy alone in patients with cancer of the esophagus. N Engl J Med 1992; 326:1593–1598.

146. Emami B, Lyman J, Brown A, Coia L, Goitein M, Munzenrider JE, Shank B, Solin LJ, Wesson M. Tolerance of normal tissue to therapeutic irradiation. Int J Radiat Oncol Biol Phys 1991; 21:109–122.

147. Coia LR, Myerson RJ, Tepper JE. Late effects of radiation therapy on the gastrointestinal tract. Int J Radiat Oncol Biol Phys 1995; 31:1213–1236.

148. Goldstein HM, Rogers LF, Fletcher GH, Dodd GD. Radiological manifestations of radiation-induced injury to the normal upper gastrointestinal tract. Radiology 1975; 117:135–140.

149. Collazzo LA, Levine MS, Rubesin SE, Laufer I. Acute radiation esophagitis: radiographic findings. Am J Roentgenol 1997; 169:1067–1070.

150. Mascarenhas F, Silvestre ME, da Costa M, Grima N, Campos C, Chaves P. Acute secondary effects in the esophagus in patients undergoing radiotherapy for carcinoma of the lung. Am J Clin Oncol 1989; 12:34–40.

151. Chabora BM, Hopfan S, Wittes R. Esophageal complications in the treatment of oat cell carcinoma with combined irradiation and chemotherapy. Radiology 1977; 123:185–187.

152. Lepke RA, Libshitz HI. Radiation-induced injury of the esophagus. Radiology 1983; 148:375–378.

153. Umsawasdi T, Valdivieso M, Barkley HT Jr, Booser DJ, Chiuten DF, Murphy WK, Dhingra HM, Dixon CL, Farha P, Spitzer G, et al. Esophageal complications from combined chemoradiotherapy (cyclophosphamide + adriamycin + cisplatin + XRT) in the treatment of non–small cell lung cancer. Int J Radiat Oncol Biol Phys 1985; 11:511–519.

154. Armstrong JG, Zelefsky MJ, Leibel SA, Burman C, Han C, Harrison LB, Kutcher GJ, Fuks ZY. Strategy for dose escalation using 3-dimensional conformal radiation therapy for lung cancer. Ann Oncol 1995; 6:693–697.

155. Armstrong J, Raben A, Zelefsky M, Burt M, Leibel S, Burman C, Kutcher G, Harrison L, Hahn C, Ginsberg R, Rusch V, Kris M, Fuks Z. Promising survival with three-dimensional conformal radiation therapy for non–small cell lung cancer. Radiother Oncol 1997; 44:17–22.

156. Mehta MP. Protection of normal tissues from the cytotoxic effects of radiation therapy: focus on amifostine. Semin Radiat Oncol 1998; 8:14–16.

157. Antonadou D, Coliarakis N, Synodinou M, Athanassiou H, Kouveli A, Verigos C, Georgakopoulos G, Panousaki K, Karageorgis P, Throuvalas N. Randomized phase III trial of radiation ± amifostine in patients with advanced stage lung cancer. Int J Radiat Oncol Biol Phys 1999; 45(3):154.

158. Antonadou D, Synodinou M, Boufi M, Sagriotis A, Paloudis S, Throuvalas N. Amifostine-reduced acute toxicity during radiochemotherapy in patients with localized advanced stage non–small cell lung cancer. Proc ASCO 2000; 19:501a.

159. Meredith R, Salter M, Kim R, Spencer S, Weppelmann B, Rodu B, Smith J, Lee

J. Sucralfate for radiation mucositis: results of a double-blind randomized trial. Int J Radiat Oncol Biol Phys 1997; 37:275–279.

160. Ng TM, Spencer GM, Sargeant IR, Thorpe SM, Bown SG. Management of strictures after radiotherapy for esophageal cancer. Gastrointest Endosc 1996; 43:584–590.

161. O'Rourke IC, Tiver K, Bull C, Gebski V, Langlands AO. Swallowing performance after radiation therapy for carcinoma of the esophagus. Cancer 1988; 61:2022–2026.

24

Supportive Care in Thoracic Oncology: Preemptive Management of Myelosuppression

Jeffrey Crawford
Duke Comprehensive Cancer Center, Durham, North Carolina

INTRODUCTION

The advent of the hematopoietic growth factors has provided the oncologist with the ability to ameliorate cytopenias in cancer chemotherapy patients (1). Clinical trials focused on anemia, neutropenia, and thrombocytopenia have taught us about the magnitude of clinical consequences associated with these laboratory abnormalities. Also, the clinical use of hematopoietic growth factors has increased our understanding of the biology of hematopoiesis, and its impact on cancer therapy. This chapter will focus on the recent state of knowledge on the use of hematopoietic growth factors in the lung cancer population as well as the potential utility of these agents in the future.

THE MANAGEMENT OF ANEMIA WITH ERYTHROPOIETIN

Anemia is prevalent among cancer patients and is related both to the underlying disease and to its treatment (2). Because lung cancer affects an older patient population who often have significant comorbid pulmonary and cardiac disease, the symptoms of anemia are often magnified in this population. Despite this, our understanding of the impact of anemia on the cancer patient was extremely naive until clinical trials focused on the treatment of anemia were performed over the last decade. Prior to this, anemia was simply considered to be part of the cancer experience, an expected cost of doing business. Clinical trials often did not even collect information on the magnitude of anemia or of need for transfusion and impact on treatment outcomes. Studies of the impact of anemia on the cancer patient and its treatment with recombinant human erythropoietin have been enlightening.

Erythropoietin was approved for clinical use in the 1980s, with the clinical indication of treatment of anemia in the renal dialysis population (3). Its use has essentially eliminated anemia as a significant problem for this patient population. It was assumed initially that the use of exogenous recombinant human erythropoietin would only benefit patients with renal failure because of the lack of endogenous erythoproietin. Subsequently, it has been demonstrated that multiple types of anemia, including cancer-related anemia and chemotherapy-induced anemia, are associated with a blunted endogenous erythropoietin response and that the use of recombinant human erythropoietin can significantly accelerate erythropoiesis (4).

The pivotal trial of recombinant human erthropoietin for the treatment of cancer-chemotherapy-related anemia was a placebo-controlled, randomized effort in patients with anemia developing in the setting of either cisplatin-containing or non–cisplatin-containing chemotherapy (5). All patients were treated with recombinant human erythropoietin at a dose of 150 units/kg subcutaneously three times a week for 12 weeks. An additional group of cancer patients with anemia who did not receive chemotherapy was treated for an 8-week period. Compared to the placebo group, the patients receiving either cisplatin-based or non–cisplatin-based chemotherapy achieved a median increase in hematocrit of 7% with an associated significant reduction in transfusion requirements. The anemic cancer patients not receiving chemotherapy did not achieve as significant an increase in hematocrit, presumably because of the shorter period of therapy. These patients also underwent an evaluation of their overall energy level and activities of daily living utilizing a linear analog scale assessment (LASA). This showed a significant increase in the patient's self-reported quality of life by this scale. Based on this randomized trial, erythropoietin was approved for treatment of anemia associated with cancer chemotherapy.

Despite the broad indication for erythropoietin, it was not widely adopted in clinical practice, which led to a series of phase IV open-label, community-based trials. Three successive trials were done with over 2000 patients in each study. The first two trials administered erythropoietin on the routine three-times-a-week schedule used in the registration trial (6,7). The third trial utilized a once-per-week dosing schedule of 40,000 units with an escalation to 60,000 units for patients who did not achieve a 1-g increase in hemoglobin in the first month (8). All three trials look remarkably similar in terms of patient outcomes. On average, more than 65% of patients responded with at least a 2-g increase in hemoglobin over the 16-week treatment. Again, a significant reduction in transfusion requirements was noted. Finally, the linear analog scale again demonstrated significant improvements in the patients' self-reported energy level, activities of daily living, and overall quality of life. These trials were also able to show that the quality-of-life improvements were directly related to improvement in hemoglobin, but in a nonlinear fashion. Although there was some improvement in quality of life between a hemoglobin of 8 and 10 g/dl, there was an even greater improvement with increase in hemoglobin from 10 to 12 g/dl, with a lesser degree of improvement above the level of 12 g/dl. Thus, achieving a hemoglobin of 12 g/dl appeared to be an optimal target.

In the Demetri trial (7), additional quality-of-life analyses were done utilizing the FACT-An (9). This demonstrated the same correlative relationship between quality-of-life measures and improvements in hemoglobin and helped validate the LASA results across all of the trials. In addition, prospective tumor responses were performed. For patients whose hemoglobin level did not improve, there was little change in quality of life despite response of the tumor to chemotherapy. However, for those who did show an improvement in hemoglobin, the quality-of-life improvement correlated with the magnitude of hemoglobin improvement. For the patients with progressive disease, however, the improvement in quality of life was significantly blunted. These data strongly suggest that both tumor response and hemoglobin response are important predictors for quality of life and are independent of one another.

While none of these three trials were placebo controlled, the power of a 7000-patient database makes the results extremely robust. Furthermore, with such a large database, analyses of subgroups of patients are ongoing to determine if particular patient subsets or disease types have a differing response. A preliminary analysis of the first two trials, which included more than 1000 lung cancer patients, suggests that lung cancer patients respond equally well in terms of these endpoints and in addition show a significant improvement in the symptom of dyspnea (10). It seems clear from this database that oncologists need to pay more attention to anemia and should specifically try to maintain patients at or above a hemoglobin of 12 g/dl. It would appear that either a three-times-a-week or once-a-week schedule is equally efficacious in this regard. Remaining questions center on the management of the patient who does not respond well to erythropoietin, and in defining what the role of iron supplementation may be (11). Most of these trials did not supplement patients with oral iron, and clinical data suggest that iron deficiency in the cancer patient population is relatively low. However, whether a functional iron deficiency might have existed that could have been treated with oral or parenteral iron to optimize the response to erythropoietin remains an area of clinical investigation.

PREVENTION OF ANEMIA

The justification for early treatment of anemic cancer patients seems clear from data showing improved quality of life. Because of the broad nature of these trials across many diseases and treatment regimens, the impact of hemoglobin improvement on actual survival rates has not been well studied. However, hemoglobin level per se has been shown to be an important prognostic factor in patients receiving radiation therapy for head and neck cancer and carcinoma of the cervix (11). The initial assumption was that patients with low hemoglobin might have more advanced disease or poorer performance status, which might compromise outcome. However, more recent studies have suggested that a more important variable is maintenance of hemoglobin during radiation, which facilitates treatment response and potentially improves survival. Whether the influence of hemoglobin is related to improvements in regional blood flow, tumor perfusion, reduction in hypoxia, or reduction in angiogenic factors, or is operational through some other mechanism is unknown at this point, but again remains an area of active clinical investigation.

In the lung cancer population the importance of chemoradiation with curative intent has been well demonstrated in both limited small cell lung cancer and stage III non–small cell lung cancer, and is discussed in detail elsewhere in this book. Whether maintenance of a normal hemoglobin through therapy could actually improve long-term outcome as well as lead to improved quality of life has not been studied. However, it appears from a pilot study done at M. D. Anderson that the use of erythropoietin at the initiation of concurrent chemotherapy and radiation can successfully prevent the development of anemia in patients with non–small cell lung cancer (12). Furthermore, two other small studies in small cell lung cancer have demonstrated that initiation of erythropoietin at the beginning of chemotherapy can lessen the development of anemia in this population (13,14).

The prevention of anemia in patients with advanced non–small cell lung cancer is the subject of an ongoing multicenter U.S. trial in patients with advanced non–small cell lung cancer receiving chemotherapy only. In this study, patients must have a normal hemoglobin above 12 g/dl to be enrolled and then are randomized to receive weekly erythropoietin or supportive care alone while receiving chemotherapy. For patients whose hemoglobins drop to ≤ 10 g/dl on the supportive-care arm, treatment with erythropoietin will be initiated. The primary objective of this study is to assess whether erythropoietin can prevent anemia in this population and if the maintenance of a normal hemoglobin impacts on quality of life compared to delayed use of erythropoietin in patients who develop significant anemia. Measures of tumor response and survival will also be obtained, although the relative magnitude of benefit of hemoglobin maintenance might presumably be less in this population than in patients with more locally advanced disease.

Until such prevention strategies are shown to be beneficial, the best approach for management of lung cancer patients is to anticipate the need for treatment when the hemoglobin level falls below 12 g/dl for patients on active chemotherapy and/or radiation treatment. In addition, aggressive management of hemoglobin may be warranted in patients undergoing neoadjuvant approaches prior to surgery. Finally, for patients with significant anemia due to the disease itself, management of the hemoglobin level may result in a significant improvement in the patient's fatigue and dyspnea even at the point when further chemotherapy or radiation may be unhelpful.

NEUTROPENIA AND INFECTION: THE ROLE OF COLONY-STIMULATING FACTORS IN PREVENTION AND TREATMENT

While the data for the use of erythropoietin to treat anemia complicating cancer chemotherapy is clear, much less data exist to support routine treatment of established neutropenia or uncomplicated febrile neutropenia with the use of colony-stimulating factors (CSFs) (15). On the other hand, a large number of randomized trials have demonstrated that the use of CSFs, as a preemptive strategy, can reduce the magnitude of neutropenia and the clinical consequences of fever and infection (1,15). Furthermore, the CSFs have played a major role in the technology of peripheral blood progenitor cell mobilization and stem cell support in use for high-dose chemotherapy (16). Although the CSFs were developed as "supportive care agents" like erythropoietin, their major clinical benefit has been in the prevention, rather than treatment, of cytopenia. The result in both standard and high-dose chemotherapy has been a reduction in infectious complications with a decrease in intravenous antibiotics and hospitalization.

A detailed discussion of the evidence supporting the use of CSFs was provided by the ASCO CSF Guidelines Committee (15) and is being updated. It will be reviewed here briefly. As mentioned, treatment of established neutropenia with CSFs has been less beneficial than prevention. This is not because of a lack of biological response to the CSF, but rather because neutropenia is a more self-limited event than anemia and generally resolves within a few days after standard chemotherapy. For patients with grade IV neutropenia (ANC less than 0.5×10^9 cells/L), the risk of developing fever and infection is approximately 10% for every day of duration (17). Thus it is not surprising that in a randomized trial in which patients who were found to have clinically asymptomatic grade IV neutropenia, after standard chemotherapy, the risk of developing febrile neutropenia was approximately 15% (18). This was not modified significantly by G-CSF because of the relatively low risk and also because the biology of the cytokine requires an adequate number of progenitor cells to achieve an adequate response. Thus the therapeutic use of the CSF in the setting of asymptomatic neutropenia in the postchemotherapy setting should be reserved for patients at high risk for complications of fever and infection. Other considerations for treatment of neutropenia with CSFs include acceleration of neutrophil recovery to insure that chemotherapy and/or radiation is given on schedule. The treatment of febrile neutropenia has been equally controversial but has been clarified by a series of clinical studies that are reviewed in detail elsewhere (1,15). Of the several randomized phase III trials evaluating growth factors, almost all have demonstrated reduction of duration of neutropenia with the use of CSF in the setting of symptomatic febrile neutropenia. A few have shown a clinical benefit in terms of reducing hospital stay or antibiotic use. Subset analyses, however, in several of these trials have suggested that patients with tissue infection or sepsis may be at a higher risk for prolonged neutropenic complications and may benefit from the use of CSFs; this may be particularly relevant to the older lung cancer population with a potential for pneumonia and postobstructive pneumonia. One other important factor observed in these clinical trials has to do with the absolute magnitude of neutropenia. While grade IV neutropenia includes all patients whose ANC drops to 0.5×10^9 cells/L, the studies that best demonstrate the benefit of CSFs have looked prospectively at populations presenting with an absolute neutrophil count of 0.1×10^9/L (19,20).

Because of the previous studies, the major focus of CSF use has been on its prevention of neutropenia and its clinical complications, rather than its treatment once it has occurred. The initial trials that led to the approval of G-CSF for the reduction in the risk of neutropenia and infection were performed in patients with small cell lung cancer receiving cyclophosphamide, adriamycin, and etoposide chemotherapy (17,21).

These studies documented a 50% reduction in the duration of neutropenia with the use of G-CSF versus placebo, and that 50% reduction in neutropenia correlated with a 50% reduction in incidence of febrile neutropenia as well as overall use of intravenous antibiotics and hospitalization. This study helped expedite the approval of G-CSF to reduce myelosuppression associated with cancer chemotherapy (17). This trial also documented that patients on placebo who had experienced febrile neutropenia during a prior cycle of chemotherapy could go on to receive full-dose chemotherapy along with G-CSF with a subsequent reduction in risk of febrile neutropenia to approximately 26%. Thus, this trial established the role of G-CSF in both primary and secondary prophylaxis of neutropenia and its complications.

Many subsequent trials confirmed the ability of G-CSF to significantly reduce the duration of neutropenia in the primary setting, but little formal study has been performed on its benefit as secondary prophylaxis (1,15). Interestingly, however, the major clinical use for G-CSF, currently, is in the setting of secondary rather than primary prophylaxis. For most standard chemotherapy regimens, routine primary prophylaxis does not appear to be necessary because the risk is relatively manageable and because of the relatively brief period of neutropenia with most standard chemotherapy regimens in otherwise good-performance-status patients. The strategy of reserving CSF for patients who have developed significant neutropenia and/or febrile neutropenia in prior cycles of therapy has been recommended to identify patients at highest risk. While this is a reasonable strategy for most standard clinical settings, the ASCO guidelines have also identified a patient population where consideration should be given either for reduction in dose of initial chemotherapy or for the use of CSF as primary prophylaxis (15). These settings would include patients with significant comorbid disease, advanced age, poor performance status, ongoing or incompletely treated infection, or other factors that might increase the risk of chemotherapy. While none of these factors have been well established in a randomized prospective trial of either standard dose reduction or primary prophylactic use of CSF, they have been clarified in work done by Talcott defining low- and high-risk populations who developed febrile neutropenia (22).

The lung cancer population, generally because of its older age and/or high likelihood of comorbid disease and/or pulmonary infections complicating treatment, represents a high-risk group. However, routine use of CSF for primary prophylaxis is not warranted for standard chemotherapy regimens used for both small cell lung cancer and non–small cell lung cancer. Careful attention should be paid to identify special populations at increased risk who might be candidates for initial use of CSF rather than to expose them to the increased risk of neutropenia and infection.

Whether preemptive CSF administration, in either the primary or secondary setting, should be utilized versus dose modification remains a controversial topic. Other chapters in this textbook have focused on evidence supporting dose intensification of chemotherapy treatments in either small cell or non–small cell lung cancer. These studies will not be reiterated here except to make a few important points. First, it is clear that in small cell lung cancer, particularly with limited stage, substandard doses of chemotherapy lead to poor outcome (23). In non–small cell lung cancer, it has only been in recent years that we have established the benefit of chemotherapy, particularly in patients with advanced disease. However, from these data, it is clear that combination chemotherapy has, in general, been superior to single-agent therapy, particularly in good-performance-status patients (24). In the lower-performance-status patient population and in the elderly with advanced non–small cell lung cancer, it remains unclear whether the combination therapy is less beneficial or simply more toxic, or both. Until clinical trials clarify this issue for patients with advanced small cell or non–small cell lung cancer, special populations deserve special treatment considerations. This may range from monotherapy in the patient of borderline performance status or combination chemotherapy with appropriate supportive care including the preemptive use of CSFs. The choice obviously depends on the clinical situation and a full discussion of the risks and benefits with the patient.

While there is prevailing sentiment that dose reduction and modification can lead to inferior outcomes in breast cancer and lymphoma, formal studies testing this issue in either small cell or non–small cell lung cancer are limited. However, given the relatively narrow therapeutic window for our agents particularly in non–small cell lung cancer, the ability to achieve "full dose" therapy particularly in potentially curative settings of limited stage small cell lung cancer and stage III non–small cell lung cancer is an appropriate goal. In this setting, the preemptive use of CSFs in either the primary or secondary setting could be considered. By contrast, dose escalation of chemotherapy above standard doses and the use of CSFs outside the setting of clinical trial is not recommended by the ASCO Guidelines Committee (15). What are the data to suggest that dose might make a difference in the management of patients with lung cancer?

Although a huge number of phase II trials have been performed, one can learn little without a phase III comparison. Of interest, for one of the most active agents in non–small cell lung cancer (paclitaxel), the most positive results have been achieved with the regimen associated with the most myelosuppression (25). While several trials have compared cisplatin and Taxol to other combinations, the trial that has shown substantial survival benefits utilized paclitaxel on a 24-h basis. In that trial, the highest survival rate was seen in the population in whom paclitaxel was increased from 135 mg/m^2 as a 24-hr infusion to 250 mg/m^2 with G-CSF support. The 1-year survival for the lower-dose paclitaxel treatment was 36% versus 39% with the higher dose of paclitaxel. Although that was not significantly different statistically, the trend was encouraging; moreover, the increase in paclitaxel dose did not result in increased myelosuppression because of the adjunctive use of G-CSF. However, the increased dose of paclitaxel was associated with a higher incidence of neurotoxicity, highlighting the observation that other nonhematological toxicities must be balanced as we escalate chemotherapy doses. In addition, alternate strategies such as weekly paclitaxel may allow dose enhancement or intensification of this drug without either rate-limiting myelosuppression or cumulative neurotoxicity.

At this point, the preemptive use of CSFs in the treatment of patients with small cell lung cancer or non–small cell lung cancer should be reserved for primary administration in the setting of high-risk patients receiving standard chemotherapy, or more commonly, as secondary prophylaxis in a patient who has received previous chemotherapy resulting in significant neutropenia or neutropenic complications, and in whom the clinical benefit of continuing full-dose chemotherapy outweighs the strategy of dose reduction. Clearly, trials that prospectively evaluate maintenance of normal dose intensity of chemotherapy with growth factors versus the strategy of dose reduction would be beneficial in future decision making. For patients who develop febrile neutropenia in the setting of cancer chemotherapy, treatment of the febrile neutropenic event with CSFs as well as antibiotics should be considered in patients with severe neutropenia (less than 0.1×10^9 neutrophils/L) or the patient with bacteremia or clinical signs of tissue infection.

INCORPORATING CSFs IN FUTURE TREATMENT STRATEGIES TO IMPROVE THE OUTCOME FOR PATIENTS WITH LUNG CANCER

As outlined above, the primary role of CSFs in clinical practice should be restricted to their use as supportive-care agents to reduce the complications of clinically effective treatment regimens. CSFs may also be extremely useful as we develop newer treatment strategies. Numerous clinical trials have taught us that CSFs alone can only modestly enhance the dose intensity of chemotherapy regimens (26). However, the use of CSFs to mobilize peripheral blood progenitor cells provides the ability to test more significant increases by five- or 10-fold in the dose intensity of conventional chemotherapy agents (1,15,16). Moreover the use of CSFs may enhance the dose density of therapy by shortening the time interval between treatments as has been done in small cell lung cancer with encouraging results (26–28). Finally, CSFs may be useful in combining multiple agents at standard doses of therapy rather than trying to increase the dose of any single agent. None of these concepts are mutually exclusive and, in fact, must be thought of in conjunction with each other. A framework by which one might determine how improved curative strategies can be developed for lung and other cancers is the concept of summation dose intensity (29).

In a review of chemotherapy regimens that have been associated with significant chance of cure, Frei et al. propose the formula shown in Figure 1.

While this formula has been best supported by treatment of hematological malignancies and germ cell tumors, the general principles may be applicable to lung cancer as well. For example, in the curable setting of stage IIIA/B inoperable non–small cell lung cancer or in the setting of limited-stage small cell lung cancer, the addition of at least two active chemotherapy agents along with radiation treatment has improved the cure rate. On the other hand, more aggressive treatment strategies in stage IV non–small cell lung cancer or extensive-stage small cell lung cancer have not been successful from a curative standpoint, although some regimens may be associated with modest improvements in survival. The

Curative Cancer Chemo- therapy	∞	≥ Three Active Agent(s) Tumor Biology	x x	Combination Chemotherapy x Full Dose Host Factors	x x	Supportive Care Toxicity

FIGURE 1 Formula for curative cancer chemotherapy. (a) Active—30% response rate; non–cross-resistant. (b) Concurrent combined administration of three or more active agents. (c) Full dose maintained in combination (i.e., nonadditive toxicity). (d) Particularly stem cells, blood products, and growth factors. (Adapted from Ref. 29.)

lung cancer population is less able to withstand the toxicities of aggressive strategies compared to a generally younger population with other cancers; in addition, our understanding of the biology of lung cancer is inferior to our understanding of the hematological malignancies. Furthermore, initial or subsequent drug resistance remains a formidable problem. Finally, most of the active agents in lung cancer unfortunately have overlapping toxicities, particularly myelosuppression. This makes the simultaneous use of several agents difficult, if one hopes to maintain the maximal beneficial dose of each agent.

Despite these limitations, this formula provides a useful framework by which future clinical trials can be developed. As observed in the study of new agents in patients with advanced non–small cell lung cancer, simply substituting one for another has not resulted in major improvements in outcome. Likewise, minor differences in dose intensity of standard chemotherapy regimens in small cell lung cancer have not yielded promising results (26). A prospective randomized trial testing the ability of preemptive management of myelosuppression to improve outcome is being explored in the current intergroup trial of extensive-stage small cell lung cancer. In this trial, patients are randomized to receive cisplatin and etoposide at standard doses versus that same regimen combined with paclitaxel and G-CSF, to ameliorate the increased neutropenia of the third agent. Strategies like this, which incorporate both the promising additional agent and the supportive care necessary to deliver those agents at their intended doses, hold promise for improving outcome in patients with lung cancer.

THE USE OF CSFs WITH CHEMOTHERAPY AND RADIATION

The ASCO guidelines flatly state that CSFs should not be used as supportive-care agents in the setting of concurrent chemotherapy/radiation therapy (15). The data to support this recommendation come from a trial of limited-stage small cell lung cancer in which patients were randomized to receive or not to receive GM-CSF after completion of a 3-day cisplatin/etoposide chemotherapy regimen, concurrent with ongoing thoracic radiation (30). In this study, patients receiving GM-CSF versus placebo had no benefit in terms of reduction of neutropenia and demonstrated an increase in thrombocytopenia. While no randomized trial of G-CSF has been performed in this setting, a small sequential study of chemotherapy/radiation therapy in non–small cell lung cancer patients, without and with G-CSF, also suggested worsening thrombocytopenia (31). Because of this very limited database, further studies are warranted to evaluate different schedules of chemotherapy/radiation and growth factor support. However, outside of clinical trials, CSFs should be avoided in the setting of primary prophylaxis of neutropenia when chemotherapy and radiation therapy are combined. Patients being treated in this setting who subsequently develop neutropenic complications may warrant the use of CSF as a form of secondary prophylaxis, but this must be done cautiously.

In this regard, it is helpful to discuss the likely reason for the paradoxical worsening of myelosuppression with the use of growth factors in the setting of combined chemotherapy and chest radiation. Of interest, coadministration of cytotoxic chemotherapy and CSFs has been conducted safely in some, but not all, studies (31). In addition, in the setting of acute lymphoblastic leukemia, patients have been randomized to receive G-CSF or no G-CSF concomitant with chemotherapy and cranial radiation (32). In this setting, G-CSF was beneficial in reducing neutropenia with no other adverse hemological or nonhemological toxlcities. What may be different between this setting and the lung cancer setting is the blood volume in the area radiation is delivered. The use of CSFs is well known to lead to mobilization of progenitor cells into the peripheral blood (1,15,16). Thoracic radiation encompasses a significant volume of the blood pool and mobilized, committed progenitor cells in this pool may be more susceptible to the cytotoxic effects of radiation in this setting. If this is a primary reason for the negative interaction of CSFs in this setting, then delay of the use of CSFs from the first to the second week of therapy might represent an alternative strategy that warrants further evaluation. Such studies are particularly promising given the importance of concurrent chemotherapy and radiation therapy early in the clinical course of both small cell and stage III non–small cell lung cancer. In addition, the use of other supportive-care agents may further enhance our ability to deliver both chemotherapy and radiation together and to reduce other limiting side effects such as mucositis and esophagitis. This would enable us to further test the Frei formula in a more curative setting of stage III non–small cell and small cell lung cancer.

THROMBOCYTOPENIA: IS THERE AN ANSWER?

As discussed previously, anemia is a common and almost universal result of the cumulative effects of chemotherapy and radiation treatment, and is significantly improved by erythropoietin, which can also improve the patient's quality of life. While neutropenia from chemotherapy is not as universal, it can be devastating in terms of febrile neutropenia and/or serious life-threatening infections. In addition, neutropenia is one of the most common dose-limiting side effects of chemotherapy treatments and its complications can be reduced with the use of CSFs. However, with standard chemotherapy, it is uncommon for thrombocytopenia to progress to the point of risk of either bleeding or need for platelet transfusion (33). It is also unusual for thrombocytopenia to be the dose-limiting toxicity of chemotherapy treatment. However, there are at least two commonly used chemotherapy agents that often cause some degree of thrombocytopenia: carboplatin and gemcitabine. By dosing carboplatin using the AUC formula, the risk of significant thrombocytopenia can be reduced substantially.

Thrombocytopenia is generally not limiting with gemcitabine by itself, but in combination with cisplatin or carboplatin, the incidence of thrombocytopenia increases substantially. Although this has not interfered with the clinical benefits of these agents in most patients, an effective agent to reduce thrombocytopenia would help support patients receiving these combinations, or enable intensification of therapy, particularly in combination with radiation.

In contrast to standard-dose chemotherapy, high-dose chemotherapy has been associated with prolonged thrombocytopenia requiring platelet support often for several days to weeks depending on the preferred regimen. None of the thrombopoietic growth factors have significantly sped platelet recovery in this setting (1,34). However, in the transition from the use of autologous bone marrow support to peripheral blood progenitor cells, generally mobilized by CSFs, there has been a significant shortening of the duration of thrombocytopenia and reduction in total platelet transfusion in this setting (1). The standard supportive-care approach for high-dose chemotherapy regimens using peripheral blood progenitor cells in lung cancer is CSF support and platelet transfusions as indicated for severe thrombocytopenia, generally less than $10,000/\mu l$. Thus far, the thrombopoietic agents have yielded little benefit in chemotherapy regimens employing either standard or high-dose therapy. Of the interleukins, use of IL-3 and IL-6 has been limited both by toxicity and by a relative lack of efficacy (34). On the other hand, IL-11 has demonstrated a reduction in thrombocytopenia and reduced the need for platelet transfusion in a randomized study of secondary prophylaxis (35). In this trial, patients who had experienced the need for platelet transfusion in a prior cycle of chemotherapy were rechallenged with the same treatments along with IL-11 or a placebo. There was a 30% reduction in the need for transfusion in the IL-11 population. Although this is a smaller incremental benefit than the benefit of G-CSF for secondary prophylaxis of neutropenia, it was sufficiently positive to result in Food and Drug Administration approval of this agent. Other prospective trials suggest that IL-11 may help support dose-intensive chemotherapy in breast cancer (36), but there are no prospective data documenting its utility in lung cancer patients as a preemptive strategy. At this point, it would seem appropriate to reserve this agent for patients who have developed severe thrombocytopenia resulting in the need for platelet support in the setting of a clinically effective chemotherapy regimen when the clinician feels that maintaining the chemotherapy dose is preferred to dose reduction. If prospective trials show benefit of IL-11 in terms of reducing radiation injury (37), a broader population of patients may be able to benefit from this cytokine.

The initial hope that thrombopoietin would help reduce dose-limiting thrombocytopenia in cancer patients has been diminished in the clinical arena (38,39). Trials of a truncated form of thrombopoietin, megakaryocyte growth and development factor (MGDF), showed encouraging acceleration of platelet recovery in dose-intensive carboplatin regimens (40). However, the development of neutralizing antibodies resulted in prolonged thrombocytopenia in a small number of lung cancer (41) patients and normal donors, leading to closure of the development program of this agent. Of interest, however, a single dose postchemotherapy seemed to be adequate to accelerate platelet recovery, perhaps because of the unique nature of megakaryocyte physiology with proplatelet and platelet formation in response to thrombopoietin. Although MGDF is no longer in development in the United States, recombinant human thrombopoietin continues to be evaluated for its potential clinical role in oncology; it is hoped that this agent will be effective in reducing thrombocytopenia and ultimately helping to support trials in which thrombocytopenia is a limiting toxicity.

FUTURE DIRECTIONS

As discussed in this chapter, several supportive-care strategies currently exist to help minimize the consequences of myelosuppression in the lung cancer patient including red cell transfusion and erythropoietin, CSFs, and antibiotics, and, when needed, platelet transfusion and IL-11. For high-dose chemotherapy strategies, autologous bone marrow support, peripheral blood cell support, and more recently, umbilical cord blood as a source of allogeneic cells remain promising strategies. The development of hematopoietic growth factors has improved our understanding of hematopoiesis and has also provided the opportunity to develop additional molecules that may be more effective than the currently available cytokines (1,16). Agents under study include stem cell factor, chimeric molecules that combine early- and late-acting factors, small molecules targeted to specific receptors, and modifications of the currently available hematopoietic growth factors.

Of all of these agents in development, one of the most promising agents appears to be pegfilgrastim (42). This is a formulation of recombinant human G-CSF or filgrastim that has been modified by the noncovalent attachment of a polyethylene glycol moiety (i.e., SD-01). The result of pegylation of filgrastim is the virtual elimination of renal clearance of the molecule. Thus, the main way in which filgrastim is cleared is by the G-CSF receptors on neutrophils. In the postchemotherapy setting, and resultant neutropenia, the half-life of the molecule is markedly prolonged. From studies done in patients with non–small cell lung cancer receiving a dose-intensive carboplatin-and-paclitaxel regimen (42), it appears that a single dose of SD-O1 is at least as effective as daily filgrastim in accelerating neutrophil recovery. Similar benefits have been observed in a phase II study of breast cancer patients receiving docetaxel and doxorubicin, and in an ongoing randomized phase III trial. In addition to the ease of administration of this agent postchemotherapy and the potential for improvement in the pharmacodynamic response, such an agent would also facilitate trials of treatment strategies that test the Frei hypothesis in patients with small cell and non–small cell lung cancer, by optimizing the means to reduce myelosuppression in future clinical trials of summation dose intensity.

REFERENCES

1. Johnston E, Crawford J. Hematopoietic growth factors in the reduction of chemotherapy toxicity. Semin Oncol 1998; 25(5):552–561.
2. Abels R. Erythropoietin for anemia in cancer patients. Eur J Cancer 1993; 29A(suppl 2):S2–S8.
3. Krantz SB. Erythropoietin. Blood 1991; 77:419–434.
4. Miller CB, Jone RJ, Piantadosi S, Abeloff MD, Spivak JL. Decreased erythropoietin response in patents with the anemia of cancer. N Engl J Med 1990; 322:1689–1692.
5. Henry Dh, Abels Ri. Recombinant human erythropoietin in the treatment of cancer and chemotherapy-induced anemia: results of double-blind and open-label follow-up studies. Semin Oncol 1994; 21(suppl 3):21–28.
6. Glaspy J, Bukowski R, Steinberg D, Taylor C, Tchekmedyian S, Vadhan-Raj S, for the Procrit Study Group. Impact of therapy with epoetin alfa on clinical outcomes in patients with nonmyeloid malignancies during cancer chemotherapy in community oncology practice. J Clin Oncol 1997; 15:1218–1234.
7. Demetri GD, Kris M, Wade J, Degos L, Cella D, for the Procrit Study Group. Quality-of-life benefit in chemotherapy patients treated with epoetin alfa is independent of disease response or tumor type: results from a prospective community oncology study. J Clin Oncol 1998; 16:3412–3425.
8. Grabilove JJ, Einhorn LH, Livingston RB, Winer E, Cleeland CS. Once weekly dosing of epoetin alfa is similar to three-times-weekly dosing in increasing hemoglobin and quality of life. Proc ASCO 1999; 2216.
9. Cella D. The functional assessment of cancer therapy-anemia (FACT-An) scale: a new tool for the assessment of outcome sin cancer anemia and fatigue. Semin Hematol 1997; 34(suppl 2):13–19.
10. Crawford J, Glaspy J, Demetri G, Gabrilove J. Epoetin alfa improves hemoglobin

levels and quality of life for lung cancer patients receiving chemotherapy. Lung Cancer 2000; 29(suppl 1):271.

11. Crawford J, Gabrilove JL. Therapeutic options for anemia and fatigue. http://www.medscape.com/Medscape/oncology/TreatmentUpdate/2000/tu02/public/toc-tu02.html.

12. Stevens CW, Lee JS, Cox J, Komaki R. Novel approaches to locally advanced unresectable non–small cell lung cancer. Radiother Oncol 2000; 55(1):11–18.

13. Zarogoulidis K, Papagiannis A, Ziogas E, Fahantidou E, Dermitzakis G, Gioulekas D, Vamvalis C. Management of chemotherapy-related anemia with low-dose recombinant human erythropoietin in patients with small cell lung cancer. Eur J Cancer 1997; 33(14):2428–2431.

14. Crawford J, Blackwell S, Shoemaker D, Pupa MR, Mulhausen T, Herndon J, Flynn J, Dempsey H. Prophylaxis of chemotherapy related anemia with recombinant human erythropoietin (epoetin alfa) in patients with small cell lung cancer (SCLC) treated with cyclophosphamide, doxorubicin and etoposide (CAE) with G-CSF. Proc ASCO 1994; 1586.

15. Ozer H, Armitage JO, Benett CL, et al. J Clin Onc 2000; 18(20):3558–3585.

16. Crawford J, Lee ME. Recombinant human granulocyte colony-stimulating factor support of cancer patient. In: Armitage JO, Antman KH, eds. High Dose Cancer Therapy, 3rd ed. Baltimore, MD: Lippincott Williams & Wilkins, 2000; 411–435.

17. Crawford J, Ozer H, Stoller R, et al. Reduction by granulocyte colony-stimulating factor of fever and neutropenia induced by chemotherapy in patients with small-cell lung cancer. N Engl J Med 1991; 325:164–170.

18. Hartmann LC, Tschetter LK, Habermann TM, et al. Granulocyte colony-stimulating factor in severe chemotherapy-induced afebrile neutropenia. N Engl J Med 1997; 336:1776–1780.

19. Aviles A, Guzman R, Garcia E, et al. Results of a randomized trial of granulocyte colony-stimulating factor in patients with infection and severe granulocytopenia. Anticancer Drugs 1996; 7:392–397.

20. Garcia-Carbonero R, Mayordomo JI, Tornamira MV, Lopez-Brea M, Rueda A, Guillem V, Arcediano A, Yubero A, Riera F, Tres A, Cortes-Funes H, Paz-Ares L. Filgrastim in the treatment of high-risk febrile neutropenia: results of a multicenter randomized phase III trial. Proc ASCO 1999; 2253.

21. Trillet-Lenoir V, Green J, Manegold C, et al. Recombinant granulocyte colony stimulating factor reduces the infectious complications of cytotoxic chemotherapy. Eur J Cancer 1993; 29A:319–324.

22. Talcott JA, Siegel RD, Finberg R, Goldman L. Risk assessment in cancer patients with fever and neutropenia: a prospective, two-center validation of a prediction rule. J Clin Oncol 1992; 10:316–322.

23. LeChevalier AR, Pignon JP, et al. Initial chemotherapy doses have a significant impact on survival in limited small cell lung cancer—results of a multicentric prospective randomized study in 105 patients. N Engl J Med 1993; 329:1848.

24. LeChavalier T, Brisgand D, Douillard J, et al. Randomized study of vinorelbine and cisplatin versus vindesine abd cisplatin versus vinorelbine alone in advanced non–small cell lung cancer: results of a European multicenter trial including 612 patients. J Clin Oncol 1994; 12:360.

25. Bonomi P, Kim K, Kusler J, Johnson D. Cisplatin-etoposide vs paclitaxel/cisplatin/ G-CSF vs paclitaxel/cisplatin in non-small cel lung cancer. Oncology 1997; 11(4 suppl 3):9–10.

26. Tjan-Heijnen VC, Postmus PE, Wagener DJ. Dose intensification of chemotherapy and the role of granulocyte colony stimulating factor and granulocyte macrophage colony stimulating factor in small cell lung cancer. Anti-cancer Drugs 1997; 8(6): 549–564.

27. Steward WP, von Pawel J, Gatzemeier U, WQOll P, Thatcher N, Koschei G, Clancey L, Verweij J, deWit R, Pfeifer W, Fennelly J, von Eiff M, Frisch J. Effects of granulocyte-macrophage colony-stimulating factor and dose intensification of V-ICE chemotherapy in small cell lung cancer: a prospective randomized study of 300 patients. J Clin Oncol 1998; 16(2):642–650.

28. Fukuoka M, Masuda N, Negoro S, Matsui K, Yana T, Kudoh S, Kusunoki Y, Takada M, Kawahara M, Ogawara M, Kodama N, Kubota K, Furuse K. CODE chemotherapy with and without granulocyte colony-stimulating factor in small cell lung cancer. Br J Cancer 1997; 75(2):306–309.

29. Frei E III, Elias A, Wheeler C, Richardson P, Hryniuk W. The relationship between high-dose treatment and combination chemotherapy: the concept of summation dose intensity. CL Cancer Res 1998; 4:2027–2037.

30. Bunn PA, Crowley J, Kelly K, et al. Chemoradiotherapy with or without granulocyte-macrophage colony-stimulating factor in the treatment of limited-stage small-cell lung cancer. A prospective phase III randomized study of the Southwest Oncology Group. J Clin Oncol 1995; 13:1632–1641.

31. Petros WP, Crawford J. Safety of concomitant use of granulocyte colony-stimulating factor or granulocyte-macrophage colony-stimulating factor with cytotoxic chemotherapy agents. Curr Opin Hematol 1997; 4(suppl 3):213–216.

32. Ottoman OG, Hoelzer D, Gracien E, Ganser A, Kelly K, Reuttzel R, Lipp T, Busch FW, Schwonzen M, et al. Concomitant granulocyte colony-stimulating factor and induction chemoradiotherapy in adult acute lymphoblastic leukemia: a randomized phase III trial. Blood 1995; 86(2):444–450.

33. Rubenstein EB, Elting L. Incorporating new modalities into practice guidelines: platelet growth factors. Oncology 1998; 12(11A):381–386.

34. Maslak P, Nimer SD. The efficacy of IL-3, SCF, IL-6, and Il-11 in treating thrombocytopenia. Semin Hematol 1998; 35(3):253–260.

35. Kaye JA. Clinical development of recombinant human interleukin-11 to treat chemotherapy-induced thrombocytopenia. Curr Opin Hematol 1996; 3(3):209–215.

36. Isaacs C, Robert NJ, Bailey FA, Schuster MW, Overmoyer B, Graham M, Cai B, Beach KJ, Loewy JW, Kaye JA. Randomized placebo-controlled study of recombinant human interleukin-11 to prevent chemotherapy-induced thrombocytopenia in patients with breast cancer receiving dose-intensive cyclophosphamide and doxorubicin. J Clin Oncol 1997; 15(11):3368–3377.

37. Redlich CA, Gao X, Rockwell S, Kelley M, Elias JA. IL-11 enhances survival and decreases TNF production after radiation-induced thoracic injury. J Immunol 1996; 157(4):1705–1710.

38. Kauschansky K. Thrombopoetin. N Engl J Med 1998; 339(11):746–754.

39. Hofmann WK, Ottmann OG, Hoelzer D. Megakaryocytic growth factors: is there a

new approach for management of thrombocytopenia in patients with malignancies? Leukemia 1999; 13(1):14–18.

40. Fanucchi M, Glaspy J, Crawford J, Garst J, Figlin R, Sheridan W, Menchaca D, Tomita D, Ozer H, Harker L. Effects of polyethylene glycol-conjugate recombinant human megakaryocyte growth and development factor on platelet counts after chemotherapy for lung cancer. N Engl J Med 1997; 336:404–409.

41. Crawford J, Glaspy J, Belani C, Garst J, Prager D, Long G, La Brecque J, Macri M, Fanucchi M. A randomized, placebo-controlled, blinded, dose-scheduling trial of pegylated recombinant human megakaryocyte growth and development factor with filgrastim supporting non-small cell lung cancer (NSCLC) patents treated with paclitaxel and carboplatin during multiple cycles of chemotherapy. Proc ASCO 1998 (abstr 285).

42. Johnston E, Crawford J, Blackwell S, et al. Randomized dose-escalation study of SD/01 compared with daily filgrastim in patients receiving chemotherapy. J Clin Oncol 2000; 18(13):2522–2528.

25

Role of Laser, Photodynamic Therapy, Cryotherapy, and Electrocautery in Endobronchial Therapy

Michael Unger

Fox Chase Cancer Center and Thomas Jefferson Medical College, Philadelphia, Pennsylvania

INTRODUCTION

Rapid technological advances in the past 40 years have greatly contributed to improved diagnostic and therapeutic modalities in lung cancer. A major advance was the introduction of the flexible bronchoscope, which became the primary diagnostic instrument by facilitating the inspection and collection of brush or needle aspiration specimens for cytology and of biopsy specimens obtained with a forceps or transbronchial needle for histology. Further refinements in instrumentation and accessories led to the development of endoscopic interventional pulmonology. Although debulking of endobronchial tumors had already been practiced for some time with the rigid bronchoscope, it was frequently associated with significant bleeding and other serious complications.

As did the flexible bronchoscope, the introduction of lasers into medicine has opened new horizons. This chapter will explore the endobronchial therapeutic armamentarium utilizing laser photoradiation therapy, cryotherapy, and endoscopic electrocautery.

LASER PHOTORADIATION THERAPY

Three essential characteristics of the laser (light amplification by stimulated emission of radiation) beam are useful in medical applications: (A) monochromaticity (specific wavelength or color of each laser); (B) coherence (three-dimensional uniformity in space and time of the beam), which significantly increases the power; and (C) low divergence, which provides a very narrow beam, permitting precise focus on a small target (1).

The first laser that was used endoscopically in upper airways was the CO_2 laser with a wavelength of 10,600 nm (in the infrared spectrum). The very high absorption coefficient in water makes this laser a superb vaporizer or cutter, but not an optimal coagulator. Owing to characteristics of this laser, initially it could be safely transmitted only through mirrors or hollow tubes like rigid scopes. The above limitations led to the development of improved CO_2 lasers and other medically useful wavelengths.

At the present time, the Nd: YAG laser has the greatest applicability in endoscopy. It produces an invisible beam of light in the near-infrared spectrum (1064 nm), and it can be transmitted through fiberoptic lightguides. The small diameter of the lightguide permits introduction through the working channel of the flexible bronchoscope, allowing performance under local anesthesia and not, as required by rigid bronchoscopy, under general anesthesia. Another significant difference between the CO_2 and the Nd: YAG laser is the increased scattering effect in the tissue with a much lower absorption coefficient in water. This permits much deeper penetration of the beam of light in soft tissue. The resultant thermal effect produces coagulation of blood vessels and devitalization of tumors. In endobronchial applications, the Nd: YAG laser can be used at a certain distance from the target tissue (noncontact technique) producing this tissue coagulation. The lightguide transmitting the laser beam through the endoscope can also be equipped with special sculpted sapphire tips, which touch the target tissue and result in the contact technique. Both techniques are complementary and used as required by given clinical circumstances.

The success of endobronchial laser photoradiation therapy is dependent upon appropriate selection of patients, adequate training and experience of the endoscopist, and the commitment of the whole team involved with patient care (2–4). Indications and contraindications for utilization of lasers for endobronchial therapy in patients with lung cancer are well defined (Tables 1 and 2). In general the same principles apply to other techniques described below.

The best results have been obtained in treating patients with primary lung malignancies or metastatic endobronchial lesions from primary tumors in other organs (colon, kidneys, thyroid, melanoma, etc.) that cause partial obstruction of major airways (trachea and bronchi). The more proximal the lesion, the more

TABLE 1 Indications for
Cancer-Related Endobronchial
Interventions

Hemoptysis
Relief of airways obstruction
Improvement of ventilation
Improvement of drainage
Relief of intractable cough
Removal of foreign body

functionally significant it becomes; thus relief of the obstruction and improved airflow results in a much better physiological improvement (5).

Developments in interventional endoscopy produced complications not previously encountered with diagnostic bronchoscopy. Most patients referred for palliative bronchoscopic procedures arrive with some degree of respiratory insufficiency. From the outset, the risks of complications related to the anesthesia are increased. Procedures done under local or general anesthesia may result in hypoxemia and hypercapnea due to hypoventilation (6). Continued monitoring throughout the procedure is mandatory. A major complication, sometimes unavoidable, is severe or fatal hemorrhage generally due to the approximation of the tumor being treated with the adjacent pulmonary artery. The thermal effect and resultant endobronchial edema may further compromise ventilation. Inappropriate use of the laser can result in severe endobronchial burns (7). Pneumothorax and pneumomediastinum have also been reported in treated patients. Patients treated under conscious sedation compared to general anesthesia have fewer complications. Otherwise, complications relating to technique do not differ when the Nd: YAG laser is used through a rigid bronchoscope under general anesthesia or through the working channel of the flexible scope under conscious sedation (8,9).

The KTP laser is another instrument producing green light with a wavelength of 532 nm, double the frequency of Nd: YAG. Green light is highly ab-

TABLE 2 Contraindications to Nd: YAG Laser Phototherapy

Bleeding diathesis
Tracheoesophageal fistula
Tracheobronchomalacia or fractured cartilagenous rings
Extrinsic compression
Total bronchial occlusion for over 4–6 weeks' duration
Ipsilateral involvement of pulmonary artery

sorbed by hemoglobin but poorly absorbed by water. Because of this absorption variation, the KTP laser is a better cutter than the Nd: YAG laser but a suboptimal coagulator. Light is transmitted through optical fibers and can be used either through the working channel of the flexible bronchoscope or through a rigid bronchoscope.

PHOTODYNAMIC THERAPY

In the visible spectrum, several lasers are utilized for photodynamic therapy (PDT). These include the argon dye laser and copper vapor and gold vapor lasers, which all produce red light in the vicinity of 630 nm.

PDT is a technique based on the combination of three components: a photosensitizer, light, and oxygen. Each contributor, individually, is nontoxic to the tissue. It is well known that neoplastic tissues have a propensity to preferentially retain certain sensitizers (10). One of the earliest tested was hematoporphyrin derivative (HpD). After intravenous injection, this photosensitizer is taken up by a variety of tissues but preferentially retained by neoplasms and the reticuloendothelial system. There is no detectable HpD in the muscles 48 hr following the injection, while the concentration in tumors remains high. At this point, amplified light of a specific wavelength (in the case of HpD, red color, 630 nm) in the presence of oxygen produces a photochemical reaction, resulting in the release of free oxygen radicals. Free oxygen radicals, by interfering with prime metabolic pathways, destroy the tissue in which they are released. Because they are produced only in the malignancies that have retained the HpD, the procedure seldom affects the surrounding normal tissue.

Several studies conducted at the Mayo Clinic and in Japan have identified the efficacy of PDT in endobronchial therapy of malignant tumors. The investigators have eradicated small, radiographically occult, bronchial malignancies with a 5-year survival, equal to that of surgical resection. Currently, the therapeutic indications for PDT are: (1) the tumor should not exceed a diameter of 2 cm, (2) its entire surface area should be easily illuminated by the activating light, and (3) there must be no peribronchial involvement (11–13). When tumors exceed this size, application of PDT does not result in cure. Cortese et al. reduced the need for surgery in 43% of patients with minimally invasive carcinoma, when treated with the PDT technique (14). On the basis of several multinational studies, the Food and Drug Administration approved the commercial form of HpD, Photofrin, for use in early carcinoma of the lung. Several other publications also dealt with the use of PDT with Photofrin in more advanced carcinomas (15). The results, although encouraging, have not shown that this technique is superior to the endobronchial use of the Nd: YAG laser or brachytherapy, in particular, in cases of extensive endobronchial tumors with associated extrinsic compression.

Limitations of photodynamic therapy include a poorly established dosimetery schedule of light delivered to the tumor, as well as lack of identification of the optimal dose of the photosensitizer. Selectivity of the Photofrin in malignant tissue does not appear to be totally specific and there remains a possibility of damage to other normal parts of the bronchus with potential formation of extensive fibrosis. Because of the delayed local reaction, treatment with PDT requires follow-up clean-up bronchoscopy to remove the necrotic eschar and debris that threaten airway patency. Skin sensitization occurs with regularity. With current photosensitizers, patients treated require protection from sunlight or any other intense light that might contain a wavelength of 630 nm. for at least 4 weeks; otherwise they risk a severe sunburn reaction.

The concept and science of PDT is fascinating and we continue to seek the ideal photosensitizer and activating energy source. Research is presently directed toward the development of other, more specific photosensitizers activated by different wavelengths, which will permit deeper and more selective tissue penetration and absorption.

CRYOTHERAPY

Interventional bronchoscopists are investigating other energies in the treatment and palliation of endobronchial obstructions. Cryotherapy cools malignant tissue and produces thrombosis of its blood supply, resulting in necrosis. Subsequent debulking of the dead tissue is required 48 hr after each treatment.

The principle of deep freezing of tissue is based on the Joule-Thompson effect (sudden expansion of gas from a high- to low-pressure region). Various rigid and flexible probes were developed for introduction through the bronchoscope to deliver the treatment endobronchially at the tumor site (16,17).

The gas most frequently used is nitrous oxide (N_2O). When N_2O (under pressure of 50 bar) is released into the probe, the external temperature at the end of the probe descends to $-40°C$. This results in the formation of an ice ball, which produces intracellular and extracellular crystallization. In the subsequent phase of thawing, further damage to the previously frozen tissues leads to their necrosis. The full effects are delayed and appear only after several hours.

Cryotherapy of endobronchial lesions had preceded pulmonological use of lasers, but has never become widely accepted. There are several disadvantages of this technique. There is no accurate way of predicting the depth of tissue destruction during the freezing phase. Although initially the cold may reduce the bleeding, the subsequent thawing phase can result in tissue fracture, with rupture of blood vessels and subsequent hemorrhage. Another complication is cold-induced bronchospasm. Repeat bronchoscopies are required to remove tissue debris and prevent airway obstruction. Proponents of this technique admit that the process is slow with no immediate recanalization of the bronchus, and cannot be applied safely when there is total luminal obstruction (18). Cryotherapy is contra-indicated in acute respiratory distress, due to severe occlusion of the trachea or main bronchi. The major advantage of cryotherapy is the lower cost of the equipment compared to laser therapies.

ELECTROCAUTERY

Endobronchial application of electrocautery is an adaptation of a well-accepted technique used extensively and safely in surgery. The high-frequency alternating electric current, transmitted beyond the tip of the bronchoscope through a probe, passes through tissue with high resistance and produces tissue coagulation, and usually bloodless debulking. The degree of necrosis depends on the voltage gradient across the probe and the targeted tissue, the duration of the cauterization pulse, and the surface area of the probe in contact with tissue. Additional effects will depend on the degree of local moisture (mucus) and the presence and amount of blood (19,20). When electrocautery is utilized in interventional pulmonology, specially grounded flexible scopes with a ceramic (not metal) tip are used to avoid electric current injury to the patient or the operator. Severe burns have occurred on occasion when this technique was used through metal rigid scopes. The disadvantage of electrocautery is the poor control of depth of penetration, and the major advantage is the low cost of the equipment.

A newer technique, monopolar coagulation, uses a noncontact approach with an argon beam coagulator. While monopolar coagulation is capable of producing superficial coagulation, there is still very limited experience with this interventional modality.

DISCUSSION

The indications for palliative endobronchial therapy are based upon a through understanding of the underlying disease process in the patient and the expected results. Patients with major obstruction in the tracheobronchial tree by an exophytic tumor could benefit from endobronchial therapy by enlarging the lumen, improving ventilation, and producing better drainage of postobstructive secretions. Endobronchial therapy can provide palliation of hemoptysis when the source of hemorrhage is within the reach of the bronchoscope. Endobronchial coagulation provides a cessation of bleeding and protects other areas of the lung from obstruction by blood clots. The largest experience has been reported using the Nd: YAG laser. Restoration of a bronchial lumen in postobstructive pneumonia will improve the resolution of the infection with additional antibiotic therapy. It may also reduce the field for potential external-beam radiation therapy and allow better tissue oxygenation, thereby improving the results of radiotherapy. Radiation therapy in treatment of lung tumors frequently results in a nonproductive cough attributed to radiation pneumonitis. Not infrequently, subsequent bronchoscopies reveal the presence of an unexpected endobronchial mass, not visible on radiographic examination, which represents destroyed, partially fibrotic, tumor. Removal of this irritating mass results in immediate relief of the symptomatic cough.

The success of endobronchial therapy improves with the proximity of the treated area. Opening of the mainstem bronchus may restore ventilation to the rest of that lung, while treatment of a lobar or segmental bronchus may improve drainage of postobstructive pneumonia, but will, in general, add little to overall ventilation. This may be mildly advantageous in patients with previous lung resection or limited ventilatory capacity.

Reports have confirmed not only subjective amelioration of symptoms reported by the patients, but also objective improvement, particularly in the treatment of exophytic lesions in the trachea or mainstem bronchi, of cough or of hemoptysis. Removal of endobronchial obstructions in malignancy will provide palliation of symptoms, using laser therapy in combination with other modalities. In the treatment of a naive patient, consolidation of laser therapy and external-beam radiation provides the best results. In patients who have already received an optimal dose of external-beam radiotherapy, consolidation of debulking and opening of the lumen and brachytherapy may further improve symptoms. If the patency of the lumen of major airways is compromised by a combination of endobronchial tumor and extrinsic compression, the exophytic part of the growth is treated first with laser therapy and then, if appropriate, a stent is placed to improve patency of the airways by relief of the extrinsic peribronchial or peritracheal compression. The success of the procedure will depend on the choice of an appropriate stent, suited to the given anatomical and clinical situation, and on the experience of the operator (21).

Except in cases of minimally invasive carcinomas where a complete response can frequently be achieved by using PDT, all other modalities previously described are directed toward local control with palliation of symptoms. Interest in PDT stimulated research in early detection of lung cancer and led to the concept of autofluorescence and its clinical application (22). Normal bronchial tissue will emit different fluorescence patterns from premalignant and malignant lesions when stimulated by light of a specific wavelength. Multicenter studies showed that the lung imaging fluorescence endoscopy (LIFE) system, as an adjunct to a regular bronchoscopy, improved the yield of detection of moderate to severe dysplasia and early minimally invasive carcinoma by a factor of 2.7 (23). Discovery of the premalignant and early neoplastic lesion and improved modalities of screening may lead to more imaginative and effective endobronchial therapeutic modalities. Further technological progress will produce different laser-driven devices. One of the most innovative is optical coherence tomography (OCT), capable of providing high-resolution histological imaging and analysis in vivo. Small probes, which can be inserted through an endoscope, have been developed for an "optical biopsy" (25). In the future we may hope for more effective screening procedures, better delineation of high-risk patients, early diagnosis of small pre-malignant and minimally invasive cancers, and effective early therapy and chemo-prevention.

At present, the overall mortality from lung cancer has not been influenced by the armamentarium of interventional pulmonary procedures such as laser pho-toradiation therapy, cryotherapy, or electrocautery. The disease-free interval can be prolonged with improvement of the quality of life in the treated patients (24). Hopefully, better screening techniques of high-risk populations and chemoprev-ention combined with early detection techniques will improve the statistics.

REFERENCES

1. Polanji TG. Physics of surgery with lasers. Clin Chest Med 1985; 6:179–204.
2. Parr GV, Unger M, Duckett JE. One hundred Neodymium: YAG laser ablations of obstructing tracheal neoplasms. Ann Thorac Surg 1984; 38:374–381.
3. Unger M, Parr GVS. The benefits of Nd: YAG applications for end stage patients. In: Tumor Diagnostick und therapie. New York: Thieme Verlag, 1986:13–16.
4. Edell EC, Cortese DA. Bronchoscopic phototherapy with hematoporphyrin deriva-tive for treatment of localized bronchogenic carcinoma: a 5-year experience. Mayo Clin Proc 1987; 62:8–14.
5. Unger M. Neodymium: YAG laser therapy for malignant and benign endobronchial obstructions. Clin Chest Med 1985; 6:277–290.
6. Duckett JE, McDonnell TJ, Unger M, Parr GV. General anesthesia for Nd: YAG laser resection of obstructing endobronchial tumours using the rigid bronchoscope. Can Anaesth Soc J 1985; 32:67–72.
7. Casey KR, Unger M. Laser bronchoscopy. In: Dixon JA, ed. Surgical Applications of Lasers. Chicago: Yearbook Medical Publishers, 1987:287–309.
8. Cortese DA. Rigid versus flexible bronchoscopy in laser bronchoscopy. Pro rigid bronchoscopic laser application. J Bronchol 1994; 1:72–75.
9. Unger M. Rigid versus flexible bronchoscopy in laser bronchoscopy: pro flexible bronchoscopic laser application. J Bronchol 1994; 1:69–71.
10. Dougherty TJ. Photosensitizers: therapy and detection of malignant tumors. Pho-tochem Photobiol 1987; 45:879–890.
11. Furuse K, Fukuoka M, Kato H, et al. A prospective phase II study on photodynamic therapy with photophrin II for centrally located early-stage lung cancer. J Clin Oncol 1993; 11:1852–1857.
12. Edell ES, Cortese DA. Photodynamic therapy in management of early superficial squamous cell carcinoma as an alternative to surgical resection. Chest 1992; 102: 1319–1322.
13. Lam S. Photodynamic therapy of lung cancer. Semin Oncol 1994; 21(suppl 15):15–19.

14. Cortese DA, Edell ES, Kinsey JH. Photodynamic therapy for early stage squamous cell carcinoma of the lung. Mayo Clin Proc 1997; 72:595–602.
15. McCaughan JS. Overview of experience with photodynamic therapy for malignancy in 192 patients. Photochem Photobiol 1987; 46:903–909.
16. Homasson JP. Bronchoscopic cryotherapy. J Bronchol 1995; 2:45–53.
17. Homasson JP, Thiery JP, Angebault M, et al. The operation and efficacy of cryosurgical nitrous oxide-driven cryoprobe. Cryoprobe physical characteristics: their effects on cell destruction. Cryobiology 1994; 31:240–304.
18. Mathur PN, Wolf KM, Busk MF, Briete M, Datzman M. Fiberoptic bronchoscopic cryotherapy in management of tracheobronchial obstruction. Chest 1996; 110:718–723.
19. Hooper RG, Jackson FN. Endobronchial electrocautery. Chest 1988; 94:595–598.
20. Sutedja TG, van Boxem TJ, Schramel FM, van Felius C, Postmus PE. Electrocautery is an excellent alternative for Nd: YAG laser to treat airway tumors. J Bronchol 1997; 4:101–105.
21. Dumon JF, Cavaliere S, Diaz-Jimenez JP, et al. Seven-year experience with the Dumon prosthesis. J Bronchol 1996; 3:6–10.
22. Lam S, MacAulay C, Leriche JD, et al. Detection of dysplasia and carcinoma in situ by lung imaging fluorescence endoscope (LIFE) device. J Thorac Cardiovasc Surg 1993; 105:1035–1040.
23. Lam S, Kennedy T, Unger M, Miller YE, Gelmont D, Rush V, Gipe B, Howard D, Lariche JC, Coldman A, Gazdar AF. Localization of bronchial intraepithelial and neoplastic lesions by fluorescence bronchoscopy. Chest 1998; 113:696–702.
24. Desai SJ, Mehta AC, Vanderbrug Medendorp S, Golish JA, Ahmad M. Survival experience following Nd: YAG laser photoresection for primary bronchogenic carcinoma. Chest 1988; 94:939–944.
25. Costas Pitris M, Brezinski ME, Bouma BE, Tearney GJ, Southern JF, Fujimoto JG. High resolution imaging of the upper respiratory tract with optical coherence tomography. A feasibility study. Am J Respir Crit Care Med 1998; 157:1640–1644.

26

Endobronchial Brachytherapy: Its Niche in Lung Cancer

Burton L. Speiser
St. Joseph's Hospital and Medical Center, Phoenix, Arizona

INTRODUCTION

Lung cancer presents the clinician with three areas of treatment failure, all of which will need significant improvement to favorably impact on the survival rates from this disease. These areas are local (which can be subdivided into the tracheobronchial tree and lung parenchyma region) and metastatic outside the thoracic cavity. Brachytherapy can be utilized to improve local control with the tracheobronchial tree for selected cases, thereby reducing the risk in one of the three areas of treatment failure.

The treatment of lung cancer by radiation has consisted primarily of the use of standard external-beam radiation. The use of endobronchial brachytherapy (EBBT) in the form of manual afterloading low-dose rate began to emerge in the early to mid-1980s. It was not until the mid- and late 1980s that high-dose rate remote afterloading brachytherapy began to be utilized in increasing numbers. At the present time it is the most prevalent means of treating endobronchial disease with brachytherapy in the world.

EBBT, however, has been used primarily for palliation, for recurrent disease. Its use for curative intent, while performed, is not as prevalent. Even less common is its use for occult carcinomas of the lung, where as the sole modality, or used in conjunction with either photodynamic therapy or limited external radiation, it can lead to high cure rates with low morbidity.

Brachytherapy was first used at the turn of the twentieth century when the Curies gave a small radium tube to Dr. Danlos for insertion into a malignancy. In the ensuing years, further progress was made in the area of brachytherapy. Kernan (1) first reported the implantation of radon 222 seeds into carcinomas of the trachea and bronchus utilizing a rigid bronchoscope. He reported on 10 cases treated with radon 222 seed implantation combined with diathermy treatment. Of interest was his comment in the report that "it was possible to destroy the tumors with diathermy and Radon implantation, and there have been no local recurrences as yet, although one case has been followed for five years." For the next 10–20 years, work was being performed on standardization of dose calculation and prescription for brachytherapy. The publication of the Manchester system of Paterson and colleagues (1934) set the foundation for brachytherapy dosimetry. This was further advanced with the publication of the manual *Radium Dosage* (2). Pool (3) reported on radon 222 used at Memorial Hospital in a total of 42 patients implanted from the time period of 1936–1960. The implanted seeds consisted of a sealed gold capillary tube filled with radon 222 gas. The technique reported by Pool "proved to benefit patients with primary tracheal tumors, and patients with bronchial stump recurrences following pulmonary resection." Radon 222 seed implantation was also used during thoracotomy with the first reported case by Graham and Singer (4).

To decrease the radiation safety problems with radon 222, efforts were made to identify radioactive isotopes of shorter half-life and lower decay energies, as well as developing afterloading techniques, to reduce medical personnel and patient exposures. Henschke (5) introduced standardized afterloading techniques with gold 198 and, subsequently, iridium 192. With the shorter half-life of iridium 192 and afterloading techniques, interstitial implantation showed a rapid increase in medical utilization, in both its range of application and its overall usage in the United States. However, in spite of this rapid increase, there were very few changes in the limited use of brachytherapy for carcinoma of the lung. Early transbronchial implantation techniques initially utilizing radon 222 and then iodine 125 through the rigid bronchoscope were difficult and associated with a considerable expenditure of physician time and effort. With the advent of the flexible bronchoscope, a new flexible applicator system was designed by Schray and colleagues (6). The use of intraluminal brachytherapy by the placement of an afterloading flexible applicator bronchoscopically was first reported in the American literature by Mendiondo et al. (7). In addition, the new neodymium-YAG laser was introduced into clinical use for treatment of tracheal and endobronchial obstructions for both primary and metastatic lung malignancies in 1984. It is this convergence of medical technologies that led to a rapid increase in the utilization of intraluminal brachytherapy utilizing the afterloading techniques, usually in concert with YAG laser photoresection.

The majority of patients diagnosed with lung malignancies present with locally advanced or metastatic disease. Those patients who are deemed resectable and undergo an attempted resection have a high risk of subsequent local recurrence. Despite treatment with external-beam radiation therapy, local recurrence still remains a problem. Even with the improved overall survival and local control for inoperable patients treated with combined radiochemotherapy, a significant rate of local tumor recurrence is still demonstrated. In one study in which patients were assessed with several bronchoscopic biopsies, the "histological" local control was only 15–17% following definitive radiotherapy or sequential radiotherapy and chemotherapy (8). This problem of local recurrence has led many to employ brachytherapy to deliver additional ionizing radiation therapy treatment in both the curative and palliative modes.

Brachytherapy is the direct application of radioactive sources to an anatomical site, such as a surgical tumor bed or within a tumor mass. Brachytherapy can be performed by implantation of radioactive sources, such as seeds within the tumor mass (interstitial brachytherapy), or by insertion of the radioactive source within the lumen of a catheter placed within the surgical bed or tumor mass (intraluminal or endobronchial brachytherapy). Brachytherapy offers the potential advantage of providing a high-dose gradient of ionizing radiation to deliver a high dose to the tumor-bearing area with a rapid relative decline in dose to the surrounding normal structures, resulting from the inverse square law of ionizing radiation. This states that the dose of radiation decreases by one divided by the square of the distance ($R_2 = R_1/D_2$).

EBBT for lung malignancies consists of the placement of a catheter into the involved bronchus, with the radiation source placed with remote or manual afterloading. Afterloaded implants can deliver either low, intermediate, or high dose rate ionizing radiation at less than 1 Gy/hr (low dose rate, LDR), 1–12 Gy/hr (intermediate dose rate, IDR), or greater than 2 Gy/min (high dose rate, HDR). A typical afterloading system utilizes hollow catheters and iridium 192 seeds embedded in nylon ribbon for LDR, or a single iridium 192 source (10 curie), which "dwells" within the lumen of the treatment catheters.

TECHNICAL ASPECTS OF REMOTE AFTERLOADING UNITS

The majority of remote afterloading units utilize high-activity radioactive sources of a small physical size, usually iridium 192, with an initial activity of 10 curie. The radioactive source is securely attached to the end of a wire cable, which is mechanically driven by a high-precision mechanism allowing for positioning of the radioactive source at specific locations within the catheter for specified periods of time. The movement of the source between these preassigned dwell positions, as well as removal of the source out of the catheter into the shielded unit's compartment, is very rapid to minimize transit time exposure. The treatment sequence for each cable/catheter, which defines the various dwell times and dwell positions, is determined by treatment-planning computers and executed under the control of an external computer that specifically drives the remote afterloading unit. The radiation dose is configured three-dimensionally to encompass the portions of the tracheal bronchial tree and carcinoma to be treated.

TREATMENT-PLANNING COMPUTER

The basics of dose calculation techniques require orthogonal radiographs taken after catheter placement with dummy seeds in place to determine catheter position. On the simulator radiographs, the seed positions are digitized from the first dwell position at the end of the catheter to the most proximal dwell position in the catheter along the dummy source seed line. Next, the treating physician defines the treatment target volume. A treatment plan is then formulated, optimizing treatment points (dwell positions) and treatment time (dwell times position). This treatment plan is evaluated in the four cardinal directions utilizing isodose lines, as well as evaluation of the patient's individual anatomy, to calculate the final prescription dose and point. New techniques using CAT scans are being tested for a better three-dimensional picture.

ENDOBRONCHIAL CATHETERS

A variety of commercial catheters are available for use. Basically, physical characteristics of each catheter must allow for easy placement and removal from the endobronchial tree and immobilization within place. It must fit through the biopsy channel of the endoscope, and the internal diameter is source compatible (most commonly used are 5 or 6 French with a 1.7- or 2-mm internal diameter, respectively). Finally, the distal end of the catheter is closed-end to prevent dummy seeds or the active source from contact with tissues and/or fluids.

The placement of the catheter is conducted assessing the cardiological and pulmonary evaluation of the patient to ensure his or her ability to satisfactorily tolerate an endobronchial procedure. Then, with a pulmonologist, the catheter can be placed in an endoscopy suite. Under constant vital sign monitoring, the use of topical anesthesia and intravenous sedation allows for bronchoscopic evaluation of the patient. Under video bronchoscopy, the malignant lesion is identified by the pulmonologist and radiation oncologist. Photographic documentation is acquired and the anatomical characteristics of the malignancy are noted, including distance from anatomical landmarks, such as bronchial branch points and carina. The extent of the malignant lesion can be further localized utilizing radiopaque markers placed on the patient's thorax corresponding to the most distal and proximal extent of the malignancy as identified by the bronchoscope and correlated under fluoroscopy. After this visual inspection and fluoroscopic confirmation, a guidewire in a catheter is placed through the biopsy channel. Its placement is confirmed visually and fluoroscopically. The bronchoscope is removed and when the catheter is positioned such that the tip is several centimeters distal to the most distal point of the malignancy, the proximal end of the catheter is secured to the nose. The guidewire is removed and replaced by a set of dummy seed sources to obtain orthogonal treatment-planning simulation films.

TREATMENT PRESCRIPTION

The prescription depth is calculated for the three-dimensional volume by multiple points perpendicular to the axis of the catheter or source train to which the minimum target dose is prescribed. The prescriptions that are reported in the literature range from 0.5 to 2 cm. To ensure treatment of the entire tumor volume with consideration for possible source or tumor movement secondary to respiratory excursions, the maximal distance from source center to margin of the malignancy must be considered during three-dimensional brachytherapy planning. A longitudinal margin of 2 cm proximal and distal to the malignant margins is commonly used. A prescription depth within the range 0.5–2 cm, which allows for effective dose distribution to encompass the tumor volume depth, without exceeding bronchial mucosa tolerance dose, is used with a recommendation that dose standardization be used (i.e., use or report the 1-cm depth from source axis for comparison to other studies).

STRATEGIES FOR TREATMENT OF OCCULT CARCINOMAS OF THE ENDOBRONCHUS

Occult carcinomas of the lung are a subpopulation defined as carcinomas diagnosed by sputum cytology, and bronchoscopy using brushings, washings, and/ or biopsy. Less commonly, patients with cough and/or hemoptysis undergo bronchoscopy and are diagnosed in that fashion without a prior sputum cytology being positive. Their defining concept is that they cannot be detected by conventional radiographic means before or immediately after the initial diagnosis.

In 1974, Sanderson et al. (9) published "Bronchoscopic Localization of Radiographically Occult Lung Cancer." In 1980, Cortese et al. (10) published their study, "Roentgenographically Occult Lung Cancer." In the same year, Martini and Melamed (11) published "Occult Carcinoma of the Lung." Initially, the treatment of choice was surgery, whether lobectomy or pneumonectomy. However, as experience with photodynamic therapy (PDT) and then EBBT increased, the "menu" of treatment modalities increased.

This subpopulation of roentgenographically occult carcinomas of the lung is associated with interesting characteristics. First, the time interval from the initial abnormal sputum cytology to bronchoscopic confirmation, as reported by the Mayo Lung Project (10), ranged from 1 to 1014 days (median, 70 days; 75th percentile, 169 days). Second, the disease is most often T_{is}, T_1 and N_0 (12) [Saito et al. (13) found that of 94 patients, 17% were T_{is} and 77% were T_1]. Third, most cases are squamous cell carcinomas; in a significant number, dysplasia initially had been the only finding (10). Fourth, adverse prognostic factors (e.g., weight loss) that predict lower survival rates are rarely present (14–16). Finally, synchronicity and metachronicity are significant. In a surgical series, Nagamoto et al. (17) reported a rate of 1.09 lesions per patient, Kato et al. (18) found 1.21 lesions per patient, and Saito et al. (13) found 1.2 lesions per patient. In the Mayo Lung Project Study (10), a metachronous rate of 5% per year was reported. Saito et al. (19) reported a rate of 0.022 lesions per patient-year; the rate was 0.041 lesions per patient-year when synchronous and metachronous tumors were combined. If a patient had a second lesion, there was a 47% probability that within 5 years, a third lesion would be identified, at a rate of 0.11 lesions per patient-year (19). The 5-year survival rate for patients with a single lesion and no evidence of synchronous or metachronous lesions was 90%. If, however, other metachronous or synchronous lesions were present, the 5-year survival rate was 59%. In 108 patients who underwent surgical resection for occult carcinoma, Nagamato et al. (17) identified 10 (9.2%) who had additional squamous cell carcinomas < 1 mm. These lesions were associated with either dysplasia or marked atypia.

Another important prognostic factor is the size of the lesion. Many studies have found that lesions ≤ 10 mm are associated with the most favorable outcomes. In a surgical study of 127 patients (20), 55 patients had lesions of this size, and no metastatic lymph nodes were identified. Of 46 patients with lesions > 10 mm but ≤ 20 mm, there were four patients (9%) with nodal metastasis. Of 26 patients with lesions that were ≥ 20 mm but ≤ 55 mm, four patients (15%) had nodal disease. Overall, for lesions > 10 mm, the incidence of nodal involvement was 11%.

In an earlier study by Saito et al. (13), extrabronchial invasion was documented by pathological analysis in 16 (17%) of 94 patients. Five (31%) of these 16 patients had metastatic spread to nodes. Only one (1%) of 78 patients had nodal disease without evidence of extrabronchial invasion. No recurrences were identified in 75 patients who had intrabronchial disease with no lymphatic spread who underwent a complete resection. Overall, the cause-specific 5-year survival rate was 93.5% (vs. 80.4% for all causes combined).

Kato et al. (18) treated 45 lesions fulfilling the criteria for occult carcinomas in 40 patients (1.13 lesions per patient). PDT was the only treatment used for 30 lesions in 20 patients, and the complete response rate was 100%. Three patients

(15%) had recurrences, one of whom (5%) died of the disease. An additional nine patients (45%) died of unrelated causes.

Considerably fewer patients with occult carcinomas have been treated with EBBT than with PDT or surgery. Sutedja et al. (21) reported two patients with T_1 squamous cell carcinoma who were treated with HDR EBBT. Three fractions of 10 Gy were delivered at a 1-cm depth. Both patients were alive without disease at follow-up examinations, at 54 and 25 months, respectively.

Tredaniel et al. (22) treated 29 patients with a diversity of lesions, whose common denominator was that their carcinomas were limited to the bronchus (radiographically occult), such that the disease could be encompassed by intraluminal brachytherapy. In contrast to other reported series, however, these patients had undergone prior treatment, which included surgery, external radiation, and/or chemotherapy. The patients were treated with HDR EBBT using a dose of 7 Gy calculated at a 1-cm depth for six fractions (42 Gy). The median actual survival of these patients had not been reached after 23 months of follow-up.

Saito et al. (13) treated 49 occult carcinomas in 41 patients (1.2 lesions per patient) with external-beam radiation using 40 Gy in 20 fractions plus EBBT of 25 Gy in five fractions. Doses were customized and the prescription point ranged between 3 mm and 9 mm in depth, based on the average diameter of the airway being treated. With a median follow-up of 24.5 months, only two patients (5%) experienced recurrences.

A prospective nonrandomized study reported by Perol (24) and co-workers (23) utilized the following selection criteria in the treatment of occult lung cancer with EBBT: All cases were proximal non–small cell lung carcinomas, ≤1 cm, in an area not previously irradiated. All lesions were roentgenographically occult, and the patients had severe chronic respiratory failure or had already had surgery or external radiation for previous lung carcinoma. An escalating-dose protocol was employed, and doses were prescribed at 1 cm. The first two patients received three fractions of 7 Gy each, the next four patients received four fractions of 7 Gy each, and the last 13 patients received five fractions of 7 Gy each. Two months after the completion of treatment, 15 (83%) of the 18 evaluable patients were locally controlled with negative biopsies. At 1 year, 12 (75%) of 16 evaluable patients revealed no evidence of disease. Actuarial 1- and 2-year survival rates were 78% and 58%, respectively, with a median survival of 28 months. Two patients who received five fractions of 7 Gy developed necrosis of the bronchial wall. Two of these patients died of hemoptysis, one with no evidence of carcinoma.

The substantial synchronous and metachronous rates and the finding of additional small lesions with dysplasia or marked atypia all lead to the concept of a ''field defect.'' It is quite likely that the entire bronchial mucosa is at risk with a high probability of more than one lesion developing. Any treatment strategy should address this basic issue. While lobectomy and/or pneumonectomy will cure a certain percentage of patients, the remaining lung will continue to be at risk. Another strategy for properly selected lesions (i.e., those ≤ 10 mm, no evidence of extrabronchial extension, and squamous cell histology) is to consider therapies designed to preserve pulmonary function (PDT or EBBT). Lesions > 10 mm or with evidence or suggestion of extrabronchial extension or nonsquamous histologies, however, should be considered for surgery, if patients are medically operable. If they are inoperable, then prophylactic nodal external radiation plus EBBT should be employed.

A suggested strategy is outlined in Figure 1. Lesions ≤ 10 mm with squamous cell histology could be randomized to the two therapeutic modalities most conserving of pulmonary function. Such a strategy would facilitate the clinical development of EBBT for occult lung cancers.

At our institution, we have treated more than 600 patients on protocols utilizing EBBT, which are described in detail later. Of these patients, only 19% were treated by the curative-intent protocol, and of these, only five (4%) met the criteria to be classified as radiographically occult carcinomas and are summarized in Table 1. The symptom index score is listed later in the chapter in Table 6. This is a semiquantitative symptom index that allows for description and scoring of the symptoms of the patients during their medical course. Five patients are included, with a total of six lesions treated, for a rate of 1.2 lesions per patient.

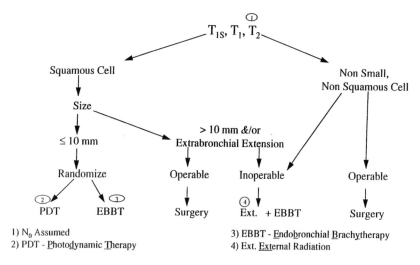

1) N_0 Assumed
2) PDT - Photodynamic Therapy
3) EBBT - Endobronchial Brachytherapy
4) Ext. External Radiation

FIGURE 1   Treatment schema for a proposed clinical trial for occult lung carcinoma with randomization between photodynamic therapy and endobronchial brachytherapy.

TABLE 1 Radiographically Occult Carcinoma in Five Patients

Patient	Disease	Symptoms	Prior Rx or med prob	Brachy/ext	Survival (days)	Status	Complications
1	T_{1s} RUL	Dyspnea 1, cough 1	PDT × 4	7.5 Gy × 3 60 Gy	202	Died-intercurrent	None
	T_1 RLL						
2	T_1 LUL	Hemoptysis 2, dyspnea 3, cough 1	COPD, severe	7.5 Gy × 3 60 Gy	1228	Alive NED	None
3	T_1 RUL	Hemoptysis 1, dyspnea 4, cough 1	COPD, severe	5 Gy × 4 60 Gy	676	Died loc. rec.	None
4	T_2 RLL	Cough 2	COPD, severe	5 Gy × 3 64 Gy	650	Alive NED	None
5	T_2 RMS	Hemoptysis 1, dyspnea 3, cough 4	COPD, severe	5 Gy × 3 64 Gy	104	Died-intercurrent	None

Two out of five patients (40%) died from intercurrent disease. One patient died of recurrence at 676 days. At the time of analysis, two of the patients were alive with no evidence of disease at 1228 and 650 days, respectively. In contrast to other reported studies, these patients were treated with a more conventional approach utilizing the current curative-intent protocol described later in detail, which allowed for the delivery of 60 or 64 Gy, with external-beam radiation given concurrently with EBBT. In this group of five patients treated with the combination of external-beam radiation and EBBT, there were no complications.

RESULTS OF ENDOBRONCHIAL BRACHYTHERAPY FOR STAGES I, II, AND III OR RECURRENT LUNG CANCER

Bronchogenic carcinoma often leads to symptoms secondary to airway involvement. These can include obstructive pneumonia, atelectasis, hemorrhage, cough, or interference with airflow. YAG laser photoresection has immediate results, but is restricted to central airways and to use by highly experienced operators. Unfortunately, conservative photo resection of the tumor without other interventions usually results in a fairly rapid reobstruction of the airway. Indeed, a recent randomized trial compared Nd-YAG laser alone versus Nd-YAG laser plus high–dose rate (HDR) brachytherapy in the management of malignant central airway disease. In a study with 29 patients, Chella et al. (24) reported that the period free from symptoms was 2.8 months with laser therapy alone (group 1) versus 8.5 months with laser/HDR branchytherapy (group 2), $p < 0.05$. Disease-free progression increased from 2.2 months in group 1 to 7.5 months in group 2 ($p < 0.05$) and the number of further endoscopic treatments reduced from 15 to 3 ($p < 0.05$). They conclude that the addition of brachytherapy to laser treatment alone significantly prolongs relief from symptoms, lessens disease progression and reduces the cost of treatment.

The principle of EBBT is that a very high dose of radiation is delivered in a short period to the tumor with sparing of normal adjacent tissues. Historically, it is of interest that as early as 1922, Yankauer (25) placed capsules of radium through a rigid bronchoscope into the region of bronchogenic carcinoma in two patients with airway obstruction. In 1933, Kernan (1) used radon seed implantation. With the advent of fiberoptic bronchoscopy, new techniques became possible. The first reported use for transbronchial implantation was by Moylan et al. (26) in 1983, using gold 198 seeds. Also in 1983, Mendiondo et al. (7) used an afterloading tube placed with the aid of the fiberoptic bronchoscope and then placed an iridium 192 source into the tube. A total of 3000 cGy delivered at a 5-mm depth was prescribed, with an average treatment time of 10 hr. Using this technique, it was noted that patients had "significant improvement" in bronchial obstruction. Schray et al. (6,27) reported on afterloading with iridium 192 in 1985 and again in 1988. A single catheter was used in 65 patients. Fifty-nine of the patients had either prior or concurrent external radiation, and 40 of the patients underwent YAG laser photoresection. Roughly 60% of the patients showed a response, 20% were stable, and 20% had progression at follow-up bronchoscopy. In the second report in 1988, 11 patients had developed either fistulas or massive hemorrhage, seven of which were felt to be secondary to treatment. It was also noted that six of the seven patients had undergone YAG photoresection and that this may have contributed to the complications.

HDR remote afterloading was first reported in the American literature by Seagren et al. (28), in 1985. All patients in this reported series had endobronchial carcinoma and had previously received a minimum external-beam radiation therapy dose equivalent to 5000 cGy prior to brachytherapy. Each patient had bronchoscopically documented disease with local symptoms and a Karnofsky performance status of 50 or greater. The HDR remote afterloading unit was a Brachyton using a 3-mm-diameter cobalt 60 source with an average strength of 0.7 Ci. The unit had the ability to oscillate the source up to a maximum of 16 cm. A single catheter was used and a dose of 1000 cGy in a single fraction was delivered at a prescription depth of 10 mm. The total time for treatment ranged between 12 and 27 min. They reported on a total of 20 patients treated between 1982 and 1983. Four patients had first received YAG laser photoresection prior to the brachytherapy procedure. Complete palliation of symptoms was seen in 25% of the patients and a partial or complete palliation of symptoms was seen in 94% of the patients. In six of these patients, palliation was long-lasting with no recurrence of symptoms. In 12 patients, these symptoms recurred or progressed, with a mean time to recurrence of 4.3 months.

Joyner and colleagues (1985) (29) first reported on the use of iridium 192 solid-wire afterloading for endobronchial treatment. They treated 14 patients with stage III non–small cell lung cancer with a combination of neodymium-YAG laser photoresection followed by endobronchial radiation and external-beam radiation therapy treatments. Brachytherapy treatment times were approximately 8–20 h to deliver 3000 cGy at a prescription depth of 5 mm. Rooney and colleagues (1984) (30) presented information on the use of HDR endobronchial treatment utilizing a Gamma Med unit with an iridium 192 source. This technique allowed for the stepping sequence of the source in up to 12 dwell positions spaced at either 0.5 or 1.0 cm. The patients were treated on a weekly basis receiving 600 cGy/week at a prescription depth of 1 cm with a maximum of five treatments. Macha et al. (31) published a report in 1987 of HDR afterloading with an iridium 192 source in which the treatment was fractionated into three treatments through a single catheter. The total dose was 1500 cGy at a 5-mm prescription depth. Patients had laser, external radiation, and/or chemotherapy and had a high complication rate.

Patients who present with atelectasis may particularly benefit from application of this approach. Reexpansion of the lung after EBBT may allow better-

TABLE 2 Compilation of Endobronchial HDR Studies

Author	Year	No. of patients	Dose (Gy)	No. of fractions	Symptoms improved (%)	X-ray improved (%)	Bronchoscopy improved (%)	Fatal hemoptysis (%)
Seagren (A1)	1985	20	10 at 10 mm	1	94	NA	100	28
Macha (A2)	1987	56	7.5 at 10 mm	3	74	88	75	7
Nori (A3)	1987	15	20 at 10 mm	3	80	88	NA	0
Burt* (A4)	1990	50	15–20 at 10 mm	1	50–86	46	88	0
Fass (A5)	1990	15	5–36 at 10 mm	1–6	75	NA	NA	0
Miller (A6)	1990	88	10 at 10 mm	3	NA	NA	80	0
Stout[a] (A7)	1990	100	15–20 at 10 mm	1	50–86	46	NA	0
Khanavkar (A8)	1991	12	8 at 5 mm	2–8	67	NA	100	50
Aygun (A9)	1992	62	5 at 10 mm	3–5	NA	36	76	15
Bedwinek (A10)	1992	38	6 at 10 mm	3	76	64	82	32
Gauwitz (A11)	1992	24	15 at 10 mm	2	88	83	100	4
Mehta (A12)	1992	31	4 at 20 mm	4†	88	71–100	85	3
Sutejda (A13)	1992	31	10 at 10 mm	3	82	NA	NA	32
Speiser (A14)	1993	144	10 at 10 mm	3	85–99	NA	80	7
		151	7.5 at 10 mm	3				8
Zajac (A15)	1993	82	10–47 at 10 mm	1–5	82	NA	74	0
Tredaniel (A16)	1994	51	7 at 10 mm	2–8	55–85	NA	84	10
Chang (A17)	1994	76	7 at 10 mm	3	79–95	NA	87	4
Gollins[b] (A18)	1994	406	10–20 at 10 mm	1 (94%) 2 (6%)	88 (H) 62 (C) 60 (D) 92 (S)	46	NA	8
Cotter (A19)	1993	65 (17 IDR, 48 HDR)	2.7–10 at 10 mm	2–4	66 (PS)	46	63	2
Goldman (A20)	1993	20	15 at 10 mm	1	37 (C) 89 (D) 100 (H)	58	55	0
Marsh (A21)	1993	12	26–53 at 10 mm; high-activity ^{125}I	1	92 (tumor response)			8
Nori (A22)	1993	32	4–5 at 10 mm	3–4	100 (H) 86 (C) 100 (P)	Local control	83	0
Pisch (A23)	1993	39	10 at 10 mm	1–2	93 (H) 80 (C) 20 (P)	NA	NA	3
Macha (A24)	1995	365	5–7.5 at 10 mm	1–6	69	NA	NA	21
Huber (A25)	1995	93	3.8 at 10 mm or 7.2 at 10 mm	4 / 2	Improved local control	NA	NA	21

Author (ref)	Year	No.	Dose	Fractions				Complications
Gustafson (A26)	1995	46	7 at 10 mm	3	74	69	92	7
Sur (A27)	1995	14	10 at 10 mm	1–2	100 (H)	NA	NA	7
Speiser[c] (A28)	1995	485 total				NA	53 (CR)	4.4 (CUR)
		47 IDR	10 at 5 mm	3	99 (H)		29 (PR)	7.3 (PAL)
		144 HDR	10 at 10 mm	3	99 (P)		82 (TR)	
		151 HDR	7.5 at 10 mm	3	86 (D)			9.1 (REC)
		143 HDR	7.5 at 10 mm	3	85 (C)			7.3 (ALL)
			5 at 10 mm	4				
Saito (A29)	1996	40	5 at 3–9 mm	5	NA	NA	100	0
Delclos (A30)	1996	81	15 at 6 mm	2	32% excellent 31% moderate 21% minimal 84% total median survival	NA	NA	0
Huber (A31)	1997	98	Ext only 60 Gy[d]	22–30	30 wk			14
		42	Ext + Int					
		56	Int 4.8 at 5 mm 5–15 Gy at 10 mm	2	43 wk			19
Corsa (A32)	1997	29		1–4	100 (H) 70 (D) 46 (C)	83	79	6.9%
Perol (A33)	1997	19	76 y at 10 mm	3–5	79% biopsy (−) actual survival 1 yr = 78% 2 yr = 58% median = 28 m			10.5%
Ornadel (A34)	1997	117	15 Gy at 10 mm	1	46 (C) 50 (I) 62 (H) 54 (PS) 46 (C) 33 (D) 20 (P) 79 (H)	43%	63%	9.4% 20% 2 yr acturial HR
Ofiara (A35)	1997	30	8 Gy at 10 mm	3				
Hennequin (A36)	1998	149	4–7 Gy at 5–15 mm	2–6	60	79%		6.7% (multivariate analysis endo-bronchiol tumor length was sig $p = 0.02$)
Total	1985–1998	3176			20–100	36–88	55–100	0–50 Mean 10.1

TABLE 2 Continued

C = cough; CR = complete response; CUR = curative; D = dyspnea; H = hemoptysis; IDR = immediate dose rate; P = pneumonia; PAL = palliative; PR = more than 50% response; PS = performance status; REC = recurrent; S = stridor; TR = CR + PR.

^a Same institution.
^b Four treatments in 2 days.
^c Speiser reporting different protocols.
^d Mean dose ~ 50Gy ± 13 Gy.

A1 Seagren SL, Harrell JH, Horn RA. High dose rate intraluminal irradiation in recurrent endobronchial carcinoma. Chest 1985; 88:810–814.

A2 Macha HN, Koch K, Stadler, et al. New technique for treating occlusive and stenosing tumours of the trachea and main bronchi: endobronchial irradiation by high dose iridium-192 combined with laser canalization. Thorax 1987; 42:511–515.

A3 Nori D, Hilaris BS, Tome M, et al. Intraluminal irradiation in bronchogenic carcinoma. Surg Clin North Am 1987; 67(5):1093–1102.

A4 Burt PA, O'Driscoll BR, Notley HM, et al. Intraluminal irradiation for the palliation of lung cancer with the high dose rate microselectron. Thorax 1990; 45:765–768.

A5 Fass DE, Armstrong J, Harrison LB. Fractionated high dose rate endobronchial treatment for recurrent lung cancer. Endocurie Hypertherm Oncol 1990; 6:211–215.

A6 Miller JI, Phillips TW. Neodymium: YAG laser and brachytherapy in the management of inoperable bronchogenic carcinoma. Ann Thorac Surg 50: 190–196.

A7 Stout R. Endobronchial brachytherapy. Lung Cancer 1993; 9:295–300.

A8 Khanavkar B, Stern P, Alberti W, et al. Complications associated with brachytherapy alone or with laser in lung cancer. Chest 1990; 99:1062–1065.

A9 Aygun C, Weiner S, Scariato A, et al. Treatment of nonsmall cell lung cancer with external beam: radiotherapy and high dose rate brachytherapy. Int J Radiat Oncol Biol Phys 1992; 23:127–132.

A10 Bedwinek J, Bruton C, Petty A, et al. High dose rate endobronchial brachytherapy and fatal pulmonary hemorrhage. Int J Radiat Oncol Biol Phys 1991; 22:23–30.

A11 Gauwitz M, Ellerbroek N, Komaki R, et al. High dose endobronchial irradiation in recurrent bronchogenic carcinoma. Int J Radiat Oncol Biol Phys 1992; 23:397–400.

A12 Mehta MP, Petereit D, Chosy L, et al. Sequential comparison of low dose rate and hyperfractionated high dose rate endobronchial radiation for malignant airway occlusion. Int J Radiat Oncol Biol Phys 1992; 23:133–139.

A13 Sutedja G, Baris G, Schaake-Koning C, et al. High dose rate brachytherapy in patients with local recurrences after radiotherapy of non–small cell lung cancer. Int J Radiat Oncol Biol Phys 1992; 24:551–553.

A14 Speiser B, Spratling L. High dose rate brachytherapy for the local control of endobronchial carcinoma. Int J Radiat Oncol Biol Phys 1993; 25: 579–588.

A15 Zajac AJ, Kohn ML, Heiser D, et al. High-dose rate intraluminal brachytherapy in the treatment of endobronchial malignancy. Radiology 1993; 187:571–575.

A16 Tredaniel J, Hennequin C, Zalcman G, et al. Prolonged survival after high-dose rate endobronchial radiation for malignant airway obstruction. Chest 1994; 105:767–772.

A17 Chang LFL, Horvath J, Peyton W, et al. High dose rate afterloading brachytherapy in malignant airway obstruction of lung cancer. Int J Radiat Oncol Biol Phys 1994; 28:589–596.

A18 Gollins S, Burt P, Barber P, et al. High dose rate intraluminal radiotherapy for carcinoma of the bronchus: outcome of treatment of 406 patients. Radiotherapy 1994; 33:31–40.

A19 Cotter GW, Larisey C, Ellingwood KE, et al. Inoperable endobronchial obstructing lung cancer treated with combined endobronchial and external beam irradiation: a dosimetric analysis. Int J Radiat Oncol Biol Phys 1993; 27-531–535.

A20 Goldman J, Bulman A, Rathmell A, et al. Physiological effect of endobronchial radiotherapy in patients with major airway obstruction. Thorax 1993; 48:110–114. A21 Marsh BR, Colvin DP, Zinreich ES, et al. Clinical experience with an endobronchial implant. Radiology 1993; 189:147–150.

A22 Nori D, Allison R, Kaplan B, et al. High dose rate intraluminal irradiation in bronchogenic carcinoma. Chest 1993; 104:1006–1011. A23 Pisch J, Villamena P, Harvey J, et al. High dose-rate endobronchial irradiation in malignant airway obstruction. Chest 1993; 104: 3721–3725.

A24 Macha HN, Wahlers B, Reichle C, et al. Endobronchial radiation therapy for obstructing malignancies: ten years' experience with iridium-192 high-dose radiation brachytherapy afterloading technique in 365 patients. Lung 1995; 173:271–280. A25 Huber R, Fischer R, Hautmann H, et al. Palliative endobronchial brachytherapy for central lung tumors. Chest 1995; 107:2:463–470.

A26 Gustafson G, Vincini F, Freedman L, et al. High dose rate endobronchial brachytherapy in the management of primary and recurrent bronchogenic malignancies. Cancer 1995; 75(9):2345–2350. A27 Sur R, Mahomed G, Pacella J, et al. Initial report on the effectiveness of high dose rate brachytherapy in the treatment of hemoptysis in lung cancer. Endocuriether Hypertherm Oncol 1995; 11:101–106.

A28 Speiser B. The role of endobronchial brachytherapy in patients with lung cancer. Clin Pulmon Med 1995; 2(6):344–352.

A29 Saito M, Yokoyama A, Kurita Y, et al. Treatment of roentgenographically occult endobronchial carcinoma with external beam radiotherapy and intraluminal low-dose rate brachytherapy. Int J Radiat Oncol Biol Phys 1996; 34:1029–1035.

A30 Delclos ME, Komaki R, Morice RC, et al. Endobronchial brachytherapy with high-dose rate remote afterloading for recurrent endobronchial lesions. Radiology 1996; 201(1):279–282.

A31 Huber RM, Fischer R, Hautmann H, et al. Does additional brachytherapy improve the effect of external irradiation? A prospective, randomized study in central lung tumors. Int J Radiat Oncol Biol Phys 1997; 38(3):533–540.

A32 Corsa P, Parisi SS, Raguso A, et al. High-dose brachytherapy in endobronchial neoplastic stenoses. Radiol Med (Torino) 1997; 94(1–2):94–99.

A33 Perol M, Caliandro R, Pommier P, et al. Curative irradiation of limited endobronchial carcinomas with high-dose rate brachytherapy. Results of a pilot study. Chest 1997; 111(5):1417–1423.

A34 Ornadel D, Duchesne G, Wall P, et al. Defining the roles of high dose rate endobronchial brachytherapy and laser resection for recurrent bronchial malignancy. Lung Cancer 1997; 16(2–3):203–213.

A35 Ofiara L, Roman T, Schwartzman K, et al. Local determinants of response to endobronchial high-dose rate brachytherapy in bronchogenic carcinoma. Chest 1997; 112(4):946–953.

A36 Hennequin C, Tredaniel J, Chevret S, et al. Predictive factors for late toxicity after endobronchial brachytherapy: a multivariate analysis. Int J Radiat Oncol Biol Phys 1998; 42(1):21–27.

tailored external-beam radiation fields. Bastin et al. (32) reported their ability to spare an average of 32% of the ipsilateral lung volume using this technique. In most of the studies described above, the procedure consisted of a single catheter for intraluminal brachytherapy. Sometimes, more than one catheter is used, such as when treating disease that straddles the carina. Additional physics factors must be taken into account, including the choice of the radioactive isotope, the dose at the prescription depth relative to the radius and inverse square law, as well as correction factors for the attenuation in water equivalent tissue versus air. Iridium 192 has the ability to be fabricated in very small physical sizes of high activity, allowing passage through catheters with an internal diameter of 1.5 mm or less. In addition, iridium 192 has virtually no significant correction for attenuation in water versus air up to a distance of 5 cm from the source. This makes iridium 192 an ideal radioactive isotope to be used within tissues with a mixed air/water density interface, such as intraluminal brachytherapy. The major drawback of iridium 192 is its relatively short half-life of 74 days, such that over a period of months, its activity changes considerably. However, this disadvantage can be addressed by frequent replacement of the sources to keep the source strength well within the HDR range.

Table 2 is a compilation of most, but not all, of the studies published on HDR remote afterloading EBBT. It covers the years 1985 to 1997 for a total of 2842 patients. The table shows the different doses used per fraction, the wide range of fractions, as well as the dose prescriptions at various depths. Of interest is that, while the variation for fatal hemoptysis is extremely large (ranging from 0 to 50%), the mean is 10.3%. This rate appears to depend on multiple factors, such as total number of patients studied, extensiveness of follow-up, and aggressiveness of the treatment. For a small series, such as that of Khanavkar et al. (33), the 50% incidence of fatal hemoptysis in 12 patients is likely not representative. Similarly, there are reports of no fatal hemoptysis, such as that of Burt et al. (12), reporting on 50 patients. However, when the same medical group updated their series and reported on a total of 406 patients (34), their rate of fatal hemoptysis was 8%. Some authors have attributed fatal hemoptysis to aggressive treatment, such as Bedwinek et al. (35), who reported a 32% rate of hemoptysis. However, Macha et al. (36) and Speiser (37) reported on 365 and 485 patients, with lower rates of fatal hemoptysis, 21% and 8%, respectively. Further information indicated that many of these cases were secondary to biological progression of the carcinoma itself, suggesting that the treatment may not have been aggressive enough.

In 1986, Speiser and Spratling developed a series of scoring systems (Tables 3–6) for selecting patients for treatment, as well as for outcome analysis. Their initial report (38) was based on experience with an IDR unit, which was a modification of a LDR unit, to allow a higher specific activity of iridium 192 for more rapid delivery of dose. In some of the LDR protocols, delivery of radia-

TABLE 3 Influence of Performance Status on Patients with Inoperable Lung Cancer

Performance status scale		
ECOG (Zubrod) (Host) (WHO)	Karnofsky	Definitions
0	100	Asymptomatic
1	80–90	Symptomatic: fully ambulatory
2	60–70	Symptomatic: in bed less than 50% of the day
3	40–50	Symptomatic: in bed more than 50% of the day but not bedridden
4	20–30	Bedridden

TABLE 4 Weight Loss Score Based on Percentage of Loss of Body Weight Within 6 Months Preceding Diagnosis

Weight loss score (WLS)	Weight loss (% of body weight)
0	0
1	1–4.9
2	5–9.9
3	10–19.9
4	>20.0

TABLE 5 Obstruction Score

Location	Percent obstruction		
	>50	10–50	<10
Trachea	10	5	2
Main stem	6	3	1
Lobar bronchi	2	1	

Atelectasis/pneumonia received additional 2 points per lobe.

TABLE 6 Symptom Index Scoring System

Score	Definition
	Dyspnea
0	None
1	Dyspnea on moderate exertion
2	Dyspnea with normal activity, walking on level ground
3	Dyspnea at rest
4	Requires supplemental oxygen
	Cough
0	None
1	Intermittent, no medication necessary
2	Intermittent, nonnarcotic medication
3	Constant or requiring narcotic medication
4	Constant, requiring narcotic medication but without relief
	Hemoptysis
0	None
1	Less than 2/week
2	Less than daily but greater than 2/week
3	Daily, bright red blood or clots
4	Decrease of Hb and/or Hct > 10%; greater than 150 cm, requiring hospitalization or transfusion
	Pneumonia/elevated temperature
0	Normal temperature, no infiltrates, WBC less than 10,000
1	Temperature greater than 38.5°C and infiltrate, WBC less than 10,000
2	Temperature greater than 38.5°C and infiltrate and/or WBC greater than 10,000
3	Lobar consolidation on radiograph
4	Pneumonia or elevated temperature requiring hospitalization

tion took as long as 60 h. The increase of iridium 192 activity allowed the treatment time to be decreased to 1.5–4 hr. This range was based on (1) shorter times when the sources were new versus longer times after the sources decayed, and (2) the use, for the first time, of multiple catheters to deliver treatment. All treatments were performed in the outpatient setting and followed a protocol outlined in the next section.

PROTOCOL

The protocol alluded to earlier in the chapter was initiated in 1986 when EBBT was transformed from LDR manual afterloading to MDR remote afterloading procedures. This was a transitory step of short duration, lasting for 9 months.

The HDR remote afterloader was, in fact, a Nucletron Selectron LDR remote afterloader that was modified to accept a longer source train and a higher level of radioactivity. The activity was typically maintained at greater than 20 mc/cm. Dose rates initially were calculated at a 5-mm depth perpendicular to the source train, and were in the range of 5–10 cGy/min.

Eligibility

Eligibility for the protocol included the following. (1) Disease must involve the trachea, mainstem, or lobar bronchi. Involvement of the segmental bronchi without involvement more proximal was not considered sufficient for entry into the protocol. (2) The central airway disease must be intraluminal, visualized, and biopsied via bronchoscopy. Patients requiring transbronchial biopsy were ineligible for the protocol. (3) Patients must have significant symptomatology within the four symptom groups consisting of cough, dyspnea, signs and symptoms of obstructive pneumonia, and/or hemoptysis.

Evaluation of the patients meeting eligibility criteria for the EBBT protocol schedule was reviewed within the context of all patients diagnosed with lung cancer in the referral area from 1986 through 1996. This involved the greater Phoenix/Maricopa County area, and based on the tumor registry, an incidence of approximately 9000 cases of lung cancer during the 10 year period was calculated. Of these, only 19% received radiation and 16% of that group, or 3% of all patients, were treated on protocol, while an additional 11% of patients receiving radiation, or 2% of all patients, were treated with brachytherapy off protocol. Thus, 27% of all patients receiving radiation, or 5% of all diagnosed lung cancer patients, received brachytherapy. For patients on the curative protocol, these figures were 3% and 0.5%, respectively.

Indications

Indications for treatment are outlined in Table 7.

Protocol 1.0: Curative Intent

To be eligible for this protocol, patients must not have had prior radiation within the thoracic area, which would preclude the adequate delivery of a full dose of external radiation. Patients must be inoperable and have a primary lung carcinoma with non–small cell histology. Stages accepted were $T_{1,2,3}$ $N_{1,2}$ M_0. These correspond to stage groupings I, II, and IIIA. Performance status using the ECOG four-tiered system must be 0, 1, or 2 and weight loss using a four-tiered weight loss system, likewise, must be 0, 1, or 2 and correspond to weight losses of 0, less than 5%, or less than 10%, respectively, of the patient's weight in the 6 months prior to diagnosis. The rational for selection of this level of weight loss is described in "Oncological Assessment Using the Four-Tiered Scoring Sys-

TABLE 7   Indications for Treatment

Indications	Exclusions	Rationale
1. Tumors must be seen and biopsied by bronchoscopy (intraluminal)	Tumors presenting with extrinsic compression of the airway as seen by bronchoscopy and the biopsy must be performed transbronchially (extraluminal)	Intraluminal brachytherapy delivers a very high dose to tumor close to the source axis; extraluminal disease due to its much greater distance from the axis would lead to unacceptable doses to the bronchial mucosa and surrounding structures
2. Tumors must be in the central airways, which are defined as the trachea, mainstem, and lobar bronchi	Tumors in peripheral airways, which are defined as segmental bronchi or beyond	Significant symptomatology is most often caused by disease in central airways; treatment of small peripheral airways leads to stenosis of those airways
3. Tumors in central airways causing significant symptomatology	Patients with significant preexisting dyspnea unrelated to carcinoma; patients with dyspnea secondary to effusion, or large extrinsic masses	Patients with symptoms secondary to disease other than central airway disease are not expected to improve with intraluminal brachytherapy
4. In situ carcinoma for inoperable patients	Patients entered into national protocols using other modes of treatment, i.e., photodynamic	Preserves lung and pulmonary function; excellent treatment for multifocal disease
5. Preop. for submucosal spread from a peripheral/central lesion	Patients should be good candidates for lobectomy or pneumonectomy	Treatment provides a clear margin for surgery

tem'' (39). Patients were treated within groups 1–4 with dose modifications as described in Table 8.

Protocol 2.0: Palliative Intent

Protocol 2.1

Eligibility for these patients includes: primary lung cancer with non–small cell histology, and stage T_4, N_3 and /or M_1 disease. These corresponded to stage

TABLE 8 Modification of Doses by Year for the Curative, Palliative, and Recurrent Protocols

Group	Year	External cGy		Internal cGy			Unit
		Dose	FXS	Dose	Depth	FXS	
Curative protocol							
1	1986–1988	6000	30	1000	5 mm	3	MDR
2	1988–1990	6000	30	1000	10 mm	3	HDR
3	1990–1992	6000	30	750	10 mm	3	HDR
4	1992–1994	6400	32	500	10 mm	3	HDR
Palliative protocol							
1	1986–1988	3750	15	1000	5 mm	3	MDR
				1000	5 mm	3	MDR
2	1988–1990	3750	15	1000	10 mm	3	HDR
				1000	10 mm	3	HDR
3	1990–1992	3750	15	750	10 mm	3	HDR
				750	10 mm	3	HDR
4	1992–1994	3750	15	500	10 mm	3	HDR
				500	10 mm	4	HDR
				750	10 mm	3	HDR
Recurrent protocol							
1	1986–1988			1000	5 mm	3	MDR
2	1988–1990			1000	10 mm	3	HDR
3	1990–1992			750	10 mm	3	HDR
4	1992–1994			500	10 mm	4	HDR

groupings IIIB and IV. In addition, the patients ineligible for protocol 1.0 because of performance scores of 3 or 4 or a weight loss of 3 or 4 (>10%, >20%) were reallocated to this protocol. Patients were treated within groups, characterized by dose, as described in Table 8.

Protocol 2.2

Primary lung cancer consisting of small cell histology, both limited and extensive, primary lung cancer with contralateral metastatic disease involving the endobronchial mucosa, and nonlung primaries with metastases primarily to the mucosa were treated within this category. Patients were treated within the group characterized by dose as described in Table 9.

TABLE 9   Grades of Radiation Bronchitis and Stenosis (RBS)

Grade	Definition
1	Fibrinoid membrane without significant luminal obstruction: no symptoms
2	Increase of exudation and fibrous membrane with mild obstructive symptoms requiring therapeutic intervention such as simple debridement or medical treatment
3	Characterized by severe inflammatory response with marked membranous exudate including fibrosis requiring multiple debridements
4	A greater degree of fibrosis resulting in stenosis with decreased luminal diameter requiring laser photoresection, balloon or bougie dilation, and/or stent placement

Protocol 3.0: Recurrent Patients

All patients who had received prior radiation for a curative intent for carcinoma of the lung were included within this category. Patients were treated within the group characterized by dose as described in Table 8. Group I patients were treated with MDR. In the palliative protocol, the brachytherapy was constant and the use of external radiation was optional at the discretion of the treating oncologist. Its use was restricted to patients with extrinsic disease that caused a significant contribution to the level of obstruction and/or symptomatology.

Results

The following results incorporate 600 patients treated in the curative, palliative, and recurrent protocols outlined previously. In each of the successive periods of the operation of the protocol, the eligibility factors for the curative, palliative, and recurrent protocols have remained constant.

All patients treated in curative protocols with external radiation received 2 Gy per fraction, and in palliative protocols, 2.5 Gy per fraction. If patients received concurrent brachytherapy and external radiation, both treatments were not given on the same day. For the curative protocol, brachytherapy was delivered during weeks 1, 3, and 5. For palliative or recurrent protocols, brachytherapy was delivered weekly for three or four fractions, depending on the protocol.

The distribution of patients into the protocol groups was as follows: curative 19%, palliative 48%, and recurrent 33%. The age distribution of the patients had a median of 68 years and a mean of 67.1 years. Most of the patients fell within the range of 60–80 years old. The gender distribution was 62% male and 38% female. The percentage of female patients increased from 28% in group 1 to 41% in group 3 and 4. The breakdown for male/female patients was similar to that of all patients presenting with carcinoma of the lung within the geographical treatment area.

Squamous cell carcinoma is by far the most common cell type, overall, in the study (49%), and even to a greater extent for those treated in the curative protocol (70%). This percentage is considerably higher than is currently being seen in newly diagnosed outpatients with lung cancer (27%). This fits with prior observations that squamous cell carcinomas tend to be more central and adenocarcinomas more peripheral.

The use of laser photoresection predated the wide use of HDR brachytherapy for airway carcinoma. In this study there was a gradual decrease in its use from an initial 32% to 16% in the latter part of the study. It is currently estimated that less than 5% of patients with central airway disease require laser photoresection.

The protocol required that to be included in this study, patients must have one or more of the four primary symptom complexes. The incidence of the symptoms in the study was: cough 99%, dyspnea 97%, hemoptysis 64%, and the signs and symptoms of obstructive pneumonia 49%. Using the four-tiered symptom index as outlined in Table 6, the severity of the symptoms was weighted and the total weighted score was subsequently normalized to 100%. Response for each symptom score is related to each brachytherapy procedure and the first follow-up bronchoscopy (Figure 2).

Hemoptysis had the most dramatic and rapid of the responses with improvements of 70%, 90%, and >99% at each intervention point. Pneumonia improvement was only slightly less dramatic with responses of 57%, 85%, and >99%. Improvement in dyspnea occurred in 36%, 54%, and 86%, respectively. Finally, improvement in cough was 32%, 52%, and 85% respectively. The improvements in hemoptysis and pneumonia were commonly seen within the first 24 hr following the first brachytherapy procedure. Patients who were admitted to the hospital with obstructive pneumonia and/or sepsis, or with severe bleeding requiring transfusion, generally had a prompt response.

In the palliative protocol, the use of concurrent external radiation with brachytherapy was optional. When the weighted responses were measured for brachytherapy only, versus brachytherapy and external radiation, the results in terms of improvement at follow-up were as follows: hemoptysis 94% and 97%, pneumonia 86% and 82%, dyspnea 54% and 48%, and cough 51% and 57%, respectively. There was no statistical difference in response for each symptom group for each of these two therapies. The use of brachytherapy only was sufficient to provide palliation without the need to add supplemental external radiation.

Airway obstruction scores, as shown in Figure 3, were analyzed in a different fashion. All of the scores were converted into median scores, which were normalized to 100%. These were obtained for each brachytherapy procedure and

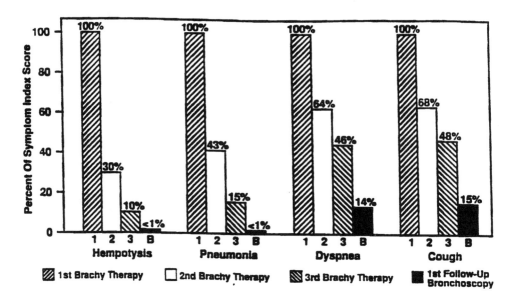

FIGURE 2 Response in the symptom index as measured by the decrease of the symptom index scores comparing the initial score at the first brachytherapy (normalized to 100%) and the scores at subsequent encounters as the percent residual.

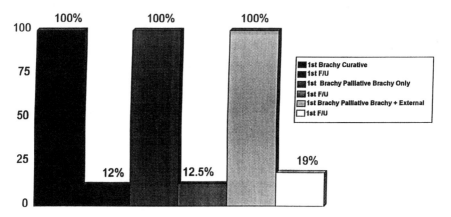

FIGURE 3 Response in the obstruction score with the mean initial score normalized to 100% at the first brachytherapy and the percent residual at the first bronchoscopic follow-up.

at the first follow-up bronchoscopy. The median score was normalized to 100% and the residual level of obstruction is expressed as a percentage. Any tissue including inflammatory tissue was included as part of the obstruction score. The curative patients and the palliative groups fared better than the recurrent group, with scores of 12%, 12.5%, and 19%, respectively (Figure 3). This is not unexpected considering that patients with recurrent carcinoma have had previous external radiation, which may select for a slightly more radioresistant carcinoma. It is interesting that the use of neither concurrent external radiation nor laser photoresection led to improved clearing of obstruction. Thus, as in the symptom index results, the addition of external radiation or laser resection did not add to clearing endobronchial disease.

The survival of patients by protocol group was, for the curative patients, 10%, and for palliative-recurrent, 5% at 5 years. The cause of death shows a significant local failure rate in all categories. These rates were 31% and 30%, respectively, for the curative and palliative-recurrent protocols. As has been seen in numerous other studies, in spite of gradually increasing doses of radiation over the last several decades, local disease continues to be a significant problem.

Survival curves for curative versus the palliative-recurrent patient illustrated in Figure 4 are calculated from the date of diagnosis and date of the first brachytherapy procedure. There was no statistically different result between these two groups when analyzed from the date of diagnosis ($p = 0.1$). However, from the date of the first brachytherapy treatment, the p value was <0.0001 comparing the curative versus the palliative-recurrent patients. The recurrent patients are self-selected by the fact that they lived long enough to develop a symptomatic recurrence. This bias was eliminated when analyzing survival by date of treatment.

COMPLICATIONS

The complication most often described when discussing endobronchial carcinoma and its treatment is fatal hemoptysis. This is defined as bleeding that most often is caused by erosion into the right or left pulmonary artery with subsequent exsanguination within the tracheal bronchial tree. This is a known complication of progression of untreated or inadequately treated carcinoma involving the tracheobronchial tree, most often in the region of the upper-lobe bronchi, owing to their proximity to the pulmonary arteries. With the advent of intraluminal treatment, it must also be considered as a possible complication of this modality.

In this study, the overall rate of fatal hemoptysis is 6% with the median time from diagnosis until death at 14 months. However, when measured from the date of the first brachytherapy until death, the median for the entire group is only 5 months. Recurrent patients, as would be anticipated, have the highest rate of fatal hemoptysis at 9% while the curative and palliative patients have rates of

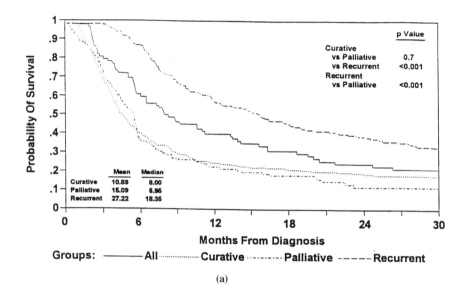

(a)

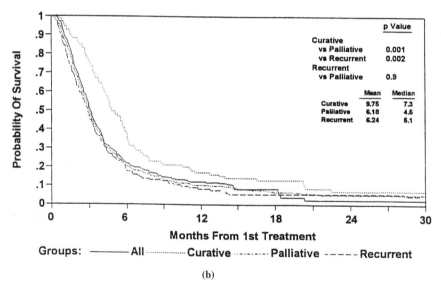

(b)

FIGURE 4   Survival cures and *p* values for curative, palliative, recurrent, and combined group measured (a) from diagnosis and (b) from date of first treatment.

5%. Of interest is that, in the different dose groups, there was an increase in fatal hemoptysis as the dose was increased from group 1 to 2. However, there was paradoxically a slight further increase in the rate of hemoptysis as the dose was initially reduced and then a decrease in the rate of fatal hemoptysis (2%) with further dose reduction. No clear dose-response relationship could be identified. In the palliative protocol, 41% of the patients were treated with brachytherapy only, and 59% with brachytherapy and external radiation. The rate of fatal hemoptysis was 5.5% in the brachytherapy only group, versus 4% in the combined group who received higher doses of radiation.

The most common side effect related to intraluminal treatment is radiation bronchitis and stenosis. This was first described by Speiser and Spratling (38). Table 9 defines the various grades of radiation bronchitis and stenosis. The incidence of radiation bronchitis and stenosis by group is 9%, 12%, 14%, and 14%, respectively. By protocol, it was 23%, 12%, and 8%, respectively, for the curative, palliative, and recurrent protocols. The rate is clearly highest in the curative patients. However, the only significant factor predicting for this response was length of follow-up. Although the true incidence of this complication is not known for patients receiving external radiation only, it appears to be a complication primarily of intraluminal brachytherapy, with its very high mucosal doses.

For palliative patients, this complication was studied in those patients receiving brachytherapy only versus those receiving brachytherapy along with concurrent external radiation, and the incidence was 17% and 10%, respectively. While the incidence was slightly higher in the brachytherapy-only group, the median time to occurrence was slightly longer in this group at 3.6 months versus 2.5 months for the patients receiving combined treatment.

MANAGEMENT OF COMPLICATIONS

The treatment of brachytherapy-related hemoptysis is the same as for hemoptysis from other causes. This includes bed rest, codeine, and/or transfusion for hemodynamic stability, avoidance and/or reversal of anticoagulants, and vascular embolization, electrocautery, or lasocautery to reduce bleeding volume.

One of the largest reported series of patients treated with palliative brachytherapy alone is from the Christi Hospital in Manchester, England (40). A total of 322 patients with inoperable non–small cell lung cancers were treated with a single fraction of HDR with a total dose of 15–20 Gy delivered intraluminally with the dose prescription 1 cm from the central axis of the catheter. Patients were evaluated 6 weeks after completing the HDR treatment regarding their symptoms, including stridor, hemoptysis, cough, dyspnea, pain, and pulmonary collapse. In addition, at various times following the brachytherapy procedure, 83 bronchoscopies were conducted on 55 patients. Massive hemoptysis leading to death occurred in 32 patients (8%). Cox multivariate analysis revealed that treatment-related factors associated with subsequent massive hemoptysis were brachytherapy dose >15 Gy, prior laser therapy, second brachytherapy treatment, and concurrent external-beam radiation therapy. Twenty of the 25 assessable deaths related to hemoptysis had recurrent and/or residual tumor suspected at the hemoptysis site. The chronology of the massive hemoptysis leading to death occurred between 9 and 12 months after completion of the HDR procedure. This was in stark contrast to deaths from all other causes, which usually occurred 3–6 months after completion of the HDR procedures (41).

Brachytherapy-related bronchitis and stenosis are managed depending on the level of severity of the reaction and/or stenosis. This can include observation for mild treatment-related bronchitis for the least symptomatic presentation, versus active treatment for its more debilitating form, with oral and/or aerosol administration of steroids, aerosol-administrated bronchodilators, codeine- or narcotic-based cough suppressants, and antifungal or antibiotic therapies as indicated. More aggressive interventional management for debilitating and/or life-threatening levels of bronchitis and/or stenosis may be managed with balloon and/or bougie dilatation, laser photoresection, bronchoscopic debridement, and/or placement of intraluminal stents.

Although lung brachytherapy has been advocated by radiation oncologists for the past 20 years, recent technological developments in the area of HDR brachytherapy, such as the design of small, high-activity, iridium 192 sources and remote afterloading machines, have prompted renewed interest in HDR endobronchial brachytherapy. The specific role of lung EBBT is not clearly defined within the standard and/or uniform community practice. There is an ongoing evolution for the selection criteria to identify those patients most likely to benefit from EBBT as part of definitive therapy. The American Brachytherapy Society (ABS) HDR consensus guidelines (42) currently state that, although EBBT has demonstrated efficacy for symptomatic relief of bronchial obstructions and hemoptysis, either alone or in combination with external-beam radiation therapy, the curative benefit of brachytherapy in addition to conventional external-beam radiation therapy and/or chemotherapy has not been proven. The ABS recommends that brachytherapy for the definitive treatment of lung cancer be done within the context of controlled clinical trials. Outside of clinical trials, the ABS suggests that brachytherapy be reserved for palliative treatments alone. Although the guidelines do not clearly state the indications for additional external-beam radiation in newly diagnosed lung cancer patients, EBBT alone is recommended for recurrences after full-dose external-beam radiation therapy treatments have been administered. No single-dose fractionation scheme has been identified, which provides for superior therapeutic ratio. Dose specifications to be prescribed have been recommended to a depth of 1 cm from the source center for uniform prescription dosimetry comparisons.

A study by the Radiation Therapy Oncology Group (RTOG) evaluated the palliation provided by external-beam radiation to patients with newly diagnosed nonmetastatic, non–small cell lung cancers (43). This study by Simpson demonstrated that a short course of external-beam radiation therapy delivering 30 Gy in 10 fractions provided relief of hemoptysis in 74% of patients, cough in 55% of patients, and dyspnea in 43% of patients. Median survival was in the range of 6 months. Compared to this RTOG study, brachytherapy alone appears to provide equivalent or improved palliation as external-beam radiation, with a similar survival outcome. Given this fact, brachytherapy may give more prompt symptomatic relief of obstructive symptoms, in a more cost-effective manner. In a small group of 19 patients treated with HDR to a total dose of 15 Gy (44), a detailed assessment with rigorous testing was performed both before and after administration of the HDR brachytherapy. This included chest x-rays, CT scan of the thorax, direct bronchoscopic evaluation, objective obstruction index scoring, 5-min walking stress tests, isotope ventilation and profusion lung scanning, and formal pulmonary function tests with maximum inspiratory and expiratory full-volume measurements. Symptomatic relief was reported in 17 of the 19 patients. Atelectasis of a collapsed lobe or lung reported in 13 patients was demonstrated to have reinstituted ventilation in nine cases by radiographic imaging. Bronchoscopic evaluation of luminal patency demonstrated improvement in 18 of the 19 patients. Isotope lung scans showed significant increase in the percentage of total lung ventilation and perfusion in the abnormal lung. This rigorous study demonstrated the high correlation between objective and subjective improvement of the presenting symptomatology in these patients. In addition, it confirmed the palliative benefit of brachytherapy, which has been described in larger groups of patients. Further prospective studies of brachytherapy and external-beam radiation therapy are clearly needed to rigorously document treatment efficacy and toxicity, as well as a cost-benefit analysis and quality of life in this setting.

CONCLUSIONS

EBBT is an excellent means of palliative treatment for patients who are symptomatic from endobronchial disease. As part of definitive therapy for curative-intent patients, however, a survival advantage is not shown. This group of patients should be randomized to external-beam radiation therapy versus external-beam plus intraluminal radiation to prospectively evaluate a possible survival advantage. Further studies will also be necessary to determine the optimal dose and number of fractions that will provide the greatest patient benefit, the lowest morbidity, and the lowest cost of treatment.

PROS AND CONS

Pro: EBBT is ideal for delivering very high doses of radiation to neoplastic tissue in or within a 1-cm radius of the main airway.

Con: Because brachytherapy doses depend on the inverse square law (that is, the dose decreases by the square of the distance), neoplastic tissue ≫ 1 cm from the airway is *not* effectively treated.

Pro: EBBT provides relief of airway obstruction to a greater extent and significantly faster than external radiation.

Con: Obstruction of airways by extrinsic compression is best treated by external radiation.

Pro: EBBT can be used in the trachea mainstem and lobar and segmented bronchi, an extent greater than feasible with the YAG laser.

Con: YAG laser works immediately (endobronchial takes 4–24 hr for a partial response) and is sometimes necessary for very bulky exophytic tumors.

Pro: For palliation of airway signs and symptoms due to intrinsic disease, EBBT provides excellent relief with minimal morbidity.

Con: Extrinsic compression such as nodal or parenchymal masses or pleural effusion can nullify benefits of brachytherapy, unless these other factors are adequately dealt with.

Pro: EBBT can cure occult cancer of the lung.

Con: Occult cancer has a high rate of synchronous lesions that must also be identified and treated.

REFERENCES

1. Kernan JD. Carcinoma of the lung and bronchus. Treatment with radon implantation and diathermy. Arch Otolaryngol 1933; 17:457–475.
2. Meredith WJ, ed. Radium Dosage, the Manchester System. Edinburgh, UK: Livingstone, 1967.
3. Pool JL. Bronchoscopy in the treatment of lung cancer. Trans Am Bronchoesoph Assoc 1961; 41:128–136.
4. Graham EA, Singer JJ. Successful removal of an entire lung for carcinoma of the bronchus. JAMA 1933; 101:1371–1374.
5. Henschke UK. Interstitial implantation in the treatment of primary bronchogenic carcinoma. Am J Roentgenol Radium Ther Nucl Med 1959; 79:981–987.
6. Schray MF, McDougall JC, Martinez A, et al. Management of malignant airway obstruction: clinical and dosimetric considerations using an iridium-192 afterloading technique in conjunction with the neodymium-YAG laser. Int J Radiat Oncol Biol Phys 1985; 11(2):403–409.
7. Mendiondo OA, Dillon M, Beach LJ. Endobronchial brachytherapy in the treatment of recurrent bronchogenic carcinoma. Int J Radiat Oncol Biol Phys 1983; 9:579–582.
8. LeChevalier T, Arriagada R, Tarayre, M, et al. Significant effect of adjuvant chemotherapy on survival in locally advanced non–small-cell lung carcinoma. J Natl Cancer Inst 1992; 84:58 (letter).

9. Sanderson D, Fontana R, Woolner L, et al. Bronchoscopic localization of radiographically occult lung cancer. Chest 1974; 65:608–612.
10. Cortese DA, Pairolero PC, Bergstraih EJ, et al. Roentgenographically occult lung cancer. J Thorac Cardiovasc Surg 1980; 86:373–380.
11. Martini N, Melamed MR. Occult carcinoma of the lung. Ann Thorac Surg 1980; 30:215–223.
12. Burt ME, Pomerantz AH, Bains MS, et al. Results of surgical treatment of stage III lung cancer invading mediastinum. Surg Clin North Am 1987; 67:997–1000.
13. Saito Y, Nagamoto N, Ota S, et al. Results of surgical treatment for roentgenographically occult bronchogenic squamous cell carcinoma. J Thorac Cardiovasc Surg 1992; 104:401–407.
14. Durci M, Komaki R, Oswald MJ, et al. Comparison of surgery and radiation therapy for non-small cell carcinoma of the lung with mediastinal metastasis. Int J Radiat Oncol Biol Phys 1991; 21:629–636.
15. Feinstein A, Wells C. A clinical-severity staging system for patients with lung cancer. Lung Med 1990; 69:1–33.
16. Maki E, Feld, R. Prognostic factors in patients with non–small cell lung cancer: a critique of the world literature. Lung Cancer 1991; 7:27–34.
17. Nagamoto N, Saito Y, Sato M, et al. Lesions preceding squamous cell carcinoma of the bronchus and multicentricity of canceration—serial slicing of minute lung cancers smaller than 1 mm. Tohoku J Exp Med 1993; 170:11–23.
18. Kato H, Kawate N, Kinoshita K, et al. Photodynamic therapy of early-stage lung cancer: a critique of the world literature. Lung Cancer 1991; 7:27–34.
19. Saito Y, Sato M, Sagawa M, et al. Multicentricity in resected occult bronchogenic squamous cell carcinoma. Ann Thorac Surg 1994; 57:1200–1205.
20. Usuda K, Saito Y, Kanma K, et al. Resected roentgenographically occult bronchogenic squamous cell carcinoma tumor size, survival, and recurrence. Nippon Geka Gakkai Zasshi 1993; 94:631–636.
21. Sutedja G, Baris G, van Zandwijk N, et al. High-dose rate brachytherapy has a curative potential in patients with intraluminal squamous cell lung cancer. Respiration 1993; 61:167–168.
22. Tredanial J, Hennequin C, Zalcman G, et al. Prolonged survival after high-dose rate endobronchial radiation for malignant airway obstruction. Chest 1994; 105:767–772.
23. Perol M, Caliandro R, Pommier P, et al. Curative irradiation of Limited endobronchial carcinomas with high-dose rate brachytherapy. Chest 1997; 111(5):1417–23.
24. Chella A, Ambrogi MC, Ribechini A, et al. Combined Nd-YAG laser/HDR brachytherapy versus Nd-YAG laser only in malignant central airway involvement: a prospective randomized trial. Lung Cancer 2000; 27(3): 169–175.
25. Yankauer S. Two cases of lung tumor treated bronchoscopically. NY Med J 1922; (June 21):741.
26. Moylan D, Strubler K, Unal A, et al. Work in progress. Transbronchial brachytherapy of recurrent bronchogenic carcinoma: a new approach using the flexible fiberoptic bronchoscope. Radiology 1983; 147:253–254.
27. Schray MF, McDougall JC, Martinez A, et al. Management of malignant airway compromise with laser and low dose rate brachytherapy. Chest 1988; 93:264–269.

28. Seagren SL, Harrell JH, Horn RA. High dose rate intraluminal irradiation in recurrent endobronchial carcinoma. Chest 1985; 88:810–814.
29. Joyner LR JR, Maran AG, Sarama R, et al. Neodymium–YAG laser treatment of intrabronchial lesions. Chest 1985; 87(4):418–427.
30. Rooney SM, Goldiner PL, Bains MS, et al. Anesthesia for the application of endotracheal and endobronchial radiation therapy. J Thorac Cardiovasc Surg 1984; 87(5): 693–697.
31. Macha HN, Kock K, Stadler M, et al. New technique for treating occlusive and stenosing tumors of the trachea and main bronchi: endobronchial irradiation by high dose iridium-192 combined with laser canalization. Thorax 1987; 42:511–515.
32. Bastin K, Mehta M, Kinsell T. Quantitative analysis of lung-sparing following endobronchial boost in stage III non–small cell lung carcinoma treated curatively. Endocuriether Hypertherm Oncol 1991; 7:225 (abstr).
33. Khanavker B, Stern P, Alberti W, et al. Complications associated with brachytherapy alone or with laser in lung cancer. Chest 1991; 99:1062–1065.
34. Burt PA, O'Driscoll BR, Notley HM, et al. Intraluminal irradiation for the palliation of lung cancer with the high dose rate microselectron. Thorax 1990; 45:765–768.
35. Bedwinek J, Bruton C, Petty A, et al. High dose rate endobronchial brachytherapy and fatal pulmonary hemorrhage. Int J Radiat Oncol Biol Phys 1991; 22:23–30.
36. Macha HN, Wahlers B, Reichle C, et al. Endobronchial radiation therapy for obstructing malignancies: ten years' experience with iridium-192 high dose radiation brachytherapy afterloading technique in 365 patients. Lung 1995; 173:271–280.
37. Speiser B. The role of endobronchial brachytherapy in patients with lung cancer. Clin Pulm Med 1995; 2(6):344–352.
38. Speiser B, Spratling L. Intermediate dose rate remote afterloading brachytherapy for intraluminal control of bronchogenic carcinoma. Int J Radiat Oncol Biol Phys 1990; 18:1443–1448.
39. Speiser B. Oncological assessment using the four-tiered scoring system. Curr Oncol 1995; 2:2:54–59.
40. Gollins S, Burt P, Barber P, et al. High dose rate intraluminal radiotherapy for carcinoma of the bronchus: outcome of treatment of 406 patients. Radiotherapy 1994; 33:31–40.
41. Gollins SW, Ryder WJ, Burt PA, et al. Massive haemoptysis death and other morbidity associated with high dose rate intraluminal radiotherapy for carcinoma of the bronchus. Radiat Oncol 1996; 39:105–116.
42. Nag S, Abitbol AA, Anderson LL, et al. Consensus guidelines for high dose rate remote brachytherapy in cervical, endometrial, and endobronchial tumors. Internat J Radiat Oncol Biol Phys 1993; 27(5):1241–1244.
43. Simpson JR. Palliative radiotherapy for inoperable carcinoma of the lung: final report of a RTOG multi-institutional trial. Internat J Radiat Oncol Biol Phys 1985; 11: 751–758.
44. Goldman J, Bulman A, Rathmell A, et al. Physiological effect of endobronchial radiotherapy in patients with major airway obstruction. Thorax 1993; 48:110–114.

27

Tumor Oxygenation and Radioresistance: From the Laboratory to the Clinic

J. Donald Chapman
Fox Chase Cancer Center, Philadelphia, Pennsylvania

R. C. Urtasun
Cross Cancer Institute, Edmonton, Alberta, Canada

INTRODUCTION

Multimodality therapy is the treatment of choice for the majority of patients with lung cancer that will be diagnosed in the year 2000. Radiotherapy is an important component of these treatments and is employed for the local control of disease (to eradicate the clonogenic cells within tumor treatment volumes), although it can also be used in a prophylactic and/or palliative role in some patients. Local tumor control is dependent upon the total dose of radiation delivered, which, in turn, determines the extent of tumor cell killing. Unfortunately, the total radiation dose that can be delivered to the thorax is limited by normal tissue toxicity expressed as both acute and late effects. These maximal tumoricidal doses are usually administered in five daily fractions or two times a day each week over 5–6 weeks. Even after the most aggressive radiation treatments of this disease utilizing the latest technologies including conformal therapy, interpatient tumor responses are heterogeneous, local-regional failures are too frequent, and the 5-year survival rates are relatively low. The mechanisms of radiation resistance that produce this heterogeneous treatment response of lung cancers have not been adequately defined.

Histology, tumor stage (extent of disease), patient performance status, and loss of weight are prognostic factors that strongly correlate with survival after lung cancer treatment (1). Other factors, such as tumor location, may also have prognostic significance. Recently, genetic factors, such as mutations in the K-ras oncogene, deletions or mutations in p53, elevated serum levels of neuron-specific enolase, and others, have been investigated as additional prognostic indicators (2). The biological genetic factors that determine lung cancer radiosensitivity and might predict for local tumor response fall into three broad categories: (1) genes that determine the intrinsic radiosensitivity of tumor clonogens, including those that regulate cell death by apoptotic versus proliferative pathways, (2) genes that determine tumor growth kinetics, and (3) tumor and host cell factors that regulate tumor angiogenesis, blood flow, and oxygen transport, the factors that ultimately define the hypoxic fraction (HF). Information about the molecular factors that determine tumor cell radiosensitivity after therapeutic dose fractions of 2 Gy is accruing rapidly from laboratory studies, but additional research is required to establish the usefulness of specific parameters for defining treatment plans and/ or beneficial modulations of tumor radiosensitivity. Likewise, while the database of tumor growth kinetics has expanded rapidly in recent years, as have available techniques of modern flow cytometry, these parameters are not routinely used to stratify patients into groups for customized therapy. And although the potential role of tumor hypoxia in predisposing to radioresistance was described initially for lung cancer (3), no one technique for measuring tumor oxygenation and hypoxia is currently accepted as a routine and accurate measurement of this tumor property in patients with lung cancer. Recently, radiodiagnostic methods for measuring tumor oxygenation and estimating radiobiological HF have been developed and some have been evaluated in lung cancer patients (4,5).

In this chapter, predictive assays of tumor response to radiotherapy under current development are briefly reviewed, with special reference to their application in the management of lung cancer. Preliminary clinical studies with radiodiagnostic markers of tumor hypoxia and radioresistance performed on patients with small cell lung cancer (SCLC) are emphasized. The identification of a significant HF in most SCLCs prompted the addition of a hypoxia-targeted therapy (etanidazole) to standard treatment regimes that resulted in improved tumor response (6). Tirapazamine, a hypoxic cell cytotoxin, when combined with cisplatin in the treatment of other lung cancers has also produced improved tumor response (7). These studies are current examples of the potential benefits that can accrue from successful translational research. They also demonstrate the long-term commitment of intellectual effort and resources that are required to successfully translate a laboratory discovery into a clinical benefit.

THE INTRINSIC RADIOSENSITIVITY OF TUMOR CLONOGENS

The success of radiotherapy (local tumor control) depends upon the eradication of clonogenic tumor cells from a treatment volume. Since the total dose that can be delivered to surrounding normal tissues and in particular to normal lung tissue is limited, the intrinsic sensitivity of tumor clonogens will have a major role in determining the ultimate success of each patient's therapy. The radiosensitivity of tumor cells in vivo depends upon their average intrinsic radiosensitivity, which is regulated by cell cycle distribution, repair potential, other genetic factors, and the fraction of clonogens that are hypoxic at the time of radiation. Cell lines derived from a variety of human tumors exhibit a wide range of radiosensitivity when irradiated under standard aerobic conditions (8–10). Analyses of their survival curves by the linear-quadratic (LQ) equation indicate that the percentage of cells killed by 2 Gy can vary from only 5–10% for the most resistant cells to 70–90% for the most sensitive cells. This heterogeneity in intrinsic radiosensitivity is demonstrated by the survival curves of selected tumor cells shown in Figure 1A. The large variation in tumor cell killing after 2 Gy results mainly from differences in their α-inactivation parameter (11), the intercept of the transformed survival curves ($-\ln(S/S_0)/D$ versus D) in Figure 1B (12).

The mechanism(s) of single-hit inactivation (α) of tumor cells by radiation has not been elucidated, but recent research suggests that compacted chromatin may be the associated molecular target and that irreparable multiply-damaged DNA sites may be the lethal lesions (13). Cells at mitosis, whose chromatin is maximally compacted, are hypersensitive to ionizing radiation and their survival curves are characterized by very large α-parameters (13,14). One feature of the genomic instability of tumor cells is an increased number of centromeres that leads to aneuploidy and also to a larger amount of compacted chromatin in interphase cells (15). These defects in DNA dispersion in interphase might increase the radiosensitivity of tumor relative to normal tissue cells, especially at the low radiation doses used in fractionated therapy. Tumor cell radiosensitivity also depends upon their genetic pathways of death and, in particular, the expression of regulators of the apoptotic mechanism (16,17). Other factors that regulate cell cycle progression, DNA repair, and intracellular signaling can also modulate the intrinsic radiosensitivity of cells derived from specific tumors (18–20). It is expected that information about the expression of several molecular factors will be required to define precisely the response of cells from specific tumors to single-dose fractions.

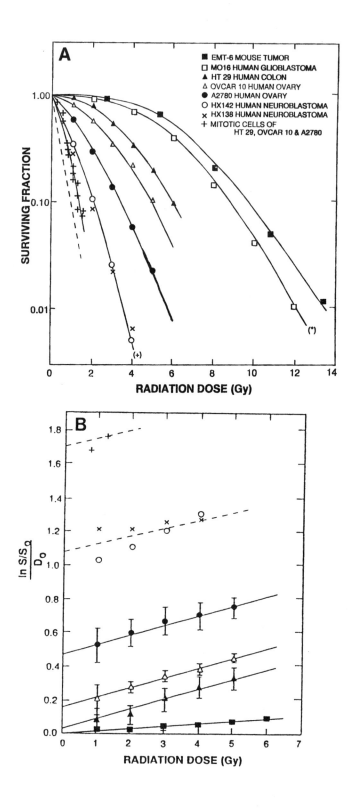

When aerobic cells in tumors are irradiated with fractionated doses of 2 Gy, their killing is well described by an exponential function whose slope is $\alpha = \ln SF_{2Gy}/2$. This description of cell inactivation in vivo presumes that the cells are of homogeneous radiation sensitivity, that there is complete repair of radiation-induced sublethal damage during the 24 h between the dose fractions, and that there is no significant increase is clonogen number (no net cell proliferation) during the treatment. When these factors are rigorously controlled in laboratory studies, this exponential equation of "effective tumor cell killing" well describes the experimental data (21,22). West and colleagues have measured the SF_{2Gy} for cells released from cervical carcinomas by a soft agar assay and found this parameter to strongly predict for tumor response to radiation treatment (23). Other studies that utilized a cell adhesive matrix (CAM) assay of cell proliferation did not find a strong correlation between intrinsic radiosensitivity and tumor response to treatment (24), although the head and neck tumors accrued to that study were treated by multimodality therapy and not by radiation alone. A major effort was undertaken to exploit the MTT assay (reduction of tetrazolium compound) of tumor cell proliferation for determining the in vitro sensitivity of tumor cells from lung cancers after treatment with chemotherapy and radiation regimens (25,26). While the drug sensitivity data generated by these studies was instructive, this assay has not found routine use as yet for defining the most appropriate therapy of specific lung tumors.

It is anticipated that the current molecular biology investigations of cell radiosensitivity will produce optimal parameters amenable for the routine and accurate measurement of intrinsic radiosensitivity of cells in individual tumors. When these become available, the relative importance of this tumor property for predicting the treatment resistance of individual lung cancers could be experimentally determined. As well, additional research will be required to define novel strategies for targeting specific mechanisms of resistance and radiosensitizing tumors (27). This property of cells in solid tumors is potentially a major determinant of treatment response and warrants intensive investigation that can be exploited for improved therapy.

THE RATE OF TUMOR GROWTH

The kinetics of tumor growth has been investigated for many years. Tumor growth rate can inform about the natural history of a specific cancer and may

FIGURE 1 (A) Radiation survival curves of various tumor cell lines irradiated aerobically as asynchronous populations with Cs-137 γ-rays. (B) Some survival data from (A) replotted as -(lnS/S₀)/D versus radiation dose. The symbols refer to the same cells shown in (A). In this transformed plot, α is the intercept of the straight line with 0 dose and β is the slope of the line.

predict for its treatment outcome. Parameters of tumor kinetics that were initially investigated included volume doubling time, mitotic index (MI), and the labeling index (LI) after the administration of a precursor of DNA synthesis. These assays along with measurements of tumor cell ploidy (chromosome number distribution) have been used to define tumor aggressiveness and progression. However, several accurate measurements of tumor volume are required over an extended time to properly estimate tumor growth rate and delay. A flow cytometer technique for measuring the potential doubling time (T_{pot}) with cells derived from a single tumor biopsy was developed and has been used to investigate tumor response to treatment (28,29). While the early research performed on head and neck carcinomas showed much promise, the ability of T_{pot} to predict for tumor response to radiotherapy and to define a subset of patients that would benefit from accelerated radiotherapy was not confirmed by larger studies (30). An accelerated fractionation scheme (CHART) was found to improve the treatment of NSCLC (31).

Several molecular markers of cell proliferation, including PCNA, Ki-67, p105, various cyclins, etc., are being investigated as potential markers of tumor proliferation kinetics (32). Some assays can be performed on fixed tissue specimens while others require fresh tissue. T_{pot} and most histological assays are all subject to the limitations associated with tumor tissue sampling. Barranco et al. (33) showed that average numerical values of tumor biology factors acquired from cancer specimens should be made with three or more biopsies obtained from different tumor sites if the average values are to be representative of the whole tumor. This is potentially a serious limitation of all studies of molecular and cell biology expression in tumors, and particularly a problem for those deep-seated tumors, like lung cancers, that cannot be readily biopsied. It is expected that tumor cell kinetics research will soon identify suitable markers of tumor proliferation that can be incorporated into several clinical studies of treatment response.

RADIOBIOLOGICAL HYPOXIC FRACTION

Mammalian cells are 2.5–3.0 times more resistant to ionizing radiation when irradiated in hypoxic relative to aerobic environments (34,35). This radiosensitizing effect of molecular oxygen is mediated by rapid free radical reactions (35) and is characteristic of all human tumor cells tested in vitro, to date. The radiobiological HF of animal tumors is defined best by the paired survival curve assay that determines the proportion of clonogens in solid tumors that express maximal (hypoxic) radioresistance (36). Unfortunately, this assay has not been adapted for use with individual tumors and, in particular, with individual human tumors. Consequently, much research effort was expended to define techniques that could quantify other tumor factors that will correlate with tumor hypoxic fraction and predict for radioresistance (37). Several novel techniques for measuring the oxygenation status of individual tumors both directly and indirectly have been reviewed recently (38,39).

The Eppendorf pO_2 microelectrode system makes direct polarographic measurements of oxygen concentration within tumor tissue along tracks determined by the operator. This device has been used to obtain oxygenation information from breast, cervix, head and neck, and brain tumors as well as from sarcomas and several normal tissues (40). Values of median pO_2 from cervical and head and neck cancers were found to strongly predict for treatment outcome (41–43). These studies confirmed the earlier postulate that low oxygen concentration in solid tumors could contribute to their resistance to treatment, and to radiotherapy in particular (3,44). Since low oxygen levels in tumors also predicted for poor response to surgery, it was postulated that hypoxic microenvironments could promote tumor cell mutation, tumor angiogenesis, and the metastatic spread of disease (45,46). Recently, with custom-made microelectrodes 12–14 cm in length, the oxygenation status was also found to be extremely variable both within and between individual prostate carcinomas (47). Tumors of similar pathological grade (Gleason 6) were found to exhibit median pO_2 values from less than 1 to as high as 30 mmHg, a variable expression that was not predicted from other tumor properties. This study has not matured to the point where median pO_2 values can be correlated with biochemical (PSA) and/or tumor response after brachytherapy treatment. While these microelectrode studies on accessible tumors clearly demonstrate the intratumor and intertumor heterogeneity of this tumor property and its potential for predicting treatment response, other assays will be required to obtain similar information from deeper tumors, such as lung cancers.

The identification of viable hypoxic cells within solid tumors by hypoxia-specific radiodiagnostics offers an attractive approach that is noninvasive (48). Drugs that contain a 2-nitroimidazole moiety are reduced by enzymes within viable cells and become bound to their molecules at rates that are inversely proportional to oxygen concentration (49). The stable adducts produced selectively in regions of low oxygen tension were proposed as positive markers of tumor hypoxia that might be detected by nuclear medicine procedures when labeled with appropriate radioisotopes (50). Several radiodiagnostics for marking hypoxic tissues have now been synthesized, radiolabeled, and evaluated in both preclinical and clinical studies by positron emission tomography (PET) and single photon emission tomography (SPECT) procedures (48). In particular, β-D-iodinated azomycin arabinofuranoside (IAZA) was labeled with iodine 123 and administered to 51 patients with tumors at different sites (5,51). Eighteen to 24 hr later, both planar and SPECT images were acquired from tumor-bearing regions and the ratio of marker activity in tumor relative to that in an equal volume of contralateral normal tissue (T/N) was determined. A T/N value of 1.1 and greater was interpreted as indicating a significant HF and, by this criterion, ~40% of all tumors investigated contained this hypoxic phenotype that may predict for radioresistance. These nuclear medicine assays of tumor hypoxia can be confounded by the pharmacokinetics of the radiolabeled marker and false positives can result from tumor hyperperfusion (48,52). In spite of these current limitations, if a reliable radiodiagnostic assay of tumor hypoxia can be developed, it would find wide application in the treatment planning of several different cancers.

IAZA was administered to 16 patients with SCLC. All patients had assays performed prior to treatment by chemoradiation and, in some cases, a second IAZA scan was obtained during or at the end of treatment. Figure 2A and 2B show planar and SPECT images, respectively, from one patient with a SCLC in the right thorax. Extensive radiolabel is observed in the thyroid (presumably resulting from the dehalogenation of the marker in vivo and the uptake of free iodine in spite of the use of Lugol's) and in the gastrointestinal tract (undergoing hepatobiliary excretion). The tumor in this patient was well visualized by the large amount of retained marker that suggests a significant HF. This uptake of marker is best viewed and quantified in the SPECT images (Figure 2B) and is seen to be heterogeneous throughout the apparent tumor volume. Although hypoxic marker uptake into contralateral "normal" tissue was used in this study as the oxygenated tissue of reference, it appears now that some normal tissue consisting of compact cells, such as thigh muscle, would have been a better reference. The ratio of radioactivity in equal voxels of tumor versus thigh muscle (T/M) could become the standard parameter for predicting significant tumor HF (48). Preclinical studies with animal tumor models indicate that T/M values can be greater than 1.0 for tumors that exhibit little or no HF (53) and that the T/M above which hypoxia is strongly indicated may be different for different tumors. Our initial clinical study with IAZA did not measure radioactivity levels in the thigh muscles of each patient but future clinical evaluations of second-generation radiodiagnostics of hypoxia should obtain such information.

Table 1 lists the lung cancer patients from whom nuclear medicine scans of tumor hypoxia have been obtained, along with information about tumor stage, pathology, volume, and specific treatment. The table also indicates those patients from whom follow-up scans with IAZA were obtained during or after treatment. Of all the human tumors investigated, SCLC showed the largest percentage of tumors with significant HF by this radiodiagnostic procedure (5,48). A similar proportion of SCLC with significant HF was observed in an earlier study that used the hypoxic marker, ^{3}H-misonidazole (54). While this result might bode poorly for their response and local control by fractionated radiation, SCLC cells are usually quite radiosensitive and they shrink rapidly during and after treatment. In fact, in those four patients that showed an initial HF and from which second IAZA scans were obtained after 3 weeks on radiation treatment (15 dose fractions), there was no significant uptake of hypoxic marker into the irradiated tumor sites. This could have resulted from the shrinkage of tumors to undetectable size, the selective killing of oxygenated cells followed by the reoxygenation of hypoxic

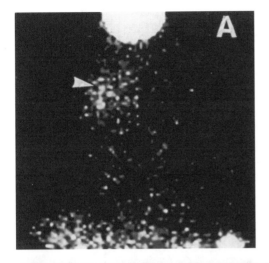

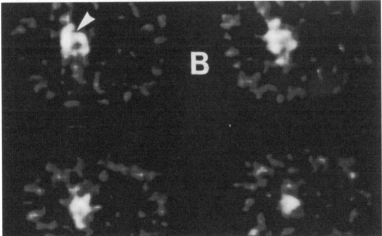

FIGURE 2   (A) A planar image of ^{123}I-IAZA 18 hr after its administration to a patient with a SCLC in the right thorax. (B) Four adjacent SPECT images through the thorax of the patient shown in (A). Heterogeneous uptake of radiolabeled hypoxic marker is clearly evident.

TABLE 1 ^{123}I-IAZA Avidity to SCLC at Initial Presentation with Pattern of Failure After Treatment

	Stage[a]	Pretreatment scan[b]	Thoracic radiation	Chemotherapy	Posttreatment scan[c]	Pattern of failure[d]
1	E	No	Yes	Yes	—	DO
2	E	No	No	Yes	—	P+D
3	L	No	Yes	Yes	—	DO
4	E	HF	Yes	Yes	Became negative	DO
5	E	HF	Yes	Yes	—	P+D
6	L	HF	Yes	Yes	Became negative	DO
7	E	HF	No	Yes	—	P+D
8	L	HF	Yes	Yes	Became negative	P+D
9	L	No	Yes	Yes	—	D
10	L	HF	Yes	Yes	—	P+D
11	L	HF	Yes	Yes	—	P+D
12	L	HF	Yes	Yes	Became negative	DO
13	L	No	Yes	Yes	—	DO
14	E	No	No	Yes	—	P+D
15	E	HF	No	Yes	—	P+D
16	L	No	Yes	Yes	—	DO

[a] E = extensive, disease outside the thorax; L = limited, disease within thorax.
[b] No = no measurable HF; HF = a measurable HF.
[c] Only performed on four patients as indicated.
[d] DO = distal only, P+D = primary and distal.

cells, or a combination of these and other processes. According to this radiodiagnostic assay, it appears that this prescribed course of fractionated radiotherapy was effective in managing the hypoxic fraction detected in these tumors prior to treatment. Unfortunately, SPECT imaging cannot readily resolve tumor volumes of <2 cm^3 and such tumor masses could still contain millions of tumor clonogens. For patients with head and neck squamous carcinomas, only 40% showed tumor IAZA avidity that was indicative of significant HF (5). For those initially IAZA-positive patients who were again scanned after 6 weeks of fractionated radiation, no diminution of IAZA avidity was observed, suggesting that the HF of these head and neck tumors had not been adequately treated. The presence of viable hypoxic cells in tumor treatment volumes at the end of therapy does not bode well for effective tumor control. The survival of viable tumor cells, even in hypoxic microenvironments, can lead to local recurrence.

While the number of patients in our IAZA study is small, the data indicate that the proportion of tumors that present with measurable HF can be different for different tumor histology (5). If this result is confirmed by larger studies and if the presence of tumor hypoxia is found to strongly predict for inferior treatment response of lung cancer, this tumor property will require quantification prior to defining treatment prescriptions. Therapy targeted to hypoxia could then be effectively administered to only those patients who are known to have a biological basis to benefit. Our data also demonstrate a potential role for radiodiagnostic markers of hypoxia for investigating human tumor reoxygenation and its kinetics.

THE RATIONAL USE OF HYPOXIC-SPECIFIC THERAPY

The validation of a new procedure that can measure tumor HF and accurately predict for treatment resistance will have little clinical value unless novel therapies are developed that are directed to overcome the specific mechanisms of resistance. In the case of tumor hypoxia, the oxygen-mimicking radiosensitizer Etanidazole was developed to overcome the radioresistance of hypoxic cells in solid tumors (55). With this in mind and since a large percentage of SCLC exhibited a measurable HF, a nonrandomized phase II study in patients with this disease was initiated in 1988 and completed in 1995 (6). In that study, 30 patients with limited-stage disease were accrued to a protocol that was identical to that used to treat a prior group of 30 patients, with the exception that Etanidazole was administered with 15 of the radiation fractions. The combination chemotherapy regimen consisted of cisplatin (25 mg/m^2/day i.v. $\times$ 3 days), etoposide (100 mg/m^2/day i.v. $\times$ 3 days) alternated with cyclophosphamide (1000 mg/m^2/day i.v. $\times$ 3 days) every 3 weeks, doxorubicin (15 mg/m^2 i.v.), and vincristine (2 mg) for a total of six cycles every 3 weeks. Radiation was initiated after the first cycle of chemotherapy and consisted of a total dose of 50 Gy in 2-Gy daily fractions over 6 weeks. Etanidazole was administered at 2 g/m^2 i.v., with three dose fractions per week (M/W/F) to a total dose of 30 g/m². Patient follow-up was for 5 years. This study reported an incidence of local thoracic failure of only 18% for the Etanidazole-treated patients relative to the 40–50% local thoracic failure rate observed in the prior 30 patients treated without the radiosensitizer as well as in another larger study (56). Furthermore, the 5-year survival with no evidence of disease was 30% for the Etanidazole group compared to the 19–20% 5-year survival reported for larger studies (56–59). These data suggest a significant therapeutic benefit when Etanidazole is added to a standard combination chemoradiation protocol used for the treatment of SCLC.

Tirapazamine (TPZ) is a chemotherapeutic agent with selective activity against hypoxic cells (60) and acts synergistically when administered in combination with cisplatin to tumor-bearing animals (61). Von Pawel and von Roemeling (7) have reported a significant survival benefit at 1 year after treatment of NSCLC patients in a phase III study with TPZ combined with cisplatin relative to cisplatin alone. The drug has a favorable safety profile and does not cause additional myelosuppression. The oxygenation status of NSCLCs has not been measured to date by microelectrodes nor by a radiodiagnostic agent like IAZA. It is interesting to speculate that if these hypoxic-specific therapies had been administered only to those patients whose lung cancers where known to contain significant HF, a larger benefit may have been realized. The relatively modest beneficial effect observed in the meta-analysis of all the clinical trials performed with the radiosensitizers misonidazole, etanidazole, and nimorazole could be explained by the significant dilution of benefit in tumors with HF from a majority of patients whose tumors had no measurable HF (62). Unless adjuvant hypoxic-specific therapy has essentially no toxicity, it would be wise to limit its use to those patients whose tumors contain significant HF and are at the greatest risk of local recurrence after standard treatment.

CONCLUSIONS

Of the several biological bases for radioresistance that have been investigated, tumor HF has commanded a large proportion of our intellectual and experimental effort (63). To this day, there is not an accurate and reliable procedure to determine this property of human cancer routinely during patient workup for treatment prescription. The Eppendorf pO_2 histograph has been used to obtain the majority of preclinical and clinical data that indicate tumor response after treatment correlates with tumor HF. This device is no longer being manufactured but the existing units should continue to provide useful clinical data for some years about the oxygenation status of accessible tumors. Our research suggests that hypoxia-specific radiodiagnostics, suitable for noninvasive diagnoses with PET and/or SPECT, is a viable possibility (48). With regard to the HF of lung cancers, a radiodiagnostic with acceptable sensitivity and specificity would be the preferred method for diagnosis.

This review of predictive assays of tumor radioresistance, and, in particular, the review of studies associated with the oxygenation status of lung cancer, attests to the relatively large commitment of intellectual effort required to translate a laboratory discovery into clinical investigation. Only after accurate predictors of tumor intrinsic radiosensitivity, growth kinetics, and HF are identified will the relative importance of these biological factors for predicting the radioresistance of individual tumors be established for cancers, including lung cancers. The adjuvant treatments required to radiosensitize individual tumors will be different and will depend upon their dominant mechanism of radioresistance. There is currently a healthy research momentum for defining predictive assays of tumor resistance and their associated biological mechanisms that can be targeted by specific therapies (64).

ACKNOWLEDGMENTS

Over the duration of this project, the research was supported by peer-reviewed funding from the National Cancer Institute of Canada, the Alberta Heritage Foundation for Medical Research, the Alberta Cancer Board, and the National Institutes of Health (USA) grants CA-06927 and CA-55893. The Fox Chase Cancer Center is also supported by an appropriation from the Commonwealth of Pennsylvania. The assistance of Pat Bateman in the preparation of the manuscript is appreciated.

REFERENCES

1. Mountain C. Prognostic implications of the international staging system for lung cancer. Semin Oncol 1988; 15:236–245.
2. van Zandwijk N, Mooi W, Rodenhuis S. Prognostic factors in NSCLC: recent experiences. Lung Cancer 1995; 12(suppl):S27–S33.
3. Thomlinson RH, Gray LH. The histological structure of some human lung cancers and the possible implications for radiotherapy. Br J Cancer 1958; 9:539–549.
4. Rasey JS, Koh WJ, Evans ML, Peterson LM, Lewellen TK, Graham MM, Krohn KA. Quantifying regional hypoxia in human tumors with positron emission tomography of [^{18}F] fluoromisonidazole: a pretherapy study of 37 patients. Int J Radiat Oncol Biol Phys 1996; 36:417–428.
5. Urtasun RC, McEwan AJ, Parliament MB, Mercer JR, Mannan RH, Wiebe LI, Morin C, Chapman JD. Measurement of hypoxia in human tumors by SPECT imaging of iodoazomycin arabinoside. Br J Cancer 1996; 74(suppl 27):209–212.
6. Urtasun RC, Palmer M, Kinney B, Belch A, Hewitt J, Hanson J. Intervention with the hypoxic tumor cell sensitizer etanidazole in the combined modality treatment of limited stage small-cell lung cancer. A one-institution study. Int J Radiat Oncol Biol Phys 1998; 40:337–342.
7. Von Pawel J, von Roemeling R. Survival benefit from Tirazone (tirapazamine) and cisplatin in advanced non–small cell lung cancer (NSCLC) patients: final results from the international phase III CATAPULT I trial. Proc ASCO 1998; 17:454a.

8. Fertil B, Malaise EP. Inherent cellular radiosensitivity as a basic concept for human tumor radiotherapy. Int J Radiat Oncol Biol Phys 1981; 1:621–629.
9. Deacon J, Peckham MJ, Steele GG. The radioresponsiveness of human tumors and the initial slope of the cell survival curve. Radiother Oncol 1984; 2:317–323.
10. Algan O, Stobbe CC, Helt AM, Hanks GE, Chapman JD. Radiation inactivation of human prostate cancer cells: the role of apoptosis. Radiat Res 1996; 146:267–275.
11. Steele GG, Deacon JM, Duchesne GM, Horwich A, Kelland LR, Peacock JH. The dose-rate effect in human tumor cells. Radiother Oncol 1987; 9:299–310.
12. Chapman JD. Biophysical models of mammalian cell inactivation by radiation. In: Meyn RE, Withers HR, eds. Radiation Biology in Cancer Research. New York: Raven Press, 1980:21–32.
13. Chapman JD, Stobbe CC, Gales T, Das IJ, Zellmer DL, Biade S, Matsumoto Y. Condensed chromatin and cell inactivation by single-hit kinetics. Radiat Res 1999; 151:433–441.
14. Biade S, Stobbe CC, Chapman JD. The intrinsic radiosensitivity of human tumor cells throughout their cell cycles. Radiat Res 1997; 147:416–421.
15. Patek E, Johannisson E, Krauer F, et al. Microfluorometric grading of mammary tumors. Anal Quant Cytol 1980; 2:264–271.
16. Sellins KS, Cohen JJ. Gene induction by γ-irradiation leads to DNA fragmentation in lymphocytes. J Immunol 1987; 139:3199–3206.
17. Dewey WC, Ling CC, Meyn RE. Radiation-induced apoptosis: relevance to radiotherapy. Int J Radiat Oncol Biol Phys 1995; 33:781–796.
18. Agarwal ML, Agarwal A, Taylor WR, Stark GR. p53 controls both the G2/M and the G1 cell cycle checkpoints and mediates reversible growth arrest in human fibroblasts. Proc Natl Acad Sci USA 1995; 92:8493–8497.
19. Bristow RG, Benchimal S, Hill RP. The p53 gene as a modifier of intrinsic radiosensitivity: implications for radiotherapy. Radiother Oncol 1996; 40:197–223.
20. Adams GE, Hasan NM, Joiner MC. The Klaas Breur Lecture: Radiation, hypoxia and genetic stimulation: implications for future therapies. Radiother Oncol 1997; 44:101–109.
21. McNally NJ, deRonde J. Effect of repeated small doses of radiation on recovery from sublethal damage by Chinese hamster cells irradiated in plateau phase of growth. Int J Radiat Biol 1976; 29:221–234.
22. Matthews JHL, Meeker BE, Chapman JD. Response of human tumor cell lines in vitro to fractionation irradiation. Int J Radiat Oncol Biol Phys 1989; 16:133–138.
23. West CML, Davidson SE, Roberts SA, Hunter RD. Intrinsic radiosensitivity and prediction of patient response to radiotherapy for carcinoma of the cervix. Br J Cancer 1993; 68:819–823.
24. Brock WA, Baker FL, Wike, JL. Cellular radiosensitivity of primary head and neck squamous cell carcinomas and local tumor control. Int J Radiat Oncol Biol Phys 1990; 18:1283–1286.
25. Gazdar AF, Oie HK. Cell culture methods for human lung cancer. Cancer Genet Cytogenet 1986; 19:5–10.
26. Tsai C-M, Ihde DC, Kadoyama C, Venzon D, Gazdar AF. Correlation of in vitro

drug sensitivity testing of long-term small cell lung cancer cell lines with response and survival. Eur J Cancer 1990:1148–1152.

27. Chapman JD, Anderson PR. Predicting and overcoming the radioresistance of individual tumors. Int J Radiat Oncol Biol Phys 1999; 44:477–479.

28. Begg AC, Hofland I, Moonen L, Bartelimk H, Schraub S, Bontemps P, LeFur R, Van Den Bogaert W, Caspers R, Van Glabbeke M, Horiot JC. The predictive value of cell kinetic measurements in a European trial of accelerated fractionation in advanced head and neck tumors: an interim report. Int J Radiat Oncol Biol Phys 1990; 19:1449–1453.

29. Hoshino T, Prados M, Wilson GB, Cho KG, Kyu-Sung L, Davis RL. Prognostic implications of the bromodeoxyuridine labeling index of human gliomas. J Neurol 1989; 71:335–341.

30. Horiot J-C, Bontemps P, van der Bogaert W, LeFur R, van den Weijngaert D, Bolla M, Bernier J, Lusinchi A, Stuschke M, Lopez-Torrecilla J, Begg AC, Pierort M, Collette L. Accelerated fractionation (AF) compared to conventional fractionation (CF) improves locoregional control in the radiotherapy of advanced head and neck cancers: results of the EORTC 22851 randomized trial. Radiother Oncol 1997; 44: 111–121.

31. Saunders M, Dische S, Barrett A, Harvey A, Gibson D, Parmar M. Continuous hyperfractionated accelerated radiotherapy (CHART) versus conventional radiotherapy in non–small-cell lung cancer: a randomized multicentre trial. Lancet 1997; 350: 161–165.

32. Fu KK, Hammond E, Pajak TF, Clery M, Doggett RLS, Byhardt RW, McDonald S, Cooper JS. Flow cytometric quantification of the proliferation-associated nuclear antigen p105 and DNA content in advanced head and neck cancers: results of RTOG 91-08. Int J Radiat Oncol Biol Phys 1994; 29:661–671.

33. Barranco SC, Perry RR, Durm ME, Werner AL, Gregorcyk SG, Bolton WE, Kolm P, Townsend Jr CM. Intratumor variability in prognostic indicators may be the cause of conflicting estimates of patient survival and response to therapy. Cancer Res 1994; 54:5351–5356.

34. Elkind MM, Swain RW, Alescio T, Sutton H, Moses WB. Cellular Radiation Biology. Baltimore: Williams & Wilkins, 1965:442.

35. Chapman JD, Dugle DL, Reuvers AP, Meeker BE, Borsa J. Studies on the radiosensitizing effect of oxygen in Chinese hamster cells. Int J Radiat Biol 1974; 26:383–389.

36. Moulder JE, Rockwell S. Tumor hypoxia: its impact on cancer therapy. Cancer Metast Rev 1987; 5:313–341.

37. Chapman JD. Tumor oxygenation. In:Bertino JR, ed. Encyclopedia of Cancer, Vol III. San Diego: Academic Press, 1997:1914–1925.

38. Chapman JD. The detection and measurement of hypoxic cells in solid tumors. Cancer 1984; 54:2441–2449.

39. Stone HB, Brown JM, Philips TL, Sutherland RM. Oxygen in human tumors: correlation between methods of measurement and response to therapy. Radiat Res 1993; 136:422–434.

40. Vaupel P, Schlenger K, Höckel M. Blood flow and tissue oxygenation of human tumors: an update. In: Erdman W, Bruley DF, eds. Oxygen Transport to Tissue, Vol. 14. New York: Plenum Press, 1992:139–151.

41. Höckel M, Knoop C, Schlenger K, Vorndran B, Baussman E, Mitze M, Knapstein PG, Vaupel P. Intratumoral pO_2 predicts survival in advanced cancer of the uterine cervix. Radiother Oncol 1993; 26:45–50.

42. Nordsmark M, Overgaard, M, Overgaard J. Pretreatment oxygenation predicts radiation response in advanced squamous cell carcinoma of head and neck. Radiother Oncol 1996; 41:31–39.

43. Brizel DM, Sibley GS, Prosnitz LR, Scher RL, Dewhirst MW. Tumor hypoxia adversely affects the prognosis of carcinoma of the head and neck. Int J Radiat Oncol Biol Phys 1997; 38:285–289.

44. Gray LH, Conger AD, Ebert M, Hornsey S, Scott OCA. Concentration of oxygen dissolved in tissues at time of irradiation as a factor in radiotherapy. Br J Radiol 1953; 26:638–648.

45. Höckel M, Schlenger K, Arad D, Mitze M, Shaffer U, Vaupel P. Association between tumor hypoxia and malignant progression in advanced cancer of the uterine cervix. Cancer Res 1996; 56:4509–4515.

46. Brizel DM, Scully SP, Harrelson JM, Layfield LJ, Bean JM, Prosnitz LR, Dewhirst MW. Tumor oxygenation predicts for the likelihood of distant metastases in human soft tissue sarcomas. Cancer Res 1996; 56:941–943.

47. Movsas B, Chapman JD, Horwitz EM, Pinover WH, Greenberg RE, Hanlon AL, Iyer R, Hanks GE. Hypoxic regions exist in human prostate carcinoma. Urology 1999; 53:11–18.

48. Chapman JD, Engelhardt EL, Stobbe CC, Schneider RF, Hanks GE. Measuring hypoxia and predicting tumor radioresistance with nuclear medicine assays. Radiother Oncol 1998; 46:229–237.

49. Chapman JD, Lee J, Meeker BE. Adduct formation by 2-nitroimidazole drugs in mammalian cells: optimization of markers for tissue oxygenation. In: Adams GE, Breccia A, Fielden EM, Wardman P, eds. Selective Activation of Drugs by Redox Processes. New York: Plenum Press, 1990:313–323.

50. Chapman JD. Hypoxic sensitizers: implications for radiation therapy. N Engl J Med 1979; 301:1429–1432.

51. Parliament MB, Chapman JD, Urtasun RC, McEwan AJ, Goldberg L, Mercer JR, Mannon RH, Wiebe LI. Non-invasive assessment of human tumor hypoxia with [123]I—iodoazomycin arabinoside: preliminary report of a clinical study. Br J Cancer 1992; 65:90–95.

52. Groshar D, McEwan AJB, Parliament MB, Urtasun RC, Goldberg LE, Hoskinson M, Mercer JR, Mannan RH, Wiebe LI,Chapman JD. Imaging tumor hypoxia and tumor perfusion. J Nucl Med 1993; 34:885–888.

53. Iyer RV, Engelhardt EL, Stobbe CC, Schneider RF, Chapman JD. Preclinical assessment of hypoxic marker specificity and sensitivity. Int J Radiat Oncol Biol. Phys. 1998; 42:741–745.

54. Chapman JD, Urtasun RC, Franko AJ, Raleigh JA, Meeker BE, McKinnon SA. The measurement of oxygenation status of individual tumors. In:Paliwel BR, Fowler JF, Herbert DE, Kinsella TJ and Orton C. Prediction of Response in Radiation Therapy: The Physical and Biological Basis. New York: American Institute of Physics, 1989: 49–60.

55. Brown DM, Parker ET, Brown JM. Structure-activity relationships of 1-substituted-

2-nitroimidazoles: effect of partition coefficient and side chain hydroxyl groups on radiosensitization in vitro. Radiat Res 1982; 90:98–108.

56. Arriagada R, Kramar A, Le Chevalier T, De Cremoux H, for the French Cancer Center's Lung Group. Competing events determining relapse-free survival in limited small cell lung carcinoma. J Clin Oncol 1992; 10:447–451.

57. Johnson BE, Bridges JD, Sobczeck M, Gray J, Linnoila RI, Gazdar AF, Hankins L, Steinberg SM, Edison M, Frame JN, Pass H, Nesbitt J, Holden D, Mulshine JL, Glatstein E, Ihde DC. Patients with limited-stage small-cell lung cancer treated with concurrent twice-daily chest radiotherapy and etoposide/cisplatin followed by cyclophosphamide, doxorubicin, and vincristine. J Clin Oncol 1996; 14:806–813.

58. Murray N, Coy P, Pater JL, Hodson I, Arnold A, Zee BC, Payne D, Kostashuk EC, Evans WK, Dixon P, Sadura A, Feld R, Levitt M, Wierzbicki R, Ayoub J, Maroun JA, Wilson KS. Importance of timing for thoracic irradiation in the combined modality treatment of limited-stage small-cell lung cancer. J Clin Oncol 1993; 11:336–344.

59. Gray JR, Sobczak ML, Hahn SM, Sullivan FJ, Johnson BE, Bridges JD. Analysis of local control in 150 limited stage small cell lung cancer patients treated with combined thoracic irradiation and multiagent chemotherapy. Proc ASCO 1995; 14: A1056 (abstr).

60. Zeman EM, Brown JM, Lemmon JJ, Hirst VK, Lee WW. SR-4233: A new bioreductive agent with high selective toxicity for hypoxic mammalian cells. Int J Radiat Oncol Biol Phys 1986; 12:1239–1242.

61. Dorie MJ, Brown JM. Tumor-specific, schedule-dependent interactions between tirapazamine (SR-4233) and cisplatin. Cancer Res 1993; 53:4633–4636.

62. Overgaard J, Horsman MR. Modification of hypoxia-induced radioresistance in tumors by the use of oxygen and sensitizers. Semin Radiat Oncol 1996; 6:10–21.

63. Finkelstein E, Glatstein E. Seduced by oxygen. Int J Radiat Oncol Biol Phys 1988; 14:205–207.

64. Bartelink H, Begg A, Martin JC, van Dijk M, van't Veer L, van der Vaart P, Verheij M. The Klaus Breur Award Lecture: Towards prediction and modulation of treatment responses. Radiother Oncol 1999; 50:1–11.

28

Economic Analysis in Lung Cancer

Craig C. Earle
Dana-Farber Cancer Institute, Harvard Medical School, Boston,
Massachusetts

Douglas Coyle
University of Ottawa, Ottawa, Ontario, Canada

William K. Evans
University of Ottawa and Cancer Care Ontario, Ottawa, Ontario, Canada

INTRODUCTION

The annual increase in medical expenditures has consistently exceeded inflation for several decades, resulting in a sharp increase in interest in health economics. In 1965 the health care industry represented about 5% of the American gross domestic product (GDP). Today that figure approaches 15% (1). While there have been important advances in medical technology over that period, increases in positive health outcomes have not occurred at the same pace.

There are several reasons for the rising cost of health care. The demographics of North America's population are changing, with the elderly representing a larger proportion of the population than ever before. Since most diseases, including lung cancer, occur primarily in the elderly, it follows that an older population incurs higher medical expenses. Technological innovation also contributes to rising costs. More can now be done, and for more people, than at any other time. Screening and preventive measures have been successful in a number of clinical circumstances, but only rarely do these strategies actually save money. Improved diagnostic technologies have come at substantial prices, and interventions are now available for conditions that were treated only with supportive care in the past.

These diagnostic and therapeutic advances bring higher expectations. Patients are becoming better informed about the latest medical advances. Many demand that a conscientious doctor apply all the resources available to arrive at a correct diagnosis, and use every intervention that has any chance of benefit. Disability or death is perceived to be due to negligence on the part of the doctor or hospital, rather than a potential outcome of disease. The American Medical Association has estimated that about 3% of all health care costs are incurred to decrease the chance of litigation. However, the true cost is likely much higher in a medical culture that is unwilling to tolerate risk and modifies its practice style to protect itself.

For these various reasons, medical expenditures are coming under increased scrutiny. To deal with rising health care costs, both public and private payers are demanding improved efficiency and "value for money" in the provision of health care services. As a result, the economic literature is growing exponentially. However, this literature is of varying quality and has spawned many as-yet-unresolved controversies.

CONTROVERSY 1: METHODOLOGICAL ISSUES

Study Design

Table 1 shows several different kinds of economic findings related to lung cancer management. Although assembled in one table, many of the component studies used very different methodologies. The type of economic study is largely determined by the denominator of its result, as illustrated in Table 1. "Cost studies" simply count the costs associated with a procedure or treated case. If the costs of two treatments are being compared to see which is the least expensive, it is a "cost-*minimization* study." Cost-minimization studies assume that the outcomes or effectiveness of the interventions are equal, and that resource utilization is the only significant difference between the options. Cost-minimization studies are not common in oncology because cancer treatments rarely produce equivalent survival or quality of life.

A "cost-*effectiveness*" analysis attempts to clarify the balance between these costs and benefits. The cost-effectiveness ratio is the average incremental

TABLE 1   The Economics of Selected Lung Cancer
Procedures

Procedure	Cost[a] denominator
Surgery, stages I and II	$9,142 per procedure
Thoracoscopic pleurodesis	$20,239 per procedure
Bleomycin pleurodesis	$7,300 per procedure
Febrile neutropenia	$1,278 per day
Terminal care, stage IV	$10,320 per case
Chemoradiotherapy, stage III	$4,687 per LYG
NVB-P vs. BSC, stage IV	$7,771 per LYG
Tax-P vs. VP-P, stage IV	$42,866 per LYG
Routine staging head CT	$70,000 per QALY

[a] 1994 U.S. dollars.
BSC = best supportive care; LYG = life years gained; NVB = vinorelbine (Navelbine); P = cisplatin (Platinol); QALY = quality-adjusted
life years; Tax = paclitaxel (Taxol); VP = etoposide (VP-16). *Source*:
Adapted from Ref. 28.

cost of an intervention divided by its average incremental benefit, such as life
years gained, cases successfully treated, or cases averted. It is calculated by the
formula:

$$\text{Cost-effectiveness} = \frac{\text{cost}_1 - \text{cost}_2}{\text{effectiveness}_1 - \text{effectiveness}_2}$$

Cost-effectiveness analysis is the most common approach to the economic
evaluation of health care (2). However, it does not necessarily assess the effects
that different strategies may have on quality of life—effects that are often important considerations in choosing cancer treatment. A "cost-*utility*" analysis is a
particular form of cost-effectiveness analysis where the outcome measure com-
bines both mortality and morbidity into a single multidimensional measure, usually a quality-adjusted life year (QALY) (3). The QALYs are the quantity of life
gained from a treatment, weighted by the quality of that life. These studies have
the advantage of being comparable across diseases, because a QALY is constant.
Finally "cost-*benefit*" studies place a dollar value on QALYs to calculate the
net cost of the intervention. Because of the difficulty in placing a credible value
on human life, these analyses are rare in medicine.

What Costs Should Be Included in an
Economic Evaluation?

There are several different types of costs, and the ones considered in a study
depend on the perspective taken. The costs of care from the perspective of an

HMO can be very different from the out-of-pocket costs that affect a patient and his/her family. Direct treatment costs are those borne by the health sector to provide treatment, such as health care provider salaries, medications, equipment, and diagnostic tests. Direct nontreatment costs are those incurred by patients and family to gain access to and participate in treatment, such as travel, parking, and accommodation near a cancer treatment center. Often these are measured by having patients complete diaries of their out-of-pocket expenses. Indirect costs include lost work time for the patient or caregiver, or the time of volunteers assisting with treatment. In accounting practice, the term "indirect cost" refers to overhead, but in health economics overhead is considered a direct cost. Many investigators use charges instead of actual economic costs in their analyses. However, charges for health care are greatly influenced by market forces, government regulations, and taxation laws (4), and often bear little resemblance to actual incremental resource expenditures (5).

Ideally, a full economic evaluation should take a broad perspective and include the costs and benefits to all sectors of society affected by an intervention. It should also consider a sufficiently long time horizon so that important downstream costs are captured, such as those from late complications. Costs and benefits can still be presented in such a way that the various stakeholders will be able to examine the results from their own perspective.

How Should We Measure Quality-of-Life Effects for Economic Evaluations?

Quality of life in economic studies is usually approximated by a utility. A utility is a measure of the preference for a given health state rated on a scale where 0 equals death and 1 equals perfect health. Several methods exist for eliciting utilities, such as the standard gamble, time tradeoff, and visual analog rating scales (6), as well as survey instruments such as the Health Utilities Index (7), the Quality of Well Being Scale (8), and the EQ-5D (EuroQoL) (9). Table 2 shows examples of utilities measured in a variety of health states.

There is controversy around whether utilities should be derived from patients, their families, health care workers, or lay people who have been given detailed scenarios describing the health state in question. Studies have shown that when patients are used, they value life very highly no matter what the quality (10). However, valuing the quality of life highly in a diseased state will make it seem less attractive to prevent or cure that disease in a cost-effectiveness analysis. Health professionals are often used to estimate utilities because they have a better understanding of the disease. However, they tend to put more weight on physical functioning than a patient would. For example, an oncologist may feel that a patient whose tumor is responding to treatment will have improved quality of

TABLE 2 Utilities Associated with Various
Health States

Health state	Utility
Perfect health	1.00
Menopausal symptoms	0.99
Side effects of antihypertensives	0.95
Mild angina	0.90
Kidney transplant	0.84
Requiring equipment to walk	0.79
Moderate angina	0.70
Hemodialysis	0.64
Severe angina	0.50
Blind	0.39
Dead	0.00
Confined to bed with severe pain	<0.00
Unconscious	<0.00

Source: Adapted from Ref. 6.

life, disregarding the potential toxicities and emotional difficulties the patient
might experience.

Recent guidelines favor lay ''jurors'' as the preferred source of utility estimates from a societal perspective (11). Since all people are potential patients,
these jurors should be sensitive to the needs of patients, yet have a perspective
on the disease relative to a normal state of health, as well as other needs within
society. The challenge is to help people who do not have direct experience with
the disease in question understand the health (disease) state properly. As a result,
any one of these sources for utility measurement is defensible but imperfect.

How Should Time Preferences Be Handled?

Costs and benefits that occur in the future should be adjusted, or discounted, to
their present value. This is because of time preference. We generally prefer to
incur benefits sooner rather than later, and costs later rather than sooner. Thus,
future costs and benefits carry less weight than current costs and benefits, and
are usually accounted for by multiplying them with a constant discount rate (usually 3% or 5%). Such adjustment has the effect of favoring therapeutic procedures
that provide immediate benefit, while rendering preventive and screening programs, which require immediate expenditure for future benefits, less attractive.
Some economists argue that benefits should also be discounted at the same rate

(11). Our next year of life is generally more valuable to us than one occurring 20 years in the future. However, empirical studies have demonstrated that people do not discount future health benefits as greatly as they do future costs (12–15).

CONTROVERSY 2: WHEN IS AN ECONOMIC ANALYSIS WARRANTED?

Economic evaluation itself is not a costless activity (16). Not every medical technology requires an economic analysis, and several factors can indicate whether such a study is appropriate. First, the more modest the difference in therapeutic effectiveness between two interventions, the more likely it is that economic issues will influence policy. For example, if a randomized study finds equivalence between two chemotherapeutic regimens for advanced non–small cell lung cancer (NSCLC), a cost-minimization study could decide which strategy is preferred.

The absolute cost of the intervention is also important. If the unit cost of a technology is small, it is unlikely to capture the attention of decision makers. For example, knowing the cost-effectiveness of using an inexpensive medication such as dexamethasone to prevent radiation-induced emesis would be unlikely to add important information to a policy decision. Similarly, if the cost of an effective treatment is large but applicable to only a small proportion of the population, an economic evaluation is unlikely to be influential, as the overall cost to the health care system would be small. Finally, political and cultural considerations must be taken into account. If a treatment is so ingrained in day-to-day practice that physicians are unlikely to change their practice regardless of the economic data, such a study may not be worth undertaking.

CONTROVERSY 3: DO SMOKERS "PAY THEIR WAY"?

Lung cancer is a largely preventable disease caused almost exclusively by tobacco smoking. Consequently, an argument has been put forward that smokers do not deserve society's help paying medical costs when they develop smoking-related illnesses. However, others have argued that this viewpoint is unfair for two distinct reasons. First, many patients who are developing lung cancer now started smoking at a time when the health risks were not known and physicians did not give advice against smoking behavior. In fact, physicians were even used in the past to promote "healthy" cigarettes, including some with asbestos filters. Furthermore, people were encouraged to smoke by governments that provided free or subsidized cigarettes during military service, and tobacco companies that manipulated nicotine levels and pH to enhance the cigarette's addictive potential.

Second, there is evidence that smokers may actually pay for the health care costs of their smoking (17–19). If only direct medical costs are considered, smoking-related illnesses, such as vascular disease and cancer, are indeed expensive to treat. However, the major factor that determines a person's total lifetime utilization of health care resources is the length of his or her life. Smokers die at a younger age than nonsmokers. As a result, smoking saves significant health care expenditures that would be incurred later in life for the treatment of the chronic diseases of aging, the use of nursing homes, and other supportive-care measures (20). Because smoking-related illnesses have their peak mortality around the time of retirement, the savings from unclaimed pensions are also significant from a societal perspective. Coupled with the cigarette taxes paid over a smoker's lifetime, these economic factors compensate for the indirect costs of lost productivity due to illness, secondhand smoke effects (most significant in children), and accidental fires.

These somewhat cynical conclusions must be interpreted with some important caveats. First, they do not take into account the enormous human costs of smoking-related illnesses. In addition, the costs of smoking occur in the present, while the "savings" from early mortality will occur in the future. Barendregt et al. (20) have shown that when a smoker quits, his/her average expenditure on medical care decreases for about 20 years. After that, costs increase because of the individual's longer life span. It takes about 25 years for these late costs to balance the immediate savings. As previously discussed, these future savings should be discounted to estimate their present value because costs and benefits in the future are generally less valuable to us. When this is done, it takes 31 years for the costs of quitting to negate the savings. Finally, many would argue that only costs and benefits that directly result from smoking-related illnesses should be considered (11). Under this assumption, smoking cessation would significantly save money. Whether these "future costs" should be included in cost-effective analyses is currently an area of methodological controversy (21).

Smoking cessation is the main form of lung cancer prevention. Intervention studies focus on restricting locations for smoking, regulating tobacco advertisement (22), and cigarette taxation (23). These approaches are modestly effective, and appear to be cost-effective (24). For example, a mass media campaign costing $759,436 over 4 years was estimated to cost $754 per smoker averted, with a cost per life year gained of $696 (25). Studies of the effect of taxation suggest that every 1% increase in cigarette price results in about a 0.5% decrease in cigarette sales (23). Young smokers are even more sensitive to any increase in price. Because the vast majority of smokers are addicted before age 20, increased taxation has been proposed as a rational method of tobacco control (22).

Behavioral interventions and nicotine-replacement therapy have also been shown to be both effective and cost-effective in different managed-care plans (26). With full insurance coverage, up to 2.8% of smokers quit each year at a cost of $1171 per user who quits. This translates into $33 per smoker, or $4.92 per enrollee per year. Interestingly, the most effective interventions occurred in plans that required copayment for these services. However, fewer people took advantage of them, so fewer quit smoking overall. This suggests that only the most motivated smokers use services when an outlay of money is required, but even the less motivated can benefit from these programs.

CONTROVERSY 4: HOW MUCH DOES LUNG CANCER TREATMENT COST?

Lung cancer is not a particularly expensive disease to treat (27). However, its frequency makes the total cost to the health care system high. It has been estimated that treating lung cancer accounts for approximately 20% of cancer care costs, and 2% of all health care costs in the United States (28). This translates into about $7.8 billion per year (28). Surgery, and to a lesser extent radiotherapy, are the only curative treatments for NSCLC. Chemotherapy can cure some patients with early-stage small cell lung cancer (SCLC). As a result, there is little controversy about applying these treatments where appropriate. However, much can still be learned about how these health services are delivered, to optimize their efficiency.

Several investigators have tried to count the costs of lung cancer management (27,29,30). Evans et al. calculated the average direct care costs over 5 years for diagnosis, treatment, follow-up, and terminal care of NSCLC in Canada to be $19,778 per case in 1988 Canadian dollars (31). The first year costs ranged from $6333 for supportive care of stage IV disease, to $17,889 for surgery and radiotherapy in early-stage lung cancer. Hospital costs were found to dominate, accounting for 77% of all costs. About one-third of the total cost was for hospitalization during the initial diagnostic workup and treatment. Terminal care accounted for about half of the total cost whether a patient received chemotherapy or not. The 5-year costs ranged from $16,501 to $23,881.

In the United States, Riley et al. determined the Medicare payments for patients aged 65 and over with various common cancers (27). They found that lung cancer was the most expensive cancer site for initial treatment at $17,518 (1990 USD) owing to high costs for hospitalization ($10,782, or 62%). However, because of the relatively short survival of lung cancer patients, it was among the least expensive in terms of total payments from diagnosis to death at $29,184.

Recently, Hillner et al. looked at the cost of lung cancer for a commercially insured cohort in Virginia (29). These patients were younger, and fees were generally higher than for those in the Medicare population studied by Riley et al. Hillner et al. found that the total cost of treatment from diagnosis to death was $47,941 (in 1992 USD), with inpatient hospital facility costs accounting for up to 65% of the total cost.

Differences in methodology, setting, and time frame make it difficult to make direct comparison between these studies. However, hospitalization consistently stands out as the major cost in all of these studies. There have been similar findings in other tumor sites (32–34). In recent years, this sort of research has led to a shift of treatment to the ambulatory setting, to the development of care maps and algorithms to expedite diagnosis (35), and to the increased use of hospices for terminal care (36).

In addition to the consistent dominance of hospital costs, one of the more important observations made in these studies has been the significant cost of supportive care. There is a common perception that advanced lung cancer can be treated with little expense by providing only symptomatic, supportive care. However, such a strategy has been found to incur significant costs, largely due to hospitalization and palliative radiotherapy. For example, Hillner et al. found that patients receiving no active treatment still incurred $26,597 in the first year after diagnosis (29). On average, these patients spent 27.6 days in hospital in the last 6 months of life.

Less work has been published on the costs associated with SCLC treatment. Evans et al. found that direct-care costs for the diagnosis and initial treatment of SCLC ranged from $18,691 (1988 Canadian dollars) for management of limited-stage disease, to only $4739 for the supportive care of patients with extensive disease who were not candidates for chemotherapy (because of their short survival times). The average total cost for treating SCLC from diagnosis to death was $25,988 (37,38). This is comparable to the $18,234 (1990 Australian dollars) for limited and $13,177 for extensive disease calculated by Rosenthal et al. (39). Again, hospitalization was the dominant cost.

CONTROVERSY 5: CAN ECONOMIC ANALYSES HELP US DEFINE RATIONAL DIAGNOSTIC STRATEGIES?

Diagnostic workup is an area of oncology where alternative approaches can have the same clinical consequences but different costs. This makes it suitable for cost-minimization studies. For example, Richardson et al. used cost-minimization methodology to develop an optimal protocol for staging SCLC patients (40). Clinical examination and biochemistry, followed sequentially by bone scan, abdominal CT, head CT, bone marrow aspirate and biopsy, CT chest, and finally pulmonary function testing, were able to avert one-third of the overall cost of staging as long as the workup was discontinued as soon as a metastasis was identified.

Several investigators have used economics to try to optimize the diagnostic strategy for NSCLC. For example, Govert et al. determined that the addition of either brushings or washings to bronchoscopic biopsy increased the sensitivity of the test at relatively low cost, but that doing both procedures was unnecessary and not cost-effective (41). Several groups have shown that CT chest with selective mediastinoscopy is more cost-effective than routine mediastinoscopy (42,43). Furthermore, there are indications that PET scanning may eventually be a cost-effective addition to CT scanning in this setting (44). However, routine CT of the head in patients without clinical evidence of metastases has been shown not to be a cost-effective staging procedure, at a cost of $70,000 per quality-adjusted life year gained (45).

CONTROVERSY 6: HOW DO WE KNOW SOMETHING IS COST-EFFECTIVE?

The value of a consumer product is usually determined by how much people are willing to pay for it. However, this "willingness to pay" approach can be problematic in health economics because medical care is generally not a discretionary purchase. A patient cannot reasonably decide to refuse lifesaving surgery because he does not think it is a good bargain. Moreover, whether something represents value for money greatly depends on the income and wealth of the person being asked.

A commonly used conceptual aid for deciding whether an intervention is cost-effective is a "league table." Named after the charts displaying the rankings of soccer teams in British newspapers, these tables allow the reader to see how a particular technology ranks in cost-effectiveness compared to others (46). Economic evaluations assume that resources are limited, and have alternative uses if not applied to the intervention in question. Policymakers must make decisions that will maximize health by getting the highest value for the money spent. Their decisions often reflect a "utilitarian" philosophy of doing the greatest good for the greatest number of people. To do this, a technology must be assessed for its efficiency relative to all other potential uses of the same resources, hence a potential role for league tables. Cost-effectiveness league tables, such as Table 3, facilitate this decision making by ranking interventions by cost per life year or cost

TABLE 3   An Example of a League Table

Medical intervention	Cost per life year gained[a]
Liver transplantation	251,000
Screening mammography, <50 years old	245,000
Zidovudine for HIV infection	87,000
Hemodialysis	53,000
Screening mammography, >50 years old	37,000
Smoking cessation counseling	1,400

[a] 1994 U.S. dollars.
Source: Adapted from Ref. 28.

per QALY gained. There are numerous other examples of league tables published across specialties (47–49), and in oncology in particular (50).

An alternative way to decide whether an intervention is cost-effective is to use a threshold. Canadian authors have proposed that interventions costing less than $20,000 (Canadian dollars) per QALY be considered definitely cost-effective, while those costing more than $20,000 but less than $100,000 per QALY are possibly cost-effective (51). Americans tend to set the threshold at approximately $50,000 (USD) per QALY (4). However, these threshold levels are relatively arbitrary. The $50,000 figure can be traced to the time when Congress, as the elected representative of American society, debated and passed the kidney act in the early 1970s, which determined that government (society) would pay for hemodialysis for patients with end-stage renal disease. As a result, hemodialysis at a cost of about $50,000 per QALY has become a standard for cost-effectiveness.

There are several methodological difficulties in using league tables, however (52). One major problem is that the constituent studies may have used different methodologies. The choice of treatment comparisons, the length of follow-up of patients, the quality-of-life or utility instrument adopted, the assumptions made, and the range and sources of costs included can affect the ranking of various technologies within a league table, leading to erroneous conclusions (52). Such Tables also may group together studies that were undertaken at different points in time. Cost-effectiveness figures can be adjusted to a base year, but this requires assumptions of constancy of relative costs, resource use, disease management, and treatment efficacy over time. Studies done in different countries may also not be comparable because of differences in health care systems. Costs for an intervention may be affected by differences in demographics and disease incidence, clinical practice patterns, and relative prices between countries. Practice patterns may be influenced by the availability of alternative treatments and diagnostic tests, as well as incentives to professionals and institutions (e.g., salary vs. fee for service) (53). For example, studies have found that the relative prices of medications and surgical procedures tend to be higher in the United States than in other countries (54,55). Because of these problems, neither league tables nor thresholds should be seen as providing accurate answers to difficult resource allocation decisions. Rather they should be seen only as an aid to inform decision makers.

CONTROVERSY 7: IS THE TREATMENT OF ADVANCED NSCLC COST-EFFECTIVE?

With this background, we can examine one of the most controversial questions in lung cancer management: is treating advanced lung cancer "worth it" (56,57)? Recent advances include the introduction of new chemotherapeutic agents and the incorporation of chemotherapy into multimodality protocols with surgery or radiotherapy. However, the survival benefits conferred by these strategies are small, and often come with nontrivial expense and toxicity (58). As a result, many have questioned whether the benefits of aggressive therapy justify the cost (57).

A seminal cost analysis performed by the National Cancer Institute of Canada on a multicenter randomized trial comparing chemotherapy with best supportive care found chemotherapy to be not only cost-effective, but also cost-saving by reducing the need for palliative radiotherapy and the length of terminal care hospitalization (59). A record linkage study of more than 600 patients in the province of Manitoba recently corroborated this finding (Statistics Canada, personal communication). This is presumably because chemotherapy had beneficial effects that reduced the need for impatient treatment and radiation. However, it is also possible that psychological factors may lead doctors and patients involved in an active treatment plan to try to avoid hospitalization. Another analysis that incorporated the quality of life of a subset of patients from the same randomized trial failed to confirm the cost savings, but still found treatment to be cost-effective (60).

The Canadian study found cost savings with chemotherapeutic agents that were relatively inexpensive and no longer in routine use. The last decade has seen the introduction of several new agents that are relatively expensive, but which provide marginal improvements in terms of either survival or toxicity (Table 4). We identified 15 economic evaluations of lung cancer treatment options with a MEDLINE search (61). These are summarized in Table 5 (55,59,60,62–72). All but one study included an evaluation of the cost-effectiveness of chemotherapeutic alternatives in lung cancer treatment (61). Despite the importance of quality-of-life effects on treatment choice, only two studies incorporated estimates of patients' quality of life into QALY (60,72). Supportive-care

TABLE 4 The Cost of Common Chemotherapeutic Drugs in Lung Cancer

Drug	Cost/dose[a]
Paclitaxel 200 mg/m^2	$1503
Carboplatin AUC 6	$707
Gemcitabine 1000 mg/m^2	$471
Vinorelbine 30 mg/m^2	$179
Cisplatin 80 mg/m^2	$26
Mannitol 12.5 mg	$4

[a] Assumes a body surface area of 1.73 m^2.
Note: Costs are given in 1996 Canadian dollars.

interventions have also been evaluated. For example, ondansetron has been shown to be cost-effective for prophylaxis against cisplatin-induced emesis (73). On the other hand, granulocyte-colony stimulating factor (G-CSF) was not found to be a cost-effective adjunct to SCLC treatment (74).

There are several different ways that investigators can integrate economic and effectiveness data in a study. One method is to collect both types of data during a clinical trial. Prospectively captured resource utilization data has the advantage that it is more likely to be complete, and the economic results will be available to decision makers at the same time as the clinical results. However, prospective data is more expensive to collect, and money can be wasted if the effectiveness of the intervention is not proven. Furthermore, care in clinical trials is often more resource intense than in routine practice. For example, trials usually take place in expensive tertiary-care teaching hospital settings, and involve more frequent monitoring with follow-up, blood tests, and imaging studies than would be done in routine care. A recent example of an economic analysis performed alongside a clinical trial is a trial of continuous hyperfractionated accelerated radiation (CHART) in locally advanced lung cancer patients (16). The investigators collected data on patients' use of hospital and community services, as well as their out-of-pocket costs for expenses such as travel for treatment. They found that CHART was more costly than conventional radiotherapy, but concluded that it may be cost-effective when its survival benefits are considered (61). They also found that collecting out-of-pocket costs incurred a significant expense, but contributed little to the final analysis (16).

To avoid such problems, many researchers use retrospective data or prospective data collected outside a clinical trial. It is often necessary to determine costs in several steps, and to use a combination of empirical data and modeling in the analysis. A recent study that incorporated economic and survival data from several sources into a decision analytical model assessed the value of multimodality therapy in locally advanced NSCLC. This analysis found that neoadjuvant chemotherapy $\pm$ radiotherapy for stage IIIA patients, as well as concurrent chemoradiotherapy for stage IIIB patients, were cost-effective, with costs ranging from \$3348 to \$14,958 per life year gained (62).

An intermediate approach is to do a post hoc analysis of resource consumption using data, such as hospital days and emergency room visits, that were collected in a clinical trial. These data can be adjusted to reflect anticipated usual care, and local costs can be allocated to the resources consumed to calculate the cost of delivering the intervention. Smith et al. used this approach when they multiplied resource utilization data from a phase III trial in advanced NSCLC by the relevant per unit costs from their local cancer center to estimate the cost-effectiveness of vinorelbine plus cisplatin (70). This combination added \$2700 in incremental costs to achieve the average 56 days of life extension found in the trial, resulting in a cost-effectiveness ratio of about \$17,700 per life year

TABLE 5 Economic Evaluations of Treatment Alternatives in Lung Cancer

Ref.	Country	Form of analysis	Disease and stage	Comparators	Main results
Coyle (61) (1997)	UK	CEA	Stage III NSCLC	CHART RT	CHART more costly than conventional treatment but cost-effective given survival benefits
Evans (62) (1997)	Canada	CEA	Stage III NSCLC	Chemo + RT Chemo + RT ± surgery	Multimodality treatment cost-effective at $3348–$14,958/LYG relative to standard treatment (radiation)
Earle (63) (1997)	Canada	CEA	Stage IV NSCLC	TAX BSC	TAX cost-effective at $4778/LYG relative to BSC
Evans (64) (1996)	Canada	CEA	Stage IV NSCLC	GEM BSC	GEM is more costly, but cost-effective relative to BSC
Palmer (65) (1996)	Italy	CEA	Stage IIIB & IV NSCLC	GEM-P MIP VP-P NVB-P	GEM-P had the lowest cost per response at 85,700,000 lira
Evans (66) (1996)	Canada	CEA	Stage IV NSCLC	NVB NVB-P VP-P VLB-P BSC	VLB-P was most cost-effective relative to BSC; however, NVB-P yielded the best survival at $5551/LYG
Doyle (67) (1996)	USA	CMA	limited & extensive SCLC	VP-P P + etoposide phosphate	Etoposide phosphate, a prodrug with shorter administration time, consumes fewer resources than standard etoposide
Copley-Merriman (55) (1996)	USA, Germany, Spain	CMA	Stage III/IV NSCLC	GEM VP-P VP-I	GEM was cost-saving compared to the other regimens when the drug costs for chemotherapy were excluded

Author (year)	Country	Analysis	Stage/type	Regimens	Comments
Copley-Merriman (68) (1996)	USA	CMA	Stage III/IV NSCLC	GEM, VP-P	If the cost of the drugs is ignored, GEM uses fewer resources than VP-P
Vergnenegre (71) (1996)	France	CEA	Stage III/IV NSCLC	M-NVB-P, M-VDS-P	Calculated that MNP cost 12,339.40 francs less per response than MVP
Koch (69) (1995)	USA	CMA	Stage III/IV NSCLC	GEM, VP-I	GEM uses fewer resources than VP-I
Smith (70) (1995)	USA	CEA	Stage III/IV NSCLC	NVB, NVB-P, VDS-P	If NVB's toxicity profile is acceptable, NVB-P is cost-effective at $17,700/LYG relative to NVB, and $15,500 compared to VDS-P
Kennedy (60) (1995)	Canada	CEA	Stage III/IV NSCLC	CAP, VDS-P, BSC	Recalculation of the Jaakkimainen et al. study incorporating health-professional-derived utilities: CAP $42,833 and VDS-P $43,496/QALY
Jaakkimainen (59) (1990)	Canada	CEA	Stage III/IV NSCLC	CAP, VDS-P, BSC	Both chemotherapy regimens cost-effective compared to BSC; CAP actually led to cost savings compared to BSC
Goodwin (72) (1988)	Canada	CEA/CUA	Extensive SCLC	CAV, CAV alternating with VP	Alternating chemotherapy cost $3370/LYG and $4495/QALY

A = doxorubicin; BSC = best supportive care; C = cyclophosphamide; CEA = cost-effectiveness analysis; CHART = continuous hyperfractionated accelerated radiotherapy; Chemo = chemotherapy; CMA = cost-minimization analysis; CUA = cost-utility analysis; GEM = gemcitabine; I = ifosfamide; LYG = life years gained; M = mitomycin; NSCLC = non–small cell lung cancer; NVB = vinorelbine; P = cisplatin; QALY = quality-adjusted life years; RT = conventional radiotherapy; SCLC = small cell lung cancer; TAX = paclitaxel; V = vincristine; VDS = vindesine; VP = etoposide.

gained. Several other studies have applied these techniques to different chemotherapy regimens in metastatic NSCLC, including newer combinations such as paclitaxel plus cisplatin (75), and have generally found them to be cost-effective (63,64,66).

This review suggests that most of the interventions physicians have adopted in lung cancer treatment are economically efficient. Furthermore, comparing these data with results in other areas of medicine indicates that lung cancer treatment is cost-effective relative to other commonly accepted medical interventions. This confirms the observation that, in general, costly but effective interventions tend to be cost-effective because of savings in the consumption of other resources.

CONTROVERSY 8: CAN HEALTH ECONOMICS GUIDE POLICY?

Policymakers have been slow to utilize economic studies when setting policy. However, this is starting to change. The decision to have Medicare pay for pneumococcal vaccination is felt to have been based on the results of a cost-effectiveness analysis (1). Both Australia and the province of Ontario (Canada) now require economic analyses to be part of new drug approval submissions (76). Perhaps the most prominent example of the use of cost-effectiveness information to make resource allocation decisions was the attempt by the state of Oregon to prioritize medical reimbursements on the basis of cost-effectiveness.

Oregon's initial attempt to use economic evaluations in policy decisions was unsuccessful largely because cost-effectiveness analyses do not take certain societal preferences into consideration. For example, economic studies may show that interventions that improve the lives of many people by a small amount, such as providing eyeglasses, are more cost-effective than potentially lifesaving interventions that benefit only a small number of people. Such counterintuitive results have prompted many to call this experiment a failure. However, Oregon continues to evolve its rank ordering of health care interventions, increasingly interpreting cost-effectiveness in the context of societal values.

Several elegant studies illustrate other societal values not accounted for in cost-effectiveness analysis (77,78). For example, society generally adheres to a ''rule of rescue'' and is willing to spend more for an intervention that has the potential to cure an illness, rather than palliate a more chronic condition. In addition, North American society generally prefers to allocate resources to the young rather than the old (79), and finds it easier to save an identifiable life, such as that of a heart transplant recipient, rather than a ''statistical'' life through a screening or prevention program. Society also favors offering treatment to sicker patients, even if the treatment is less effective than an alternative that could be given to the less ill (80). Obviously, economic analyses alone cannot be used to make policy. They can only inform the debate about how society should allocate its resources.

CONCLUSION

The exercise of economic analysis is important because it requires investigators to explicitly value and balance the effectiveness of an intervention with its cost and effect on quality of life. However, health economics is a relatively young science facing many complex dilemmas. The ''product,'' health care, is a poorly defined service with an uncertain outcome. It is usually no more concrete than a probability of an uncertain benefit, with another probability of undesirable side effects. Moreover, even these estimates of effectiveness may not be generalizable to the real world if they come from clinical trials in highly selected populations. It is also unclear who the ''consumer'' is. It can be any combination of the patient, the insurer, government, or society. This affects the perspective taken in the analysis. Perhaps the most important departure of health economics from classic microeconomics is the ''agency effect.'' Physicians, acting as ''agents'' for patients, largely determine the consumption of health care resources, but do not pay for it themselves. Depending on the physician's reimbursement arrangement, the incentive may be to either under- or overutilize resources. Finally, the true ''cost'' of a health care service is usually not apparent as its cost is distorted by insurance, taxes, and subsidies. Charges and reimbursements are notoriously poor proxies for cost. Moreover, it is often debated whether costs such as capital costs, lost wages, or leisure time should be included in economic analyses. Methodologically, controversy exists in almost every aspect of a cost-effectiveness study, and the analytical techniques are far from standardized.

Despite these challenges, an impressive body of health economic literature has developed in recent years. Studies in lung cancer generally show that in selected patients, current treatments are both effective and cost-effective relative to other health care interventions. Acknowledging these results, recent practice guidelines have incorporated economic considerations when recommending chemotherapy for metastatic NSCLC (81,82).

Consequently, the weight of evidence suggests that any attempts to restrict access to lung cancer treatments cannot be justified on economic grounds.

REFERENCES

1. Gold MR, Siegel JE, Russell LB, Weinstein MCE. Cost-Effectiveness in Health and Medicine. New York: Oxford University Press, 1996.
2. Williams C, Coyle D, Gray A, Hutton J, Jefferson T, Karlsson G, Kesteloot K, Uylde Groot C, Wait S. European School of Oncology advisory report to the Commis-

sion of the European Communities for the "Europe Against Cancer Programme" cost-effectiveness in cancer care. Eur J Cancer 1995; 31A:1410–1424.

3. Gudex C, Kind P. The QALY Toolkit. Centre for Health Economics Discussion Paper 38. University of York, 1988.

4. Hayman J, Weeks J, Mauch P. Economic analyses in health care: an introduction to the methodology with an emphasis on radiation therapy. Int J Radiat Oncol Biol Phys 1996; 35:827–841.

5. Finkler SA. The distinction between costs and charges. Ann Intern Med 1982; 96: 102–109.

6. Torrance GW, Feeny D. Utilities and quality-adjusted life years. Int J Technol Assess Health Care 1989; 5:559–575.

7. Torrance GW, Furlong W, Feeny D, Boyle M. Multi-attribute preference functions. Health Utilities Index. Pharmacoeconomics 1995; 7:503–520.

8. Kaplan RM, Anderson JP. A general health policy model: update and applications. Health Serv Res 1988; 23:203–235.

9. Euroqol Group. EuroQol—a new facility for the measurement of health related quality of life. Health Policy 1990; 16:199–208.

10. Slevin ML, Stubbs L, Plant HJ, Wilson P, Gregory WM, Armes PJ, Downer SM. Attitudes to chemotherapy comparing views of patients with cancer with those of doctors, nurses, and general public. Br Med J 1990; 300:1458–1460.

11. Siegel JE, Weinstein MC, Russell LB, Gold MR. Recommendations for reporting cost-effectiveness analyses. JAMA 1996; 276:1339–1341.

12. Parsonage M, Neuberger H. Discounting and health benefits. Health Econ 1992; 1: 71–79.

13. Coyle D, Tolley K. Discounting of health benefits in the pharmacoeconomic analysis of drug therapies: an issue for debate? Pharmacoeconomics 1992; 2:153–162.

14. Cairns J. Discounting and health benefits: another perspective. Health Econ 1992; 1:76–79.

15. Sheldon TA. Discounting in health-care decision-making—time for a change. J Public Health Med 1992; 14:250–256.

16. Drummond MF, Coyle D. The role of pilot studies in the economic evaluation of health technologies. Int J Technol Assess Health Care 1998; 14:405–418.

17. Manning WG, Keeler EB, Newhouse JP, Sloss EM, Wasserman J. The taxes of sin. Do smokers and drinkers pay their way? JAMA 1989; 261:1604–1609.

18. Leu RE, Schaub T. Does smoking increase medical care expenditure? Soc Sci Med 1983; 17:1907–1914.

19. Goodwin PJ, Shepherd FA. Economic issues in lung cancer: a review. J Clin Oncol 1998; 16:3900–3912.

20. Barendregt JJ, Bonneux L, van der Maas PJ. The health care costs of smoking. N Engl J Med 1997; 337:1052–1057.

21. Meltzer D. Accounting for future costs in medical cost-effectiveness analysis. J Health Econ 1997; 16:33–64.

22. MacKenzie TD, Bartecchi CE, Schrier RW. The human costs of tobacco use. N Engl J Med 1994; 330:975–980.

23. Peterson DE, Zeger SL, Remington PL, Anderson HA. The effect of state cigarette tax increases on cigarette sales, 1955 to 1988. Am J Public Health 1992; 82:94–96.

24. Phillips CJ, Prowle MJ. Economics of a reduction in smoking: case study from Heartbeat Wales. J Epidemiol Commun Health 1993; 47:215–223.

25. Secker-Walker RH, Worden JK, Holland RR, Flynn BS, Detsky AS. A mass media programme to prevent smoking among adolescents: costs and cost-effectiveness. Tobacco Control 1997; 6:207–212.

26. Curry SJ, Grothaus LC, McAfee T, Pabiniak C. Use and cost effectiveness of smoking-cessation services under four insurance plans in a health maintenance organization. N Engl J Med 1998; 339:673–679.

27. Riley GF, Potosky AL, Lubitz JD, Kessler LG. Medicare payments from diagnosis to death for elderly cancer patients by stage at diagnosis. Med Care 1995; 33:828–841.

28. Desch CE, Hillner BE, Smith TJ. Economic considerations in the care of lung cancer patients. Curr Opin Oncol 1996; 8:126–132.

29. Hillner BE, McDonald MK, Desch CE, Smith TJ, Penberthy LT, Maddox P, Retchin SM. Costs of care associated with non–small cell lung cancer in a commercially insured cohort. J Clin Ocol 1998; 16:1420–1424.

30. Coy P, Schaafsma J, Schofield JA, Nield JA. Comparative costs of lung cancer management. Clin Invest Med 1994; 17:577–587.

31. Evans WK, Will BP, Berthelot J-M, Wolfson MC. Diagnostic and therapeutic approaches to lung cancer in Canada and their costs. Br J Cancer 1995; 72:1270–1277.

32. Hurley SF, Huggins RM, Snyder RD, Bishop JF. The cost of breast cancer recurrences. Br J Cancer 1992; 65:449–455.

33. Barr R, Furlong W, Henwook J, Feeny D, Wevener J, Walker I, Brain M. Economic evaluation of allogeneic bone marrow transplantation: a rudimentary model to generate estimates for the timely formulation of clinical policy. J Clin Oncol 1996; 14:1413–1420.

34. Covens A, Boucher S, Roche K, Macdonald M, Pettitt D, Jolain B, Souetre E, Riviere M. Is paclitaxel and cisplatin a cost-effective first-line therapy for advanced ovarian carcinoma? Cancer 1996; 77:2086–2091.

35. Smith TJ, Desch CE, Hillner BE. Ways to reduce the cost of oncology care without compromising the quality. Cancer Inves 1994; 12:257–265.

36. Emanuel EJ, Emanuel LL. The economics of dying. The illusion of cost savings at the end of life. N Engl J Med 1994; 330:540–544.

37. Evans WK, Will BP, Berthelot J-M, Wolfson MC. Estimating the cost of lung cancer diagnosis and treatment in Canada: the POHEM model. Can J Oncol 1995; 5:408–419.

38. Evans WK, Earle CC, Berthelot J-M, Will BP, Houle C, Flanagan B. The cost and cost-effectiveness of small cell lung cancer treatment in Canada. Proc ASCO 1997; 16:Abstr 1503.

39. Rosenthal MA, Webster PJ, Gebski VJ, Stuart-Harris RC, Langlands AO, Boyages J. The cost of treating small cell lung cancer. Med J Aust 1992; 156:605–610.

40. Richardson GE, Venzon DJ, Phelps R, Edison M, Brown M, Frame JN, Ihde DC, Johnson BE. Application of an algorithm for staging small-cell lung cancer can save one third of the initial evaluation costs. Arch Intern Med 1993; 153:329–337.

41. Govert JA, Kopita JM, Matchar D, Kussin PS, Samuelson WM. Cost-effectiveness

of collecting routine cytologic specimens during fiberoptic bronchoscopy for endoscopically visible lung tumor. Chest 1996; 109:451–456.

42. Black WC, Armstrong P, Daniel TM. Cost effectiveness of chest CT in T_1 N_0 M_0 lung cancer. Radiology 1988; 167:373–378.

43. The Canadian Lung Oncology Group. Investigation for mediastinal disease in patients with apparently operable lung cancer. Ann Thorac Surg 1995; 60:1382–1389.

44. Gambhir SS, Hoh CK, Phelps ME, Madar I, Maddahi J. Decision tree sensitivity analysis for cost-effectiveness of FDG-PET in the staging and management of non–small cell lung carcinoma. J Nucl Med 1996; 37:1428–1436.

45. Colice GL, Birkmeyer JD, Black WC, Littenberg B, Silvestri G. Cost-effectiveness of head CT in patients with lung cancer without clinical evidence of metastases. Chest 1995; 108:1264–1271.

46. Mason J, Drummond MF, Torrance GW. Some guidelines on the use of cost effectiveness league tables. Br Med J 1993; 306:570–572.

47. Williams AH. Economics of coronary artery bypass grafting. Br Med J 1985; 291: 326–329.

48. Maynard A. Developing the health care market. Econ J 1990; 101:1277–1286.

49. Schulman KA, Lynn LA, Glick HA, Eisenberg JM. Cost-effectiveness of low-dose zidovudine therapy for asymptomatic patients with human immunodeficiency virus (HIV) infection. Ann Intern Med 1991; 114:798–802.

50. Smith TJ, Hillner BE, Desch CE. Efficacy and cost-effectiveness of cancer treatment: rational allocation of resources based on decision analysis. J Natl Cancer Inst 1993; 85:1460–1474.

51. Laupacis A, Feeny D, Detsky A, Tugwell P. How attractive does a new technology have to be to warrant adoption and utilization? Tentative guidelines for using clinical and economic evaluations. Can Med Assoc J 1992; 146:473–481.

52. Drummond MF, Torrance GW, Mason J. Cost-effectiveness league tables: more harm than good? Soc Sci Med 1993; 37:33–40.

53. Drummond MF. Comparing cost-effectiveness across countries. The model of acid-related disease. Pharmacoeconomics 1994; 5:60–67.

54. Drummond MF, Bloom BS, Carrin G, Hillman AL, Hutchings HC, Knill-Jones RP. Issues in the cross-national assessment of health technology. Int J Technol Assess Health Care 1992; 8:671–682.

55. Copley-Merriman C, Martin C, Johnson N, Sacristan JA, Drings PA, Bosanquet N. Economic value of gemcitabine in non-small cell lung cancer. Semin Oncol 1996; 23, Suppl 10:90–98.

56. Ruckdeschel JC. Is chemotherapy for metastatic nonsmall-cell lung cancer "worth it"? J Clin Oncol 1990; 8:1293–1296.

57. Tannock IF, Boyer M. When is cancer treatment worthwhile? N Engl J Med 1990; 323:989–990.

58. Thatcher N, Ranson M, Lee M, Niven R, Anderson H. Chemotherapy in non–small cell lung cancer. Ann Oncol 1995; 6:S83–S95.

59. Jaakkimainen L, Goodwin PJ, Pater J. Counting the costs of chemotherapy in a National Cancer Institute of Canada randomized trial in non–small cell lung cancer. J Clin Oncol 1990; 8:1301–1309.

60. Kennedy W, Reinharz D, Tessier G, Contandriopoulos A-P, Trabut I, Champagne

F, Ayoub J. Cost utility of chemotherapy and best supportive care in non–small cell lung cancer. Pharmacoeconomics 1995; 8:316–323.

61. Coyle D, Drummond MF. Costs of conventional radical radiotherapy versus continuous hyperfractionated accelerated radiotherapy (CHART) in the treatment of patients with head and neck cancer or carcinoma of the bronchus. Clin Oncol 1997; 9:313–321.

62. Evans WK, Will BP, Berthelot J-M, Earle CC. The cost of combined modality interventions for stage III non–small cell lung cancer. J Clin Oncol 1997; 15:3038–3048.

63. Earle CC, Evans WK. A comparison of the cost of paclitaxel versus best supportive care in stage IV non–small cell lung cancer. Cancer Prevent Control 1997; 1:282–288.

64. Evans WK. Cost-effectiveness of gemcitabine in stage IV non–small cell lung cancer: an estimate using the POpulation HEalth Model lung cancer module. Semin Oncol 1997; 24 (2 suppl 7):S7-56–S7-63.

65. Palmer AJ, Brandt A. The cost-effectiveness of four cisplatin-containing chemotherapy regimens in the treatment of stages IIIB and IV non–small cell lung cancer: An Italian perspective. Monaldi Arch Chest Dis 1996; 51:279–288.

66. Evans WK, Chevalier T. The cost-effectiveness of Nevelbine alone or in combination with cisplatin in comparison to standard therapies in stage IV non–small cell lung cancer. Eur J Cancer 1996; 32A:2249–2255.

67. Doyle JJ, Dezii CM, Sadana S. A pharmacoeconomic evaluation of cisplatin in combination with either etoposide or etoposide phosphate in small cell lung cancer. Semin Oncol 1996; 23 (suppl 13):51–60.

68. Copley-Merriman C, Corral J, King K, Whiteside R, Voi M, Dorr FA, McDonald RC. Economic value of gemcitabine compared to cisplatin and etoposide in non–small cell lung cancer. Lung Cancer 1996; 14:45–61.

69. Koch P, Johnson N, van Schaik J, Andersen S, Blatter J, Bosanquet N, Copley-Merriman C, Drings PA. Gemcitabine: clinical and economic impact in inoperable non–small cell lung cancer. Anti-Cancer Drugs 1995; 6(suppl 6):49–54.

70. Smith TJ, Hillner BE, Neighbors DM, McSorley PA, Le Chevalier T. An economic evaluation of a randomized clinical trial comparing vinorelbine, vinorelbine plus cisplatin, and vindesine plus cisplatin for non-small cell lung cancer. J Clin Oncol 1995; 13:2166–2173.

71. Vergnenegre A, Perol M, Pham E. Cost analysis of hospital treatment—two chemotherapic regimens for non-surgical non–small cell lung cancer. Lung Cancer 1996; 14:31–44.

72. Goodwin PJ, Feld R, Evans WK, Pater J. Cost-effectiveness of cancer chemotherapy: an economic evaluation of a randomized trial in small-cell lung cancer. J Clin Ocol 1988; 6:1537–1547.

73. Stewart DJ, Dahrouge S, Coyle D, Evans WK. Costs of treating and preventing nausea and vomiting in patients receiving chemotherapy. J Clin Oncol 1999; 17: 344–351.

74. Nichols CR, Fox EP, Roth BJ, Williams SD, Loehrer PJ, Einhorn LH. Incidence of neutropenic fever in patients treated with standard-dose combination chemotherapy for small-cell lung cancer and the cost impact of treatment with granulocyte colony-stimulating factor. J Clin Oncol 1994; 12:1245–1250.

75. Earle CC, Evans WK. Cost-effectiveness of paclitaxel plus cisplatin in advanced non–small cell lung cancer. Br J Cancer 1999; 80(5/6):815–820.
76. Guidelines for Preparation of Economic Analysis in Submission to Drug Programs Branch for Listing in the Ontario Benefit Formulary/Comparative Drug Index. Toronto: Ontario Ministry of Health, 1991.
77. Ubel PA, DeKay ML, Baron J, Asch DA. Cost-effectiveness analysis in a setting of budget constraints—is it equitable? N Engl J Med 1996; 334:1174–1177.
78. Ubel PA, Loewenstein G. Public perceptions of the importance of prognosis in allocating transplantable livers to children. Med Decision Making 1996; 16:234–241.
79. Lewis PA, Charney M. Which of two individuals do you treat when only their ages are different and you can't treat both? J Med Ethics 1989; 15:28–32.
80. Ubel PA, Loewenstein G. Distributing scarce livers: the moral reasoning of the general public. Soc Sci Med 1996; 42:1049–1055.
81. Lopez PG, Stewart DJ, Newman TE, Evans WK. Chemotherapy in stage IV (metastatic) non–small-cell lung cancer. Cancer Preven Control 1997; 1:18–27.
82. American Society of Clinical Oncology. Clinical practice guidelines for the treatment of unresectable non–small-cell lung cancer. J Clin Ocol 1997; 15:2996–3018.

Index